HOWARD M. LEIBOWITZ, M.D.

Professor and Chairman
Department of Ophthalmology
Boston University School of Medicine
Ophthalmologist-in-Chief
Boston University Medical Center
Boston, Massachusetts

and seventeen contributing authors

CORNEAL DISORDERS
CLINICAL DIAGNOSIS AND MANAGEMENT

W.B. SAUNDERS COMPANY
1984

Philadelphia   *London*   *Toronto*

Mexico City   *Rio de Janeiro*   *Sydney*   *Tokyo*

W. B. Saunders Company: West Washington Square
Philadelphia, PA   19105

1 St. Anne's Road
Eastbourne, East Sussex BN21 3UN, England

1 Goldthorne Avenue
Toronto, Ontario M8Z 5T9, Canada

Apartado 26370—Cedro 512
Mexico 4, D.F., Mexico

Rua Coronel Cabrita, 8
Sao Cristovao Caixa Postal 21176
Rio de Janeiro, Brazil

9 Waltham Street
Artarmon, N.S.W. 2064, Australia

Ichibancho, Central Bldg., 22-1 Ichibancho
Chiyoda-Ku, Tokyo 102, Japan

Library of Congress Cataloging in Publication Data

Leibowitz, Howard M.

Corneal disorders.

1. Cornea—Diseases.   I. Title. [DNLM: 1. Corneal diseases.   2. Cornea—Surgery.   3. Contact lenses. WW 220
   C8135]

RE336.L38 1984   617.7′19   83–4614

ISBN 0–7216–5727–3

Corneal Disorders: Clinical Diagnosis and Management   ISBN   0-7216-5727-3

Last digit is the print number: 9   8   7   6   5   4   3   2   1

To my wife
Ann Galperin Leibowitz
With admiration
And
With love

CONTRIBUTORS

JAMES V. AQUAVELLA, M.D.
Clinical Professor of Ophthalmology, University of Rochester School of Medicine and Dentistry; Ophthalmologist, Strong Memorial Hospital, Rochester, New York
Corneal Edema; Donor Material for Penetrating Keratoplasty: Short-Term and Intermediate-Term Preservation; Therapeutic Uses of Hydrophilic Contact Lenses in Corneal Disease

SOHRAB DAROUGAR, M.D., D.T.M.H., M.R.C. Pathology
Professor of Public Health Ophthalmology, Institute of Ophthalmology, University of London; Honorary Consultant, Moorfields Eye Hospital, London, England
Corneal Manifestations of Ocular Chlamydial Infections

DONALD J. DOUGHMAN, M.D.
Professor and Chairman, Department of Ophthalmology, University of Minnesota, Minneapolis, Minnesota
Donor Material for Penetrating Keratoplasty: Long-Term Corneal Preservation in 37° C Organ Culture

STEVEN P. DUNN, M.D.
Assistant Clinical Professor, Department of Surgery, Division of Ophthalmology, Michigan State University, East Lansing, Michigan; Attending Ophthalmologist, William Beaumont Hospital, Royal Oak, Michigan; Sinai Hospital of Detroit, Detroit, Michigan
Altering the Contour of the Cornea: Keratorefractive Surgery

JOSEPH A. ELIASON, M.D.
Assistant Professor of Surgery (Ophthalmology), Stanford University Medical School, Stanford, California
Rationale for Selection of Suturing Technique in Penetrating Keratoplasty

GEORGE E. GARCIA, M.D.
Associate Clinical Professor of Ophthalmology, Boston University School of Medicine; Assistant Clinical Professor of Ophthalmology, Harvard Medical School; Associate Chief of Ophthalmology, Massachusetts Eye and Ear Infirmary, Boston, Massachusetts
Contact Lens Fitting in Keratoconus and Following Keratoplasty

GLENN J. GREEN, M.D.
Attending Surgeon in Ophthalmology, St. Luke's Hospital, Newburgh, New York; Associate Attending Surgeon in Ophthalmology, Horton Hospital, Middletown, New York
Superficial Punctate Keratopathy

JOHN E. HARRIS, M.D., Ph.D.
Professor Emeritus of Ophthalmology, University of Minnesota Medical School, Minneapolis, Minnesota
Donor Material for Penetrating Keratoplasty: Long-Term Corneal Preservation in 37° C Organ Culture

JAY H. KRACHMER, M.D.
Professor, Department of Ophthalmology, University of Iowa, Iowa City, Iowa
Altering the Contour of the Cornea: Keratorefractive Surgery

ALLAN KUPFERMAN, Ph.D.
Associate Professor of Pharmacology and Ophthalmology, Boston University School of Medicine, Boston, Massachusetts
Use of Corticosteroids in the Treatment of Corneal Inflammation; Antibiotics

PETER R. LAIBSON, M.D.
Professor of Ophthalmology, Thomas Jefferson University School of Medicine; Director of Cornea Service, Attending Surgeon, Wills Eye Hospital, Philadelphia, Pennsylvania
Corneal Dystrophies; Anterior Corneal Dystrophies and Corneal Erosions; Herpes Zoster Ophthalmicus

RONALD A. LAING, Ph.D.
Associate Professor of Ophthalmology and Physiology, Boston University School of Medicine, Boston, Massachusetts
Specular Microscopy

v

HOWARD M. LEIBOWITZ, M.D.
Professor and Chairman, Department of Ophthalmology, Boston University School of Medicine; Ophthalmologist-in-Chief, Boston University Medical Center, Boston, Massachusetts
Keratoconus; Specular Microscopy; Superficial Punctate Keratopathy; Inflammation of the Cornea: Basic Principles; Use of Corticosteroids in the Treatment of Corneal Inflammation; Antibiotics; Bacterial Keratitis; Operative Procedures in Penetrating Keratoplasty

JAMES P. McCULLEY, M.D.
Professor and Chairman, Department of Ophthalmology, University of Texas Health Science Center at Dallas, Southwestern Medical School; Chief of Service, Parkland Memorial Hospital and Dallas Children's Medical Center; Consultant, Dallas Veterans Administration Hospital, Dallas, Texas
Chemical Injuries of the Eye; Rationale for Selection of Suturing Technique in Penetrating Keratoplasty

THOMAS E. MOORE, JR., M.D.
Clinical Professor, Department of Ophthalmology, University of California, San Francisco; Attending Ophthalmologist, R. K. Davies Medical Center, San Francisco General Hospital, and University of California, San Francisco, San Francisco, California
Chemical Injuries of the Eye; Keratoplasty

DENIS M. O'DAY, M.D.
Professor of Ophthalmology, Director of Corneal and External Disease Service, Vanderbilt University School of Medicine; Active Staff, Vanderbilt University Hospital, Nashville, Tennessee
Antiviral Agents; Antifungal Agents; Herpes Simplex Keratitis; Fungal Keratitis

ROBERT H. POIRIER, M.D.
Clinical Professor, Department of Ophthalmology, University of Texas Health Science Center; Active Staff, Methodist Hospital, San Antonio, Texas
The Corneal Limbus; Corneal Manifestations of Ocular Chlamydial Infections

IRVING M. RABER, M.D., F.R.C.S.(C.)
Assistant Professor of Ophthalmology, Presbyterian–University of Pennsylvania Medical Center, University of Pennsylvania School of Medicine; Chief, Corneal and External Disease Service, Department of Ophthalmology, Scheie Eye Institute, Presbyterian–University of Pennsylvania Medical Center, and Hospital of the University of Pennsylvania, Philadelphia, Pennsylvania
Herpes Zoster Ophthalmicus

GULLAPALLI N. RAO, M.D.
Associate Clinical Professor of Ophthalmology, Assistant Clinical Professor, Center for Brain Research, University of Rochester Medical Center; Director, Rochester Eye Bank Laboratory; Senior Associate Attending Ophthalmologist, Strong Memorial Hospital, Rochester, New York
Donor Material for Penetrating Keratoplasty: Short-Term and Intermediate-Term Preservation

MERLYN M. RODRIGUES, M.D., Ph.D.
Head, Section on Clinical Eye Pathology, National Eye Institute, National Institutes of Health, Bethesda, Maryland
Corneal Dystrophies

LINDA A. SMITH, B.S.
Electron Microscopist, Albany Medical College of Union University, Albany, New York
Donor Material for Penetrating Keratoplasty: Long-Term Cryopreservation

RICHARD S. SMITH, M.D.
Professor and Chairman, Department of Ophthalmology, Albany Medical College of Union University; Chairman, Department of Ophthalmology, Albany Medical Center Hospital, Albany, New York
Epithelial Downgrowth; Donor Material for Penetrating Keratoplasty: Long-Term Cryopreservation

R. DOYLE STULTING, M.D., Ph.D.
Assistant Professor of Ophthalmology, Emory University School of Medicine, Atlanta, Georgia
Diagnosis and Management of Tear Film Dysfunction

GEORGE O. WARING, III, M.D., F.A.C.S.
Professor of Ophthalmology, Emory University School of Medicine, Atlanta, Georgia
Corneal Structure and Pathophysiology; Congenital and Neonatal Corneal Abnormalities; Corneal Dystrophies; Diagnosis and Management of Tear Film Dysfunction; Operative Procedures in Penetrating Keratoplasty

PREFACE

The cornea is a remarkable tissue. It functions as a fine optical element and yet is sufficiently strong to act as the most vulnerable portion of the outer wall of the eye. It is exposed for much of each day and yet is able to maintain the smooth outer surface necessary for retinal image formation by continuously replacing its surface epithelium and, with the aid of the lids and lacrimal apparatus, by maintaining a tear film on its surface. It withstands repeated distortion by rubbing hands and gratifyingly returns to the original shape. It is regularly in contact with microbial agents and other noxious materials in our environment and yet generally manages to defend itself extremely well. When things do go awry, it lends itself to surgical replacement. And where else can one find a tissue that ages so gracefully?

Regrettably, however, a wide variety of disorders can affect the cornea adversely. Most can produce a substantial visual deficit, but many are amenable to therapy. Choosing the optimal treatment regimen requires that one arrive at a correct diagnosis, often a difficult undertaking. Because of its relatively simple structure, the response of the cornea to an exogenous or endogenous insult is limited, and, owing to its transparency and the subtleness of some abnormal findings, pathology can be difficult to discern and define. All too often the diagnosis is not evident after careful examination. Add to this the relative infrequency with which many corneal disorders are encountered and one can begin to appreciate the problem of teaching the vagaries of corneal disease.

Nonetheless, this book attempts to do just that: teach corneal disease. More precisely, since this discipline can probably be truly learned only by repeated clinical observation under the guidance of an experienced mentor, this book is a teaching adjunct. It concentrates on clinically relevant topics and makes no attempt to be encyclopedic. Where relevant, basic science is discussed, but with an aim to enhancing an understanding of the pathophysiology of the disease, the clinical problems it produces, and the optimal manner in which to cope with these problems.

Our primary goal has been to produce a practical text written by a number of recognized authorities in a format that would lend itself to periodic updating. To ensure its usefulness as a practical reference, we have departed from the norm somewhat in its organization. For instance, since diagnosis of corneal infections and the agents used to treat them are very different matters in a clinical setting, we discuss bacterial keratitis and antibiotics in separate chapters and handle herpetic keratitis and antiviral agents as well as mycotic keratitis and antifungal agents in similar fashion. Likewise, a wide variety of disparate disorders is discussed in the chapter on the corneal limbus because that is where they are encountered by the clinician. The same is true for superficial punctate keratopathy. Considerable effort has been expended in describing the surgical aspects of corneal disease, including a complete step-by-step, how-to atlas of penetrating keratoplasty, a representative compendium of the surgical techniques used by the many authorities contributing to this book. Though considered experimental, a discussion of the status of the various types of "refractive" corneal surgery is offered.

Compilation of this text was a task of far greater magnitude requiring more years than the editor had anticipated. Needless to say, it was not done alone. Each of the contributors had loyal and invaluable support personnel. I became well acquainted with several of these people via the telephone as they bore the brunt of my wrath but always loyally defended the errant author, promising faithfully, "The manuscript will be in the mail shortly." I acknowledge their efforts and express my sincerest thanks to all. In my own office, Barbara Luca, Dorothy Williams, Joanne Shionis, Elaine McBride, and Barbara Hartsell typed and retyped as chapters were perennially altered and updated. I thank them not only for the accuracy of their efforts but also for their constant good humor in the face of not-always-reasonable demands. My colleagues, Romeo K. Chang, M.D., and Benjamin Y. P. Lee, M.D., helped in various stages of preparing this book and have my thanks and appreciation.

Finally, I must acknowledge the help of my administrative assistant and secret weapon, Laurien Enos. From start to finish she organized and reorganized the project, corrected misplaced commas with a vengeance, proofread well into the night on many occasions, insisted that all chapters appear as if English were the author's native language "even it I have to rewrite it myself" (which often she did), transported manuscripts between Boston and Cape Cod each July (there were several), gave up vacation time to keep the project vaguely on schedule, and, in short, spared no effort to preserve my sanity. Her heart is in this book and she deserves special thanks.

CONTENTS

I

THE NORMAL CORNEA

Corneal Structure and Pathophysiology

GEORGE O. WARING, III, M.D.

INTRODUCTION

This chapter presents a working model of the cornea that integrates corneal structure and function and helps the ophthalmologist interpret clinical observations in anatomic and physiologic terms. It presents neither a superficial survey directed to the beginning student of ophthalmology nor a reference source chock full of quantitative details; each of these is available elsewhere.[1-3] Rather, its purpose is to construct a coherent picture of how the cornea protects the intraocular contents, retains its transparency, and acts as the major refracting surface of the eye.

Major advances in corneal anatomy[4] and physiology have occurred in the last 30 years. In 1950[5] no one had studied the cornea with the electron microscope, the epithelium and endothelium were thought to have similar functions, and the major sources of corneal nutrition were thought to be the limbal blood vessels and the tear film. Now we dissect the cornea at the molecular level. We look between the leaves of the cell wall with freeze fracture microscopy; we identify specific molecules with monoclonal antibodies; and we assay nanomolar quantities of actively transported materials. This increased understanding leads us to more effective management of patients with corneal disease.

FUNCTIONS OF THE CORNEA

The cornea has two major functions: protection of the intraocular contents and refraction of light. To accomplish these two functions the cornea must maintain its strength and transparency, no mean task for an avascular connective tissue.

Contrary to the layman's concept that the eyeball is a delicate structure, the corneoscleral connective tissue shell can withstand considerable blunt force before rupturing and can resist lacerating assaults, both accidental and surgical. The major structural component of the cornea is the collagenous connective tissue stroma, which is confluent with the sclera at the limbus.

The tear-air interface forms the first and most powerful refracting surface of the eye, accounting for about 48 of the 60 diopters (80 per cent) of the eye's total power. Thus, the corneal surface must remain smooth and the eyelids must spread the tears uniformly over the epithelium, since the slightest distortion degrades the geometric image received by the retina. The cornea must also remain transparent. It is remarkable that this epithelium-lined connective tissue has a specialized structure and function that maintain consistent optical clarity. Any opacity in the cornea will scatter light, degrading the optical image.

One can consider the cornea fancifully as a sandwich dipped in nutritious soup (Fig. 1-1). Two surface layers, the epithelium and endothelium, contain a central filling, the stroma; all three layers are nourished by the tears, aqueous humor, and limbal vessels. More precisely, the structure of the cornea fits that of many other tissues: the surface layers of

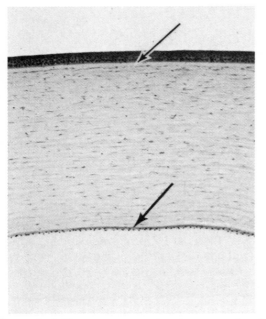

Figure 1–1. Human cornea showing normal epithelium, Bowman's layer (upper arrow), stroma, Descemet's membrane (lower arrow), and endothelium (H&E, × 80). (From Rodrigues, M. M., Waring, G. O., Hackett, J., and Donohoo, P.: Cornea. In Duane T. D., and Jaeger, E. A. (eds.): *Biomedical Foundations of Ophthalmology*. Vol. 1. Hagerstown, Md., Harper & Row, 1982, Chapter 8.)

cells (the epithelium and endothelium) rest on basement membranes (the epithelial basement membrane and Descemet's membrane) that lie on a layer of connective tissue (the stroma).

The five-layered stratified squamous epithelium maintains a smooth optical surface and blocks the penetration of water and solutes from the tears into the stroma. In the stroma proteoglycan molecules hold the collagen fibrils in orderly lamellar array to maintain optical clarity. To accomplish this the proteoglycans must remain relatively dehydrated. The endothelium performs this dehydrating function by blocking the flow of aqueous humor into the stroma and by removing water from the stroma.

To nourish the cornea, the tear film conveys oxygen and the aqueous humor provides amino acids, carbohydrates, and lipids; the limbal vessels may play a small nutritive role.

OPTICAL FUNCTIONS OF THE CORNEA

The clinician who deals with corneal disease considers the optical properties of the cornea from two points of view: (1) image formation on the retina based on geometric optics and (2) intensity discrimination of the retinal image, based on the amount of light scattering.

Image Formation

Refracting Power of the Cornea

The tear-air interface is the most powerful refracting surface in the eye, accounting for about 80 per cent of the total refracting power. The curvature of the tear film surface reflects that of the underlying cornea. The central 3 mm. of the cornea is spherical, and this is the portion that is considered in discussing the physiologic optics of the cornea.

The refractive power of the cornea is determined by both its index of refraction, 1.376, which is assumed to be the same across all corneal layers, and its radius of curvature, which averages 7.7 mm. on the central anterior surface and, because the central cornea is thinner than the peripheral cornea, averages 6.8 mm. posteriorly. The anterior corneal power is about +49 diopters and the posterior power about −6 diopters, for an average total corneal power of 43 diopters.[6] However, like most biologic variables, normal corneal power varies as a bell-shaped distribution, from +39.00 to +47.00 diopters.[7]

Corneal curvature contributes little to refractive ametropias, since it usually falls within the normal range for individuals with both myopia and hyperopia. Thus, individuals with structurally normal corneas usually do not become hyperopic or myopic because of abnormal corneal curvature.[7]

Keratometry

A keratometer measures central corneal curvature, in most cases by measuring the size of the image reflected from the anterior surface. The steeper the cornea, the smaller the image; the flatter the cornea, the larger the image. The image size is converted to corneal curvature, which is read from the scale on the keratometer. Two keratometer images (mires) are reflected from points about 1.5 mm. on either side of the visual axis. Thus, the keratometer samples corneal curvature at only two paracentral spots. Different brands of keratometers use different size zones of reflection (0.1 to 0.4 mm.) and different size separations of the two images (2.0 to 3.6 mm.), so it is not surprising that different instruments record different radii of curvature for the same cornea.

Most practitioners think of the cornea in terms of its power in diopters rather than its shape in radii, so most keratometers give readings in diopters. The instrument must convert from radius of curvature to diopters using an assumed refractive index of 1.3200 to 1.3375, because this gives a reading of the total corneal power (the anterior surface minus the posterior surface) rather than a reading of the power of the anterior surface alone. Different brands of keratometers use different indices of refraction, increasing the variability from one instrument to another.

The average radius of curvature measured by a keratometer ranges from 7.2 to 8.4 mm. The shorter the radius of curvature, the steeper the cornea and the more refracting power it has. The practitioner can easily conceptualize this by tying a pencil to a piece of string, changing the length of the string (the radius of curvature), and seeing that the pencil describes increasingly steep arcs as the length of the string decreases.

Corneal Topography

With the slit lamp the cornea appears spherical, as if it had the same radius of curvature from limbus to limbus in all meridians, but it is really an aspheric surface composed of compound curves that are different in different meridians. The cornea becomes flatter paracentrally and peripherally, increasing the radius of curvature about 2 mm. paracentrally and about 4 mm. peripherally. The changes occur more rapidly along the nasal portion of the cornea than along the temporal portion.

These facts are important in fitting hard contact lenses, where the shape of the back of the lens needs to approximate that of the corneal surface itself, and in interpreting the results of refractive corneal surgery like radial keratotomy or wedge resections, where incisions in the peripheral cornea effect changes in the central curvature.

The clinician can measure the topography of the cornea in two ways:

1. Using a standard keratometer to survey the cornea, changing the direction of the patient's fixation.[8] This approach is practical in fitting contact lenses and in diagnosing early keratoconus, where there is steepening of the cornea inferotemporally.

2. Using a keratoscope to project a series of concentric rings onto the corneal surface.[9, 10] This method uses the principles of contour mapping to measure corneal curvature: the closer the lines are together, the steeper the curvature. By taking a photograph of the ring pattern and comparing it with patterns of known corneal steepness, the clinician can quantitate variations in corneal topography (Fig. 1–2).

Figure 1–2. Photokeratoscope shows the uniform topography of a normal cornea *(A)* and the distortion produced by keratoconus *(B)*.

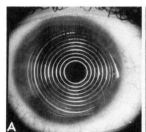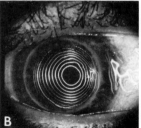

The layers of the cornea that maintain its curvature and topography are unknown. Bowman's layer is a compact acellular feltwork of fine collagen fibrils and probably contributes substantially to corneal shape. Further research is necessary to define the roles of the lamellar stroma and the elastic Descemet's membrane.

Astigmatism

If corneal curvature varies from one meridian to another, corneal astigmatism is present. If the meridians of maximum and minimum curvature are at right angles to each other, the astigmatism is regular, and light is focused at two lines that are perpendicular to each other, separated by the interval of Sturm. Since most adult corneas with astigmatism are steeper in the vertical meridians (30 degrees to either side of the vertical axis), this pattern is called with-the-rule astigmatism. An easy way to remember this is to recall the common medical abbreviation "c̄" for the Latin cum, with, the "c" bringing to mind the steep vertical with-the-rule curvature. With advancing age astigmatism against the rule becomes more common.

Irregular astigmatism occurs when the meridians of greatest and least curvature are not at 90-degree angles to each other or when there is variable curvature along a single meridian.

The clinician can use simple images to help patients understand these variations in corneal shape: a basketball for a spherical cornea, a football for regular astigmatism, and a deflated basketball or football for irregular astigmatism.

Control of Astigmatism at Surgery. The combination of operating microscopes, fine sutures and needles, delicate instruments for less traumatic handling of tissue, and improved eye banking techniques have fostered technical success in both cataract and corneal surgery. No longer is the surgeon concerned primarily about a clear corneal transplant or a secure cataract wound. Today the most common complication of cataract and corneal surgery is postoperative astigmatism.

Most ophthalmic surgeons think that the major determinants of postoperative astigmatism are the regularity of the wound and the tension of the sutures, such that a wound that is smooth and uniform across its entire extent and sutures that exert equal tension across the wound will be most likely to yield minimal postoperative astigmatism. However, the details of how these two factors determine the shape of the cornea are unknown.

The concept of wound compression—i.e., a suture compresses the tissue, reducing the linear amount of tissue present on that meridian—helps us understand and manage corneal astigmatism postoperatively.[11] The steepest meridian lies in the axis of the tightest suture or in the area of the wound where tissue has been excised. If the tightest suture is tied at 12 o'clock, the cornea will be steepest in the 90 degree meridian. This is especially true when elastic nylon or polypropylene sutures are used. Likewise, if tissue is absent at 12 o'clock, because of an elliptical keratoplasty trephine cut[12] or because of an irregular cataract wound incision, the steepest meridian postoperatively will probably be at 90 degrees. This is because the tight sutures pull the tissues together and compress the wound, which decreases the chord length across the cornea, increases sagittal depth of the cornea over the central anterior chamber, and increases the central corneal curvature in that meridian.

This is the opposite of what one thinks intuitively, since a tight suture brings forth the image of pulling the tissue flat, as one would pull a carpet taut when it is nailed down at one wall and is stretched toward the other. Indeed, the area adjacent to the suture is flattened. But the suture is not pulling against a fixed opposite side; it is compressing the tissue in that meridian and increasing the corneal curvature. To visualize this, take a calling card and arch it between your thumb and forefinger to simulate the cornea arched over the anterior chamber, press down on one end of the card with a finger of your other hand to simulate a tight suture compressing tissue, and observe the increased curvature of the card.

Intraoperatively the surgeon may use an operating keratometer to help control astigmatism. Using either a qualitative approach, in which a circle is projected on the cornea and observed to be either round (spherical) or elliptical (astigmatic), or a quantitative approach, in which keratometry mires are overlapped with the usual quantitative reading of corneal power, the surgeon can adjust the tightness of the sutures to achieve a spherical cornea after the wound is healed.[13] In cataract surgery most surgeons leave the vertical meridian about 1.00 to 1.50 diopters steep, since wound healing produces some flattening in this direction. In keratoplasty it is most desirable to leave circular mires, indicating equal tension all around the wound.

Postoperatively the surgeon can also control astigmatism. He can cut a tight suture in the steep meridian to flatten the cornea. Likewise, if the wound is already healed, he can make a paralimbal relaxing incision centered in the steep meridian and covering about three clock hours to relieve some of the tissue compression and flatten that meridian. Alternatively, he can resect an arcuate wedge of tissue about 1.0 mm. wide and about three clock hours long, centered on the flat meridian, and by resuturing the wound, compress the tissue and steepen the flat meridian.[14]

Unfortunately, even in the face of a smooth, uniform incision and properly placed and tied sutures, corneal astigmatism may persist postoperatively because of forces created during wound healing, a process over which the clinician has little control.

Treatment of Astigmatism with Contact Lenses. A contact lens placed on the surface of the cornea creates a new tear-air interface and can be used to mask both regular and irregular astigmatism. A hard contact lens is most effective since it holds its own shape, whereas a soft contact lens will mold to the underlying cornea. A hard contact lens can be used diagnostically to distinguish the effect of surface irregularity from that of corneal opacification on visual acuity. Thus, in patients with corneal scars a hard contact lens that creates a new surface will eliminate much of the astigmatism. Ofttimes this is all that is necessary to obtain good visual acuity, in spite of the stromal scars.

Glare and Light Scattering

Glare can be defined colloquially as light where it shouldn't be. Opacities in the ocular media sometimes reduce visual acuity not by distorting the geometric image but by producing light scattering within the globe that reduces intensity discrimination of images on the retina.[15]

The most common clinical example of this is the posterior subcapsular cataract, in which the patient has good visual acuity in the dim illumination of the examining room but is incapacitated in bright lights. Similar circumstances occur in the cornea, particularly if a stromal scar from trauma or inflammation lies adjacent to the visual axis. Although good visual acuity can be obtained, often with the aid of a contact lens, the patient functions poorly because of glare.

There are two approaches to managing this problem: one is to provide sunglasses that effectively filter out most of the incident light (especially effective are those with ultraviolet and infrared filters), and the other is to perform keratoplasty to remove the opacity.

The amount of image destruction by light scattering is roughly proportionate to the distance of the object from the translucent irregular surface. This has been called the "nude in the shower phenomenon," in which the presumably lascivious observer can detect only the vague shape of the voluptuous nude who stands at a distance from the shower door. As the body moves closer and closer to the door, the observer can see increasing amounts of detail. In an ophthalmic setting this principle explains the circumstance in which the ophthalmologist has a good view of the fundus through a scarred cornea because the fundus is only 24 mm. away, but the patient has poor distance acuity because the object is a greater distance from the opaque cornea.

CORNEAL EPITHELIUM

Functions of the Epithelium

The corneal epithelium has three major functions: (1) formation of a mechanical barrier to foreign material and microorganisms; (2) creation of a smooth, transparent optical surface to which the tear film can adsorb; and (3) maintenance of a barrier to the diffusion of water, solutes, and drugs.

Structure of the Epithelium

The corneal epithelium is a five- to seven-layer thick stratified squamous epithelium that is organized more orderly than stratified squamous epithelia elsewhere in the body. This arrangement is a prerequisite for formation of a smooth transparent optical surface.

The epithelium consists of three types of epithelial cells and four other types of cells. The three epithelial cells include the single layer of columnar-shaped basal cells, two layers of wing-shaped cells, and the three layers of superficial squamous cells. In general, normal epithelial growth begins in the basal cells, where mitotic activity occurs. Dividing basal cells become the wing-shaped cells that migrate superficially as flattening squamous cells and ultimately lose their attachments to the cornea and slough into the tear film. In addition, there are neurons, melanocytes, modified macrophages (Langerhans cells), and occasional leukocytes within the epithelium. The Langerhans

cells are macrophages normally located in the peripheral corneal epithelium. They probably play a role in ocular hypersensitivity and immunologic phenomena by processing antigens and presenting them to lymphocytes and therefore may participate in limbal immunologic phenomena like Mooren's ulcer and possibly in corneal transplant rejection.[17]

Corneal epithelial cells contain organelles designed primarily for protein synthesis, like endoplasmic reticulum and Golgi apparatus. The corneal epithelium turns over about once a week, and there must be a high production of structural molecules for this purpose. Mitochondria are sparse, indicating that energy-requiring metabolic processes are less important in the epithelium. The large amount of filamentous material in the cytoplasm attests to the epithelium's structural role (tonofilaments) and its role in migration and healing (contractile filaments).[18]

Epithelium—Tear Film Interaction

The plasma membrane of the epithelial cell is a typical unit membrane consisting of a lipid bilayer that contains protein macromolecules. This lipid surface is hydrophobic; as a result, the aqueous tear film, left to its own devices, would bead up on the corneal surface like raindrops on a newly waxed car. However, the goblet cells in the conjunctiva and other epithelial cells produce mucin that spreads directly over the epithelial surface and decreases surface tension so that the aqueous component of the tears can spread over and adsorb to the epithelial surface and maintain an intact tear film for 20 to 30 seconds between blinks. Abnormalities of the mucin layer or the epithelial surface will cause the tear film to break up rapidly into dry spots after the resurfacing effect of a blink.

Since the preocular tear film is hypertonic to corneal stroma, it osmotically draws water out of the stroma. In the presence of decreased endothelial function the tear film may play a more noticeable role in corneal dehydration. When evaporation of the tears during waking raises the osmolarity, more water is drawn out of the cornea, but when the osmolarity falls during sleep, less fluid is removed from the stroma. Thus, patients with disorders like Fuchs' endothelial dystrophy and aphakic corneal edema experience blurred vision on awakening, which may clear in a few hours as the tear osmolarity rises. This is the basis for the use of hypertonic agents to treat corneal edema.[19]

Squamous Cells

By the time the epithelial cells have migrated from the basal to the squamous layer, they have undergone considerable morphologic transformation. The superficial squamous cells have unique features important in corneal function.

Spread over the surface of the epithelium is a layer of glycoprotein. This protein-sugar complex probably has two constituents: mucin from the tear film that decreases surface tension, and glycolipids and glycoproteins in the plasma membrane that send branching arms of polymerized sugars out over the cell surface. These glycoproteins may play a role in the adhesive properties of the cell during wound healing and desquamation.

The surface of the squamous cells is not smooth but contains myriad projections in the form of fingerlike microvillae and ridgelike microplicae. These projections create a corrugated surface that may help stabilize the tear film, may increase absorption of metabolites, and may increase the amount of plasma membrane available for elongation during migration (Figs. 1–3 to 1–5).

In addition to the usual desmosomal (macula adherens) intercellular junctions (Fig. 1–5), the superficial squamous cells are zippered together by zonulae occludentes—tight junctions that

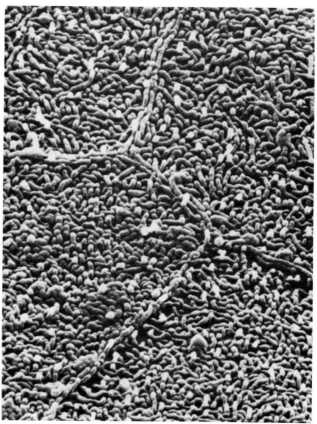

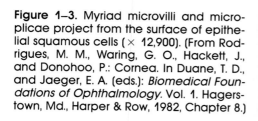

Figure 1–3. Myriad microvilli and microplicae project from the surface of epithelial squamous cells (× 12,900). (From Rodrigues, M. M., Waring, G. O., Hackett, J., and Donohoo, P.: Cornea. In Duane, T. D., and Jaeger, E. A. (eds.): *Biomedical Foundations of Ophthalmology.* Vol. 1. Hagerstown, Md., Harper & Row, 1982, Chapter 8.)

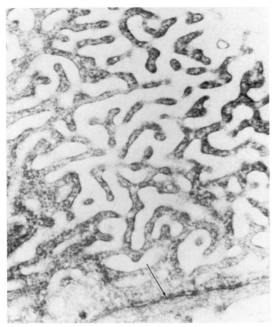

Figure 1–4. Tangential section across surface corneal epithelial cell shows the maze of microplicae and microvillae. The zonula occludens junctions (arrow) are the primary structures that create the barrier function of the corneal epithelium (× 10,200).

is not clear; (2) accumulations of glycogen granules, which provide a reserve energy source for the epithelium; and (3) numerous contractile proteins like actin, which attach to plasma membranes and microprojections and which act as a cytoskeleton and enhance migration.[21]

The stratified squamous epithelium of the cornea does not produce a surface layer of keratin. However, the cells are capable of producing keratin, as demonstrated by the presence of keratohyalin filaments in the normal epithelium and of the appearance of surface keratin in Vitamin A deficiency.

Wing Cells

The multisided wing cells interdigitate with each other, their plasma membranes meshing like pieces of a jigsaw puzzle (Fig. 1–6). They adhere with large numbers of desmosomal attachments

encircle the cells and consist of adhesion of the two adjacent plasma membranes. The zonulae occludentes create a formidable barrier. Not only do they block the penetration of microorganisms, except for those such as the gonococcus and herpes simplex virus, that have the ability to parasitize the epithelial cell directly, but they also block the flow of fluid, electrolytes, and metabolites from the tears to the stroma. This blockade assists in keeping the stroma dehydrated. It also blocks nutrients that might be present in the tear film, so the cornea must obtain its sugars and amino acids primarily from the stroma.

The superficial squamous epithelial cells are not mere passive barriers, however, since they also contain an active chloride pump, at least in the rabbit. This pump may play a small role in corneal deturgescence.[20]

The squamous cells have three characteristic intracytoplasmic findings: (1) a prominent Golgi apparatus with numerous vesicles, the function of which

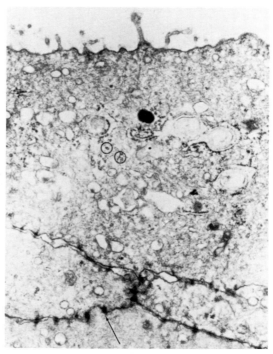

Figure 1–5. Cross-section of surface corneal epithelial cell shows microvillae and microplicae on the surface, glycogen granules in the cytoplasm (circles), and many desmosomal attachments (arrow) (× 5500).

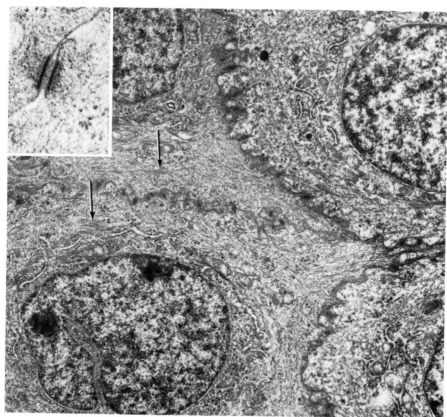

Figure 1–6. Wing cells exhibit prominent interdigitations and desmosomes. The cytoplasm contains numerous tonofilaments (arrows), rough endoplasmic reticulum, scattered mitochondria, and ribosomes (× 13,800). Inset shows desmosomal connection between wing cells (× 49,500). (From Rodrigues, M. M., Waring, G. O., Hackett, J., and Donohoo, P.: Cornea. In Duane, T. D., and Jaeger, E. A. (eds.): *Biomedical Foundations of Ophthalmology.* Vol. 1. Hagerstown, Md., Harper & Row, 1982, Chapter 8.)

that consist of sheaves of cytoplasmic tonofilaments converging on a focal thickened plaque in the plasma membrane, extending across the intercellular space, where an additional adhesive substance is present, and attaching to the adjacent cell. The interdigitation and desmosomes produce tenacious adhesion that allows the epithelium to form large bullae in corneal edema or to fall off in sheets in recurrent epithelial erosion.

Fluid can accumulate in the epithelium both intracellularly and extracellularly. Intracellular fluid expands the cell into a small round vesicle, and extracellular fluid accumulates between the cells, which remain attached by the desmosomes. These little pockets of fluid produce a microcystic texture that resembles a layer of dewdrops and act as a diffraction grating to set up interference fringes that create the halos described by patients with epithelial edema.

Basal Cells

A row of columnar basal cells line up in single file along the basement membrane. Their plasma membranes interdigitate less and they have fewer desmosomal attachments than the wing cells. Cytoplasmic organelles are sparse. Tonofilaments are scattered throughout (Fig. 1–7).

Hemidesmosomes along the basal plasma membrane provide points of attachment (Fig. 1–8). These focal spot-welds consist of intracytoplasmic tonofilaments that extend across plaque-like

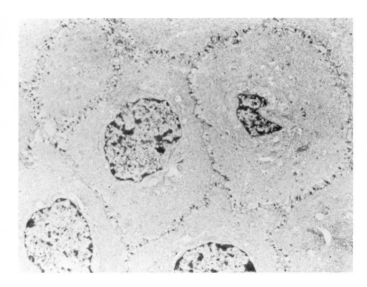

Figure 1–7. Section through basal corneal epithelial cells parallel to the basement membrane shows cells in regular array with desmosomal attachments.

thickenings through the basement membrane to Bowman's layer. Any clinician who has tried to remove a normal epithelium with either a moist Q-tip or a scalpel blade can attest to the tenacity of the adhesion.

Epithelial Basement Membrane

The basement membrane is similar to that of any epithelial basement membrane. Secreted by the basal epithelial cells, it has an amorphous appearance on transmission electron microscopy and forms the orderly scaffold on which the epithelium rests.

During healing the surface of the basement membrane contains glycoproteins, such as fibronectin and laminin, that play a role in the migration and adhesion of epithelial cells.[22]

Abnormalities of the basement membrane appear in disorders such as recurrent corneal epithelial erosion, epithelial basement membrane dystrophy (map-dot-fingerprint dystrophy), and diabetes mellitus, where abnormal adhesion of the epithelium and abnormal secretion of basement membrane fre-

Figure 1–8. The hemidesmosomes (arrows) are present along the basal cell membrane and connect the basal epithelium (E) and basement membrane (asterisks) with Bowman's layer (BL) (× 10,800). Inset shows thickening of the epithelial basement membrane (asterisk) adjacent to the hemidesmosomes. (From Rodrigues, M. M., Waring, G. O., Hackett, J., and Donohoo, P.: Cornea. In Duane, T. D., and Jaeger, E. A. (eds.): *Biomedical Foundations of Ophthalmology.* Vol. 1. Hagerstown, Md., Harper & Row, 1982. Chapter 8.)

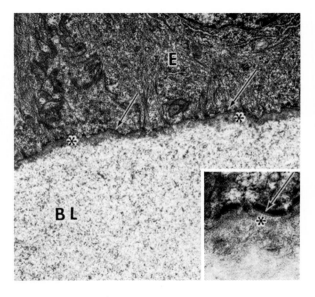

quently result in an irregular surface with blurred vision and sometimes painful erosion.[23]

Metabolism of Corneal Epithelium

Although epithelial metabolism may appear uninteresting to the clinician, the millions of individuals who wear contact lenses bring the ophthalmologist face to face with the epithelium's ability to survive the hypoxic assault of a piece of plastic skidding across its surface. One can conceptualize corneal metabolism by remembering that the cornea breathes oxygen from the tears and eats nutrients from the aqueous.

Delivery of Oxygen to the Cornea

Atmospheric oxygen dissolves in the tear film and diffuses into the cornea across the epithelium. Under normal waking conditions more than enough oxygen is available.[24] The epithelium requires a minimum of 7 to 15 mm. Hg partial pressure of oxygen in tears to remain clear, and with the eyes open the oxygen tension in tears is about 155 mm. Hg. With the eyes closed oxygen diffuses into the tears from the conjunctival capillaries, and still provides an environment of 55 mm. Hg. Of course, this oxygen must diffuse across the epithelium through the stroma and to the endothelium even though there is a contribution of oxygen to the aqueous humor from iris and ciliary body capillaries.

Epithelial Nutrition and Metabolism

The epithelium utilizes glucose as a primary source of energy and amino acids as building blocks, both of which diffuse from the aqueous humor across the endothelium and stroma.[25] These metabolites do not enter from the tears because the epithelial barrier prevents their diffusion and because there are only small amounts of glucose and amino acids in the tears. The aqueous origin of nutrients can be demonstrated clinically by inserting an impermeable membrane into the stroma. The membrane blocks the flow of water into the epithelium, decreasing epithelial edema, and also blocks the flow of nutrients, causing the epithelium in front of the membrane to gradually lose its glycogen stores, slough, and leave a sterile ulcer.[26] This process can be prevented by drilling holes in the membrane or by using permeable hydrophilic materials that allow passage of nutrients.[27]

The squamous epithelial cells have large stores of glycogen that provide an energy reserve. The epithelium metabolizes glucose through two major pathways. The first is the familiar tricarboxilic acid (Krebs) cycle, which produces carbon dioxide, water, and the all-important ATP that provides phosphate for active metabolic processes. The other pathway is the hexosemonophosphate shunt, which produces NADPH (nicotinamide adenine dinucleotide phosphate) which performs a number of functions in the epithelium, including potentiation of the tricarboxilic acid cycle, conversion of pyruvate to lactate in anaerobic metabolism, synthesis of fatty acids that can be used in plasma membrane construction, synthesis of RNA by the incorporation of ribose, and the reduction of glutathione, which, in addition to other functions, helps to neutralize free radicals that may arise in the epithelium. Under hypoxic conditions, such as those induced by a malfitting contact lens, the epithelium can metabolize glucose anaerobically by way of the Embden-Myerhof pathway, resulting in the production of ATP and lactic acid.

Effect of Contact Lens on Corneal Epithelium

A contact lens may have multiple effects on the epithelium: metabolic, traumatic, and thermal.[28] Above all, a contact lens must allow adequate oxygenation of the cornea.

Contact lenses ride on the tear film that separates them from the epithelium. Hard or semiflexible contact lenses that contain methyl methacrylate move during a blink, allowing circulation of tears beneath the lens, replenishing oxygen supplies. If such a lens does not move, oxygen in the underlying tear film decreases to zero in about 15 seconds. This explains why patients who blink poorly develop problems with hard contact lens wear. For hydrophilic contact lenses, the oxygen transmission across the contact lens increases as the thickness decreases and as the water content increases. There is less tear flow beneath soft contact lenses than hard contact lenses. Silicone lenses are highly oxygen-permeable but are hydrophobic and more difficult to fit. The transmission of oxygen across a soft contact lens is estimated by the equation $j = Dk \div L$, where j = oxygen flux, D = diffusion coefficient, k = the proportionality constant, and L = the thickness of the lens.[29]

Contact lenses traumatize the epithelium and may raise epithelial temperature. Left unchecked, these processes damage epithelial cells, producing intercellular and intracellular edema, with resulting blurred vision, halos, and painful punctate epithelial erosions.

Under conditions of trauma and increased temperature and decreased oxygen, epithelial glycogen supplies decrease and anaerobic metabolism produces increased lactic acid. The lactic acid diffuses into the stroma, raising its osmolarity and possibly having a toxic effect on the endothelium, with resultant stromal edema. The effect of these toxic products can be demonstrated clinically by scraping the epithelium off the cornea and gluing a methyl methacrylate lens onto the corneal surface with cyanoacrylate adhesive. Although no oxygen reaches the cornea from the tear film under these circumstances, stromal edema does not occur, probably because there are no products of anaerobic metabolism.

Individuals with tear film dysfunction, such as keratoconjunctivitis sicca, will experience difficulties wearing contact lenses. Not only will there be insufficient tear film to float the plastic gently over the corneal surface, but there will also be deficient tear film to convey oxygen to the epithelium and underlying cornea and insufficient tears to keep a hydrophilic lens from drying out.

BOWMAN'S LAYER AND STROMA

Functions of Bowman's Layer and Stroma

The connective tissue of the cornea performs three functions:

1. Protection. The collagen fibrils that are the major constituents of these tissues make the cornea tough, so that it provides protection to intraocular contents.

2. Determination of shape. Like many other connective tissues in the body, Bowman's layer and the stroma play a structural role by maintaining a fixed shape of the cornea so that it can perform its optical function.

3. Transparency. Unlike most other connective tissues in the body, the cornea must remain transparent.

Bowman's Layer

Bowman's layer is a compact feltwork of fine, randomly oriented collagen fibrils that lies between the epithelial basement membrane and the cellular stroma. This acellular, 12 μm. thick tissue probably helps maintain corneal shape. When the cornea swells, it protrudes posteriorly, not anteriorly, because of the elasticity of Descemet's membrane and the ungiving nature of Bowman's layer.

Bowman's layer is probably produced by the basal epithelial cells, but these cells cannot regenerate it, so in diseases like keratoconus or corneal trauma breaks in Bowman's layer fill with cellular scar tissue that creates permanent opacities.

Corneal Stroma

Structural Components of Stroma

Stromacytes (keratocytes) synthesize the extracellular matrix of the stroma. Collagen fibrils of uniform diameter are stacked in orderly sheets that form approximately 200 lamellae. Proteoglycans, which consist of a protein core with glycosaminoglycan side chains, are the molecules that hold the collagen fibrils in orderly array. These molecules also contain the water in the stroma. Other macromolecules, like glycoproteins, are also present around the collagen molecules and stroma.

Cells in the Stroma

It seems reasonable to call the predominant cell in the stroma a stromacyte rather than a keratocyte since the word more precisely indicates its location in the stroma, whereas the term keratocyte might refer to any cell in the cornea. The flat stromacytes lie between the collagen lamellae and extend five to seven cell processes that touch adjacent stromacytes (Fig. 1–9).[4]

The most prominent intracellular structure is the large nucleus. The cytoplasm contains fine filaments and some organelles, but the organelles do not reflect a high degree of metabolic or synthetic activity. Glycogen particles in the cytoplasm are used as energy stores in this avascular tissue. The small amount of rough endoplasmic reticulum makes the stromacyte structurally different from an ordinary fibroblast, which contains much rough endoplasmic reticulum for protein synthesis. In some pathologic conditions the amount of rough endoplasmic reticulum in the stromacyte increases.

The plasma membrane is smooth but contains focal thickened zones, outside of which fine fibrils and basal lamina substance accumulate, reaching larger proportions in pathologic conditions. There are no connections between the collagen fibrils or proteoglycans and the plasma membrane. The stromacyte is not a phagocytic cell and cytoplasmic lysosomes are rare, although intracellular particles of lipid and debris occasionally appear.

The stromacytes can migrate, and in the area of a corneal wound they accumulate around the margin of the wound, where they act more like fibroblasts and leave a cell-free zone a small distance from the wound.

The histiocytes normally present in the stroma lie flattened between the collagen lamellae like the stromacytes and are probably the main phagocytic cell in the stroma. The presence of lysosomes distinguishes them from stromacytes. Polymorphonuclear leukocytes, plasma cells, and lymphocytes also appear in the normal stroma.

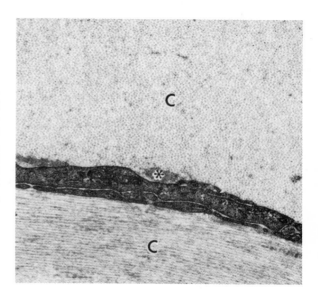

Figure 1–9. Corneal stromal fibroblast surrounded by collagen fibrils (C) in cross and longitudinal section. Patches of granular material (asterisk) are present adjacent to the fibroblast (× 30,000). (From Rodrigues, M. M., Waring, G. O., Hackett, J., and Donohoo, P.: Cornea. In Duane, T. D., and Jaeger, E. A. (eds.): *Biomedical Foundations of Ophthalmology.* Vol. 1. Hagerstown, Md., Harper & Row, 1982, Chapter 8.)

Collagen in the Stroma

The major extracellular material in the corneal stroma is collagen. The collagen fibrils, which apparently stretch from limbus to limbus, form an orderly array in the flat lamellae, where they stack in an orthogonal pattern, with the fibrils of one lamella running approximately at right angles to those in adjacent lamellae (Fig. 1–9). In the anterior stroma the lamellae are not as discrete, since bundles of fibrils interdigitate from one lamella to another. In the posterior stroma the lamellae are more discrete. The clinician can observe this biomicroscopically: the anterior third of the stroma has a slightly grayer appearance than the posterior two thirds. During lamellar keratoplasty the dissection in the posterior stroma is easier where the layers are more defined than in the anterior stroma.

The individual collagen fibrils have a structure similar to collagen fibrils elsewhere in the body.[30] They consist of monomer units of tropocollagen, each consisting of three protein chains wound together in a helical pattern. The tropocollagen units are then assembled end to end in microfibrils, which are cross-linked to form the collagen fibrils. The staggered arrangement of the tropocollagen units creates the characteristic 64 nm. banded pattern seen by transmission electron microscopy. The collagen fibrils are 22 to 32 nm. in diameter, manifest a uniform diameter in the center of the cornea, and vary in size nearer the limbus.

The human corneal stroma contains three different types of collagen,[31] each distinguished according to the biochemical composition of the three protein chains that form the tropocollagen molecule. The predominant collagen is type I, which is the collagen most commonly present in the tissues like the dermis of the skin. There is also some type III collagen, which is characteristically present in tissues that support epithelia. Some type IV collagen, characteristic of basement membranes, may also be present.

Proteoglycans in the Stroma

Unlike other connective tissues, the cornea must remain transparent. This occurs because the regular architecture of the cornea allows light to pass through with minimal disruption.[32] The molecules responsible for maintaining the uniform spacing of the collagen fibrils are the proteoglycans, also referred to as acid mucopolysaccharides. These molecules consist of a central protein core from which glycosaminoglycans extend like bristles from a hairbrush. The glycosaminoglycan molecules are sugars in which repeating disaccharide units form a long polymer chain. The proteoglycan molecules align themselves between the collagen fibrils, and the glycosaminoglycan arms link to the collagen fibrils, holding them apart by a fixed distance of approximately 30 to 60 nm. The exact mechanism by which they accomplish this is unknown, but the glycosaminoglycans are negatively charged, and the repulsive forces within the molecules may be responsible for maintaining the regular structure.

Two glycosaminoglycans are present in normal human stroma: (1) keratan sulfate, which contains both galactose and glucosamine, and (2) chondroitin sulfate B (dermatan sulfate), which contains both galactosamine and glucuronic acid. The protein cores of these two proteoglycans are also different.

The glycosaminoglycans play an important role in stromal hydration. The normal corneal stroma is about 78 per cent water by weight. If more water enters the stroma, as in endothelial dysfunction, the glycosaminoglycan molecules take up the water and swell. This swelling increases corneal thickness, which can be measured clinically by optical or ultrasonic pachymetry. This displaces the collagen fibrils, disrupting their regular alignment and light transmission through the stroma, so that light is scattered and the stroma appears opaque.

Other Material in the Stroma

Glycoproteins are present in the corneal stroma, associated with the proteoglycan molecules. These molecules may aid communication between cells. Elastic-type fibrils occasionally appear in the stroma. Lipids and degenerated material accumulate in the peripheral cornea and may form the corneal arcus.

Corneal Transparency

An exposition of how light traverses the cornea to form a clear image on the retina quickly involves one in mathematical formulations. We explain the phenomenon here in simpler conceptual terms.[15]

When light strikes tissues of nonuniform structure, it is scattered in different directions. This light scattering is observed clinically as opacification of the tissue. Since the cornea consists of tissues that have different indices of refraction, one might expect light scattering; however, only about 1 per cent of light is scattered in the cornea. The reason for this is that the changes in the index of refraction within the cornea occur over distances that are less than half the wave length of light, so that the light makes its way through this structure without interference. One can conceptualize this by considering that the light wave has a limit to its resolution; it cannot detect variations that are less than half its wavelength. Since half the wavelength of visible light is about 200 nm., and since the diameter of the collagen fibrils is 30 nm. and the distance between them about 60 nm., the light passes through the stroma relatively undisturbed. Two analogies help explain this. If one rubs the surface of a finely finished sculpture, it feels very smooth, and yet a scanning electron micrograph would show considerable surface irregularity. Likewise, a basketball rolling down a driveway will not be deflected by small pieces of gravel, but will bounce wildly among potholes. Similarly, the light waves make their way through the normal cornea, unable to detect the small variations in the indices of refraction that are present.

Under pathologic conditions collagen fibrils more than 200 nm. in diameter appear and lakes of edema fluid occur, scattering the light waves and creating a corneal opacity.

CORNEAL ENDOTHELIUM

Population of Endothelial Cells and Aging

The endothelium is the most posterior layer of the cornea and consists at birth

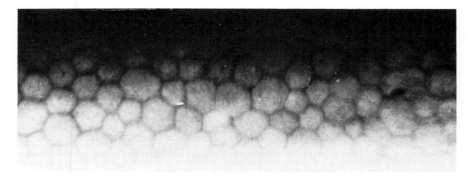

Figure 1–10. Endothelial specular photomicrograph of a normal 27-year-old male shows mosaic pattern with hexagonal cells showing only slight variation in size and shape.

of approximately 350,000 cells (approximately 3000 cells per mm.[2]) arranged in a continuous monolayer 4 to 6 μm. thick.[35] It forms a uniform paving-stone mosaic of closely opposed polygonal cells with five to seven sides, the cells being about 20 μm. in diameter with 250 μm.[2] surface area (Figs. 1–10 and 1–11). The endothelial population is uniformly distributed over the cornea[34] and is symmetrical in both eyes of an individual. In the peripheral cornea the cells become progressively more irregular as they merge with the trabecular endothelium.

In the early years of life cell densities can vary from about 2000 to 4000 cells per mm.[2,35] As the endothelial cells age, some die and disappear. Unfortunately, the human endothelium does not have the capacity to divide rapidly enough to replace aging or injured endothelial cells, so they must enlarge, reorganize, and migrate to maintain the intact monolayer.[36] Although mitosis of the human endothelium has been demonstrated in tissue culture[37] by the cells' ability to incorporate tritiated thymidine, the adult human endothelium must be considered a nonreplicating tissue for clinical purposes.

While some cells enlarge in reponse to aging or disease, other cells remain the same size, so the original homogeneous endothelial population gradually becomes heterogeneous. Between the ages of 5 and 50, the range of normal endothelial cell densities becomes wider, from 1000 to 3500 cells per mm.[2], and by age 80 the range is from 900 to 4000 cells per mm.[2,35,38] This variation makes sense, since individuals are born with different numbers of endothelial cells and these cells age at different rates. Therefore, even though the endothelial cell density generally decreases with age, one cannot look at an endothelial photograph and accurately predict an individual's age. Similarly, although most corneal transplant surgeons think a younger donor cornea is preferable, no study has demonstrated a correlation between donor age and graft clarity.

To accurately describe normal endothelial cell aging or the endothelial response to disease or trauma, measurement of three variables is helpful: (1) cell size in terms of cell density (cells per mm.[2]) or mean cell area (μm.[2]), (2) the spread of cell size in terms of the standard deviation or the coeffecient of variation, and (3) the heterogeneity or asymmetry of the population in terms of the coefficient of skewness.[39]

Endothelial cell density does not correlate well with endothelial function. As the cells enlarge, they can maintain a functional capacity that keeps the cornea clear. However, as the cell density drops below 500 cells per mm.[2], the functional reserve is minimal and corneal edema is likely to appear.[42]

Descemet's Membrane and the Posterior Collagenous Layer

Descemet's membrane is the normal basement membrane of the corneal endothelium and is composed of predominantly type IV collagen and glycopro-

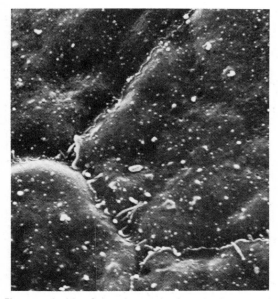

Figure 1–11. Scanning electron micrograph showing intercellular junctions (× 8100). (From Rodrigues, M. M., Waring, G. O., Hackett, J., and Donohoo, P.: Cornea. In Duane, T. D., and Jaeger, E. A. (eds.): *Biomedical Foundations of Ophthalmology.* Vol. 1. Hagerstown, Md., Harper & Row, 1982, Chapter 8.)

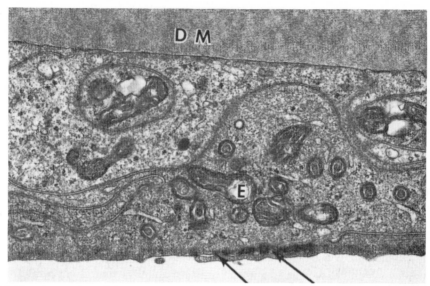

Figure 1–12. The corneal endothelial cells (E) are characterized by numerous mitochondria with a longitudinal orientation of cristae and by abundant free ribosomes. Junctional complexes are indicated by arrows. The posterior portion of Descemet's membrane (DM) appears normal (× 30,000). (From Rodrigues, M. M., Waring, G. O., Hackett, J., and Donohoo, P.: Cornea. In Duane, T. D., and Jaeger, E. A. (eds.): *Biomedical Foundations of Ophthalmology.* Vol. 1. Hagerstown, Md., Harper & Row, 1982, Chapter 8.)

teins, including fibronectin. It stains positive with PAS. The fibronectin may play a role in maintaining the endothelium in a uniform monolayer and in attaching it to Descemet's membrane.

Normal Descemet's membrane has two morphologic components seen by transmission electron microscopy, an anterior portion secreted in utero that manifests a 110-nm. vertical banded pattern and is approximately 3 μm. thick, and a posterior homogeneous nonbanded layer that thickens with age, becoming 10 to 12 μm. thick in the latter decades of life.

Descemet's membrane forms a scaffolding on which the endothelial cells spread themselves (Fig. 1–12) and serves as a barrier to the penetration of leukocytes and blood vessels into the corneal stroma but does not form a barrier to the passage of water and small molecules.

When Descemet's membrane is broken, whether intentionally at surgery or as part of a disease process like the acute breaks that occur in keratoconus, it retracts and coils toward the stroma like a watch spring. To heal this wound the remaining endothelial cells must migrate back over the dehiscence and secrete a new basement membrane.

This production of a new extracellular matrix by an injured healing endothelium is a nonspecific response. The rough endoplasmic reticulum and Golgi apparatus play a role in its production. The tissue produced usually is an abnormal collagenous tissue that accumulates posterior to the normal pre-existing Descemet's membrane, and such a tissue has been described in over 30 corneal disorders. The tissue has been called a retrocorneal fibrous membrane or a thickened Descemet's membrane, but the general descriptive term posterior collagenous layer (PCL) of the cornea sets this tissue apart as a distinct senescent or pathologic entity rather than confusing it with the normal Descemet's membrane.[41] Clinically this abnormal tissue appears as a gray sheet on the back of the cornea that may take on discrete forms like cornea guttata and posterior corneal ridges.

As Descemet's membrane and the posterior collagenous layer accumulate in the posterior cornea, they create an archaeologic record of the endothelial

cells' life experience. This record can be studied by transmission electron microscopy.

Maintenance of Corneal Transparency

The corneal stroma naturally imbibes water because of two forces (Fig. 1–13): (1) the glycosaminoglycans exert an osmotic pressure called the swelling pressure (approximately 60 mm. Hg) that pulls water into the stroma,[42] and (2) the intraocular pressure forces aqueous humor into the stroma. The endothelium counteracts this hydrophilic tendency and maintains corneal transparency in two ways: its barrier function decreases the flow of water into the stroma, and its pump function transports water out of the stroma.

Pump-Leak Model of Corneal Endothelium

The endothelial barrier is leaky; some water normally passes across it into the stroma (Figs. 1–14 and 1–15). However, the leak rate normally equals the ability of the endothelium to pump water back out of the stroma, so the stromal water content remains relatively constant at about 78 per cent by weight and the corneal thickness remains relatively constant at approximately 0.57 mm. At first glance the leaky endothelial barrier may seem inefficient, but when we consider that the nutrients for the entire cornea come from the aqueous and diffuse across the endothelium, the situation makes better sense.[43] Some of the nutrients may be actively transported across the endothelium in pinocytotic vesicles.

Barrier Function of Endothelium

The endothelial cells are attached to each other at their apical margins by junctional complexes, which consist of focal tight junctions, maculae occludentes, with no intercellular space and gap junctions with a 3-nm. interspace (Fig. 1–12). These junctions do not form a tight barrier to the passage of small molecules and water, as the zonulae

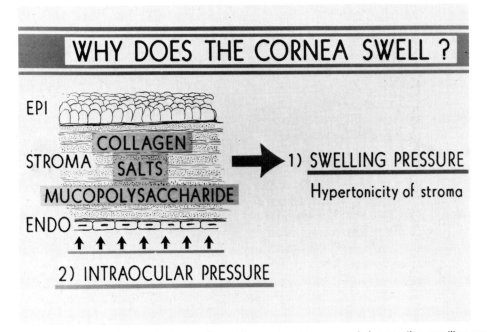

Figure 1–13. Drawing illustrates two forces that drive water into corneal stroma: the swelling pressure created by the glycosaminoglycans in the stroma and the intraocular pressure. (From Waring, G. O., Bourne, W. M., Edelhauser, H. F., and Kenyon, K. R.: The corneal endothelium. Normal and pathologic structure and function. Ophthalmology 89:531, 1982.)

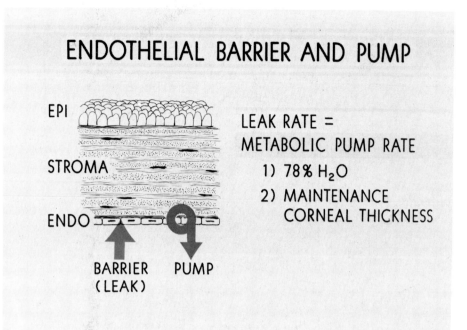

Figure 1-14. Drawing illustrates two endothelial functions that maintain corneal deturgescence: the leaky barrier and the metabolic pump. (From Waring, G. O., Bourne, W. M., Edelhauser, H. F., and Kenyon, K. R.: The corneal endothelium. Normal and pathologic structure and function. Ophthalmology *89*:531, 1982.)

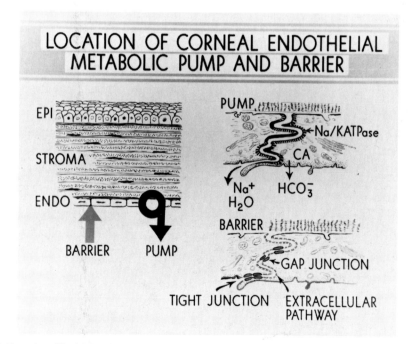

Figure 1-15. Drawing illustrates location of corneal endothelial pump ATPase in the lateral plasma membranes, where it catalyzes transport of ions and of apical junctional complexes that create barrier function. (From Waring, G. O., Bourne, W. M., Edelhauser, H. F., and Kenyon, K. R.: The corneal endothelium. Normal and pathologic structure and function. Ophthalmology *89*:531, 1982.)

occludentes of the surface epithelial cells do. Therefore the barrier is leaky.

The intercellular junctions depend on calcium for their integrity, and calcium-free solutions will reduce the barrier function resulting in increased stromal edema.[44] Intracellular glutathione also helps to maintain intact junctions, and oxidation of this substance will lead to increased stromal thickness (Fig. 1–16).[45]

Drugs and irrigating solutions can damage the barrier function. Those with a pH outside of the tolerable range of 6.8 to 8.2 will damage the plasma membrane. Preservatives, such as thimerosal and benzalkonium chloride, that function as antimicrobials, and sodium bisulfite, which acts as an antioxidant in epinephrine solutions, will break down the endothelial barrier if they are present in too high a concentration.[46]

Pump Function of Endothelium

The first evidence that an active metabolic pump played a role in maintaining corneal transparency was the observation that corneal clarity was temperature-dependent. Lowering the temperature inhibits endothelial metabolic function and results in stromal swelling, and restoration of a physiologic temperature can restore corneal clarity.[47]

The endothelial pump consists of enzymes located in the lateral plasma membrane that catalyze the movement of ions from the stroma to the aqueous humor, creating an osmotic gradient that draws water out of the stroma (Fig. 1–15). These enzymes are ATP-dependent (Fig. 1–16). The many mitochondria in the cytoplasm metabolize glucose, both aerobically and anaerobically, to provide this ATP. The ATPase that catalyzes the transport of bicarbonate ions into the aqueous humor is currently thought to be the major factor in the endothelial pump, although the active transport of sodium and potassium ions may also play a role.[49]

A number of factors can alter this pump function (Fig. 1–17). Inhibition of ATPase with ouabain will produce corneal swelling. A bicarbonate-free solution or the inhibition of endothelial carbonic anhydrase, which produces the bicarbonate ion, will also produce corneal swelling. However, disruption of the barrier function will result in a great deal more corneal swelling than disruption of the pump function.

Intraocular Pressure and the Endothelium

If the endothelium is functioning normally, elevated intraocular pressure may compress the stroma. For example, if a penetrating keratoplasty appears quite clear and compact on the first postoperative day, the surgeon should suspect elevated intraocular pressure. If the endothelial function is marginal, an elevated intraocular pressure will drive fluid across the endothelium, creating epithelial edema, as in acute angle-closure glaucoma. If endothelial function is poor, elevated intraocular pressure will produce stromal and epithelial edema. A low intraocular pressure will often produce a thick, edematous cornea without epithelial edema because of the loss of the compressive effect.

Intraocular Irrigating Solutions

Surgeons must select an intraocular irrigating solution that will not damage the corneal endothelium.[50] Such a solution should contain:

	mM/liter
Sodium	160
Potassium	5
Calcium	1
Magnesium	1
Chloride	130
Bicarbonate	25
Phosphate	3
Dextrose	5
Glutathione disulfide	0.3
pH	7.2–7.4
Osmolality	305

Many medications may be used safely intraocularly. Antibiotics that may be

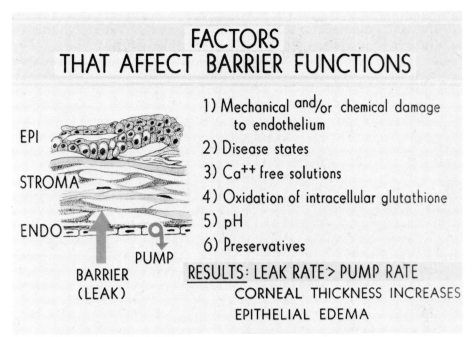

FACTORS
THAT AFFECT BARRIER FUNCTIONS

EPI

STROMA

ENDO

PUMP

BARRIER
(LEAK)

1) Mechanical and/or chemical damage to endothelium
2) Disease states
3) Ca^{++} free solutions
4) Oxidation of intracellular glutathione
5) pH
6) Preservatives

<u>RESULTS</u>: LEAK RATE > PUMP RATE
CORNEAL THICKNESS INCREASES
EPITHELIAL EDEMA

Figure 1–16. Drawing emphasizes factors that decrease barrier function so that the leak of fluid into the stroma exceeds removal of fluid by the pump, resulting in corneal edema. (From Waring, G. O., Bourne, W. M., Edelhauser, H. F., and Kenyon, K. R.: The corneal endothelium. Normal and pathologic structure and function. Ophthalmology *89*:531, 1982.)

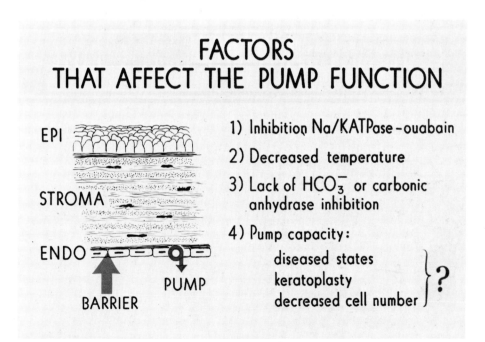

FACTORS
THAT AFFECT THE PUMP FUNCTION

EPI

STROMA

ENDO

PUMP

BARRIER

1) Inhibition Na/KATPase – ouabain
2) Decreased temperature
3) Lack of HCO_3^- or carbonic anhydrase inhibition
4) Pump capacity:
   diseased states
   keratoplasty
   decreased cell number } ?

Figure 1–17. Drawing emphasizes factors that decrease function of the metabolic pump, resulting in excess water remaining in the stroma. (From Waring, G. O., Bourne, W. M., Edelhauser, H. F., and Kenyon, K. R.: The corneal endothelium. Normal and pathologic structure and function. Ophthalmology *89*:531, 1982.)

used safely include gentamicin, chloromycetin, erythromycin, penicillin G, and oxacillin. Phenylephrine can damage the endothelium, but epinephrine seems safe[51, 52] if it does not contain high levels of the antioxidant sodium bisulfite. The preservatives thimerosal, benzalkonium chloride and chlorhexidine cause severe endothelial damage and should not be used intraocularly.[53, 54]

REFERENCES

1. Edelhauser, H. F., Van Horn, D. L., and Records, R. E.: Cornea and sclera. In Records, R. E. (ed.): *Physiology of the Human Eye and Visual System*. Hagerstown, Md., Harper & Row, 1979, pp. 68–97.
2. Edelhauser, H. F., Van Horn, D. L., and Records, R. E.: Cornea and sclera. In Duane, T. D., and Jaeger, E. A. (eds.): *Biomedical Foundations of Ophthalmology*. Vol. 2. Hagerstown, Md., Harper & Row, 1982, Chapter 4.
3. Maurice, D. M.: The cornea and sclera. In Davson, H. (ed.): *The Eye*. Vol 1. New York, Academic Press, 1969, pp. 489–600.
4. Kuwabara, T.: Current concepts in anatomy and histology of the cornea. Cont Intraoc Lens Med J 4:101, 1978.
5. Cogan, D. G.: Applied anatomy and physiology of the cornea. Trans Amer Acad Ophthalmol Otolaryngol 55:329, 1951.
6. Ruben, M. (ed.): *Contact Lens Practice*. Baltimore, Williams & Wilkins, 1975.
7. Sorsby, A.: Biology of the eye as an optical system. In Duane, T. D., and Jaeger, E. A. (eds.): *Clinical Ophthalmology*. Vol. 1. Hagerstown, Md., Harper & Row, 1982, Chapter 34.
8. Sampson, W. G., and Soper, J. W.: Keratometry. In Girard, L. J. (ed.): *Corneal Contact Lenses*. St. Louis, C. V. Mosby Co., 1970, pp. 65–92.
9. Doss, J. D., Hutson, R. L., Rowsey, J. J., and Brown, D. R.: Method for calculation of corneal profile and power distribution. Arch Ophthalmol 99:1261, 1981.
10. Rowsey, J. J., Reynolds, A. E., and Brown, R.: Corneal topography. Arch Ophthalmol 99:1093, 1981.
11. Jaffe, N. S., and Clayman, H. M.: The pathophysiology of corneal astigmatism after cataract extraction. Trans Amer Acad Ophthalmol Otolaryngol 79:615, 1975.
12. Perlman, E. M.: An analysis and interpretation of refractive errors after penetrating keratoplasty. Ophthalmology 88:39, 1981.
13. Colvard, D. M., Kratz, R. P., Mazzocco, T. R., and Davidson, B.: Clinical evaluation of the Terry surgical keratometer. Amer Intraoc Implant Soc J 6:249, 1980.
14. Krachmer, J. H., and Fenzl, R. E.: Surgical correction of high postkeratoplasty astigmatism. Arch Ophthalmol 98:1400, 1980.
15. Miller, D., and Benedek, G.: *Intraocular Light Scattering*. Springfield, Ill., Charles C Thomas, 1973.
16. Thoft, R. A., and Friend, J. (eds.): *The Ocular Surface*. Boston, Little, Brown, 1979.
17. Rodrigues, M. M., Rowden, G., Hackett, J., and Bakos, I.: Langerhans cells in the normal conjunctiva and peripheral cornea of selected species. Invest Ophthalmol Vis Sci 21:759, 1981.
18. Gipson, I. K., and Keezer, L.: Effect of cytochalasins and colchicine on the ultrastructure of migrating corneal epithelium. Invest Ophthalmol Vis Sci 22:643, 1982.
19. Foulks, G. N.: Treatment of recurrent corneal erosion and corneal edema with topical osmotic colloidal solution. Ophthalmology 88:801, 1981.
20. Candia, O. A., and Podos, S. M.: Inhibition of active transport of chloride and sodium by vanadate in the cornea. Invest Ophthalmol Vis Sci 20:733, 1981.
21. Gipson, I. K., and Anderson, R. A.: Actin filaments in normal and migrating corneal epithelial cells. Invest Ophthalmol Vis Sci 16:161, 1977.
22. Fujikawa, L. S., Foster, C. S., and Colvin, R. B.: Basement membrane components in rabbit corneal epithelial wounds. Invest Ophthalmol Vis Sci 20(Suppl):38, 1981 (abstract).
23. Fogle, J. A., Green, W. R., and Kenyon, K. R.: Anterior corneal dystrophy. Amer J Ophthalmol 77:529, 1974.
24. Rosco, W. R., and Hill, R. M.: Corneal oxygen demands: a comparison of the open- and closed-eye environments. Amer Optom Physiol Opt 57:67, 1980.
25. Friend, J.: Biochemistry of ocular surface epithelium. In Thoft, R. A., and Friend, J. (eds.): *The Ocular Surface*. Boston, Little, Brown, 1979, pp. 73–91.
26. Dohlman, C. H., Refojo, M. F., and Rose, J.: Synthetic polymers in corneal surgery. I. Glyceryl methacrylate. Arch Ophthalmol 77:252, 1967.
27. McCarey, B. E., and Andrews, D. M.: Refractive keratoplasty with intrastromal hydrogel lenticular implants. Invest Ophthalmol Vis Sci 21:107, 1981.
28. Mishima, S.: Corneal physiology under contact lenses. In Gasset, A. R., and Kaufman, H. E. (eds.): *Soft Contact Lens*. St. Louis, C. V. Mosby Co., 1972, pp. 19–36.
29. Fatt, I.: Gas transmission properties of soft contact lenses. In Ruben, M. (ed.): *Soft Contact Lenses: Clinical and Applied Technology*. New York, John Wiley & Sons, 1978, pp. 83–110.
30. Klintworth, G. K.: The cornea—structure and macromolecules in health and disease. A review. Amer J Pathol 89:719, 1977.
31. Newsome, D. A., Gross, J., and Hassel, J. R.: Human corneal stroma contains 3 distinct collagens. Invest Ophthalmol Vis Sci 22:376, 1982.
32. Borcherding, M. S., Blacik, L. J., Sittig, R. A., Bizzell, J. W., Breen, M., and Weinstein, H. G.: Proteoglycans and collagen fibre organization in human corneoscleral tissue. Exp Eye Res 21:59, 1975.
33. Waring, G. O., Bourne, W. M., Edelhauser, H. F., and Kenyon, K. R.: The corneal endothelium. Normal and pathologic structure and function. Ophthalmology 89:531, 1982.
34. Sturrock, G. D., Sherrard, E. S., and Rice, N. S. C.: Specular microscopy of the corneal endothelium. Brit J Ophthalmol 62:809, 1978.

35. Hiles, D. A., Biglan, A. W., and Fetherolf, E. C.: Central corneal endothelial cell counts in children. Amer Intraoc Implant Soc J 5:292, 1979.

36. Van Horn, D. L., and Hyndiuk, R. A.: Endothelial wound repair in primate cornea. Exp Eye Res 21:113, 1975.

37. Simonsen, A. H., Sorensen, K. E., and Sperling, S.: Thymidine incorporation by human corneal endothelium during organ culture. Acta Ophthalmol 59:110, 1981.

38. Hoffer, K. J., and Kraff, M. C.: Normal endothelial cell count range. Ophthalmology 87:861, 1980.

39. Waring, G. O., Krohn, M. A., Ford, G. E., and Rosenblatt, L. S.: Individual corneal endothelial cell size correlates poorly with age. Invest Ophthalmol Vis Sci 19 (Suppl):263, 1980.

40. Mishima, S.: Clinical investigations on the corneal endothelium. Am J Ophthalmol 93:1, 1982.

41. Waring, G. O.: Posterior collagenous layer of the cornea. Ultrastructural classification of abnormal collagenous tissue posterior to Descemet's membrane in 30 cases. Arch Ophthalmol 100:122, 1982.

42. Elliott, G. F., Goodfellow, J. M., and Wollgar, A. E.: Swelling studies of bovine corneal stroma without bounding membranes. J Physiol 298:453, 1980.

43. Thoft, R. A., Friend, J., and Dohlman, C. H.: Corneal glucose flux. II. Its response to anterior chamber blockade and endothelial damage. Arch Ophthalmol 86:685, 1971.

44. Stern, M. E., Edelhauser, H. F., Pederson, H. J., and Staatz, W. D.: Effects of ionophores X537A and A23187 and calcium-free medium on corneal endothelial morphology. Invest Ophthalmol Vis Sci 20:497, 1981.

45. Edelhauser, H. F., Van Horn, D. L., Miller, P., and Pederson, H. J.: Effect of thiol-oxidation of glutathione with diamide on corneal endothelial function, junctional complexes, and microfilaments. J Cell Biol 68:567, 1976.

46. Green, K., Hull, D. S., Vaughn, E. D., et al.: Rabbit endothelial response to ophthalmic preservatives. Arch Ophthalmol 95:2218, 1977.

47. Harris, J. E.: Symposium on the cornea. Introduction: factors influencing corneal hydration. Invest Ophthalmol 1:151, 1962.

48. Hodson, S.: The endothelial pump of the cornea. Invest Ophthalmol Vis Sci 16:589, 1977.

49. Hull, D. S., Green, K., Boyd, M., and Wynn, H. R.: Corneal endothelium bicarbonate transport and the effect of carbonic anhydrase inhibitors on endothelial permeability and fluxes and corneal thickness. Invest Ophthalmol Vis Sci 16:883, 1977.

50. Edelhauser, H. F., Gonnering, R., and Van Horn, D. L.: Intraocular irrigating solutions: a comparative study of BSS plus and lactated Ringer's solution. Arch Ophthalmol 96:516, 1978.

51. Olson, R. J., Kolodner, H., Riddle, P., and Escapini, H., Jr.: Commonly used intraocular medications and the corneal endothelium. Arch Ophthalmol 98:2224, 1980.

52. Coles, W. H.: Effects of antibiotics on the in vitro rabbit corneal endothelium. Invest Ophthalmol 14:246, 1975.

53. Van Horn, D. L., Edelhauser, H. F., and Prodanovich, G.: Effect of the ophthalmic preservative thimerosal on rabbit and human corneal endothelium. Invest Ophthalmol Vis Sci 16:273, 1977.

54. Green, K., Livingston, V., and Bowman, K.: Chlorhexidine effects on corneal epithelium and endothelium. Arch Ophthalmol 98:1273, 1980.

II

DEVELOPMENTAL AND STRUCTURAL ABNORMALITIES

Congenital and Neonatal Corneal Abnormalities

2

GEORGE O. WARING, III, M.D.

The practicing ophthalmologist rarely sees corneal abnormalities in the newborn infant. When he does, he often feels anxious because of the child's potential lifelong blindness and because of his own difficulty in making a proper diagnosis. This concise survey of neonatal corneal abnormalities emphasizes practical clinical diagnosis and management.

EXAMINATION OF THE NEONATAL CORNEA

The ophthalmologist can gain much pertinent information from examination of the infant in the office or nursery (Figs. 2–1 to 2–7). If the child is hungry prior to the examination, a bottle or pacifier will help keep him quiet. After the instillation of topical anesthetic and placement of an infant eyelid speculum or small Koeppe lens, the hungry infant will become quiet while sucking on the pacifier or bottle in the parent's lap. The ophthalmologist can then obtain much of the information listed in Table 2–1.[1]

A portable slit lamp provides the most information about the anterior segment and allows the ophthalmologist to make a careful drawing of anterior segment abnormalities.[2] Measurement of corneal diameter with calipers provides a baseline for detection of later enlargement from infantile glaucoma, and measurement of the diameter of a corneal opacity helps in selection of the size of a corneal graft. Electronic or pneumatic tonometry determines intraocular pressure through a scarred cornea without disturbing the supine child, but in eyes with hypertrophic scarred corneas, the ophthalmologist must estimate the pressure by palpation. A portable contact B-scan ultrasound instrument rapidly detects vitreoretinal abnormalities, although quantitative A-scan ultrasound may be necessary to define their structure. Retinal and afferent visual pathway function may be estimated by a bright-flash photopic electroretinogram and the visually evoked potential, using periorbital and occipital electrodes and a signal averager.[3]

A well-equipped ophthalmology facility can perform all the examinations in about 2 hours and the results are immediately available, so that the ophthalmologist can usually make an accurate diagnosis, decide about possible visual rehabilitation, and give the family a general prognosis for useful vision. Detailed examination of the anterior chamber angle or fundus may, of course, require general anesthesia; often, however, the corneal abnormality prevents visualization of these structures.

ABSENCE OF THE CORNEA AND CRYPTOPHTHALMOS

Total absence of the cornea is extremely rare, but a more common abnormality, cryptophthalmos, may be seen in office practice. In this disorder, facial skin replaces the eyelid and covers the orbit,

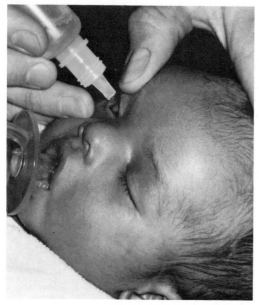

Figure 2-1. Ocular examination of the neonate in the office begins with bilateral instillation of a topical anesthetic.

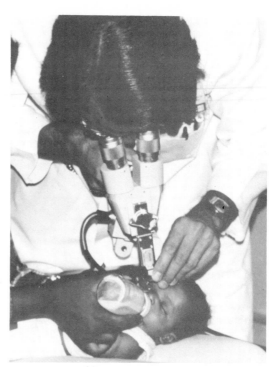

Figure 2-3. Portable slit lamp with fiberoptic illumination and zoom optics permits detailed anterior segment examination and photography.

obliterating the underlying cornea[4] (Fig. 2-8). It usually occurs sporadically as part of a systemic syndrome with dyscephaly, syndactyly, and urogenital abnormalities, but autosomal recessive inheritance may occur.[5] In bilateral cases, if B-scan ultrasonography reveals an apparently normal posterior segment to the underlying globe, eyelid reconstruction and possible keratoplasty may be at-

tempted, although the chance of success is remote.

MEGALOCORNEA AND ANTERIOR MEGALOPHTHALMOS

The cornea of the newborn measures about 10 mm. in horizontal diameter and reaches the adult average measurement of 11.75 mm. by age 2 years. If the horizontal diameter of the cornea is 12 mm. or more in the neonate or 13 mm. or more in the adult, megalocornea is present.

Megalocornea occurs in three patterns: (1) simple megalocornea unassociated with other abnormalities; (2) anterior megalophthalmos with megalocornea, iris and angle abnormalities, lens subluxation, and early cataract formation; and (3) buphthalmos in infantile glaucoma. In keratoglobus, a generalized corneal thinning results in a protuberant cornea that appears enlarged clinically but usually has a normal diameter (Table 2-2).

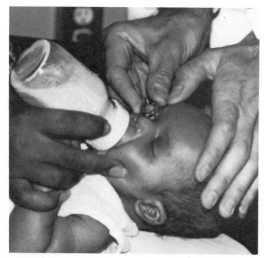

Figure 2-2. A hungry infant will not object to the placement of a pediatric eyelid speculum or small Koeppe lens.

Text continued on page 36

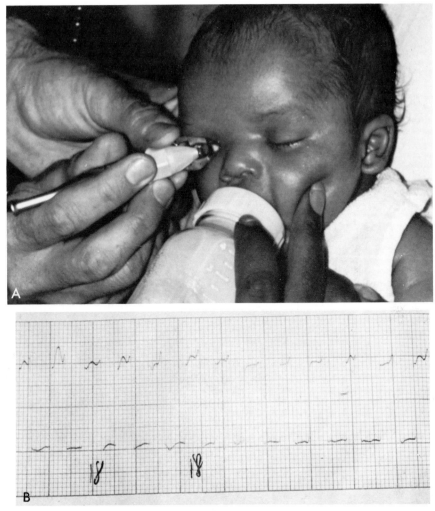

Figure 2–4. *A,* Electronic MacKay-Marg tonometry accurately measures ocular pressure through most scarred corneas. Lifting lid speculum prevents artificial elevation of ocular pressure. *B,* Only consistent readings of good waveform accurately reflect ocular pressure.

Figure 2–5. Measurement of corneal diameter provides a baseline to detect corneal enlargement from infantile glaucoma, and measurement of opacity diameter helps determine keratoplasty size.

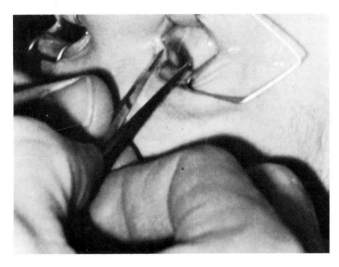

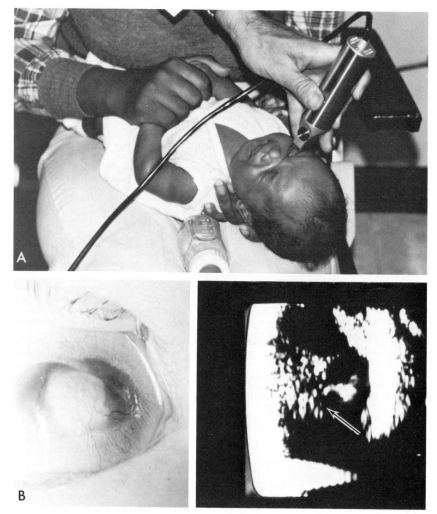

Figure 2–6. *A,* Contact B-scan ultrasound rapidly reveals vitreoretinal abnormalities, even in an uncooperative infant. *B,* Behind the congenitally scarred cornea (left), B-scan ultrasound (right) shows extensive vitreoretinal echoes (arrow).

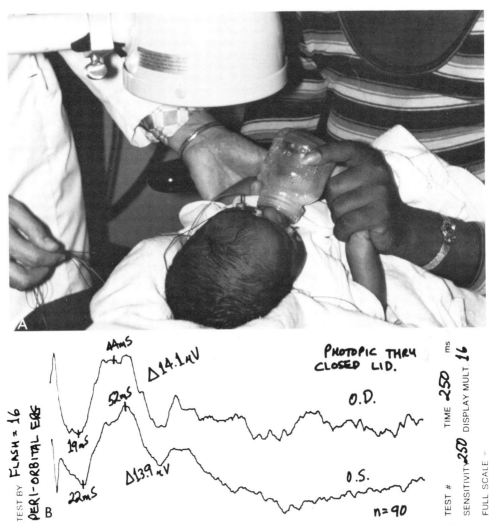

Figure 2–7. *A,* Bright flash electroretinogram can be recorded through closed eyelids with periorbital electrodes and summating apparatus. Likewise, visually evoked potentials can be measured in infants. *B,* Electroretinogram recorded from periorbital electrodes in infant with bilateral Peters' anomaly reveals normal amplitude and latency.

Table 2–1. EVALUATION OF NEONATAL CORNEAL ABNORMALITY*

Evaluation	Instruments (Portable)	Record
Eyelid and tear function	Hand light Schirmer strip	Eyelid and lash anatomy Tear production

Biomicroscopy	Kowa II portable slit lamp or
	  operating microscope
	35-mm. camera
		Frontal and cross-section drawing of
		  anterior segment
		Photographs

Corneal diameter measurement	Caliper	Diameter of cornea and opacity
Ophthalmoscopy	Mydriatics Indirect ophthalmoscope	Vitreoretinal and optic disc appearance
Refraction	Retinoscope	Estimates of refractive error in mild opacities
Tonometry	Electronic or pneumatic tonometer	Repeatable accurate intraocular pressure readings
	Palpation	Estimated pressure if cornea grossly distorted
Gonioscopy	Koeppe lens; Kowa II slit lamp or Kowa fundus camera	Angle drawing Goniophotography
Ultrasonography	Contact B-scan	Acoustical clarity of vitreous and retina
	A-scan or B-scan with water bath	Position of iris and lens; globe diameter

Afferent visual pathway	Electroretinogram—periorbital
	  electrodes
		Summated response to multiple bright
		  flashes

	Visually evoked potential apparatus	Summated response to multiple bright flashes

*See Reference 1.

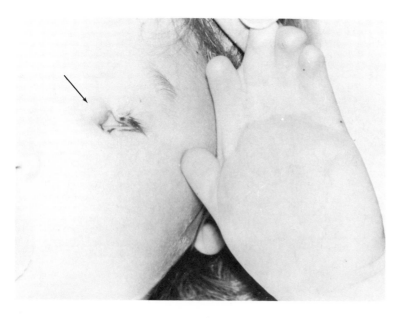

Figure 2–8. Partial cryptophthalmos and syndactyly. Medial eyelids are absent and skin fuses to cornea (arrow). Medial portion of eyebrow is also absent, and hair stream extends down to orbit.

Table 2–2. DIFFERENTIAL DIAGNOSIS OF ENLARGED CORNEA

	Simple Megalocornea	Anterior Megalophthalmos	Primary Infantile Glaucoma with Buphthalmos	Keratoglobus (Ehlers-Danlos Type VI A)
Inheritance	Autosomal dominant (?)	X-linked recessive	Sporadic	Autosomal recessive
Time of appearance	Congenital	Congenital	First year of life	Usually congenital
Bilaterality	Bilateral Symmetrical	Bilateral Symmetrical	Unilateral or bilateral Asymmetrical	Bilateral Symmetrical
Natural history	Nonprogressive	Nonprogressive	Progressive	Nonprogressive
Corneal clarity	Clear	Clear or mosaic dystrophy	Diffuse edema; tears in Descemet's membrane	Clear; acute central edema
Intraocular pressure	Normal	Elevated in some adults	Elevated	Normal
Corneal diameter	13–18 mm.	13–18 mm.	13–18 mm.	10–12 mm. (occasionally > 13 mm.)
Corneal thickness	Normal	Normal	Thick	Thin
Keratometry	Normal	Normal	Flat	Steep
Gonioscopy	Normal	Excess mesenchymal tissue	Abnormal mesenchymal tissue	Normal
Major ocular complications	None	Lens dislocation Cataract < 40 years Secondary glaucoma	Optic nerve damage Late corneal edema	Corneal rupture from minor trauma Acute corneal edema Amblyopia
Associated systemic disorders	None	Occasionally Marfan's and other skeletal abnormalities	None consistent	Hyperextensible joints Hearing loss Tooth discoloration

Simple Megalocornea

A clear cornea with normal thickness that has a diameter 13 mm. or more may be present in a normal globe. This is nonprogressive and may be autosomal dominant, although few pedigrees have been reported.[6, 7]

Anterior Megalophthalmos

In this X-linked recessive disorder, abnormalities occur throughout the anterior segment, sometimes associated with skeletal, neurologic, and dermatologic abnormalities.[8] The cornea is usually clear but may contain a mosaic stromal opacity. Although corneal curvature is usually normal, the enlarged cornea produces a deep anterior chamber. The anterior iris stroma is often hypoplastic (Fig. 2–9), and full thickness iris holes may occur along with diffuse pigment dispersion. Excess mesenchymal tissue may occupy the angle, and elevated intraocular pressure occurs more frequently than normal. Iridodonesis re-

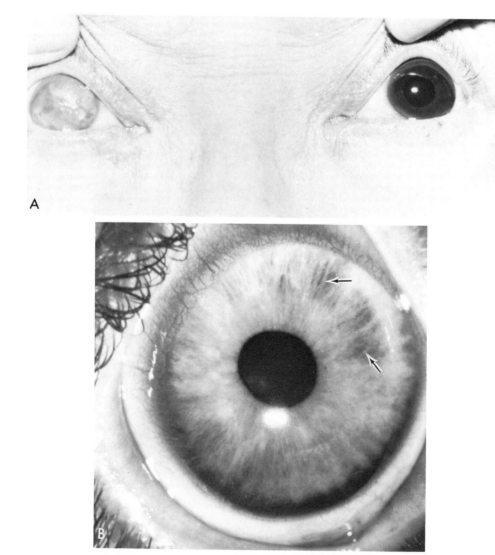

Figure 2–9. Anterior megalophthalmos. *A*, Both corneas measure 15 mm. horizontal diameter. This 45-year-old man developed bilateral early cataracts and subluxated lenses and is now surgically aphakic, with aphakic corneal edema in the right eye. *B*, Cornea 15 mm. in diameter manifests normal clarity. Pupil is slightly oval, and focal areas of iris stromal atrophy (arrows) are present. Lens was clear and in normal position in this 27-year-old patient.

flects the lens subluxation that occurs commonly, and cataracts frequently appear before age 40.[9]

These patients should have lifelong examinations to detect elevated intraocular pressure and early lens opacity. Cataract extraction is more hazardous in anterior megalophthalmos than in a normal eye (Fig. 2–9A), since the lens is dislocated and since the surgery occurs at an earlier age; the surgeon should be prepared to perform a mechanical anterior vitrectomy. Management of the elevated intraocular pressure is similar to that of chronic open-angle glaucoma.

KERATOGLOBUS

Keratoglobus is a generalized thinning and anterior protrusion of the cornea that occurs bilaterally as an autosomal recessive condition, often associated with blue sclerae and hyperextensible hand and ankle joints.[10–13] It may be part of the Ehlers-Danlos syndromes, as Type VI A.[14] Corneal diameter is usually normal, although sometimes it reaches 13 to 16 mm. The cornea is about one third of normal thickness and arches steeply over the anterior chamber (Fig. 2–10), with keratometry readings often over 50 diopters. Faint stromal opacification may occur, and spontaneous central breaks in Descemet's membrane, similar to those in acute hydrops of keratoconus, may appear at any time. This acute corneal edema clears gradually and spontaneously over weeks to months and requires no treatment.

Early recognition of the disorder, which often is suggested by the blue sclera, is important, since careful refraction may reduce the amblyopia that results from the refractive errors. Whether or not lamellar keratoplasty helps to reduce amblyopia in the more severely involved eyes is unknown.

The most serious aspect of this disorder is the fragility of the cornea and sclera. Rupture of these tissues may occur following minimal blunt trauma. Until the child matures enough to protect his own eyes, careful parental coun-

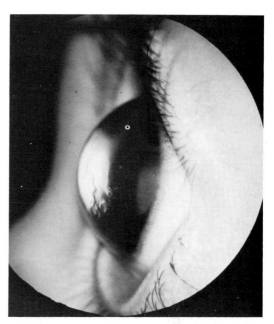

Figure 2–10. In keratoglobus, diffusely thin cornea protrudes anteriorly.

seling, provision of an unusually safe environment, and enforced wearing of protective spectacles or eyeguards are mandatory.

MICROCORNEA

Microcornea usually measures 7 to 10 mm. in horizontal diameter but may be as small as 4 mm.[15] It may occur as an isolated abnormality[16] or accompany other anterior segment anomalies like aniridia and anterior chamber cleavage abnormalities. Microcornea is part of nanophthalmos or "pure microphthalmos," a condition in which a reduction in global dimensions is the only structural abnormality,[17] as well as microphthalmos, a term generally used to signify a small, abnormal globe (Fig. 2–11). This wide variety of manifestations makes generalities about microcornea difficult. In some instances, microcornea may be familial. In eyes with an indistinct scleralized limbus, measurement of the true corneal diameter is difficult, and transillumination will highlight the ciliary ring, allowing more accurate measurements. Although the radius of curvature is usually large and the cornea is usually

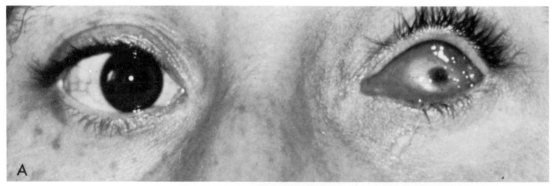

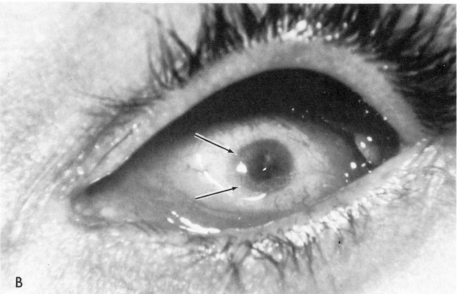

Figure 2–11. Microcornea in microphthalmos. *A,* Cornea 4 mm. in diameter is part of small globe with multiple abnormalities. *B,* Peripheral scleralization (arrows) makes exact measurement of horizontal corneal diameter difficult.

flat, the refractive error varies from hyperopia to myopia. Glaucoma may occur more frequently; lifelong follow-up will detect a rise in intraocular pressure before optic nerve damage occurs.

NEONATAL CORNEAL OPACITIES

The ophthalmologist who examines an uncooperative infant with corneal opacities often feels "stumped," and this reaction provides him with an acronym to help remember the differential diagnosis of the neonatal cloudy cornea (Table 2–3). Infantile glaucoma and Peters' anomaly are the most common.

SCLEROCORNEA

Sclerocornea is not a discrete diagnostic entity, since ophthalmologists apply the term to a broad spectrum of corneal disorders.[18] The common feature is the peripheral, white, vascularized cornea that blends with the sclera, obliterating the limbus and scleral sulcus. The center of the cornea is clearer than the periphery. It usually appears sporadically, either unilaterally or bilaterally, without consistent systemic abnormalities. Sclerocornea falls into four groups, but the distinctions are not clear-cut: (1) isolated sclerocornea; (2) sclerocornea plana (cornea plana); (3) peripheral sclerocornea with anterior chamber

Table 2–3. STUMPED: Acronym for the Differential Diagnosis of Neonatal Cloudy Cornea

S	Sclerocornea
T	Tears in Descemet's membrane
	Infantile glaucoma
	Birth trauma
U	Ulcer
	Herpes simplex virus
	Bacterial
	Neurotrophic
M	Metabolic (rarely present at birth)
	Mucopolysaccharidoses
	Mucolipidoses
	Tyrosinosis
P	Posterior corneal defect
	Posterior keratoconus
	Peters' anomaly
	Staphyloma
E	Endothelial dystrophy
	Congenital hereditary
	Posterior polymorphous
	Congenital hereditary stromal dystrophy
D	Dermoid, central

cleavage abnormality; and (4) total sclerocornea.

Isolated Sclerocornea

In isolated sclerocornea, other ocular abnormalities are absent, and histopathologic examination should demonstrate collagen fibrils with a diameter and arrangement similar to that of sclera.[19, 20]

Sclerocornea Plana

This bilateral disorder manifests a flat cornea with keratometry readings of about 38 diopters or less. Amblyopia and strabismus are often present, sometimes accompanied by aniridia, cataracts, or infantile glaucoma. The central cornea is usually clear, but the peripheral cornea blends with the adjacent sclera, rendering measurement of the true corneal diameter difficult.

Peripheral Sclerocornea with Anterior Chamber Cleavage Abnormalities

About 80 per cent of eyes with Rieger's syndrome and many eyes with Peters' anomaly manifest an indistinct corneoscleral limbus, sometimes called scleralization of the cornea.[21] When most of the cornea is opaque, the distinction between Peters' anomaly with its central corneal opacity and sclerocornea with its slightly clearer central zone may be difficult. A histopathologic distinction also may be difficult, since some cases of clinical Peters' anomaly have a thin Descemet's membrane over the posterior surface, while other clinical cases of sclerocornea have posterior defects in Descemet's membrane.[22–24] In either case, the management is similar.

Total Sclerocornea

When the entire cornea is opaque and vascularized, precise clinical diagnosis is difficult (Fig. 2–12).

The clinical appearance of sclerocornea is variable.[25] A peripheral rim may extend 1 or 2 mm. into the cornea with a fairly distinct central margin. Irregular areas of grayish-white tissue may spread from the peripheral opacity into the midperipheral cornea. A diffusely opaque cornea, more dense in the periphery, may be surfaced with a network of anastomosing vessels.

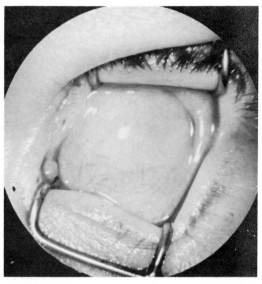

Figure 2–12. Total sclerocornea. White, vascularized, scleralike tissue replaces entire cornea. Penetrating keratoplasty revealed lens and iris adherent to posterior surface of sclerocornea.

The characteristic histopathologic finding is one of disorganized bundles of vascularized collagenous tissue that contains fibrils 70 to 150 nm. in diameter. These are much larger than the normal corneal fibril (25 to 30 nm.).[20]

TEARS IN THE ENDOTHELIUM AND DESCEMET'S MEMBRANE

Tears or breaks in the endothelium and Descemet's membrane occur after birth trauma or in infantile glaucoma and produce corneal edema. The cornea and sclera of infants are more elastic and distensible than those of adults, so that elevation of intraocular pressure, whether acute as in birth trauma or chronic as in infantile glaucoma, distends the infant globe, exceeds the elasticity of Descemet's membrane, and produces tears that allow the stroma to imbibe aqueous with resultant stromal and epithelial edema.

Most ophthalmologists will not see an acute case of ocular birth trauma, since elective cesarean section and improved prenatal care have greatly reduced complicated forceps deliveries. When they do occur, there is periorbital ecchymosis and diffuse corneal edema. Careful slit lamp examination may be necessary to detect the refractile edges of the breaks in Descemet's membrane. As the young endothelium heals over the tears, corneal edema disappears and a series of parallel, vertical or oblique, refractile, posterior corneal ridges (Haab's striae) appears (Fig. 2–13). These ridges occur in pairs, each representing one side of the break in Descemet's membrane. They become prominent because the regenerating endothelium lays down new layers of thickened basement membrane over the coiled edge of the original break (Fig. 2–14).

In infantile glaucoma, corneal epithelial and stromal edema is the most common presenting sign in the first 5 days of life;[26] the enlarged cornea and globe of buphthalmos generally are not present in the immediate postpartum period. Removal of the edematous epithelium with a cotton applicator or application of a Koeppe lens enhances the view of the underlying tears. The tears assume a random distribution, often lying circumferential to the limbus and then turning in serpentine fashion toward the center of the cornea. Each tear has two edges, which are roughly parallel. After treatment lowers the intraocular pressure, the overlying corneal edema clears and the edges of the underlying tears assume their prominent refractile appearance because of the excess basement membrane produced by the healing endothelium.

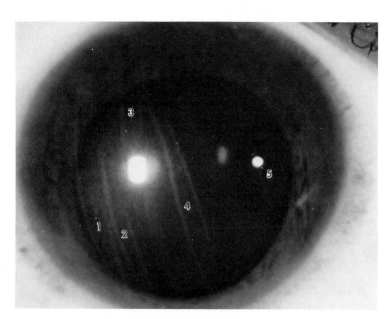

Figure 2–13. Tears in Descemet's membrane after birth trauma. Juvenile endothelium has resurfaced the cornea, which is now clear. Each of five vertical tears (1–5) is bounded by two parallel refractile ridges.

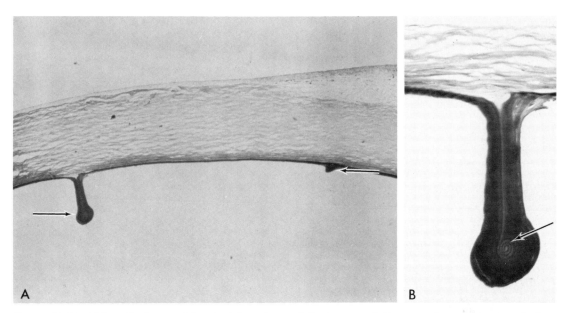

Figure 2–14. Histopathology of healed tear in endothelium and Descemet's membrane. *A,* Two prominent ridges of newly produced collagenous tissue protrude into anterior chamber (arrows). These correspond to the two edges of the tear seen clinically. Endothelium has resurfaced the tear between these two edges and produced new basement membrane. (PAS, × 4.) *B,* High power view of one of the ridges reveals a central core of original Descemet's membrane coiled like watch spring (arrow) that is surrounded by layers of regenerated basement membrane with an irregular knobby surface. (PAS, × 256.) (From Waring, G. O., Laibson, P. R., and Rodrigues, M. M.: Clinical and pathologic alterations of Descemet's membrane: With emphasis on endothelial metaplasia. Surv Ophthalmol *18*:325, 1974. Used with permission of the Survey of Ophthalmology.)

In the second and third decade of life, the endothelium previously stressed by birth trauma or infantile glaucoma may decompensate, with resulting corneal edema that requires penetrating keratoplasty to restore vision (Fig. 2–15).[27] High corneal astigmatism may also be present.

CORNEAL ULCERS

Corneal ulcers rarely occur at birth, but herpes simplex keratitis, bacterial keratitis, neurotrophic keratitis, and tyrosinosis may present in the neonatal period. Tyrosinosis is discussed in the following section on metabolic corneal opacities.

Two cases of congenital herpes simplex keratitis have been reported.[28, 29] In both infants, the disease was characterized by a purulent exudate, a conjunctival membrane, a geographic central epithelial defect, and stromal opacities.

The latter occupied the central cornea, whereas the periphery generally was clearer and slightly vascularized (Fig. 2–16). Ocular involvement may also be present in about 10 per cent of neonates with systemic herpes simplex infection, and it appears 1 to 5 weeks postpartum as conjunctivitis, keratitis, chorioretinitis, optic neuritis, or cataracts. Unfortunately, topical silver nitrate prophylaxis is ineffective.[30] The ophthalmologist must have a high index of suspicion to make the diagnosis. Conjunctival scrapings may reveal giant cells or intranuclear inclusions typical of herpes simplex, and bacterial cultures usually show no growth. However, as more rapid methods of viral diagnosis, such as fluorescein antibody or peroxidase antibody staining, become available in community hospital laboratories, the ophthalmologist will have more precise tools to make the diagnosis. Under these circumstances, he will scrape the conjunctiva, place the epithelial cells on a

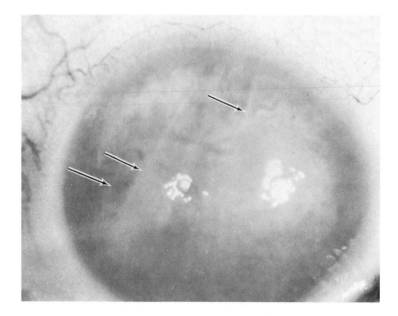

Figure 2–15. This cornea that had been damaged by forceps at birth and had remained clear for three decades developed late corneal edema at age 35. Edema partially obscures edges of tears in Descemet's membrane (arrows).

glass microscope slide, and send them to the laboratory for rapid viral diagnosis.

Management includes the early institution of topical antiviral therapy. Since neither of the reported congenital cases responded to idoxuridine, topical vidarabine 3 per cent ointment five times daily or trifluorothymidine 1 per cent solution hourly is the treatment of choice.

Bacterial corneal ulcers are exceed-

ingly rare at birth and seldom appear in the neonate. In the late 19th and early 20th centuries, bacterial ophthalmia neonatorum commonly produced corneal ulceration and blindness, but the advent of topical 1 per cent silver nitrate prophylaxis and of many effective topical antibiotics has virtually eliminated corneal ulceration in this age group. Ulcers caused by *Pseudomonas* species are an exception, since *Pseudomonas* bacteria may act as opportunists to cause a

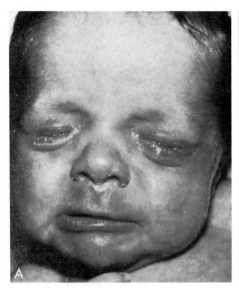

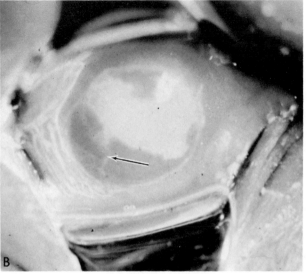

Figure 2–16. Neonatal herpes simplex keratitis. *A,* Bilateral eyelid edema in infant with moderately severe mucopurulent discharge. (Courtesy of Andrew Nahmias, M.D.) *B,* Fluorescein stain of cornea reveals geographic epithelial defect with dendritic extension (arrow). (Courtesy of Walter Stark, M.D.)

diffuse corneal abscess that may be associated with endophthalmitis, septicemia, and death.[31]

In exceptional circumstances, congenital sensory neuropathy may be associated with central nonmicrobial corneal ulceration.

Infants of mothers who had rubella in the first trimester of pregnancy may manifest corneal opacities from three different causes at birth, although none of these has been carefully defined: (1) transient corneal edema, possibly from viral keratitis; (2) corneal edema that may result from elevated intraocular pressure; and (3) corneal edema associated with anterior segment anomalies like Peters' anomaly.

Spirochetes in the cornea in infants with congenital syphilis probably do not produce a neonatal keratitis. Syphilitic interstitial keratitis appears in the second decade of life and probably is immunologically mediated.

METABOLIC CORNEAL OPACITIES

Corneal opacities of metabolic cause generally appear after the neonatal period, since maternal enzymes have been available to the child in utero. These opacities may give the first clue to the systemic disease.[32, 33]

Mucopolysaccharidoses, Mucolipidoses, and Sphingolipidoses

The rarity of these disorders and the obscurity of the constantly changing nomenclature render them difficult for ophthalmologists to understand. We cover here only the major points about corneal opacification in these disorders. Details are available elsewhere.[14, 34, 35]

These are lysosomal storage diseases in which deficiency of lysosomal enzymes allows abnormal accumulation of complex carbohydrates within keratocytes. Most of the disorders are autosomal recessive. There are three groups:

1. Systemic mucopolysaccharidoses (disorders of catabolism of glycosaminoglycans), which commonly cause corneal opacities. The prototype disorder is Hurler's syndrome (MPS I-H) or gargoylism, with its characteristic dwarfism, extreme lumbar kyphosis (hunchback), and excess glycosaminoglycans in the urine.

2. Mucolipidoses (abnormalities of glycoprotein catabolism), which sometimes cause corneal opacities. The prototype disorder is GM_1 gangliosidosis type I (generalized gangliosidosis), with its dwarfing and skeletal abnormalities but with normal glycosaminoglycans in the urine.

3. Sphingolipidoses (abnormalities of glycosphingolipid catabolism), which are not manifested by diffuse corneal opacities. The prototype syndrome is Tay Sachs' disease, in which there is neither skeletal abnormality nor excess glycosaminoglycan excretion but rather visceral storage of glycosphingolipids.

Corneal opacities are not present at birth in most of these disorders, but diffuse symmetrical corneal clouding becomes apparent within the first few years of life. The severity of the corneal clouding varies; it is severe in some types, like MPS I-H Hurler and I-S Scheie, and clinically insignificant in other types, like MPS II Hunter. All the mucopolysaccharidoses and mucolipidoses in which corneal histology has been studied have demonstrated abnormal storage substances in their keratocytes, even when corneal opacities were clinically absent. For practical purposes, the clinician needs to know the disorders in which readily detectable corneal opacities appear early in life, since this is where confusion with infantile glaucoma and congenital hereditary endothelial dystrophy occurs. Thus, MPS I-H Hurler and MPS I-S Scheie, GM_1 gangliosidosis I, and mucolipidosis IV are the important entities, since corneal opacification may appear in the first months of life in these disorders. By the time corneal opacities appear in the other disorders, the systemic aspects of the syndrome have become apparent.

The corneal opacities consist of a diffuse gray stromal haze peppered with fine punctate dots. The epithelium and endothelium generally appear normal. Visual acuity may be surprisingly good, since opacification occurs in the peripheral posterior stroma first.

Histopathologically, storage of excess glycosaminoglycans and glycolipids in membrane-bound vacuoles causes enlargement of stromal keratocytes. These large keratocytes probably produce the white stromal dots seen clinically. The diffuse gray haze is probably caused by extracellular storage material and by disruption of the collagen lamellar architecture.[35]

Glycosaminoglycan Accumulation in Bowman's Layer

Two infants have been reported who exhibited bilateral, diffuse, gray congenital corneal opacities associated with accumulation of excess glycosaminoglycans in an irregularly thickened Bowman's layer without evidence of systemic mucopolysaccharidoses or mucolipidoses.[36]

Congenital thickening of Bowman's layer without histopathologically detectable abnormal substances may also produce opacification of the cornea.[63]

Hypertyrosinemia Type II

There are at least six different disorders of tyrosine metabolism in man. One of them, persistent hypertyrosinemia Type II (Oregon Type), is a rare condition in which deficiency of hepatic cytosol tyrosine aminotransferase produces elevated levels of plasma and urine tyrosine with varying combinations of mental retardation, hyperkeratoses of the palms and soles, and central corneal epithelial opacities (Richner-Hanhart syndrome). Within the first weeks to months of life, the affected child develops photophobia secondary to central gray corneal epithelial lesions that manifest irregular sharp pointed margins similar to the branching of herpes simplex epithelial keratitis. These lesions

fluctuate spontaneously and remain unaffected by topical medications.[33, 37] Occasionally, ulceration occurs. Treatment with a diet low in phenylalanine and tyrosine produces healing of the corneal epithelium, reduction of the painful keratoses on the palms and soles, and improvement in psychomotor ability. A rat model for this disorder has been described with needle-shaped crystals of tyrosine in the corneal epithelium.[38, 39]

POSTERIOR CORNEAL DEFECT

Disorders in this group of congenital abnormalities are manifested by a central or paracentral corneal opacity overlying a focal attenuation or absence of the endothelium and Descemet's membrane. These disorders are part of the group known as mesenchymal dysgenesis of the anterior ocular segment (or anterior chamber cleavage syndrome).[40, 41] Because the variety of abnormalities in this group is confusing, we have devised a descriptive anatomic stepladder classification that categorizes the disorders from simple to more complex forms (Fig. 2–17, Table 2–4). In general, there are four clinical groups: (1) posterior keratoconus, a posterior corneal depression with minimal overlying opacity; (2) a corneal opacity with iris strands adhering to its margins; (3) a corneal opacity with adherent iris strands and corneolenticular contact or cataract, commonly associated with vitreoretinal abnormalities; and (4) corneal staphyloma. Sporadic cases occur most commonly and the opacity is usually bilateral. The glaucoma, present in about half of the cases,[21] appears most frequently in the first 6 years of life as the nonbuphthalmic infantile form.

Posterior Keratoconus

A focal sharply circumscribed central depression indents the posterior cornea with a faint overlying lamellar stromal opacity (Fig. 2–18). Sometimes, the depression covers the entire posterior

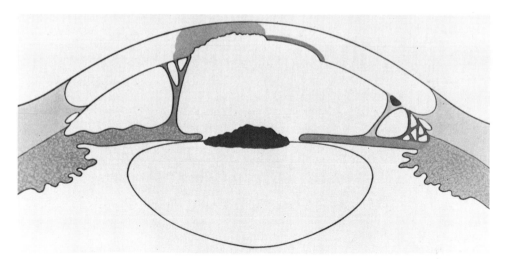

Figure 2–17. Composite illustration of anatomic findings in mesenchymal dysgenesis of the anterior ocular segment (anterior chamber cleavage syndrome). Stepladder classification in Table 2–4 demonstrates spectrum of anatomic combinations and terms by which they are commonly known. (Modified from Reese, A. B., and Ellsworth, R. M.: The anterior chamber cleavage syndrome. Arch Ophthalmol *75*:307, 1966.)

Table 2–4. MESENCHYMAL DYSGENESIS OF THE ANTERIOR OCULAR SEGMENT: STEPLADDER CLASSIFICATION

Posterior Keratoconus	Peters' Anomaly*†			Posterior Embryotoxon	Axenfeld's Anomaly*	Rieger's Syndrome*	Irido-gonio-dys-genesis*	Anterior Chamber Cleavage Syndrome*
Posterior corneal depression	Posterior corneal defect and opacity	Posterior corneal defect and opacity	Posterior corneal defect and opacity					Posterior corneal defect and opacity
		Iris adhesions to opacity margin	Iris adhesions to opacity margin					Iris adhesions to opacity margin
			Lens apposition to opacity					Lens apposition to opacity
				Prominent Schwalbe's ring	Prominent Schwalbe's ring	Prominent Schwalbe's ring		Prominent Schwalbe's ring
					Iris strands to Schwalbe's ring	Iris strands to Schwalbe's ring	Iris strands to Schwalbe's ring	Iris strands to Schwalbe's ring
					Hypoplastic anterior iris stroma	Hypoplastic anterior iris stroma	Hypoplastic anterior iris stroma	Hypoplastic anterior iris stroma

*May have developmental glaucoma.
†von Hippel's Internal Corneal Ulcer, if inflammatory.
From Waring, G. O., Rodrigues, M. M., and Laibson, P. R.: Anterior chamber cleavage syndrome. A stepladder classification. Surv Ophthalmol *20*:3, 1975. Used with permission of the Survey of Ophthalmology.

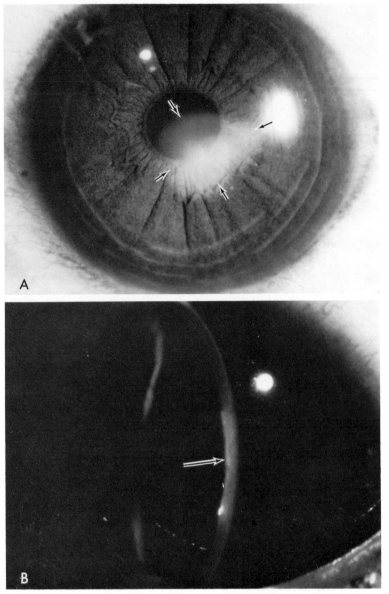

Figure 2–18. Posterior keratoconus. *A,* Central nebular opacity (arrows) overlies focal posterior corneal indentation. *B,* Slit view shows faint opacity and slight posterior corneal indentation (arrow).

cornea.[8] The disorder has no relationship to the common ectatic degenerative form of keratoconus, and it rarely becomes apparent in infancy. The ophthalmologist usually detects it during routine examination because of an abnormal retinoscopic reflex or mild amblyopia. It has been described by Haney and Falls[62] as part of a syndrome along with hypertelorism, flat bridge of nose, brachydactyly, webbed neck, stunted growth, and mental retardation. A small degree of irregular anterior corneal astigmatism, detected best by keratometry, may be present, and this may reduce vision enough to produce mild amblyopia. If the posterior indentation is severe enough, it may cause regular astigmatism as well; this can be corrected by a contact lens or spectacles. Histopathologically,[42, 43] there is focal thinning of the corneal stroma with irregularity of the collagen lamellae. A multilaminar Descemet's membrane occupies the posterior indentation.

Peters' Anomaly

Three anatomic components comprise this anomaly: a posterior corneal defect with overlying corneal opacity, keratoiridial adhesions to the edge of the defect, and corneolenticular contact or cataract.

In general, the central cornea appears more opaque than the periphery. The opacity may be a small discrete paracentral white spot, a discrete round central disc (Fig. 2–19A), a paracentral white arc paralleling the limbus, a tongue-shaped peninsula that extends in from the limbus, a central avascular leukoma with fingerlike connections to the limbus (Fig. 2–20), a central elevated mass that simulates a corneal dermoid, or a diffusely vascularized corneal opacity

Figure 2–19. Peters' anomaly. *A,* Focal, central, moderately dense corneal opacity extends to limbus at 5 o'clock meridian. *B,* Gonioscopic view shows coarse iris strands (arrows) reaching to the margin of a central posterior corneal defect. Inset: Sketch shows corneal opacity, posterior corneal defect, and iris attached to margin of opacity. (From Waring, G. O., Rodrigues, M. M., and Laibson, P. R.: Anterior chamber cleavage syndrome. A stepladder classification. Surv Ophthalmol *20:*3, 1975. Used with permission of the Survey of Ophthalmology.)

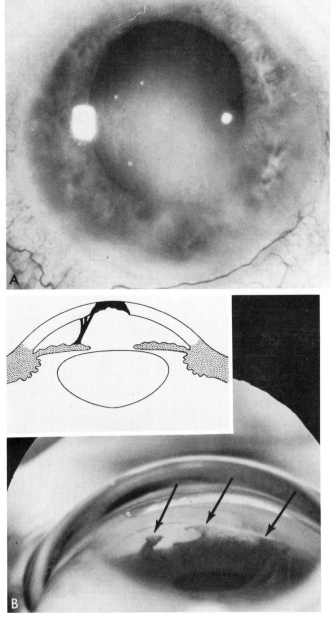

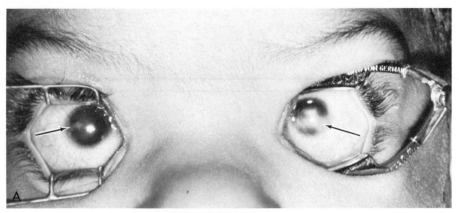

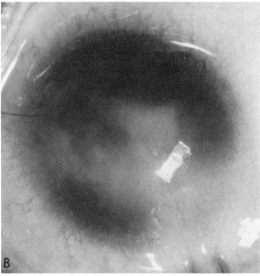

Figure 2–20. Peters' anomaly. *A,* Right cornea manifests faint nebular central opacity with connection to limbus at 9 o'clock (arrow). Left eye shows dense central corneal opacity (arrow). *B,* Corneal opacity in left eye has geographic configuration with extensions to limbus at 9 o'clock and 5 o'clock. Keratoiridial adhesions present behind opacity.

that resembles sclerocornea. The iris strands usually extend from the collarette to the margin of the opacity and may appear as fine filaments, wide strands, focal cords, or fenestrated sheets (Fig. 2–19B). The anterior chamber is often shallow. The density of the opacity will dictate how much anterior segment detail the ophthalmologist can see.

The histopathologic picture is equally variable (Fig. 2–21).[41, 44–47] Stromal scarring usually is present, but some lamellar pattern may be preserved. The pos-

Figure 2–21. Peters' anomaly. *A,* Extensive corneal opacity with superior and inferior scleralization. *B,* Keratoplasty button demonstrates peripheral Descemet's membrane (c), central absence of Descemet's membrane and endothelium (d), and iridocorneal adhesion (e). (PAS, × 4.) *C,* In paracentral cornea, abnormal collagenous tissue is present posterior to Descemet's membrane, giving a multilaminar, split appearance (arrow). It gradually disappears more centrally. (PAS, × 256.) *D,* Corneal endothelium and Descemet's membrane are absent centrally, where a fusiform fibrous plaque is present (arrows). (PAS, × 256.) *E,* An iris strand adheres to the edge of posterior corneal defect (large arrow). Superficial fibrous tissue and vascularization (scleralization) are present (small arrow). (PAS, × 64.) (From Waring, G. O., Rodrigues, M. M., and Laibson, P. R.: Anterior chamber cleavage syndrome. A stepladder classification. Surv Ophthalmol *20*:3, 1975. Used with permission of the Survey of Ophthalmology.)

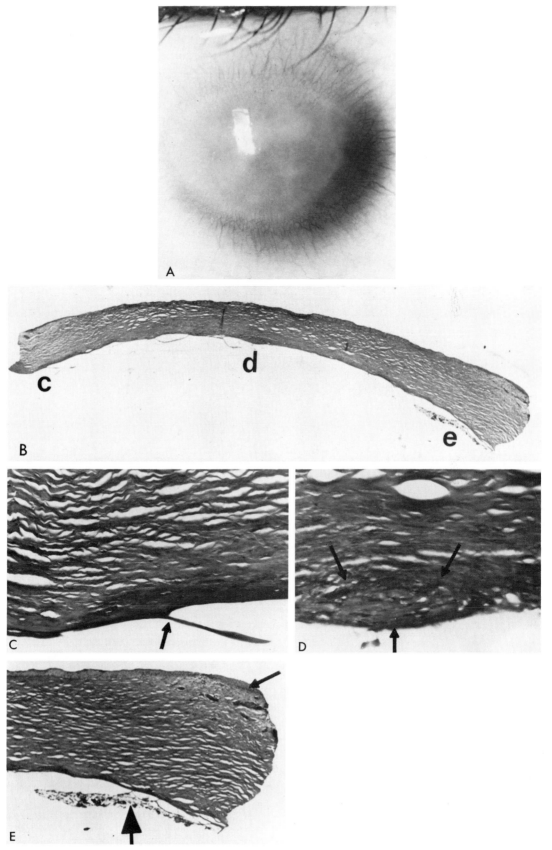

Figure 2–21. *See legend on opposite page*

terior stromal defect varies from a shallow saucer to a crater. Peripherally, Descemet's membrane and the endothelium may be normal, but Descemet's membrane becomes thinner paracentrally. In most cases it disappears, along with the endothelium, within the posterior corneal defect, which is occupied by fibrous tissue. Descemet's membrane and the endothelium also are absent where iris strands adhere to the posterior stroma.

If corneolenticular adhesion, corneolenticular contact, or cataract is present, vitreoretinal abnormalities and systemic abnormalities occur more frequently.[44, 45] A variety of lenticular abnormalities occurs. A clear ectopic lens may move back and forth;[46] a lens adherent to the cornea may separate spontaneously into the posterior chamber;[48] a small stalk may connect the lens to the underlying cornea (Fig. 2–22);[49] an hourglass-shaped lens may occupy the pupil; and a shrunken lens may adhere firmly to the posterior cornea. Histopathologically, the lens capsule is usually intact, although adhesion of the corneal stroma to lens cortex sometimes occurs.

Corneal Staphyloma

This is the most severe form of posterior corneal defect (Fig. 2–23).[50, 51] The thin, scarred, vascularized cornea that protrudes between the eyelids has a bluish color because it is lined by uveal tissue. Intraocular pressure is usually elevated.

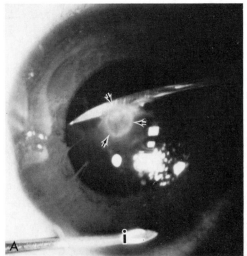

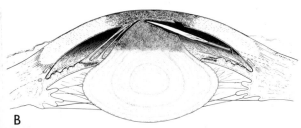

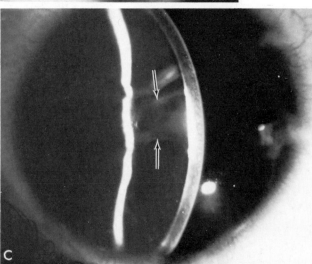

Figure 2–22. Congenital corneolenticular adhesion. *A,* Photograph during surgery demonstrates corneal opacity with underlying corneolenticular adhesion (arrows). Knife is about to separate lens from cornea. Anterior chamber irrigation tube is indicated by i. *B,* Illustration of corneolenticular adhesion, keratoiridial adhesions, and knife separating lens from cornea. *C,* Slit lamp photograph taken 8 years after surgery shows healed posterior corneal defect (arrows) with slight overlying opacity. (Reprinted with permission from the Ophthalmic Publishing Company. From Waring, G. O., and Parks, M. M.: Successful lens removal in congenital corneolenticular adhesion (Peters' anomaly). Amer J Ophthalmol *83:*526, 1977.)

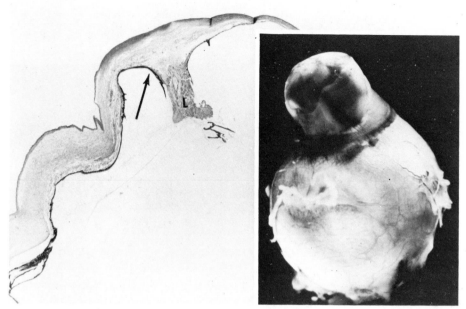

Figure 2–23. Corneal staphyloma. Inset: enucleated globe demonstrates marked ectasia of entire cornea. Main figure: Cornea is focally thinned and vascularized with adherent shrunken lens (L). Ciliary processes extend from the posterior surface of lens. Atrophic iris (arrow) lines cornea and lens stalk. (H and E, × 4.) (From Waring, G. O., Rodrigues, M. M., and Laibson, P. R.: Anterior chamber cleavage syndrome. A stepladder classification. Surv Ophthalmol *20*:3, 1975. Used with permission of the Survey of Ophthalmology.)

Rarely, the cornea develops a hypertrophic keloid scar.[52]

Mesenchymal Dysgenesis of the Anterior Ocular Segment

Congenital abnormalities of the iris and iridocorneal angle may accompany posterior corneal defects in a variety of combinations (Fig. 2–17). Some forms are a prominent Schwalbe's ring (posterior embryotoxon), iris strands to a prominent Schwalbe's ring (Axenfeld's anomaly), and Rieger's syndrome (prominent Schwalbe's ring with iris strands and hypoplasia of the anterior iris stroma) (Fig. 2–24).

CORNEAL DYSTROPHIES

Three corneal dystrophies exhibit diffuse cloudiness at birth: congenital hereditary endothelial dystrophy, congenital hereditary stromal dystrophy, and

posterior polymorphous dystrophy. These are discussed in more detail in Chapter 3.

Congenital Hereditary Endothelial Dystrophy

This disorder, which may be either autosomal dominant or autosomal recessive, exhibits bilaterally symmetrical full thickness stromal edema, with corneal thickness two to three times normal. The edema may remain stationary, but it usually progresses slowly.[53]

Congenital Hereditary Stromal Dystrophy

This autosomal dominant disorder has recently been distinguished from the congenital endothelial dystrophy, and exhibits bilaterally symmetrical, central, anterior stromal, flaky-feathery opacities from birth. Corneal thickness is normal, and this disorder is not progressive.[54]

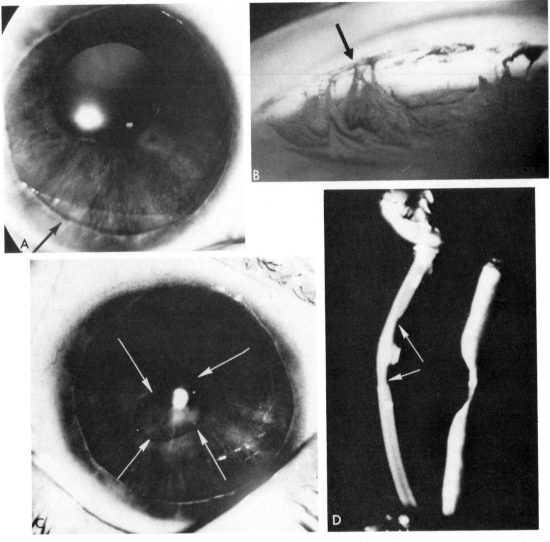

Figure 2–24. Rieger's syndrome with posterior keratoconus. *A,* Left eye demonstrates prominent Schwalbe's ring (arrow), thin anterior iris stroma, and corectopia. *B,* Gonioscopy of left eye demonstrates broad iris strands sweeping up angle recess to prominent Schwalbe's ring (arrow). *C,* Right eye shows prominent Schwalbe's ring with attached iris strands and central, focal posterior keratoconus (arrows). *D,* Slit lamp photograph of right eye demonstrates focal posterior keratoconus (arrows). Slit beam is seen posteriorly on iris and pupil. (From Waring, G. O., Rodrigues, M. M., and Laibson, P. R.: Anterior chamber cleavage syndrome. A stepladder classification. Surv Ophthalmol *20:*3, 1975. Used with permission of the Survey of Ophthalmology.)

Posterior Polymorphous Dystrophy

Congenital corneal edema is one form of posterior polymorphous dystrophy and appears as a diffuse corneal haze at birth without corneal thickening. It is autosomal dominant, and family members exhibit the more characteristic appearance of posterior polymorphous dystrophy: grouped vesicles, refractile geographic lesions, scalloped bands, and peripheral iridocorneal adhesions.[55, 56]

CENTRAL CORNEAL DERMOID

Dermoid tumors comprise about 20 per cent of epibulbar tumors excised in childhood.[57] These tumors are choristomas because they contain histologically normal tissue like fat, hair follicles, sebaceous glands, and sweat glands in an abnormal location. When a dermoid occupies the central cornea as an isolated mass or when it replaces the entire cornea, the diagnosis may be difficult, since

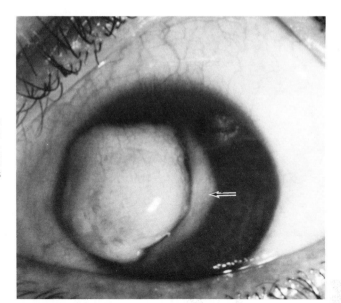

Figure 2–25. Central corneal dermoid is vascularized, moderately elevated, and sharply circumscribed. Arc of lipid in anterior stroma is separated from dermoid by clear zone (arrow). Surface hair is absent.

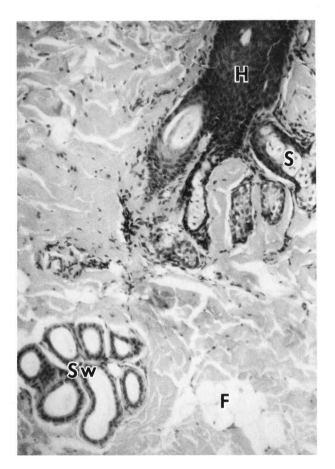

Figure 2–26. Biopsy of corneal dermoid demonstrates hair follicle (H), sebaceous gland (S), sweat glands (Sw), and fat (F) enmeshed in connective tissue.

the tumor mimics a vascularized posterior corneal defect (Peters' anomaly), a corneal keloid, and a corneal staphyloma. Transillumination of the globe will help in differential diagnosis, since the staphyloma will transmit light. A- or B-scan ultrasonography performed through a water bath will also help define anterior segment anatomy and detect a thickened cornea.

The discrete, slightly elevated, whitish-yellow tumors sometimes are rimmed by a lipoidal stromal infiltrate, separated from it by a clear zone (Fig. 2–25). Since many dermoids occupy only the anterior stroma, a biopsy demonstrating hair follicles and sweat and sebaceous glands (Fig. 2–26) will allow the corneal surgeon to plan a lamellar keratoplasty as the most efficacious form of treatment. He should, of course, be prepared to perform penetrating keratoplasty in every case.[58–60]

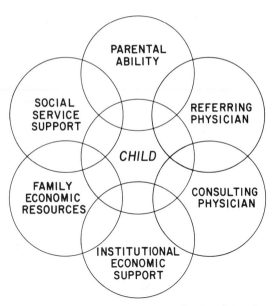

Figure 2–27. Venn diagram emphasizes interplay of socioeconomic factors that affect successful keratoplasty in children. (From Waring, G. O., and Laibson, P. R.: Keratoplasty in children. In Kwitko, M. L. (ed.): *Surgery of the Infant Eye*, 1979. Courtesy of Appleton-Century-Crofts, Publishing Division of Prentice-Hall, Inc., Englewood Cliffs, N.J.)

KERATOPLASTY IN INFANTS WITH OPAQUE CORNEAS[1, 61]

Keratoplasty in infants is most commonly performed for posterior corneal defect (Peters' anomaly), sclerocornea, and corneal dermoid. Since corneal opacification in infancy will produce severe amblyopia, the surgeon must decide promptly whether or not to perform anterior segment surgery with keratoplasty. The infant with dense, bilateral corneal opacities should receive a corneal transplant in the first months of life to minimize visual deprivation and the chance of irreversible amblyopia. A child with a unilateral corneal opacity and a contralateral normal eye has less need for surgery. Since effective treatment of amblyopia after removal of congenital monocular opacities, whether in the cornea or in the lens, is difficult to achieve, and since the probability of a persistently clear corneal graft is less than 50 per cent, the ophthalmologist must weigh surgical and social morbidity against the chances of improved vision.

Neonatal corneal opacities compose three groups with different prognoses for penetrating keratoplasty:

1. Avascular corneas with diffuse corneal edema or central corneal opacity and a clear periphery have about a 50 per cent chance of clarity at 2 years.

2. Eyes with densely vascularized corneas, often accompanied by keratoiridial or corneolenticular adhesions, have about a 10 per cent chance of being treated successfully by keratoplasty.

3. Eyes with vitreoretinal disorganization demonstrated by ultrasound are usually inoperable.

The surgeon must carefully consider other ocular abnormalities likely to influence the success of a corneal graft. Abnormal tear production or eyelid abnormalities like distichiasis may damage the epithelium of the graft, creating a nonhealing epithelial defect. Elevated intraocular pressure, present so commonly in congenital anomalies, may be difficult to measure accurately through the corneal opacity and may plague the surgeon postoperatively. Control of elevated pressure preoperatively by filtering procedure, cyclocryotherapy, or medication will improve the chance of prolonged graft clarity.

The success of corneal grafts in children depends on psychosocial factors as much as medical factors (Fig. 2–27). An unstable family or inadequate socioeconomic circumstances are grounds for avoiding keratoplasty in young children. Parents will cooperate more when they have had detailed preoperative discussions with the ophthalmologist, when they have received direct instruction in topical medical delivery, when they fully understand the need for long-term patching to treat amblyopia, and when

they are well instructed about proper use of spectacles and contact lenses. A responsible adult must be able to perform a careful daily examination for signs of corneal graft rejection, like circumcorneal injection and graft edema. The physician who personally enlists social service support and garners adequate economic support to cover costs of the surgery and postoperative care will enhance the likelihood of prolonged graft clarity. Referring and consulting ophthalmologists must communicate frequently and clearly to insure careful follow-up of the child.

Details of keratoplasty in infants are discussed elsewhere.[61]

REFERENCES

1. Waring, G. O., and Laibson, P. R.: Keratoplasty in infants and children. Trans Amer Acad Ophthalmol Otolaryngol 83:OP283, 1977.
2. Waring, G. O., and Laibson, P. R.: A systematic method of drawing corneal pathologic conditions. Arch Ophthalmol 95:1540, 1977.
3. Uchida, K., Mitsuyu-Tsuboi, M., and Honda, Y.: Studies on skin-electrode ERG in the closed-eye state. J Ped Ophthalmol Strab 16:62, 1979.
4. Waring, G. O., and Shields, J. A.: Partial unilateral cryptophthalmos with syndactyly, brachycephaly, and renal anomalies. Amer J Ophthalmol 79:437, 1975.
5. Francois, J.: Syndrome malformatif avec cryptophtalmie. Acta Genet Med Gemellol 18:18, 1969.
6. Roger, G. L., and Polomeno, R. C.: Autosomal-dominant inheritance of megalocornea associated with Down's syndrome. Amer J Ophthalmol 78:526, 1974.
7. Wood, W. J., Green, W. R., and Marr, W. G.: Megalocornea: A clinico-pathologic clinical case report. Md State Med J 23:57, 1974.
8. Collier, M.: Le keratocone posterieur. Arch Ophthalmol (Paris) 22:376 and 475, 1962.
9. Vail, D. T.: Adult hereditary anterior megalophthalmos sine glaucoma: A definite disease entity. Arch Ophthalmol 6:39, 1931.
10. Judisch, G. F., Waziri, M., and Krachmer, J. H.: Ocular Ehlers-Danlos syndrome with normal lysyl hydroxylase activity. Arch Ophthalmol 94:1489, 1976.
11. Biglan, A. W., Brown, S. I., and Johnson, B. L.: Keratoglobus and blue sclera. Amer J Ophthalmol 83:225, 1977.
12. Greenfield, G., Stein, R., Romano, A., et al.: Blue sclerae and keratoconus: Key features of a distinct heritable disorder of connective tissue. Clin Genet 4:8, 1973.
13. Hyams, S. W., Dar, H., and Neumann, E.: Blue sclerae and keratoglobus. Ocular signs of a systemic connective tissue disorder. Brit J Ophthalmol 53:53, 1969.
14. McKusick, V. A.: *Mendelian Inheritance in Man.* 5th ed. Baltimore, Johns Hopkins Press, 1978.

15. Dinno, N. D., Lawwill, T., Leggett, A. E., Shearer, L., and Weisskopf, B.: Bilateral microcornea, coloboma, short stature and other skeletal anomalies— A new hereditary syndrome. Birth Defects 12:109, 1976.
16. Batra, D. V., and Paul, S. D.: Microcornea with myopia. Brit J Ophthalmol 51:57, 1967.
17. Cross, H. E., and Yoder, F.: Familial nanophthalmos. Amer J Ophthalmol 81:300, 1976.
18. Howard, R. O., and Abrahams, I. W.: Sclerocornea. Amer J Ophthalmol 71:1254, 1971.
19. Wood, T. O., and Kaufman, H. E.: Penetrating keratoplasty in an infant with sclerocornea. Amer J Ophthalmol 70:609, 1970.
20. Kanai, A., Wood, T. C., Polack, F. M., and Kaufman, H. E.: The fine structure of sclerocornea. Invest Ophthalmol 10:687, 1971.
21. Alkemade, P. P. H.: *Dysgenesis Mesodermalis of the Iris and the Cornea.* Assen, Netherlands, Van Gorcum, 1969.
22. Friedman, A. H., Weingeist, S., Brackup, A., and Marinoff, G.: Sclerocornea and defective mesodermal migration. Brit J Ophthalmol 59:683, 1975.
23. Rodrigues, M. M., Calhoun, J., and Weinreb, R.: Sclerocornea with an unbalanced translocation $(17_p, 10_q)$. Amer J Ophthalmol 78:49, 1974.
24. Brown, S. I.: Corneal transplantation of the infant cornea. Trans Amer Acad Ophthalmol Otolaryngol 78:461, 1974.
25. Goldstein, J. E., and Cogan, D. G.: Sclerocornea and associated congenital anomalies. Arch Ophthalmol 67:761, 1962.
26. Costenbader, F. D., and Kwitko, M. L.: Congenital glaucoma: A review of seventy-seven consecutive eyes. J Ped Ophthalmol 4:9, 1967.
27. Spencer, W. H., Ferguson, W. J., Jr., Shaffer, R. N., and Fine, M.: Late degenerative changes in the cornea following breaks in Descemet's membrane. Trans Amer Acad Ophthalmol Otolaryngol 70:973, 1966.
28. Nahmias, A. J., Visintine, A. M., Caldwell, D. R., and Wilson, L. A.: Eye infections with herpes simplex viruses in neonates. Surv Ophthalmol 21:100, 1976.

29. Hutchison, D. S., Smith, R. E., and Haughton, P. B.: Congenital herpetic keratitis. Arch Ophthalmol 93:70, 1975.

30. Wilkie, J. S., Easterbrook, M., Coleman, V., and Stevens, T.: Credé prophylaxis and neonatal corneal infection with herpesvirus. Arch Ophthalmol 91:386, 1974.

31. Burns, R. P., and Rhodes, D. H.: Pseudomonas eye infection as a cause of death in premature infants. Arch Ophthalmol 65:517, 1961.

32. Scheie, H. G., Hambrick, G. W., Jr., and Barness, L. A.: A newly recognized forme fruste of Hurler's disease (gargoylism). Amer J Ophthalmol 53:753, 1962.

33. Burns, R. P.: Soluble tyrosine aminotransferase deficiency: An unusual cause of corneal ulcers. Amer J Ophthalmol 73:400, 1972.

34. McKusick, V. A.: *Heritable Disorders of Connective Tissue.* 4th ed. St. Louis, C. V. Mosby Co., 1972, pp. 292–371.

35. Kenyon, K. R.: Ocular ultrastructure of inherited metabolic disease. In Goldberg, M. A. (ed): *Genetic and Metabolic Eye Disease.* Boston, Little, Brown, 1974, pp. 139–185.

36. Rodrigues, M. M., Calhoun, J., and Harley, R. D.: Corneal clouding with increased acid mucopolysaccharide accumulation in Bowman's membrane. Amer J Ophthalmol 79:916, 1975.

37. Sundmacher, R.: Bilaterale pseudokeratitis dendritica (Richner-Hanhart Syndrom). Klin Mbl Augenheilk 170:84, 1977.

38. Burns, R. P., Gipson, I. K., and Murray, M. J.: Keratopathy in tyrosinemia. In Bergsma, D., Bron, A. J., and Cotlier, E. (eds): *The Eye and Inborn Errors of Metabolism.* Birth Defects: Original Article Series 12:169, 1976.

39. Gipson, I. K., and Anderson, R. A.: Response of the lysosomal system of the corneal epithelium to tyrosine-induced cell injury. J Histochem Cytochem 25:1351, 1977.

40. Reese, A. B., and Ellsworth, R. M.: The anterior chamber cleavage syndrome. Arch Ophthalmol 75:307, 1966.

41. Waring, G. O., Rodrigues, M. M., and Laibson, P. R.: Anterior chamber cleavage syndrome. A stepladder classification. Surv Ophthalmol 20:3, 1975.

42. Wolter, J. R., and Haney, W. P.: Histopathology of keratoconus posticus circumscriptus. Arch Ophthalmol 69:357, 1963.

43. Krachmer, J. H., and Rodrigues, M. M.: Posterior keratoconus. Arch Ophthalmol 96:1867, 1978.

44. Townsend, W. M., Font, R. L., and Zimmerman, L. E.: Congenital corneal leukomas. II. Histopathologic findings in 19 eyes with central defect in Descemet's membrane. Amer J Ophthalmol 77:192, 1974.

45. Townsend, W. M., Font, R. L., and Zimmerman, L. E.: Congenital corneal leukomas. III. Histopathologic findings in 13 eyes with noncentral defect in Descemet's membrane. Amer J Ophthalmol 77:400, 1974.

46. Stone, D. L., Kenyon, K. R., Green, W. R., and Ryan, S. J.: Congenital central corneal leukoma (Peters' anomaly). Amer J Ophthalmol 81:173, 1976.

47. Kupfer, C., Kuwabara, T., and Stark, W. J.: The histopathology of Peters' anomaly. Amer J Ophthalmol 80:653, 1975.

48. Hagedoorn, A., and Velzeboer, C. M. J.: Postnatal partial spontaneous correction of a severe congenital anomaly of the anterior segment of an eye. Arch Ophthalmol 63:685, 1959.

49. Waring, G. O., and Parks, M. M.: Successful lens removal in congenital corneolenticular adhesion (Peters' anomaly). Amer J Ophthalmol 83:526, 1977.

50. Olson, J. A.: Congenital anterior staphyloma. Report of two cases. J Ped Ophthalmol 8:177, 1971.

51. DeLong, P.: Congenital anterior staphyloma. Trans Ophthalmol Soc UK 31:315, 1933.

52. Smith, H. C.: Keloid of the cornea. Trans Amer Ophthalmol Soc 38:519, 1940.

53. Maumenee, A. E.: Congenital hereditary corneal dystrophy. Amer J Ophthalmol 50:1114, 1960.

54. Witschel, H., Fine, B. S., Grützner, P., and McTigue, J. W.: Congenital hereditary stromal dystrophy of the cornea. Arch Ophthalmol 96:1043, 1978.

55. Cibis, G. W., Krachmer, J. A., Phelps, C. D., and Weingeist, T. A.: The clinical spectrum of posterior polymorphous dystrophy. Arch Ophthalmol 95:1529, 1977.

56. Levenson, J. E., Chandler, J. W., and Kaufman, H. E.: Affected asymptomatic relatives in congenital hereditary endothelial dystrophy. Amer J Ophthalmol 76:967, 1973.

57. Elsas, F. J., and Green, W. R.: Epibulbar tumors in childhood. Amer J Ophthalmol 79:1001, 1975.

58. Wood, D. J., and Scott, R. S.: Dermo-lipoma of the cornea. Trans Ophthalmol Soc UK 45:112, 1925.

59. Zolog, N., Schneider, I., and Atanasescu, F.: Fibrome congenital de la cornee. Ann Oculist (Paris) 195:289, 1962.

60. Henkind, P., Marinoff, G., Manas, A., and Friedman, A.: Bilateral corneal dermoids. Amer J Ophthalmol 76:972, 1973.

61. Waring, G. O., and Laibson, P. R.: Keratoplasty in children. In Kwitko, M. L. (ed): *Surgery of the Infant Eye.* New York, Appleton-Century-Crofts, 1979, pp. 197–215.

62. Haney, W. P., and Falls, H. F.: The occurrence of congenital keratoconus posticus circumscriptus in two siblings presenting a previously unrecognized syndrome. Am J Ophthalmol 52:53, 1961.

63. Ohrloff, C., and Olson, R.: Personal communication, 1983.

Corneal Dystrophies | 3

GEORGE O. WARING, III, M.D.
MERLYN M. RODRIGUES, M.D., Ph.D.
PETER R. LAIBSON, M.D.

Corneal dystrophies are rare disorders. With the exception of epithelial basement membrane dystrophy and Fuchs' endothelial dystrophy, most general ophthalmologists seldom see corneal dystrophies or have experience with keratoplasty as treatment for corneal dystrophy. Although corneal dystrophies generally present a distinctive clinical and histochemical appearance, transmission electron microscopy is the most precise current method of diagnosis. Therefore, we suggest that the corneal surgeon place a small piece of tissue in electron microscopy fixative immediately after removal of the host button and send it to the pathology laboratory for processing, so the tissue remains available for future ultrastructural examination.

We summarize here the clinically relevant features of corneal dystrophies, leaving fine details to more extensive reviews.[1-7]

DEFINITION AND CLASSIFICATION

Table 3–1 characterizes corneal dystrophies. Corneal dystrophies are inherited as autosomal dominant traits, except for three autosomal recessives: macular dystrophy, some cases of congenital hereditary endothelial dystrophy, and some cases of posterior polymorphous dystrophy. Thus, the clinician can expect about half the family members to be affected and should examine available relatives to counsel family members about both their visual expectations and the probability of having affected offspring. Because of this autosomal dominant pattern, corneal dystrophies manifest wide variations in severity (variable expressivity), not only among unrelated individuals but also within families and even between two eyes of the same patient.

By conventional definition, corneal dystrophies are primary corneal diseases unassociated with prior inflammation or with systemic diseases. Fabry's disease, for example, usually manifests whorl-shaped superficial cornea verticillata, which was initially considered a corneal dystrophy but is now regarded as part of the systemic disease.[8]

Most dystrophies become apparent by age 20, but epithelial basement membrane dystrophy and Fuchs' endothelial dystrophy do not appear until age 30 to 50. Since corneal dystrophies progress slowly, many affected younger individuals remain asymptomatic. Most dystrophies affect only the central cornea, although Meesmann's, fleck, macular, and congenital hereditary endothelial dystrophies extend to the limbus.

Table 3–2 classifies dystrophies according to the primary corneal layer affected and distinguishes the dystrophies that often reduce visual acuity from those that do not.

When corneal dystrophies in different families resemble each other in some features but remain distinctive in others, it is difficult to know whether to lump

Table 3–1.   CHARACTERISTICS OF CORNEAL DYSTROPHIES

Characteristic	Exceptions
Autosomal dominant hereditary	Macular (autosomal recessive) Congenital hereditary endothelial (may be autosomal recessive) Posterior polymorphous (rarely autosomal recessive) Pre-Descemet's and polymorphic stromal "dystrophies" (not inherited)
No associated systemic disease	Central crystalline (occasional hyperlipidemia and genu valgum)
Cornea otherwise normal (primary disease)	
Onset by age 20	Epithelial basement membrane (map-dot-fingerprint) (age 30–40) Fuchs' endothelial (age 40–50)
Bilateral	Rare unilateral cases occur in most types
Central	Meesmann's Fleck Macular } (extend to limbus) Congenital hereditary endothelial Congenital hereditary stromal
Slowly progressive	Posterior polymorphous } (some cases stable) Congenital hereditary endothelial
Primarily involvement of single corneal layer	Macular (stroma and endothelium)

them into a single group or to split them into discrete entities. We prefer to lump dystrophies with similar characteristics together but remain aware that subsequent studies may differentiate them.

The epithelial dystrophies and those involving Bowman's layer are considered in Chapter 8; they are covered here to ensure continuity and to provide a complete, albeit brief, discussion of the corneal dystrophies.

EPITHELIAL DYSTROPHIES

Epithelial dystrophies are characterized by intraepithelial cysts and multiple layers of subepithelial basement membrane and fibrillar tissue. They usually reduce visual acuity less severely than the stromal and endothelial dystrophies.

Epithelial Basement Membrane Dystrophy

Patients with epithelial basement membrane dystrophy are seen frequently in office practice with corneal epithelial erosions.[9, 10] Also called map-dot-finger-

Table 3–2.   CLASSIFICATION OF CORNEAL DYSTROPHIES

Primary Corneal Layer Affected	Vision Often Reduced	Vision Often Spared
Epithelium	Epithelial basement membrane (map-dot-fingerprint) dystrophy	Meesmann's juvenile epithelial dystrophy
Bowman's layer	Reis-Bücklers' ring-shaped dystrophy	Anterior mosaic dystrophy
Stroma	Granular dystrophy Lattice dystrophy Macular dystrophy Central crystalline dystrophy Congenital hereditary stromal dystrophy	Central cloudy dystrophy Fleck (speckled) dystrophy Pre-Descemet's "dystrophy"* Polymorphic stromal "dystrophy"*
Endothelium and Descemet's membrane	Fuchs' endothelial dystrophy Posterior polymorphous dystrophy Congenital hereditary endothelial dystrophy	Nonprogressive cornea guttata

*Inheritance not established; probably corneal degenerations.

print dystrophy[11] or Cogan's microcystic dystrophy,[12] it occurs bilaterally and is probably autosomal dominantly inherited.[13] Most patients are asymptomatic, but between ages 20 and 40 about 10 per cent of affected individuals develop transiently blurred vision or painful recurrent epithelial erosions, often with severe acute unilateral ocular pain upon awakening in the morning. The margin of the upper eyelid is violaceous and edematous, blepharospasm is severe, the epithelium appears loose and wrinkled, and a brownish granular edema occupies the underlying anterior stroma. Although the erosions may recur spontaneously, they usually stop after 1 to 3 years even though the dystrophic lesions persist.

The maps, dots, and fingerprints composing this dystrophy are difficult to see with the slit lamp unless the physician searches specifically for them in retro-illumination and broad tangential illumination. Observation of moving debris in the tear film helps to keep the epithelium in focus.

The map pattern (Fig. 3–1) appears as diffuse gray geographic patches that contain oval clear zones. The gray sheets have a single sharp edge and gradually become less visible as one moves away from this discrete margin. White intraepithelial microcysts often appear within the gray map area. Broad tangential illumination reveals these changes best, and the fluorescein-stained tear film breaks up quickly over these map areas.[14]

Numerous types of superficial corneal lines have been described, the most common being fingerprint lines—fine,

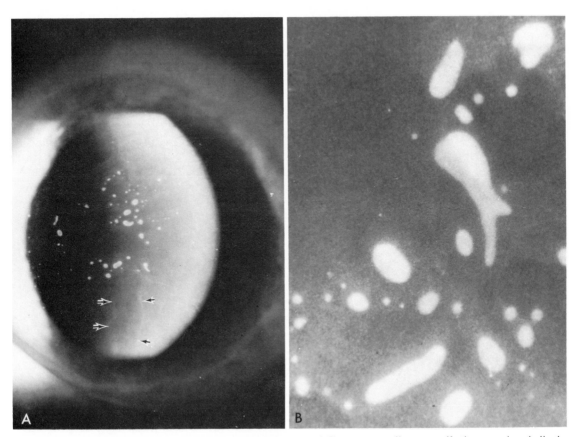

Figure 3–1. Epithelial basement membrane dystrophy. *A,* The map pattern manifests gray sheets that create sharp lines (arrows) surrounding clearer zones. The dot pattern manifests variably sized, ameboid-shaped, white intraepithelial microcysts that usually lie in the gray zone of the maps. *B,* High-powered photomicrograph of intraepithelial microcysts of Cogan demonstrates their gray color and discrete configuration against the somewhat granular background of the map pattern.

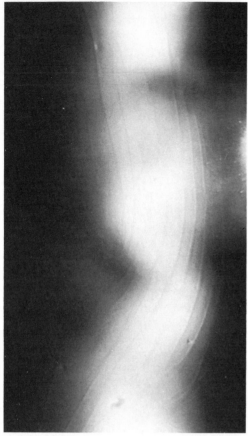

Figure 3–2. Epithelial basement membrane dystrophy, fingerprint pattern. In retroillumination the fingerprint lines form a roughly parallel configuration of refractile ridges.

roughly parallel clusters of refractile lines that form a curvilinear pattern seen only in retroillumination (Fig. 3–2). Other types of superficial corneal lines appear gray in direct illumination and occur less commonly.[15]

The major histopathologic alteration in the map and fingerprint changes is a thick epithelial basement membrane, part of which extends into the epithelium as a multilaminar, sometimes corrugated sheet of fibrillar and basement membrane–like material[9, 10, 16, 17] (Fig. 3–3).

Two types of dystrophic epithelial dots occur:[18, 19]

1. The large ameba-shaped gray microcysts of Cogan cluster like an archipelago in the central cornea, usually in association with map changes (Fig. 3–1). They seldom stain with fluorescein.

Histopathologically, these are intraepithelial cystic aggregations of degenerating cells, most commonly located beneath an intraepithelial sheet of basement membrane material (Fig. 3–3). Sometimes they migrate forward to break through the epithelial surface, where they produce a foreign-body sensation and stain with fluorescein.[16, 17, 20]

2. The blebs of Bron and Brown[9] are small, clear, round dots that cluster closely together and are apparent only in retroillumination. A continuous layer of fibrillogranular material between the epithelial basement membrane and Bowman's layer apparently forms these blebs.[21]

The basic disorder that causes epithelial basement membrane dystrophy is probably an abnormal basement membrane synthesis within the epithelium itself. These intraepithelial sheets block the forward migration of epithelium so that the trapped cells degenerate to form the intraepithelial cysts. The basal epithelium adheres poorly to the abnormal basement membrane, resulting in epithelial erosions.[22]

Management of the symptomatic patient is difficult. Blurred vision from mild irregular astigmatism can be aggravated in dry or windy circumstances like skiing or sailing. Topical 5 per cent sodium chloride ointment at bedtime and drops during the day may decrease the epithelial edema and irregularity. If the blurred vision is severe, the central epithelium can be gently removed with a moist cotton applicator or scalpel blade, and the regenerating epithelium may not manifest the dystrophy.

More severe and incapacitating are the epithelial erosions. If the epithelium is not too loose, instillation of a hypertonic ointment, a cycloplegic agent, and a prophylactic antibiotic, followed by a firm pressure patch and systemic analgesics, will render the patient comfortable and promote epithelial healing. The pressure patch should remain undisturbed for 48 hours. If re-epithelialization is slow, the patch may need to be changed every other day for a week or bilateral patches may be required. If the epithelium is

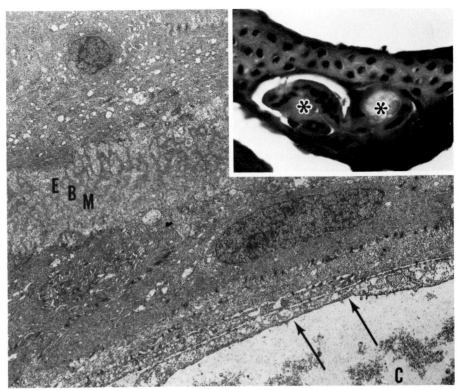

Figure 3–3. Histopathology of epithelial basement membrane dystrophy, dot pattern. Inset shows intraepithelial cysts that contain degenerated epithelial cells (asterisks). (H and E, × 500.) Electron micrograph shows portion of cyst (C) surrounded by degenerating subepithelial cells (arrows) and thickened anomalous intraepithelial basement membrane (EBM). (× 7,000.)

extremely redundant and loose, it can be gently removed with a moist cotton applicator. Large sheets of epithelium may loosen during this debridement, and the physician should avoid removing it all the way to the limbus, since conjunctival epithelium resurfaces the cornea less well than corneal epithelium. Removing the epithelium in a slightly eccentric pattern will prevent the central irregularity in the healed defect from overlying the visual axis.

A loosely fit, flat, thin, high-water-content soft contact lens will help decrease recurrence of the erosion. After the initial application of the lens, a period of moderately severe ocular inflammation and corneal edema may occur, but the lens may be left in place while the patient is carefully observed and treated with low-dose steroids and cycloplegics. After a few days the cornea will adjust to the hypoxic insult of the lens, which should be left in place for

approximately 3 months to promote reattachment of the epithelium to its basement membrane. Nocturnal hypertonic ointments and daytime instillation of hypertonic solutions will supplement the soft contact lens.

Meesmann's Juvenile Epithelial Dystrophy

This bilaterally symmetrical, autosomal dominant dystrophy appears during the first year of life as tiny epithelial vesicles that remain asymptomatic until middle age. The vesicles then spread throughout the corneal epithelium to create an irregular astigmatism that transiently blurs vision. They also can break through the epithelial surface and cause intermittent irritation and photophobia.[23] The characteristic lesions are tiny, round or oval blebs that appear as discrete gray dots in focal illumination and

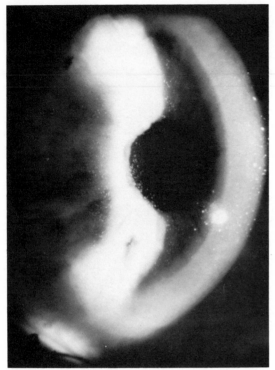

Figure 3–4. Meesmann's juvenile epithelial dystrophy. Tiny round or oval intraepithelial blebs appear as discrete gray dots in focal illumination and as transparent tiny vesicles in retroillumination. (Courtesy of J. Krachmer, M.D.)

as transparent tiny vesicles in retroillumination (Fig. 3–4). They affect the entire corneal epithelium but congregate in the palpebral fissure. In some instances fine wormlike lines accompany the vesicles.

Histopathologically, the vesicles correspond to intraepithelial cysts (really pseudocysts) that are most prominent in the anterior epithelium and contain degenerated cell debris. The cysts and the large amount of glycogen that is present in the basal epithelial cells probably reflect rapid epithelial turnover and are not specific findings for the disorder. The characteristic ultrastructural finding in Meesmann's dystrophy is intracytoplasmic "peculiar substance," a fibrillogranular material surrounded by cytoplasmic filaments,[23, 24] the nature of which is unknown.

Since most individuals remain asymptomatic, management is not difficult. Removal of the epithelium is followed by reappearance of the vesicles, although superficial keratectomy results in re-epithelialization without recurrence of the dystrophy.[23]

BOWMAN'S LAYER DYSTROPHIES

Reis-Bücklers' Ring-Shaped Dystrophy

This autosomal dominant, bilaterally symmetrical, central corneal dystrophy appears in the first few years of life as a reticular superficial corneal opacification associated with painful epithelial erosions.[25] The frequency of the erosions declines as central subepithelial opacities appear in a ring-shaped or fishnet pattern (Fig. 3–5), but visual acuity falls, primarily because of the accompanying irregular astigmatism. Variants of this disorder include the anterior membrane dystrophy of Grayson and Wilbrandt[26] and the honeycomb dystrophy of Thiel and Behnke.[27]

The histopathologic correlate of the swirling and ring-shaped opacities is fibrocellular connective tissue that fragments the epithelial basement membrane and replaces Bowman's layer (Fig. 3–6). Fingers of this tissue indent the basal epithelium, corresponding to the ridges in the epithelium seen clinically. The characteristic ultrastructural findings in this abnormal tissue are short, curled microfibrils that taper toward the ends.[28] The exact nature of these fibrils is unknown. The destruction of the epithelial basement membrane diminishes the epithelial attachments and accounts for the recurrent erosions.[22]

Management of the epithelial erosions is similar to that described for epithelial basement membrane dystrophy. As superficial opacification becomes more severe, superficial keratectomy may improve visual acuity,[29] but lamellar or penetrating keratoplasty may be necessary in advanced cases.[30] Superficial opacification may recur in the graft.

Anterior Mosaic Dystrophy

This bilaterally symmetrical dystrophy appears as central, gray, polygonal opacities separated by clear spaces that

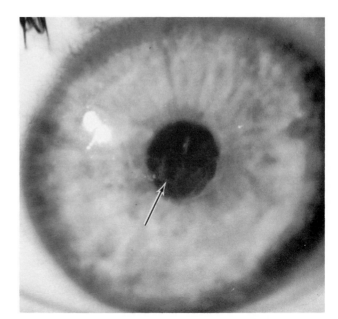

Figure 3–5. Reis-Bücklers' ring-shaped dystrophy. Subepithelial irregular gray lines (arrow) form a ring or fishnet pattern in the central cornea.

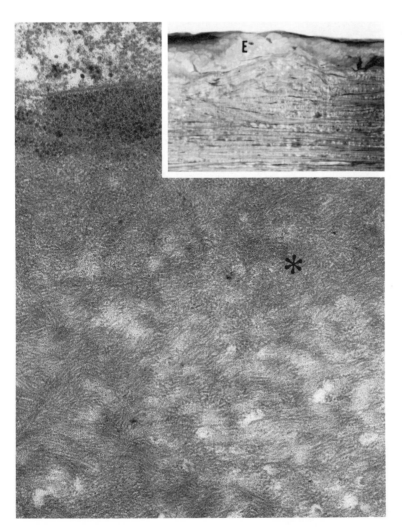

Figure 3–6. Histopathology of Reis-Bücklers' ring-shaped dystrophy. Inset shows thin, irregular epithelium (E) with absent basement membrane. Irregular connective tissue replaces Bowman's layer. (Toluidine blue, × 200.) Electron micrograph of the region of Bowman's layer shows short, curled, electron dense filaments (asterisk) characteristic of Reis-Bückler's dystrophy. (× 61,132.)

impart a crocodile-skin appearance to Bowman's layer (anterior crocodile shagreen).[31] It may accompany X-linked recessive anterior megalophthalmos.[32] No histopathologic studies are available. It should be distinguished from the sporadic degenerative crocodile shagreen that affects either the central posterior stroma or the peripheral stroma and from the post-traumatic mosaic degeneration that may be related to band keratopathy.

STROMAL DYSTROPHIES

In stromal corneal dystrophies an abnormal substance appears within the keratocytes or among the collagen fibrils.

The substance may be an excess amount of a normal metabolite, such as the glycosaminoglycans in macular dystrophy; a material not usually present, such as the amyloid in lattice dystrophy; or an unknown substance, such as hyaline in granular dystrophy.

Granular Dystrophy

This bilaterally symmetrical, autosomal dominant, central corneal dystrophy is characterized by white spots in the central superficial stroma during the first decade of life. The opacities usually do not become dense enough to obstruct vision until the fourth or fifth decade. The discrete, white, round to oval, gran-

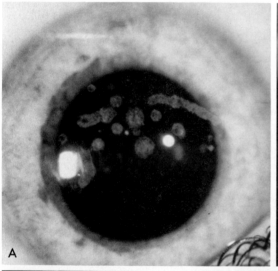

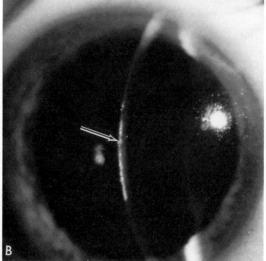

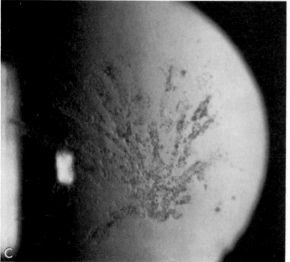

Figure 3–7. Granular dystrophy. *A,* Discrete, white, round-to-oval granular opacities occupy the relatively clear central stroma. *B,* Slit view shows the opacities lying predominantly in the anterior stroma (arrow). *C,* In retroillumination the refractile granular opacities form chains that radiate from the central cornea.

ular opacities lie in the relatively clear stroma and form a variety of configurations, including arcuate chains and straight lines (Fig. 3–7). The individual granular lesion may appear solid white with irregular borders, crumblike with fine dots, or ring-shaped with a punched-out center. At about age 40, a diffuse, irregular, ground-glass haze may appear in the superficial stroma. The epithelial surface remains smooth and corneal erosions are rare.

Histopathologically, focal aggregates of eosinophilic material occupy all levels of the stroma (Fig. 3–8A) but are concentrated anteriorly and may break through dehiscences in Bowman's layer. They characteristically stain bright red with Masson's trichrome.[33] These hyaline deposits contain microfibrillar proteins and probably phospholipids.[33a] Discrete electron-dense, rod-shaped, crystallike, rhomboidal structures compose the lesion ultrastructurally (Fig. 3–8B).[34, 35] In general, the adjacent collagen fibrils appear normal. Some keratocytes exhibit degeneration.

When the opacities become dense and subepithelial connective tissue appears, penetrating keratoplasty is indicated. Approximately 85 per cent of these grafts are clear after 1 year. However, granular dystrophy recurs in corneal grafts 1 to 19 years postoperatively, appearing as white granular spots within a diffuse haze in the superficial stroma.[36]

Lattice Dystrophy

This autosomal dominant, bilaterally symmetrical, central corneal dystrophy exhibits a highly variable clinical picture. Therefore, careful family studies must be done before reports of isolated or unilateral cases can be accepted.[37] In the first or second decade, small refractile lines, white dots and dashes, or a faint central haze appears in the central stroma. The characteristic translucent lattice lines vary from a few small comma-shaped flecks to a dense network of large, irregular, ropy cords that sometimes contain white dots within them

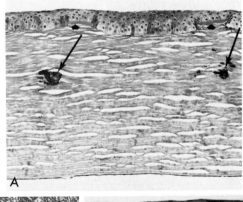

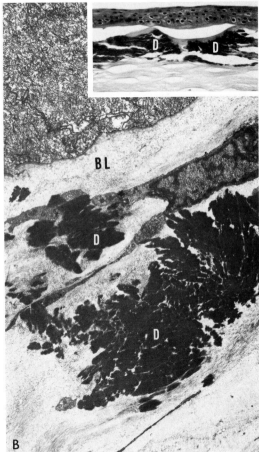

Figure 3–8. Histopathology of granular dystrophy. *A,* Focal deposits of hyaline material stained red with Masson's trichrome (long arrows). Only focal fragments of Bowman's layer remain (short arrows). The corneal stroma between the granular deposits, Descemet's membrane, and endothelium are normal. (Masson's trichrome, × 200.) *B,* Inset shows superficial deposits (D) of hyaline material forming vertical stacks that extend to Bowman's layer. (Masson's trichrome, × 200.) Electron micrograph shows irregular, elongated, somewhat rhomboid, electron-dense deposits that involve the superficial stroma just beneath Bowman's layer (BL). The overlying epithelium and basal lamina are intact. (× 13,800.)

(Fig. 3–9). In direct illumination they appear gray with irregular margins and take on the refractile character of a plastic rod in retroillumination. Lattice lines fluoresce under ultraviolet light.[37] Flake-like, fluffy, white discrete dots appear between the lattice lines and in some cases may resemble granular corneal dystrophy. A central, indistinct, subepithelial, round, white opacity may be present early and may become progressively denser.

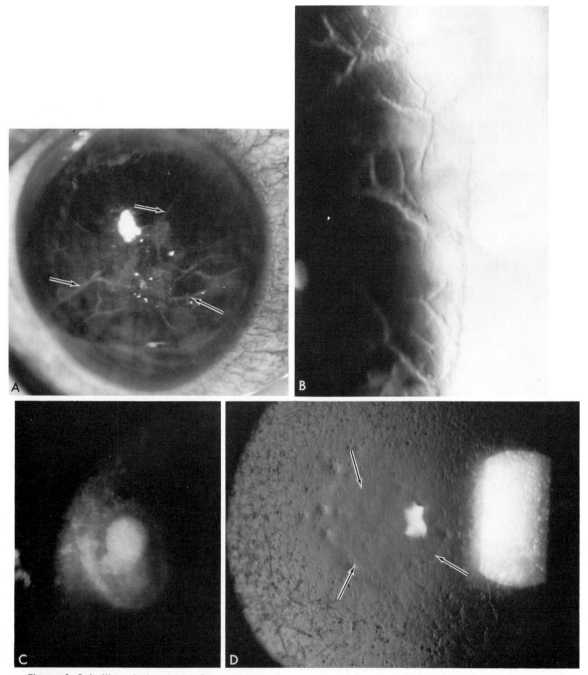

Figure 3–9. Lattice dystrophy. *A,* Coarse lattice lines (arrows) branch dichotomously toward the center of the cornea, where subepithelial opacification has occurred. Corneal surface is irregular because of epithelial erosions. *B,* In retroillumination the lattice lines appear like refractile ropy cords. *C,* Central oval opacities often occur in lattice corneal dystrophy, as seen in this broad tangential slit lamp photomicrograph. *D,* In retroillumination fine lattice lines take on a spicule configuration surrounding the central gray opacity (arrow), which has an irregular, slightly nodular appearance.

As these opacities increase, epithelial erosions appear, creating irregular astigmatism and reduced visual acuity. Indeed, some individuals in families with lattice dystrophy manifest recurrent epithelial erosions without clinically identifiable stromal involvement.[37] In the absence of epithelial erosions, the dystrophic lesions affect vision minimally.

The white dots and lattice lines consist of amyloid in the corneal stroma[33, 38] in the form of fusiform deposits that push aside the collagen lamellae to create a light microscopic pattern like water currents in a river flowing around a bridge piling. Deposits are most dense anteriorly but occupy the entire stroma (Fig. 3–10). Numerous histochemical findings confirm the presence of amyloid, the most important being the pink to orange staining with Congo red, the demonstration of alternate red and green color when the lesion is viewed in green light through a rotating polarizing filter (dichroism), the demonstration of an intermittent yellowish-green color against a black background when the lesion is viewed through two rotating polarizing filters (birefringence), and the greenish-yellow fluorescence when specimens stained with thioflavine T are viewed in ultraviolet light. The characteristic ultrastructural lesion is a feltlike mass of short, delicate, nonbranching fibrils without periodicity (Fig. 3–10).

Subepithelial deposits of amyloid,

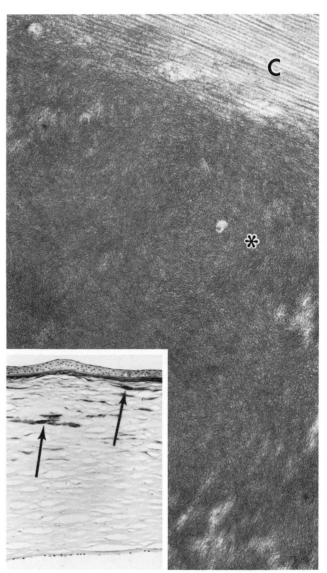

Figure 3–10. Histopathology of lattice dystrophy. Inset shows fusiform shaped deposits of amyloid that stain pink with Congo red (arrows). (Congo red, × 200.) Electron micrograph shows myriad of electron-dense filaments (asterisk) characteristic of amyloid adjacent to stromal collagen fibrils (C). (× 30,000.)

collagen fibrils, and fibroblasts disrupt Bowman's layer and produce fragmentation of the epithelial basement membrane. This may correspond to the superficial portion of the central, round, diffuse opacity seen clinically, and the disrupted epithelial basement membrane may account for the frequent epithelial erosions.[22]

The amyloid in lattice dystrophy has no connection with systemic amyloidosis or with primary or secondary amyloid degeneration of the cornea. The latticelike lines have no relationship to corneal nerves except in an atypical type of lattice dystrophy.[39] The amyloid is of the A protein type, rather than of the immunoglobulin type, and probably results from abnormal keratocyte synthesis.[40]

Treatment of the epithelial erosions includes topical hypertonic solutions and ointments, intermittent pressure patching, epithelial debridement, and soft contact lenses, as described in the section on epithelial basement membrane dystrophy earlier in this chapter. Penetrating keratoplasty has a good prognosis and should be performed when the visual acuity falls below acceptable levels or when the recurrent erosions are incapacitating. Lattice dystrophy may recur in the corneal graft 2 to 14 years postoperatively.

Macular Dystrophy

Macular dystrophy is an exception to many of the generalities concerning corneal dystrophies. It is an autosomal recessive disease that extends to the corneal periphery and involves more than one layer of the cornea at its onset. Both the stroma and the endothelium are affected.

The disorder can occur in offspring with no prior family history, since asymptomatic carriers who are unaware they have the gene may marry each other. It is bilaterally symmetrical and becomes apparent within the first decade of life as a superficial corneal cloudiness studded by small, irregular, rounded, gray-white anterior stromal patches (Fig. 3–11). The opacification gradually extends to the limbus and to the deep stroma, and by age 20 to 30 the surface irregularity and stromal opacification reduce vision enough to require penetrating keratoplasty. As the disorder progresses, Descemet's membrane becomes grayer and develops guttate excrescences that are difficult to see clinically. Epithelial erosions are infrequent.

The stromal opacities correspond to accumulation of excess glycosaminoglycan (acid mucopolysaccharide), probably corneal keratan sulfate, within most stromal keratocytes and diffusely among

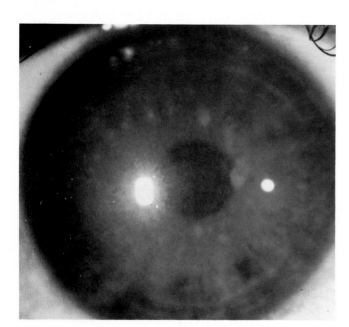

Figure 3–11. Macular dystrophy. Focal gray spots lie in a diffuse haze in the early stages of the disorder.

the collagen fibrils[41, 42] (Fig. 3–12). These deposits, which stain blue with colloidal iron and Alcian blue, are also present in Descemet's membrane and the endothelium. Ultrastructurally, the variably sized membrane-bound vacuoles distend many keratocytes up to two or three times their normal size (Fig. 3–12). The vacuoles contain both fibrillogranular material, presumably the corneal keratan sulfate, and lamellar bodies that may represent glycolipid. Ruptured keratocytes deposit vacuoles and clumps of fibrillogranular material in the extracellular stroma. The posterior nonbanded zone of Descemet's membrane is honeycombed with spaces containing the fibrillogranular material and lamellar bodies that extend into focal guttate excrescences. Endothelial cells contain vacuoles similar to those in the keratocytes.[43]

The basic abnormality in macular dystrophy probably resides in the enzymes that catabolize corneal keratan sulfate or other glycosaminoglycans. Accumulation of this material in the rough endoplasmic reticulum, Golgi vesicles, and lysozomes produces the membrane-bound vacuoles. When these vacuoles fill the keratocyte, they rupture, releasing the material into the stroma. The endothelial cells are also primarily affected and deposit the material in Descemet's membrane as it is produced.[44] In tissue culture Klintworth[41] could not distinguish between glycosaminoglycan production in normal keratocytes and keratocytes from macular dystrophy.

Penetrating keratoplasty is usually

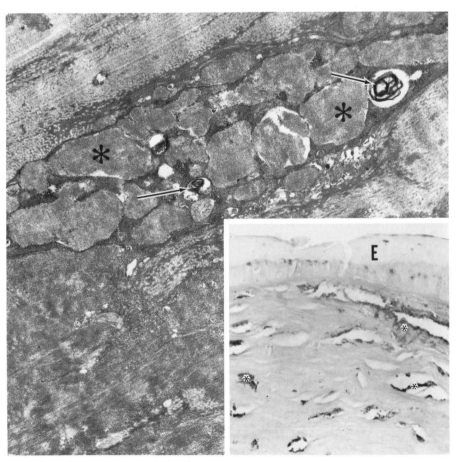

Figure 3–12. Histopathology of macular dystrophy. Inset shows increased accumulation of stromal glycosaminoglycans (asterisks) both intracellularly and extracellularly. These stain blue with colloidal iron. E = epithelium. (Colloidal iron, × 330.) Electron micrograph shows a keratocyte swollen with membrane-bound vacuoles that are filled with fibrillogranular material (asterisks) and lamellar bodies (arrows). Outside the keratocyte some fibrillogranular material lies interspersed among the collagen fibrils. (× 16,545.)

performed earlier for macular dystrophy than for the other stromal dystrophies. Opacities recur in the graft less commonly than in lattice or granular dystrophies,[45] but when they appear from 1.5 to 11 years postoperatively, they correspond to intracellular and extracellular stromal deposits of glycosaminoglycan.[46]

Central Crystalline Dystrophy (of Schnyder)

In this rare bilateral, autosomal dominant dystrophy, anterior stromal crystals appear in the first year of life but remain asymptomatic and often go undetected until a dense corneal arcus and diffuse central opacification appear in the third or fourth decade. The clinical appearance varies widely, with some members of a family manifesting a few faint crystals, some demonstrating only the dense early corneal arcus, and others having the full-blown central round corneal opacity. The central opacity consists of fine, minute, needlelike crystals that glisten yellow, red, blue, and green like slivers of fiberglass against a diffuse gray stromal haze. The opacity is usually round and forms either a solid disc or a clear-centered ring. The crystals may be randomly oriented or may palisade around the periphery.[47] The uninvolved stroma remains clear (Fig. 3–13).

The crystals are cholesterol and are manifested histopathologically as rectangular spaces with notched corners randomly oriented among the normal collagen fibrils (Fig. 3–14). Round empty spaces among the collagen fibrils probably represent neutral fat deposits. To perform histochemical staining on these fatty substances, the surgeon must request frozen sections of the corneal tissue, since fat solvents used in histologic preparations dissolve lipids. Oil red O stains the globular neutral fats red, while the Schultz method stains cholesterol crystals blue-green. The dense corneal arcus and limbal girdle are histopathologically similar to those found in normal aging.

Central crystalline dystrophy has two frequent systemic associations, hyperlipidemia and genu valgum, and is therefore an exception to the definition of corneal dystrophy as an isolated corneal disorder. Of 26 reported patients with crystalline dystrophy who have had serum lipid measurements, ten have had elevated cholesterol.[48] No direct association exists between the crystalline dystrophy and any of the six clinical types of hyperlipidemia. Within a single family individuals may manifest only crystalline dystrophy, both the crystalline dystrophy and the hyperlipidemia, or hyperlipidemia alone. Therefore, the abnormal systemic lipid metabolism and

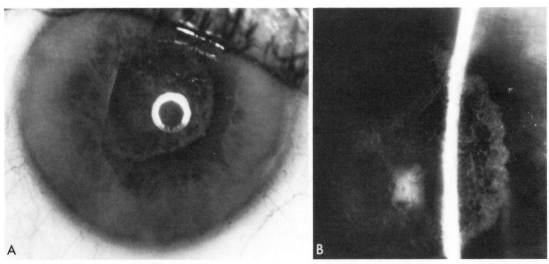

Figure 3–13. Central crystalline dystrophy of Schnyder. *A,* Gross view. *B,* Higher magnification of central crystalline opacity.

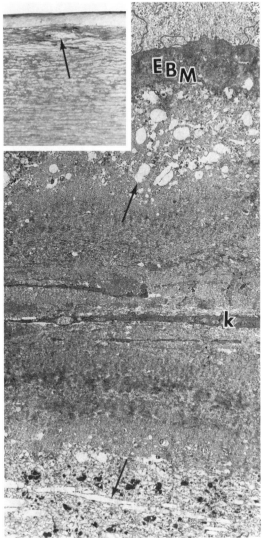

Figure 3–14. Histopathology of central crystalline dystrophy. Inset shows globular and slitlike spaces in the superficial stroma that previously contained lipid (arrow). (Toluidine blue, × 200.) Electron micrograph shows thickened epithelial basement membrane (EBM) with subjacent vacuoles in the region of Bowman's layer. The anterior stroma contains vacuoles and elongated crystal-like spaces (arrows). K = keratocyte. (× 9,000.)

the crystalline corneal deposits are not integral parts of the same disease, since the two may occur independently. The ophthalmologist who examines a patient with central crystalline dystrophy should screen for hyperlipidemia by ordering tests of fasting serum cholesterol and triglyceride.

Central crystalline dystrophy infrequently reduces vision enough to require keratoplasty. Crystalline material may recur in the graft.[47]

Fleck Dystrophy

This autosomal dominant dystrophy, also called speckled or mouchetée dystrophy of Francois and Neetens,[3] may be congenital and does not affect visual acuity. Although the condition is bilateral, extreme asymmetry may occur. The discrete, flat, gray-white, dandrufflike specks extend throughout the otherwise clear stroma, sparing Bowman's layer and reaching the limbus (Fig. 3–15). The individual flecks form a discrete white ring like a wreath and appear refractile in retroillumination. The disorder is sometimes associated with punctate cortical lens opacities[49] and central cloudy corneal dystrophy.[50]

The flecks correspond to isolated keratocytes filled with excess glycosaminoglycan (which stain blue with Alcian blue and appear ultrastructurally as membrane-bound vacuoles containing fibrillogranular material) and to isolated keratocytes filled with lipids (which stain black with Sudan black B and appear ultrastructurally as membrane-bound vacuoles containing lamellar bodies).[51] Ultrastructurally, the keratocytes resemble those in macular corneal dystrophy. No treatment is necessary.

Central Cloudy Dystrophy (of Francois)

This bilaterally symmetrical, nonprogressive, autosomal dominant dystrophy does not reduce visual acuity. The central, oval, stromal opacity is most dense posteriorly and consists of a cluster of multiple small, fuzzy, marginated gray areas that manifest a slightly polygonal shape and are separated by clearer crack-like zones[52] (Fig. 3–16). The posterior central location differentiates it from the similar-appearing mosaic degeneration (crocodile shagreen) that affects Bowman's layer. The gray opacities probably correspond to the sawtooth-like configuration of the stromal collagen lamellae.[52a]

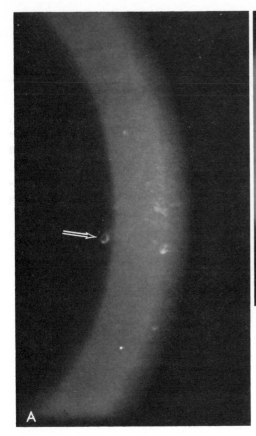

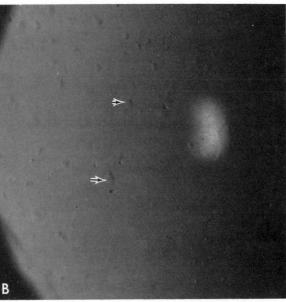

Figure 3–15. Fleck dystrophy. *A*, In slit view the individual flecks are discrete, white, and wreath-shaped (arrow). *B*, Retroillumination accentuates the refractile flecks (arrows).

Pre-Descemet's "Dystrophy"

Although these gray dots deep in the corneal stroma probably represent a corneal degeneration, they commonly carry the name "dystrophy," and we discuss them here for clarity. The spots usually occur bilaterally and symmetrically, but no more than two members of a single family have been described as having them. They become increasingly apparent after age 30, another suggestion that they might be degenerative, and they do not reduce visual acuity.

The discrete, minute opacities appear as linear or punctate gray specks manifesting a variety of forms, including dendrites with three or four arms, boomerangs with angular extensions, circles, commas, and worm shapes.[53] All types may occur together and may occupy the central or the peripheral deep stroma. They correspond to isolated abnormal deep stromal keratocytes that contain unsaturated neutral fats and phospholipids in vacuoles.[54]

Two other types of pre-Descemet's opacities include cornea farinata, a fine flourlike dusting of the deep corneal stroma that is probably a normal aging change and does not affect visual acuity, and the fine spots associated with systemic diseases like X-linked recessive ichthyosis.[55]

Polymorphic Amyloid Degeneration

This bilaterally symmetrical disorder, also called polymorphic stromal dystrophy, appears after age 50, is sporadic, and is sometimes classified with the pre-Descemet's "dystrophies." We discuss it here for completeness. Gray-white, snowflakelike flecks and irregularly beaded filamentous opacities occupy the posterior third of the stroma. They appear to indent Descemet's membrane and create refractile irregularities against the red fundus reflection.[56] The opacities consist of focal deposits of amyloid in the posterior cornea.[57] The disorder does not affect visual acuity.

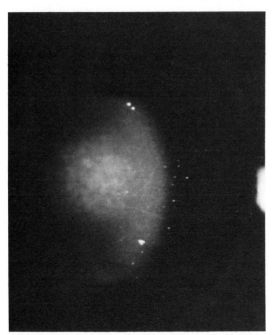

Figure 3–16. Central cloudy dystrophy. The clustered nebular stromal opacities stand out in broad oblique illumination.

Posterior Amorphous Dystrophy

This corneal dystrophy has been described in one family with autosomal dominant, bilaterally symmetrical, corneal opacification and thinning.[58] The disorder appears in the first decade of life, remains asymptomatic, and progresses slowly to a corneal thickness of about 0.3 mm. with minimal corneal astigmatism. Gray sheets form indistinct lamellae at various levels of the deep stroma across the entire cornea. No histopathology has been reported.

Congenital Hereditary Stromal Dystrophy

This autosomal dominant disorder exhibits bilaterally symmetrical, central, anterior stromal, flaky-feathery opacities that are present at birth.[59] Normal corneal thickness and absence of both epithelial edema and thickening of Descemet's membrane distinguish this clinically from congenital hereditary endothelial dystrophy. The disorder is nonprogressive but is often accom-

panied by searching nystagmus and esotropia. Histopathologically, the stroma consists of alternating layers of tightly packed and loosely packed collagen fibrils of about 15 nm. diameter, which is about half of normal diameter. The prognosis for a clear penetrating keratoplasty is good, although amblyopia usually limits visual acuity to 20/200.

ENDOTHELIAL DYSTROPHIES

Endothelial dystrophies have two major clinical and histopathologic characteristics:

1. The stressed endothelial cell produces excess collagen posterior to Descemet's membrane, a tissue we call the posterior collagenous layer (PCL) of the cornea. Clinically, this tissue appears as thickening of Descemet's membrane that is manifested as cornea guttata, polymorphic excrescences, or gray sheets. Ultrastructurally, it corresponds to the deposit of abnormal basement membrane or fibrillar collagenous tissue between the original Descemet's membrane and the dystrophic endothelial cells.

2. With breakdown of the endothelial barrier and pump functions, stromal and epithelial edema occur and reduce visual acuity.

Fuchs' Endothelial Dystrophy

Cornea guttata are focal, clinically refractile accumulations of collagen posterior to Descemet's membrane and are commonly called warts or excrescences of Descemet's membrane. Primary cornea guttata may occur in small numbers as part of normal aging,[60] in confluent patches as a reflection of a mildly dystrophic endothelium,[61] or in the company of corneal edema as Fuchs' endothelial dystrophy. Secondary cornea guttata occur after inflammatory, toxic, or traumatic insult to the endothelium.[62]

Fuchs' dystrophy is probably inherited as an autosomal dominant, although only three pedigrees have been reported with sufficient information for genetic analysis.[63] Relatives over age 40 of individuals with confluent cornea guttata manifest cornea guttata more frequently than the normal population.[61] However, the female-to-male ratio may be as high as 4 to 1, a distribution unusual in an autosomal dominant disease. Fuchs' endothelial dystrophy is bilateral but may be asymmetric. Cornea guttata preceding Fuchs' dystrophy may appear around age 30, but corneal edema seldom appears before age 50, an exception to the generality that corneal dystrophies appear early in life.

The clinical and histopathologic progression of Fuchs' dystrophy is complex, and it can best be divided into three stages, which usually span 10 to 20 years.[64] In the first stage the asymptomatic patient manifests central, irregularly distributed guttate excrescences and geographically arranged fine pigment dusting (Fig. 3–17). The guttate excrescences interrupt the endothelial mosaic and produce irregular cell borders by pushing the endothelial nuclei into dumbbell or sickle shapes and by thinning the overlying epithelial cells. Even though individual endothelial cells enlarge up to 1000 μm^2 (normal 400 μm^2) and lose their characteristic hexagonal shape, they usually maintain an intact covering of the posterior corneal surface. Clinical specular microscopy demonstrates the guttate excrescences as black spots disrupting the endothelial mosaic (Fig. 3–18). As the disorder progresses, Descemet's membrane may appear gray and thickened. By light microscopy, Descemet's membrane appears multilaminar on PAS stain and ultrastructurally manifests deposits of abnormal basement membrane on the posterior surface of the original Descemet's membrane. This abnormal material characteristically contains 110-nm. banded wide-spacing material in addition to finer collagen fibrils and amorphous background material. This is the material that constitutes the guttate wart (Fig. 3–19). Endothelial cells contain phagocytosed pigment granules.

In the second stage the patient develops stromal and epithelial edema with symptoms of glare and hazy vision. When mild, the stromal edema is limited to the pre-Descemet's and subepithelial area and is accompanied by mild epithelial bedewing. As the edema increases, the stroma thickens centrally, the opacity spreads peripherally, and the epithelium develops bullae that correspond to intraepithelial and subepithelial lakes of fluid (Fig. 3–20). As stromal edema increases, Descemet's membrane develops

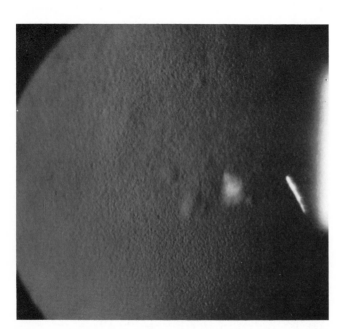

Figure 3–17. Cornea guttata. In retroillumination the discrete guttate excrescences appear as a pattern of refractile dots against a beaten metal background.

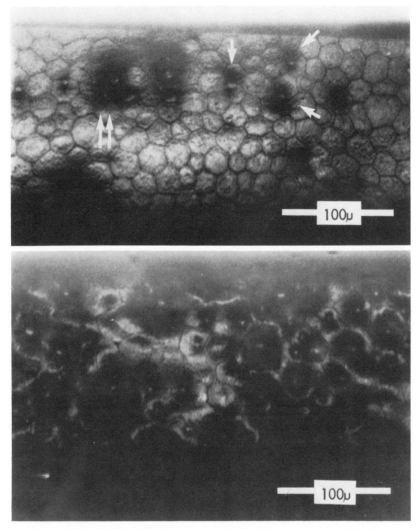

Figure 3–18. Central guttata in Fuchs' dystrophy. *A,* Individual excrescences (single arrows) and larger lesions, probably formed by the coalescence of individual excrescences (double arrow). *B,* Advanced guttate changes; many of the excrescences have coalesced and obscure the great majority of endothelial cells. (Courtesy of Ronald A. Laing, Ph.D., and Howard M. Leibowitz, M.D.)

folds. The endothelium consists of both normal and degenerating cells; the degenerating cells have fibroblast-like qualities.[65] Layers of fibrillar collagen appear posterior to the abnormal banded material, forming a loose-knit feltwork that accounts for the increased grayness of Descemet's membrane clinically and for the multilaminar appearance by light microscopy. These new layers of collagen bury the guttate excrescences so that no protrusions are present on the posterior corneal surface.

In the third phase subepithelial connective tissue appears centrally. This is an avascular tissue that does not migrate in from the periphery like a pannus but arises in the central cornea. Clinically, it appears as an irregular, dense, gray, swirling sheet of scar tissue. Histologically, it consists of active fibroblasts and of large and small collagen fibrils between Bowman's layer and the epithelium. In some areas connective tissue septa extend into the epithelium. In advanced cases the stromal edema and epithelial bullae gradually disappear as the stroma scars, and the patient becomes more comfortable even though the visual acuity is severely reduced.

In the early stages the patient experiences a foreign body sensation and blurred vision upon awakening, since decreased nocturnal tear evaporation makes the tears more dilute and they draw less fluid from the cornea osmotically. Topical hypertonic sodium chloride ointment instilled upon retiring and the early morning use of a hair dryer to dehydrate the corneal epithelium will decrease the time during which this blurriness persists. Hypertonic drops, such as 5 per cent sodium chloride, instilled during the day will help to decrease the epithelial edema. A loosely fitting, thin, flat, high-water-content soft contact lens will decrease the irregular astigmatism and the pain from ruptured epithelial bullae. However, when stromal edema further decreases vision, the soft contact lens will not improve visual acuity. Since elevated intraocular pressure will force more fluid into the stroma across the compromised endothelium, appropriate pressure reduction with carbonic anhydrase inhibitors and topical miotics, epinephrine, or β-adrenergic blocking drugs may decrease cor-

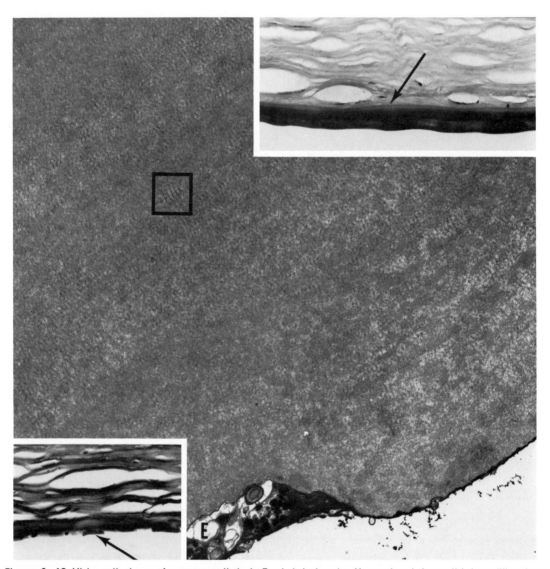

Figure 3–19. Histopathology of cornea guttata in Fuchs' dystrophy. Upper inset shows thick multilaminar Descemet's membrane with buried guttate warts. (PAS, × 380.) Lower inset shows anvil-shaped guttate excrescences that protrude into the anterior chamber (arrow). Endothelial cells are atrophic. (PAS, × 380.) Electron micrograph of guttate excrescence shows wide-spacing material with macroperiodicity of about 110 nm. (box) interspersed throughout amorphous basement membrane–like material. Endothelium (E) appears degenerated. (× 10,650.)

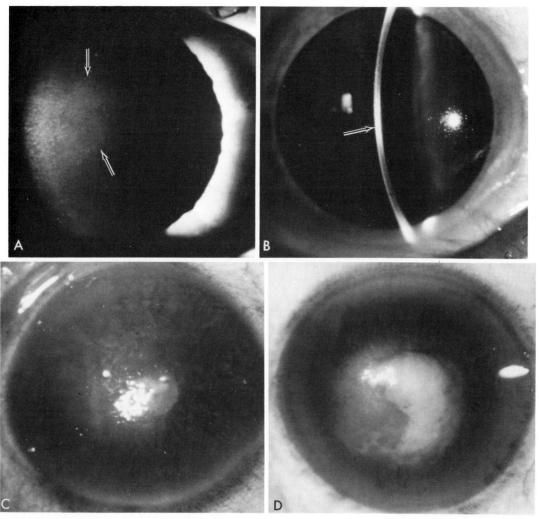

Figure 3–20. Fuchs' endothelial dystrophy. *A,* Diffuse, central, irregular gray patch of thickened Descemet's membrane is outlined by pigment granules (arrows). *B,* Slit view shows central mild corneal edema (arrow). *C,* As endothelial function decreases, epithelial edema becomes apparent, manifest here as a broken corneal light reflection. *D,* In a more advanced stage central subepithelial fibrosis and stromal scarring occur.

neal edema. MacKay-Marg tonometry or pneumotonometry is probably more accurate in measuring intraocular pressure through an edematous cornea than Goldmann applanation tonometry.

As visual acuity falls, penetrating keratoplasty should be performed. Corneal grafts for Fuchs' dystrophy account for about 10 per cent of all corneal grafts, and if the graft is performed before the process reaches the peripheral cornea, about 80 per cent will remain clear for 2 years.[66] Keratoplasty in eyes with narrow angles should include lens removal to avoid angle closure with the formation of peripheral anterior synech-

iae. Patients with both Fuchs' endothelial dystrophy and cataract will do well with a combined penetrating keratoplasty and cataract extraction.[67] Those with advanced painful bullous keratopathy in whom keratoplasty and soft contact lens therapy are inappropriate will often regain comfort after a conjunctival flap or cautery of Bowman's layer.

Posterior Polymorphous Dystrophy

A variety of terms have described this entity, including posterior polymorphous dystrophy of Schlicting, hereditary deep dystrophy, grouped vesicles, Schnyder's posterior herpes, and hereditary corneal edema.[68] All of these abnormalities occur in families with posterior polymorphous dystrophy. Theodore was among the earliest observers to document that this disorder is inherited as an autosomal dominant trait.[69] However, its expression is highly variable, and seemingly it may sometimes exhibit autosomal recessive inheritance. Posterior polymorphous dystrophy is almost always bilateral, though it may be asymmetrical.

The disorder is probably congenital, since cases of congenital corneal edema[70–72] occur in families with posterior polymorphous dystrophy.[68, 72] Since it does not usually reduce visual acuity, affected individuals are often identified during routine ophthalmologic examination or as part of family studies. Although it has been described as stationary, the disorder can progress slowly to produce diffuse ground-glass stromal edema with secondary corneal degeneration that requires keratoplasty.

The simplest form of the disorder is grouped vesicles, 2 to 20 small, discrete, round lesions with the optical quality of blisters, surrounded by a diffuse gray halo. A sporadic, unilateral form of posterior corneal vesicles also occurs, unrelated to posterior polymorphous dystrophy.[72a] Larger geographic lesions, a more severe form of grouped vesicles, create a variety of patterns on the posterior cornea. They protrude posteriorly in a narrow slit beam, form gray patches in broad tangential illumination, and appear refractile in retroillumination. Some of them contain round empty spots (Fig. 3–21). A broad band about 1 mm. wide is a distinctive lesion in posterior polymorphous dystrophy and extends across the posterior corneal surface as two translucent, scalloped, elevated, roughly parallel ridges. They also appear gray in direct illumination and refractile in retroillumination. Diffuse irregular thickening of Descemet's membrane without guttate excrescences may occur, giving a beaten metal ap-

pearance on specular reflection and in retroillumination.

Individuals in one family manifested posterior polymorphous dystrophy and the anterior chamber cleavage syndrome.[73] Elevated intraocular pressure may be present.[73] In some cases, broad peripheral iridocorneal adhesions[74] occupy the peripheral 1 mm. of the posterior cornea, sometimes accompanied by a glassy membrane that extends onto the surface of the iris to produce ectropion of the iris pigment epithelium. Corneal edema overlies these adhesions. No histopathologic studies of this iris abnormality have been described.

The posterior corneal abnormalities correspond to deposits of collagenous tissue on the posterior surface of a very thin original Descemet's membrane. By light microscopy they appear as fusiform bundles of tissue and by electron microscopy as multilaminar fibrillar tissue consisting either of abnormal basement membrane with 110-nm. banded wide-

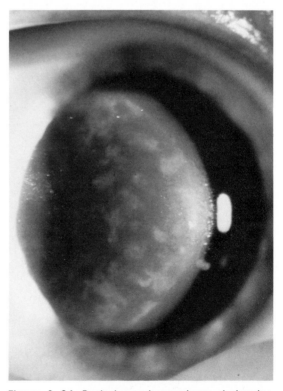

Figure 3–21. Posterior polymorphous dystrophy. Discrete gray geographic thickenings of Descemet's membrane sometimes contain clear vesicular areas.

spacing collagen or of a loose feltwork of small and large collagen fibrils. The histopathologic basis for the unusual polymorphic and vesicular lesions is irregularities and craters at the level of Descemet's membrane. A distinctive ultrastructural abnormality in posterior polymorphous dystrophy is the epithelial-like morphology of the multilayered cells surfacing the posterior cornea.[73] They exhibit numerous surface microvillae, abundant intracellular keratofibrils, multiple desmosomes instead of the usual apical junctions, minimally interdigitated cell borders, and sparse organelles. The cells stain with antisera prepared against human epidermal keratin.[73a] However, epithelial-like cells are not always present in posterior polymorphous dystrophy and may occur in other disorders[75] (Fig. 3–22).

Most patients with posterior polymorphous dystrophy are asymptomatic. Those with mild stromal or epithelial edema may obtain comfort and some improvement of vision from hypertonic solutions or soft contact lenses. When the edema is severe enough, penetrating keratoplasty should be used to restore visual acuity.[68]

Congenital Hereditary Endothelial Dystrophy

This disorder originally was considered a variant of luetic interstitial keratitis and later took its place among the stromal dystrophies as congenital macular corneal opacity (now called congenital hereditary stromal dystrophy[59]). Ultrastructural studies have demonstrated the dystrophic endothelium and Descemet's membrane that provide the basis for the appellation congenital hereditary endothelial dystrophy.[76–79] Congenital autosomal recessive and juvenile autosomal dominant forms have been distinguished.[80]

The bilaterally symmetrical edematous corneas have a diffuse, gray-blue, ground-glass appearance occasionally studded with focal gray spots (Fig. 3–23). The corneas are two to three times

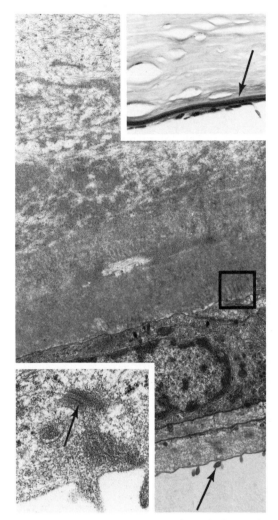

Figure 3–22. Histopathology of posterior polymorphous dystrophy. Upper inset shows thin multilaminar Descemet's membrane (arrow) with multilayered cells on its posterior surface. Electron micrograph shows epithelial-like cells with many surface microvillae (arrow) lining posterior cornea. The thin, irregular Descemet's membrane consists of fine fibrils anteriorly and of widespacing material (box) immersed in amorphous basement membrane–like material posteriorly. ($\times$ 10,800.) Lower inset shows desmosome between two cells (arrow) with microvillae protruding into the anterior chamber. ($\times$ 53,000.)

normal thickness, and individuals with dense opacification early in life often develop nystagmus and esotropia. Discomfort is unusual, since the fine epithelial edema does not form bullae.[79] Although the stromal edema sometimes remains stable, it usually progresses gradually over 5 to 10 years with secondary changes like band keratopathy.

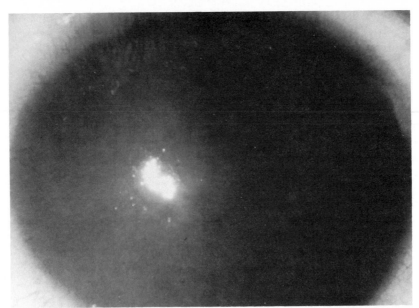

Figure 3–23. Congenital hereditary endothelial dystrophy. The diffuse ground-glass edema is associated with a corneal thickness two or three times normal.

Table 3–3. CONGENITAL CORNEAL DYSTROPHIES

Characteristics	Congenital Hereditary Endothelial Dystrophy		Posterior Polymorphous Dystrophy (Congenital Corneal Edema)	Congenital Hereditary Stromal Dystrophy
Inheritance	Autosomal recessive	Autosomal dominant	Autosomal dominant	Autosomal dominant
Laterality	Bilateral	Bilateral	Bilateral	Bilateral
Time of appearance of opacity	At birth	First or second year	At birth or within first year	At birth
Other signs or symptoms	None	Photophobia, tearing	None	None
Progression	Minimal	Slowly progressive	Slowly progressive	None
Corneal thickness	2–3 times normal	2–3 times normal	Probably normal	Normal
Location of opacity	Diffuse	Diffuse	Diffuse	Central
Appearance of opacity	Ground-glass, few white maculae	Ground-glass, few white maculae	Ground-glass	Ground-glass, flaky, feathery
Nystagmus	Frequent	Infrequent	?	Frequent
Histopathology				
Epithelium	Mild edema		Mild edema	Normal
Bowman's layer	Intact or fragmented		Fragmented or intact	Normal
Stroma	Edema, some large collagen fibrils (700 nm. diameter)		Edema, some large collagen fibrils (700 nm. diameter)	Small diameter collagen fibrils (15 nm.) form alternating loose and compact lamellae
Descemet's membrane	Thin original Descemet's membrane covered by acellular feltwork of 30 nm. diameter collagen fibrils		Thin original Descemet's membrane covered by multilaminar collagen tissue	Normal, anterior banding not prominent
Endothelium	Often atrophic		Epithelial-like: many microvillae, desmosomes, tonofilaments	Normal

During the neonatal period, the clinician may mistake this disorder for congenital glaucoma without buphthalmos and perform glaucoma surgery.[81] Absence of inflammation and photophobia, absence of elevated pressure by electronic or pneumatic tonometry, and absence of progressive corneal enlargement make congenital glaucoma less likely. Both posterior polymorphous dystrophy and congenital hereditary endothelial dystrophy may manifest diffuse corneal clouding at birth, but corneal thickness is usually normal in posterior polymorphous dystrophy, whereas it is two to three times normal in congenital hereditary endothelial dystrophy (Table 3–3).

Histopathologically, the epithelium varies in thickness and the stroma demonstrates fluid pockets with variably sized collagen fibrils that form irregular lamellae. The endothelium and Descemet's membrane exhibit the major abnormalities, and descriptions have varied.[76a] In one eye enucleated from a newborn infant,[76, 82] the area of Descemet's membrane consisted of multiple layers of fine filamentous material similar to that seen in the developing fetus, and endothelial cells were sparse. Generally the original Descemet's membrane is thick and characterized by normal 110-nm. banding. Collagen tissue appears posterior to it and consists of a feltwork of small and large collagen fibrils interspersed among small amounts of basement membrane–like material (Fig. 3–24). Guttate excrescences are absent. Although the endothelium functions well enough in utero to produce an original Descemet's membrane, its malfunction early in life is demonstrated by the thick posterior collagenous material and the severe stromal edema.

If the edema is mild and remains stationary, little therapy is necessary, since epithelial erosions seldom occur. However, if corneal opacification is moderately severe, early keratoplasty will diminish the density of the amblyopia and may prevent nystagmus and esotropia. Unfortunately, corneal grafts performed for congenital hereditary endothelial dystrophy often gradually opacify

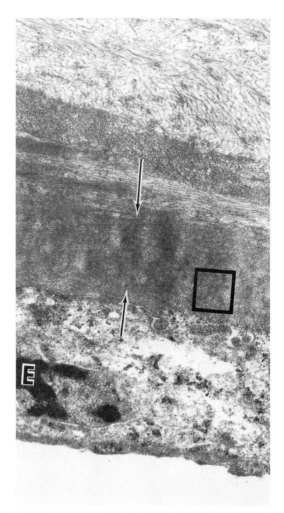

Figure 3–24. Histopathology of congenital hereditary endothelial dystrophy. Electron micrograph shows thin Descemet's membrane (between arrows) with overlying degenerating endothelial cell (E). This is an unusual case, since Descemet's membrane is usually thick in this disorder. (× 11,000.)

months to years after surgery;[76, 81] however, recent reports have been more encouraging.

OTHER DYSTROPHIES

We have omitted reports of isolated individuals and of a few members in a family said to have a corneal dystrophy. For example, annular endothelial dystrophy, characterized by posterior peripheral flat, ring-shaped opacities, has been described in a mother and daughter.[83]

Attentive clinicians undoubtedly will discover more corneal dystrophies.

REFERENCES

1. Bron, A. J., and Tripathi, R. C.: Corneal disorders. In Goldberg, M. F. (ed.): *Genetic and Metabolic Eye Diseases.* Boston, Little, Brown, 1974, pp. 281–323.
2. Duke-Elder, S., and Leigh, A. G.: Diseases of the outer eye. In Duke-Elder, S. (ed.): *System of Ophthalmology.* Vol. VIII, Part 2. St. Louis, C. V. Mosby Co., 1965, pp. 921–976.
3. Francois, J.: Heredofamilial corneal dystrophies. In *Symposium on Surgical and Medical Management of Congenital Anomalies of the Eye,* Transactions of the New Orleans Academy of Ophthalmology. St. Louis, C. V. Mosby Co., 1968, pp. 114–156.
4. Malbran, E. S.: Corneal dystrophies: A clinical, pathological, and surgical approach. Amer J Ophthalmol 74:771, 1972.
5. Polack, F. M.: Contributions of electron microscopy to the study of corneal pathology. Surv Ophthalmol 20:375, 1976.
6. Waring, G. O., Rodrigues, M. M., and Laibson, P. R.: Corneal dystrophies. I. Dystrophies of the epithelium, Bowman's layer, and stroma. Surv Ophthalmol 23:71, 1978.
7. Waring, G. O., Rodrigues, M. M., and Laibson, P. R.: Corneal dystrophies. II. Endothelial dystrophies. Surv Ophthalmol 23:147, 1978.
8. Francois, J.: Cornea verticillata. Doc Ophthalmol 27:235, 1969.
9. Bron, A. J., and Brown, N. A.: Some superficial corneal disorders. Trans Ophthalmol Soc UK 91:13, 1971.
10. Laibson, P. R.: Microcystic corneal dystrophy. Trans Amer Ophthalmol Soc 74:488, 1976.
11. Trobe, J. D., and Laibson, P. R.: Dystrophic changes in the anterior cornea. Arch Ophthalmol 87:378, 1972.
12. Cogan, D. G., Donaldson, D. D., Kuwabara, T., and Marshall, D.: Microcystic dystrophy of the corneal epithelium. Trans Amer Ophthalmol Soc 62:213, 1964.
13. Laibson, P. R., and Krachmer, J. H.: Familiar occurrence of dot (microcystic), map, fingerprint dystrophy of the cornea. Invest Ophthalmol 14:397, 1975.
14. Guerry, D.: Observations on Cogan's microcystic dystrophy of the corneal epithelium. Trans Amer Ophthalmol Soc 63:320, 1965.
15. Brown, N. A., and Bron, A. J.: Superficial lines and associated disorders of the cornea. Amer J Ophthalmol 81:34, 1976.
16. Cogan, D. G., Kuwabara, T., Donaldson, D. D., and Collins, E.: Microcystic dystrophy of the cornea. A partial explanation for its pathogenesis. Arch Ophthalmol 92:470, 1974.
17. Rodrigues, M. M., Fine, B., Laibson, P., and Zimmerman, L.: Disorders of the corneal epithelium— A clinicopathologic study of dot, geographic, and fingerprint patterns. Arch Ophthalmol 92:475, 1974.
18. Bron, A. J., and Tripathi, R. C.: Cystic disorders of the corneal epithelium. I. Clinical aspects. Brit J Ophthalmol 57:361, 1973.
19. Bron, A. J., and Tripathi, R. C.: Cystic disorders of the corneal epithelium. II. Pathogenesis. Brit J Ophthalmol 57:376, 1973.
20. Broderick, J. D., Dark, A. J., and Peace, G. W.: Fingerprint dystrophy of the cornea: A histologic study. Arch Ophthalmol 92:483, 1974.
21. Dark, A. J.: Bleb dystrophy of the cornea: Histochemistry and ultrastructure. Brit J Ophthalmol 61:65, 1977.
22. Fogle, J. A., Kenyon, K. R., Stark, W. J., and Green, W.R.: Defective epithelial adhesion in anterior corneal dystrophies. Amer J Ophthalmol 79:925, 1975.
23. Burns, R. P.: Meesmann's corneal dystrophy. Trans Amer Ophthalmol Soc 66:530, 1968.
24. Fine, B. S., Yanoff, M., Pitts, E., and Slaughter, F. D.: Meesmann's epithelial dystrophy of the cornea. Amer J Ophthalmol 83:633, 1977.
25. Rice, N. S. C., Ashton, N., Jay, B., and Black, R. K.: Reis-Bücklers' dystrophy. A clinico-pathological study. Brit J Ophthalmol 52:577, 1968.
26. Grayson, M., and Wilbrandt, H.: Dystrophy of the anterior limiting membrane of the cornea (Reis-Bücklers' Type). Amer J Ophthalmol 61:345, 1966.
27. Thiel, H. J., and Behnke, H.: Eine bisher unbekannte subepitheliale hereditäre Hornhautdystrophie. Klin Monatsbl Augenheilk 150:862, 1967.
28. Griffin, D. G., and Fine, B. S.: Light and electron microscopic observations in a superficial corneal dystrophy. Probable early Reis-Bücklers' type. Amer J Ophthalmol 63:1659, 1967.
29. Wood, T. O., Fleming, J. C., Dotson, R. S., and Cotten, M. S.: Treatment of Reis-Bücklers' corneal dystrophy by removal of subepithelial fibrous tissue. Amer J Ophthalmol 85:360, 1978.
30. Hall, P.: Reis-Bücklers' dystrophy. Arch Ophthalmol 91:170, 1974.
31. Pouliquen, Y., Dhermy, P., Presles, D., and Tollard, M. F.: Dégénérescence en Chagrin de crocodile de Vogt ou dégénérescence en mosaique de Valerio. Arch Ophtalmol (Paris) 36:395, 1976.
32. Malbran, E., D'Alessandro, C., and Valenzuela, J.: Megalocornea and mosaic dystrophy of the cornea. Ophthalmologica 149:161, 1965.
33. Jones, S. T., and Zimmerman, L. E.: Macular dystrophy of the cornea (Groenouw Type II). Amer J Ophthalmol 47:1, 1959.
33a. Rodrigues, M. R., Streeten, B. W., Krachmer, J. H., Laibson, P. R., Salem, N., Passonneau, J., and Chock, S.: Phospholipid and microfibrillar protein in granular corneal dystrophy. Invest Ophthalmol Vis Sci 24(Suppl):274, 1983.
34. Iwamoto, T., Stuart, J. C., Srinivasan, B. D., et al.: Ultrastructural variations in granular dystrophy of the cornea. Albrecht von Graefes Arch Klin Exp Ophthalmol 194:1, 1975.
35. Kanai, A., Yamaguchi, T., and Nakajima, A.: The histochemical and analytical electron microscopic studies of the corneal granular dystrophy. Acta Soc Ophthalmol Jap 81:145, 1977.
36. Rodrigues, M. M., and McGavic, J. S.: Recurrent corneal granular dystrophy: A clinico-pathologic study. Trans Amer Ophthalmol Soc 73:306, 1975.
37. Dark, A. J., and Thompson, D. S.: Lattice dystrophy of the cornea. A clinical and microscopic study. Brit J Ophthalmol 44:257, 1960.
38. Klintworth, G. K.: Lattice corneal dystrophy. An inherited variety of amyloidosis restricted to the cornea. Amer J Pathol 50:371, 1967.
39. Meretoja, J.: Comparative histopathological and clinical findings in eyes with lattice corneal dystrophy of two different types. Ophthalmologica 165:15, 1972.

40. Wheeler, G. E., and Eiferman, R. A.: Immunohistochemical identification of the AA protein on lattice dystrophy. Invest Ophthalmol Vis Sci 20(Suppl):115, 1981.

41. Klintworth, G. K., and Smith, C. F.: Macular corneal dystrophy: Studies of sulfated glycosaminoglycans in corneal explant and confluent stromal cell cultures. Amer J Pathol 89:167, 1977.

42. Klintworth, G. K., and Vogel, F. S.: Macular corneal dystrophy—An inherited acid mucopolysaccharide storage disease of the corneal fibroblast. Amer J Pathol 45:565, 1964.

43. Snip, R., Kenyon, K., and Green, W.: Macular corneal dystrophy. Ultrastructural pathology of corneal endothelium and Descemet's membrane. Invest Ophthalmol 12:88, 1973.

44. Francois, J., Victoria-Transoco, V., Maudgal, P.C., and Victoria-Ihler, A.: Study of the lysosomes by vital stains in normal keratocytes and in keratocytes from macular dystrophy of the cornea. Invest Ophthalmol 15:599, 1976.

45. Herman, S. J., and Hughes, W. F.: Recurrence of hereditary corneal dystrophy following keratoplasty. Amer J Ophthalmol 75:689, 1973.

46. Robin, A. L., Green, W. R., Lapsa, T. P., Hoover, R. E., and Kelley, J. S.: Recurrence of macular corneal dystrophy after lamellar keratoplasty. Amer J Ophthalmol 84:457, 1977.

47. Delleman, J. W., and Winkelman, J. E.: Degeneratio corneae cristallinea hereditaria: A clinical, genetical, and histological study. Ophthalmologica 155:409, 1968.

48. Bron, A. J., Williams, H. P., and Carruthers, M. E.: Hereditary crystalline stromal dystrophy of Schnyder. I. Clinical features of a family with hyperlipoproteinaemia. Brit J Ophthalmol 56:383, 1972.

49. Purcell, J. J., Jr., Krachmer, J. H., and Weingeist, T. A.: Fleck corneal dystrophy. Arch Ophthalmol 95:440, 1977.

50. Gillespie, F., and Covelli, B.: Fleck (mouchetée) dystrophy of the cornea: Report of a family. South Med J 56:1265, 1963.

51. Nicholson, D. H., Green, W. R., Cross, H. E., Kenyon, K. R., and Massof, D.: A clinical and histopathological study of Francois-Neetens speckled corneal dystrophy. Amer J Ophthalmol 83:554, 1977.

52. Bramsen, T., Ehlers, N., and Baggesen, L. H.: Central cloudy corneal dystrophy of Francois. Acta Ophthalmol 54:221, 1976.

52a. Krachmer, J. H., Dubord, P. J., Rodrigues, M. M., and Mannis, M. J.: Corneal posterior crocodile shagreen and polymorphic amyloid degeneration. Arch Ophthalmol 101:54, 1983.

53. Grayson, M., and Wilbrandt, H.: Pre-Descemet's dystrophy. Amer J Ophthalmol 64:276, 1967.

54. Curran, R. E., Kenyon, K. R., and Green, W. R.: Pre-Descemet's membrane corneal dystrophy. Amer J Ophthalmol 77:711, 1974.

55. Sever, R. J., Frost, P., and Weinstein, G.: Eye changes in ichthyosis. JAMA 206:2283, 1968.

56. Thomsitt, J., and Bron, A. J.: Polymorphic stromal dystrophy. Brit J Ophthalmol 59:125, 1975.

57. Mannis, M. J., Krachmer, J. H., Rodrigues, M. M., and Pardos, G. J.: Polymorphic amyloid degeneration of the cornea. Arch Ophthalmol 99:1217, 1981.

58. Carpel, E. F., Sigelman, R. J., and Doughman, D. J.: Posterior amorphous corneal dystrophy. Amer J Ophthalmol 83:629, 1977.

59. Witschel, H., Fine, B. S., Grützner, P., and McTigue, J.W.: Congenital hereditary stromal dystrophy of the cornea. Arch Ophthalmol 96:1043, 1978.

60. Lorenzetti, D. W. C., Uotila, M. H., Parikh, N., and Kaufman, H. E.: Central corneal guttata. Incidence in the general population. Amer J Ophthalmol 64:1155, 1967.

61. Krachmer, J. H., Purcell, J. J., Young, C. W., and Bucher, K. D.: Corneal endothelial dystrophy: A study of 64 families. Arch Ophthalmol 96:2036, 1978.

62. Waring, G. O., Font, R. L., Rodrigues, M. M., and Mulberger, R. D.: Alterations of Descemet's membrane in interstitial keratitis. Amer J Ophthalmol 81:773, 1976.

63. Cross, H. E., Maumenee, A. E., and Cantolino, S. J.: Inheritance of Fuchs' endothelial dystrophy. Arch Ophthalmol 85:268, 1971.

64. Stocker, F. W.: The Endothelium of the Cornea and its Clinical Implications. 2nd ed. Springfield, Ill., Charles C Thomas, 1971, pp. 79–109.

65. Iwamoto, T., and DeVoe, A.: Electron microscopic studies on Fuchs' combined dystrophy: I. Posterior portion of the cornea. Invest Ophthalmol 10:9, 1971.

66. Stocker, F. W., and Irish, A.: Fate of successful cornea graft in Fuchs' endothelial dystrophy. Amer J Ophthalmol 68:820, 1969.

67. Arentsen, J. J., and Laibson, P. R.: Penetrating keratoplasty and cataract extraction. Combined vs nonsimultaneous surgery. Arch Ophthalmol 96:75, 1978.

68. Cibis, G. W., Krachmer, J. A., Phelps, C. D., and Weingeist, T. A.: The clinical spectrum of posterior polymorphous dystrophy. Arch Ophthalmol 95:1529, 1977.

69. Theodore, F. H.: Congenital type of endothelial dystrophy. Arch Ophthalmol 21:626, 1939.

70. Kanai, A.: Further electron microscopic study of hereditary corneal edema. Invest Ophthalmol 10:545, 1971.

71. Kanai, A., Waltman, S., Polack, F. M., and Kaufman, H. E.: Electron microscopic study of hereditary corneal edema. Invest Ophthalmol 10:89, 1971.

72. Levenson, J. E., Chandler, J. W., and Kaufman, H. E.: Affected asymptomatic relatives in congenital hereditary endothelial dystrophy. Amer J Ophthalmol 76:967, 1973.

72a. Pardos, G. J., Krachmer, J. H., and Mannis, M. J.: Posterior corneal vesicles. Arch Ophthalmol 99:1573, 1981.

73. Grayson, M.: The nature of hereditary deep polymorphous dystrophy of the cornea. Its association with iris and anterior chamber dysgenesis. Trans Amer Ophthalmol Soc 72:516, 1974.

73a. Rodrigues, M. M., Newsome, D. A., Krachmer, J. H., and Sun, T. T.: Posterior polymorphous dystrophy of the cornea: Cell culture studies. Exp Eye Res 33:535, 1981.

74. Cibis, G. W., Krachmer, J. A., Phelps, C. D., and Weingeist, T. A.: Iridocorneal adhesions in posterior polymorphous dystrophy. Trans Amer Acad Ophthalmol Otolaryngol 81:770, 1976.

75. Johnson, B.L., and Brown, S.I.: Posterior polymorphous dystrophy: A light and electron microscopic study. Brit J Ophthalmol 62:89, 1978.

76. Kenyon, K. R., and Antine, B.: The pathogenesis of congenital hereditary endothelial dystrophy of the cornea. Amer J Ophthalmol 72:787, 1971.

76a. Stainer, G. A., Akers, P. H., Binder, P. S., and Zavala, E. V.: Correlative microscopy and tissue culture of congenital hereditary endothelial dystrophy. Am J Ophthalmol 93:456, 1982.

77. Kenyon, K. R., and Maumenee, A. E.: The histological and ultrastructural pathology of congenital hereditary corneal dystrophy: A case report. Invest Ophthalmol 7:475, 1968.

78. Kenyon, K. R., and Maumenee, A. E.: Further studies of congenital hereditary endothelial dystrophy of the cornea. Amer J Ophthalmol 76:419, 1973.

79. Maumenee, A. E.: Congenital hereditary corneal dystrophy. Amer J Ophthalmol 50:1114, 1960.

80. Judisch, G. F., and Maumenee, I. H.: Clinical differentiation of recessive congenital hereditary endothelial dystrophy and dominant hereditary dystrophy. Amer J Ophthalmol 85:606, 1978.

81. Keates, R. H., and Cvintal, T.: Congenital hereditary corneal dystrophy. Amer J Ophthalmol 60:892, 1965.

82. Antine, B.: Histology of congenital corneal dystrophy. Amer J Ophthalmol 69:964, 1970.

83. Francois, J., and Evens, A.: Heredo-dystrophie annulaire de l'endothelium corneen. J Genet Hum 9:78, 1960.

Appendix

For the resident in training or the general ophthalmologist faced with a patient with a rare corneal dystrophy and seeking information to assist him in making a diagnosis, "one picture is worth a thousand words." Therefore, as a supplement to Dr. Waring's discussion and illustrative material, the editor has collaborated with medical illustrator Mark Lefkowitz to produce a series of drawings depicting the characteristics of the various corneal dystrophies. In effect, these are composite drawings; a given patient may not show all of the abnormalities presented for a given dystrophy. In figures illustrating deep dystrophies (e.g., Plates 9, 10, 11, and 14), the anterior appearance of the abnormality has been depicted in the three-quarter view although it may not actually be visible from this vantage. We hope this appendix provides a useful reference that is readily available for clinical use.

HOWARD M. LEIBOWITZ

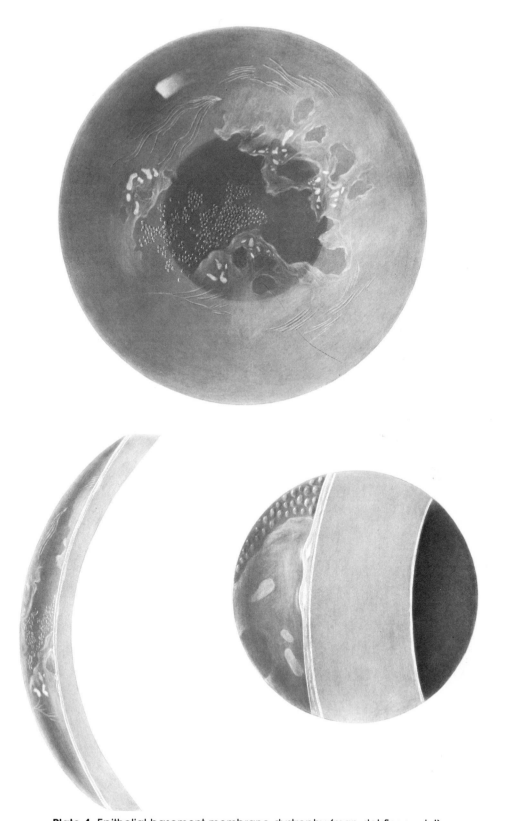

Plate 1. Epithelial basement membrane dystrophy (map-dot-fingerprint).

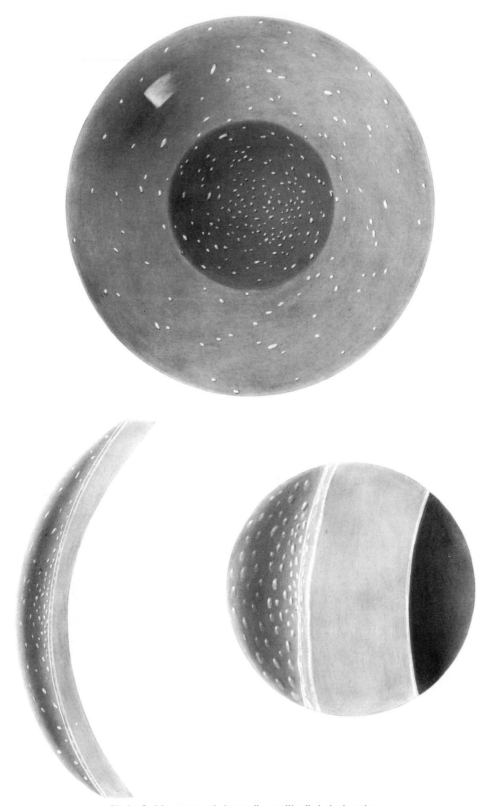

Plate 2. Meesmann's juvenile epithelial dystrophy.

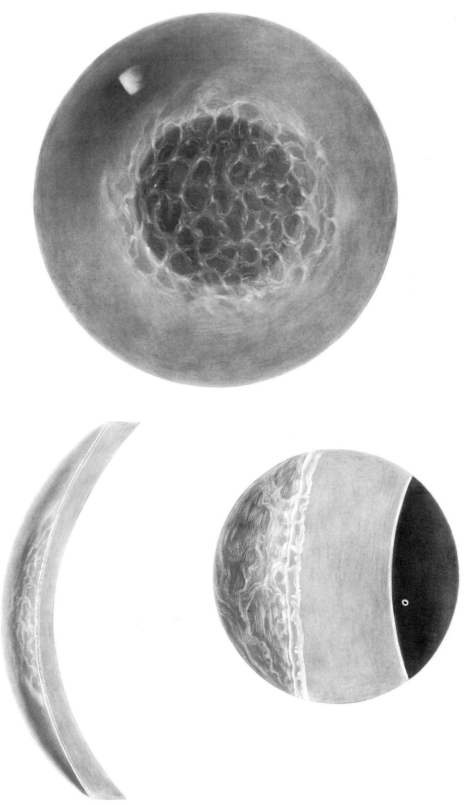

Plate 3. Reis-Bücklers' ring-shaped dystrophy.

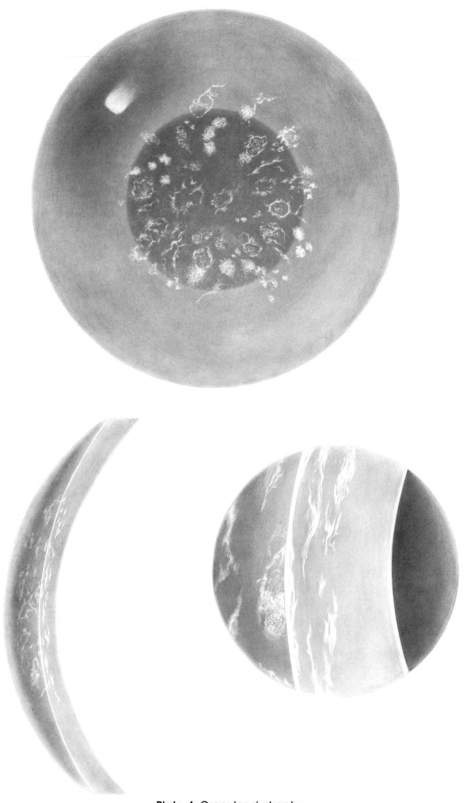

Plate 4. Granular dystrophy.

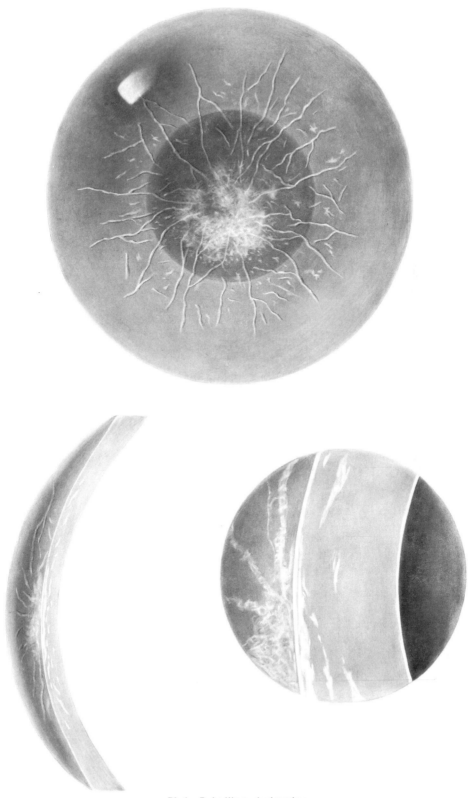

Plate 5. Lattice dystrophy.

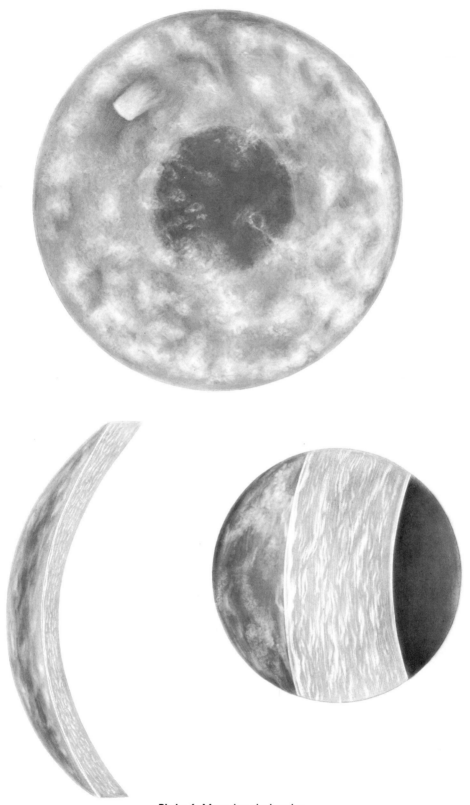

Plate 6. Macular dystrophy.

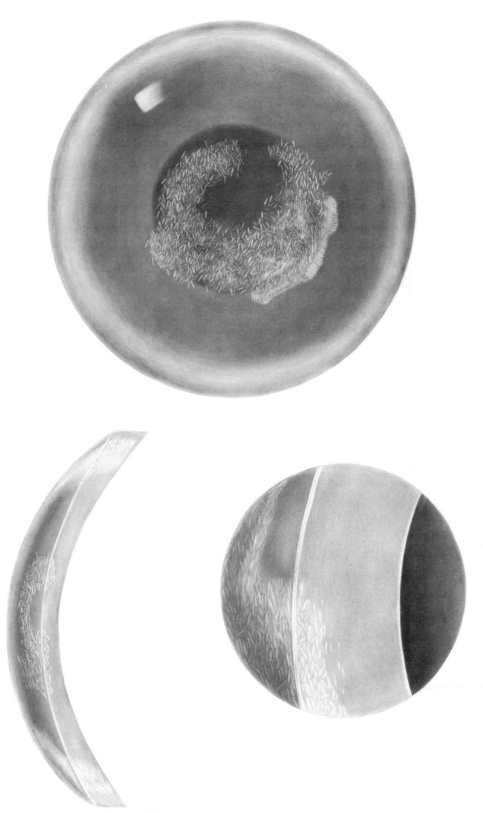

Plate 7. Central crystalline dystrophy (of Schnyder).

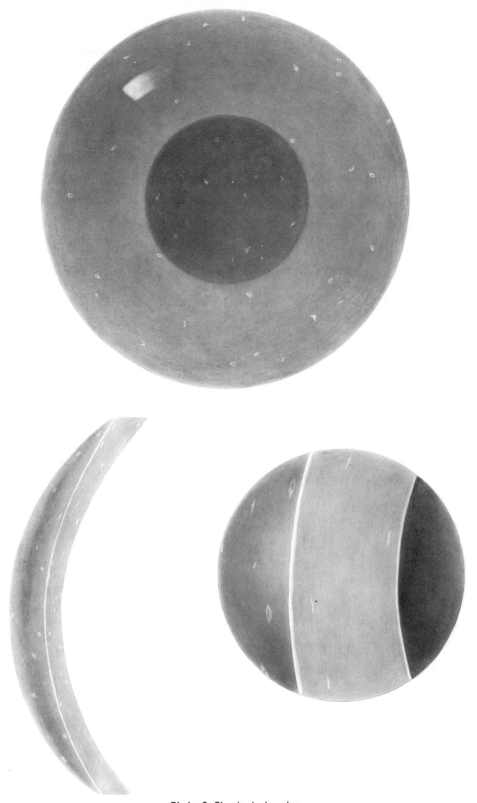

Plate 8. Fleck dystrophy.

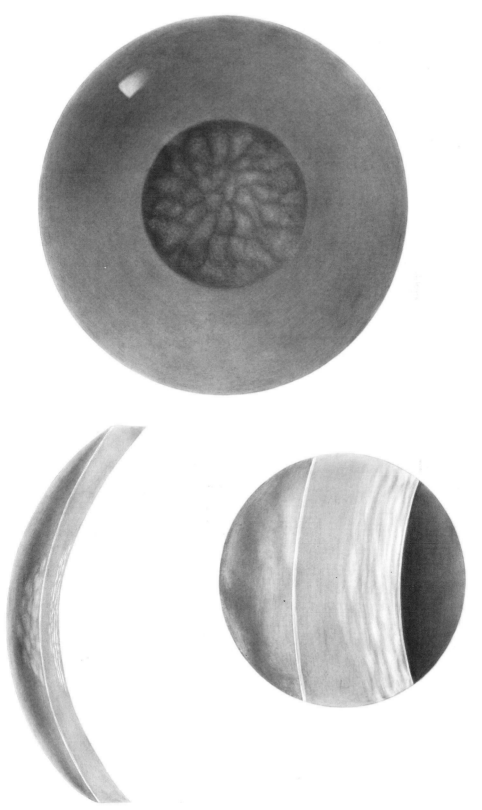

Plate 9. Central cloudy dystrophy (of Francois).

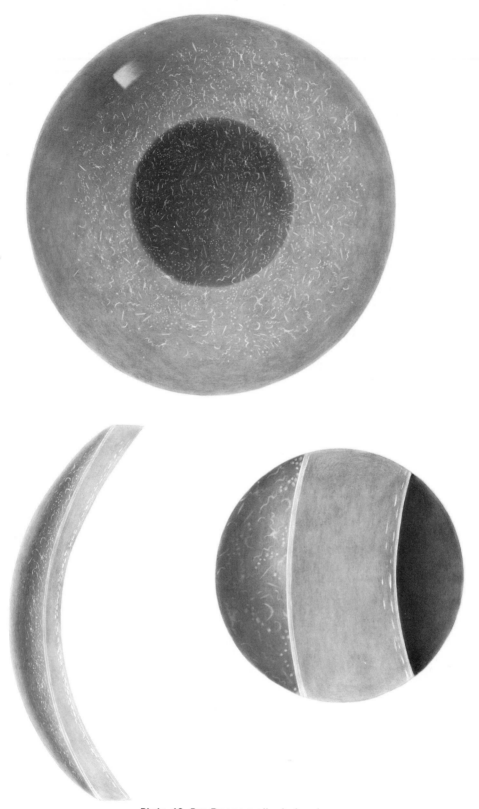

Plate 10. Pre-Descemet's dystrophy.

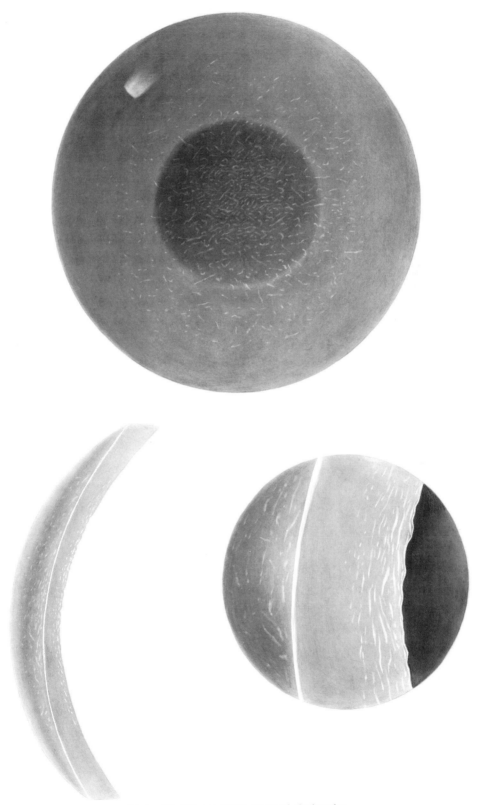

Plate 11. Polymorphic stromal dystrophy.

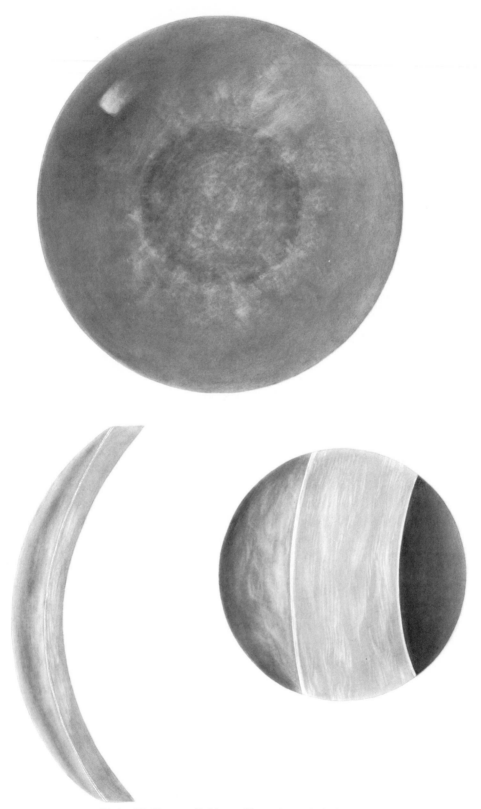

Plate 12. Congenital hereditary stromal dystrophy.

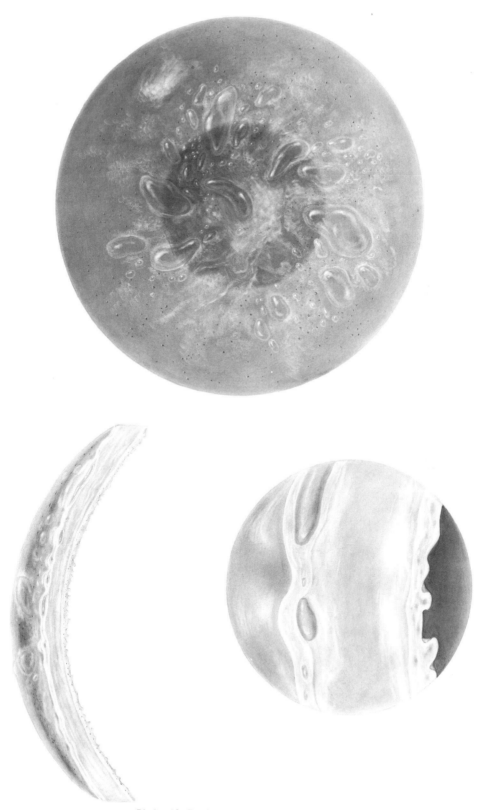

Plate 13. Fuchs' endothelial dystrophy.

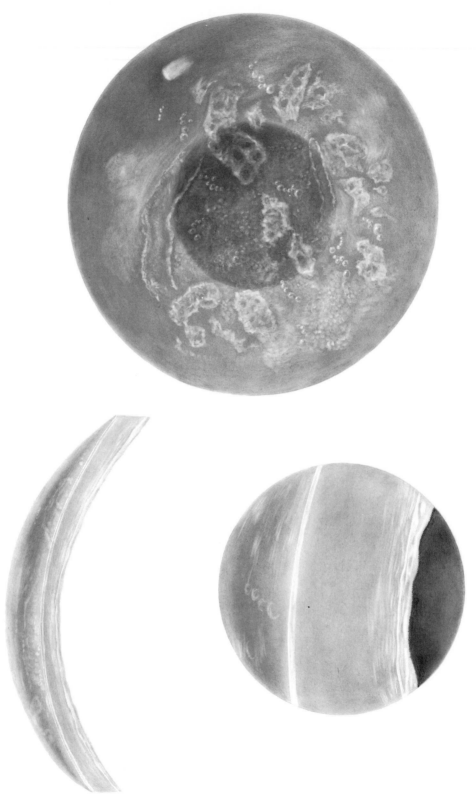

Plate 14. Posterior polymorphous dystrophy.

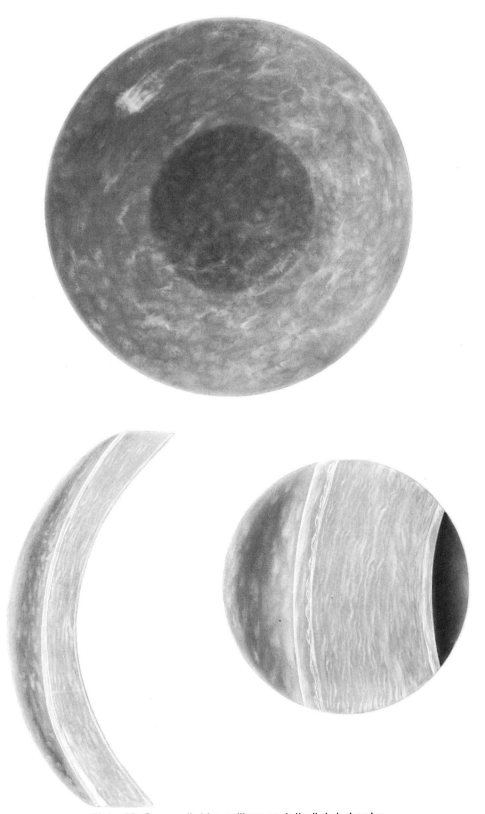

Plate 15. Congenital hereditary endothelial dystrophy.

4 Keratoconus

HOWARD M. LEIBOWITZ, M.D.

Keratoconus is an entity characterized by ectasia of the cornea. In the absence of involvement of the tissue by inflammatory processes, a conelike anterior protrusion of the cornea occurs, generally involving the central and inferior paracentral areas. This results in the development of a high degree of irregular, myopic astigmatism, causing considerable visual impairment. The etiology of the entity is not known.

In the great majority of cases keratoconus occurs bilaterally, although the condition may be considerably more pronounced or appear considerably earlier in one eye of a given individual than in the other. It is said to occur more frequently in females than in males, with some reported series showing the entity to be twice as prevalent among females.[1, 2] However, it is of interest that, although Amsler reported a greater prevalence of keratoconus among females in his overall series of 600 cases (59.2 per cent), he pointed out that he had encountered the entity more frequently in males in the last 116 cases he had examined.[3] Sixty-two per cent of Buxton's series of 140 cases were in males.[4] Among the cases seen by this author during the past 15 years, the condition also has been more prevalent among males. It is not known whether or not this reflects a true shift in the sexual prevalence of keratoconus.

The condition commonly first presents during the second decade. Many of the cases slowly and gradually progress in severity, but the rate of progression and the length of time that the entity remains actively progressive tend to vary considerably. The ectasia may progress slowly but continuously for 5 to 10 years and then stabilize permanently, or periods of progression may alternate with periods of varying length during which the ectatic process appears to have arrested. Cases also are encountered in which the ectasia remains stationary after its initial appearance. It is uncommon for the condition to progress once the affected individual has attained the age of 40. The factors governing progression and stabilization of keratoconus are not known.

Biochemical abnormalities have been found in corneas with keratoconus.[5, 6] These include decreased levels of glucose-6-phosphate dehydrogenase, relative decreases in hydroxylation of lysine and glycosylation of hydroxylysine, decreased total collagen, and relatively increased structural glycoprotein. Examination of reducible collagen crosslinks in corneas with keratoconus reveals that lysinonorleucine is present in amounts far greater than that found in normal, age-matched corneas.[7] This was interpreted to imply that the rate of collagen synthesis in keratoconus does not differ from normal but, rather, that the character of the corneal collagen in this entity is unusual. Unfortunately, these findings are insufficient to allow us to construct a unified thesis about the etiology of keratoconus. No causal relationship has been established between any of these abnormalities and the clinical pathology, and available data do not permit us to define keratoconus as a specific biochemical disorder.

Hereditary transmission of keratoconus has been reported,[3, 8] but the mode of transmission is not clear. Dominant, recessive, and irregular transmission all appear to have been documented. The situation is complicated by the fact that minimal forms of the disease often are not recognized and that the gene for keratoconus seems to have a rather feeble penetrance and a great variability of expression. In any event, hereditary transmission is by no means universal.

CLINICAL CHARACTERISTICS

In the more advanced cases of keratoconus the entity can be diagnosed by gross inspection (Fig. 4–1). When viewed from the side, it is readily apparent that the cornea has assumed the shape of a truncated cone. In such cases the diagnosis can be confirmed by raising the upper lids while the patient looks downward, so that the lower lid margins are angulated by the cone (Munson's sign), facilitating observation of the abnormality in corneal curvature (Fig. 4–2). Most schematic drawings depict these advanced cones as round or nipple-shaped. Its base has a relatively small diameter; thus, the ectasia encompasses a limited portion of the total cornea (Fig. 4–3A). Despite its relatively small size, it can achieve a marked degree of anterior protrusion. The apex of this type of cone lies below but close to the visual axis, most commonly in the lower nasal quadrant. There is also an

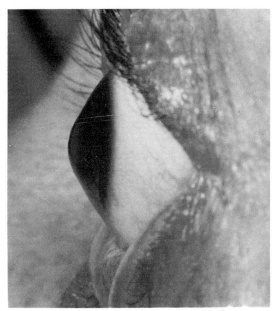

Figure 4–1. Profile of cornea in keratoconus.

oval or sagging type of cone, whose base is horizontally oval and whose apex most often lies in the lower temporal quadrant (Fig. 4–3B). This type usually is larger (both in its diameter and in its degree of protrusion), its apical center tends to be farther from the visual center of the cornea, and it generally extends farther into the inferior corneal periphery than the round type. However, the studies of Amsler[9–12] have demonstrated that keratoconus encompasses a complete continuum in the degree of alteration of corneal curvature, ranging from a rudimentary form or so-called forme fruste to the obvious corneal cone. The

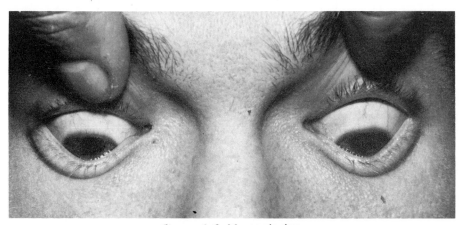

Figure 4–2. Munson's sign.

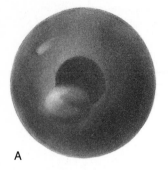
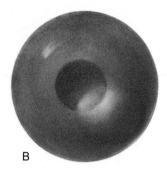

A   B

Figure 4–3. Shape of corneal cones in keratoconus. *A*, Round or nipple-shaped. *B*, Oval or sagging shape.

first sign probably is the development of marked astigmatism, which may (or may not) progress until the more characteristic signs of the disorder are present.

From a practical standpoint, mild forms of keratoconus are detected by looking for distortion of the rings of Placido's disk or the keratometer mires in the image on the anterior corneal surface, or by observation of abnormalities of the red reflex with the direct ophthalmoscope or the streak retinoscope. Basically, the Placido disk is a circular white disk with black concentric circles that decrease in size from the periphery to the center. An observation hole is situated in the center of the disk. Among currently available instruments the most useful is a modern adaptation of the Placido disk, the self-illuminated Klein keratoscope (Fig. 4–4A). This contains a +6.00 diopter lens in the center of the illuminated Placido target. In use, the examiner approaches the patient's eye, observing the cornea through the lens while the patient maintains fixation on the center of the target. At a distance equal to the focal length of the lens (approximately 9 cm.) the reflected image of the target is clearly seen on the anterior corneal surface. The examiner notes whether or not the image is distorted (Fig. 4–4B). Irregularities in the reflection of the illuminated rings near the corneal center and distortion of the horizontal axis suggest early keratoconus. When the circles of the Placido disk image are close together, the slope of the cornea is greater than when they are far apart. In keratoconus the circles commonly are wide apart in the superior and nasal sector of the cornea but tend to be closer together in the inferior temporal portion.

Angulation of the horizontal axis of the image of the Placido disk was said by Amsler to be a pathognomonic sign of keratoconus; he never observed this angulation in cases of conventional astigmatism. This was the sign upon which he based his diagnosis of the mildest type of keratoconus. Amsler's keratoconus of the first degree had an angle of only 1 to 3 degrees between the two sides of the horizontal axis. This minimal degree of angulation can only be assessed on a photograph taken with a sophisticated instrument designed for this purpose, such as Amsler's photokeratoscope. Since these instruments are not in widespread use and since patients with such mild keratoconus have astigmatic vision that can be corrected with spectacles, it is unlikely that many of the milder cases are diagnosed unless they progress.

Mild forms of keratoconus can also be detected by observation of distortion of the keratometer mires on the anterior corneal surface. A lack of parallelism of the images of the mires of the Javal keratometer was cited by Amsler as possibly the earliest sign of keratoconus. With the Javal instrument, the two corneal images are irregular and unequal, and the two main axes are not perpendicular in the rudimentary forms of keratoconus (Fig. 4–5A). With the Bausch and Lomb keratometer, asymmetric astigmatism of early keratoconus is manifested by inclination of the mires and/or the appearance of an eccentric apex[4] (Fig. 4–5B). At times the inclination of the mires cannot be corrected by rotating

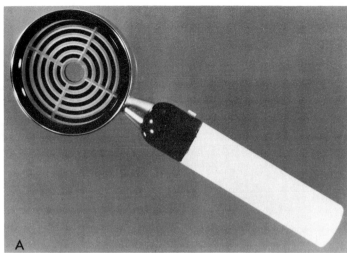

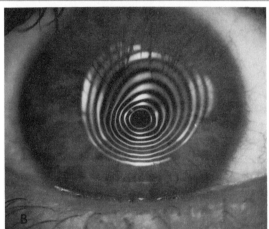

Figure 4–4. *A,* Klein keratoscope. *B,* Distortion of the image of Placido target keratoconus. (*B* courtesy of George O. Rich, O.D.)

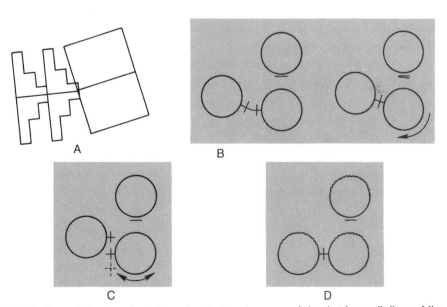

Figure 4–5. Distortion of the keratometer mires in keratoconus. *A,* Lack of parallelism of the mires of the Javal keratometer. *B,* Inclination of the mires of the Bausch and Lomb keratometer. *C,* Inclination of the plus mires that cannot be corrected by rotation of the axis. The plus mire "jumps" from one side to the other when alignment is attempted. *D,* Irregular astigmatism of keratoconus manifested by a waviness or blurriness of the mires that cannot be eliminated by focusing.

the axis of the keratometer; the plus mire jumps from one side to the other and cannot be aligned (Fig. 4–5C). Irregular astigmatism is manifested by waviness or blurriness of the outline of the image of the keratometer mires (Fig. 4–5D). When the cone becomes moderately advanced, the mires appear unequal in size.

As the degree of keratoconus progressed somewhat, Amsler classified it as second-degree keratoconus. Keratoconus of the second degree had an angle of 4 to 8 degrees between the two sides of the horizontal axis on photographs of the Placido disk image (Fig. 4–6). Direct ophthalmoscopy and streak retinoscopy are helpful adjuncts for detecting these still mild forms of the disease. Observation of the dilated pupil with both instruments yields a characteristic red reflex. With a +6.00 diopter lens in place in the direct ophthalmoscope and with the patient roughly an arm's length away from the examiner, there is a dark, round shadow in the corneal midperiphery due to total internal reflection of the light, separating the central bright red fundus reflex from a red reflex in the corneal periphery. With the retinoscope (plain mirror), there is a scissors motion of the shadow. The center of the pupil is clearly illuminated and the shadow moves in the direction opposite

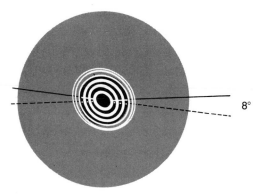

Figure 4–6. Keratoconus of the second degree (Amsler) manifested by an angle of 8 degrees between the two sides of the horizontal axis of the Placido disk image.

the mirror. The periphery is less clearly defined and the shadow moves in the same direction as the mirror. The two areas are separated by a circular shaded zone. Attempts to examine the fundus with the direct ophthalmoscope often yield a hazy view of fundus details and a finding of parallax. The size, location, and relative contour of the cone can be documented by photographing the red reflex with a fundus camera.[13]

With continued progression of the condition, several typical signs can be seen with the slit-lamp biomicroscope (Fig. 4–7). Corneal transparency is retained, but the apex of the cone protrudes anteriorly and is often accom-

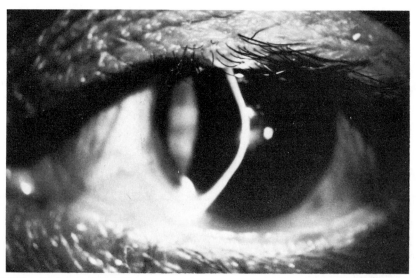

Figure 4–7. Slit-lamp view of keratoconus showing anterior protrusion of cone, apical scarring, and stromal thinning at the apex of the cone.

panied by thinning of the corneal stroma. Stromal thinning increases gradually from the base of the cone toward the apex, where the thinning reaches its maximum (Fig. 4–8). These changes may be quite pronounced, and in advanced cases the stroma at the apex of the cone may be reduced to 20 per cent of its normal thickness. Thin, vertical stress lines become visible in the deeper stromal layers of the cornea, and occasionally characteristic ruptures in Descemet's membrane occur in the more advanced cases. Corneal nerves may become increasingly visible. Ruptures in Bowman's membrane also occur in advanced cases and produce superficial linear scars. Fleischer's ring, a brownish-yellow or greenish line formed by the deposition of iron in the basal epithelium, may form an incomplete circle that partially outlines the base of the cone. It is said to occur in about 50 per cent of cases[14] and may be present in the early stages of keratoconus prior to the development of advanced corneal changes. The endothelial reflex becomes readily visible in the peak of the cone because of the increased concavity and irregularity of the posterior corneal surface. In later stages the apex of the cone becomes hypesthetic and may show considerable scarring over a period of time

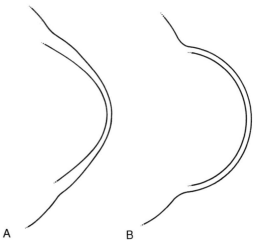

Figure 4–8. Configuration of the protruding cornea. *A,* Keratoconus. Apex of the cone protrudes anteriorly and stromal thinning increases gradually from the base of the cone toward its apex. *B,* Keratoglobus. Cornea is enlarged and thinning is generalized.

(Fig. 4–9). The portion of the cornea actually involved by the cone can perhaps best be documented by photographing the red reflex through a dilated pupil with a fundus camera[13] (Fig. 4–10).

Bron and coworkers[15, 16] have described fibrillar structures lying just beneath the corneal epithelium of keratoconus patients. These fibrillary lines are fine, white, curved, and slightly wavy.

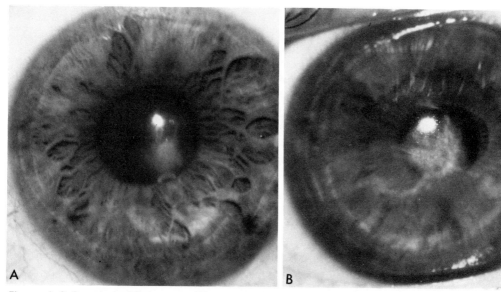

Figure 4–9. Scarring of the apex of the cone. *A,* Moderate apical scarring. *B,* More advanced apical scarring.

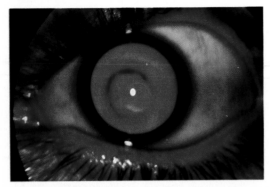

Figure 4–10. Red reflex outlining that portion of the cornea involved by the cone.

Individual fibrils are identical to similar structures seen in the normal cornea both in their subepithelial location and in their biomicroscopic characteristics. However, the fibrils in keratoconus differ in their grouping and distribution in the cornea and in their relative prominence. Generally the fibrils in the conical cornea are more easily seen than the comparable structures in the normal cornea. Nonetheless, they are not visible in all keratoconus patients but tend to be most readily evident when Fleischer's ring is dense and fully developed. They tend to lie in concentric bundles at the internal margin of Fleischer's ring, and most fibrils in keratoconus are found within the confines of Fleischer's ring. In the normal eye, fibrils tend to be topographically related to the Hudson-Stähli line. Since both Fleischer's ring and the Hudson-Stähli line are produced by visible intraepithelial accumulations of iron, there is a strong suggestion that identical processes are involved in the pathogenesis of these structures in the normal and in the conical cornea. In both instances communications may be found between these subepithelial fibrils and nerve fibers in the stroma, an observation that supports the conclusion that the fibrils are subepithelial nerve arborizations. However, no specific relationship between the visibility of nerves in the corneal stroma and the extent or visibility of the subepithelial fibrils has been demonstrated. It must be concluded that the exact nature of these fibrils and the factors influencing their formation are not known.

Virtually the only clinical symptom is a painless loss of vision, usually gradual and progressive in nature. This is due to irregular myopic astigmatism, and it becomes increasingly difficult to correct the visual deficit even partially with spectacles. However, the patient can often improve the visual acuity of the affected eye by partially closing his lids and squinting, in effect converting the palpebral fissure into a stenopeic slit. When opacities develop at the apex of the cornea, this maneuver ceases to be effective and vision continues to deteriorate. Some patients complain of photophobia in addition to visual loss.

HISTOPATHOLOGY

Histopathological examination of corneal disks removed from conical corneas at the time of penetrating keratoplasty confirms the clinical observation that the tissue is thinner centrally than peripherally and that it gradually and progressively becomes thinner as one approaches the apex of the cone. While all layers of the cornea ultimately may show microscopic alterations, the earliest changes occur in the superficial layers of the cornea. The basal layer of the epithelium is involved at a relatively early stage. At a time when the superficial layers of the epithelium frequently are normal, especially at the base of the cone, some of the basal cells are pale and edematous and contain pyknotic nuclei. There is disorganization of their cytoplasmic organelles, especially the endoplasmic reticulum. In more advanced stages of keratoconus the cell membrane may break up; the basal cells eventually disappear, leaving only one or two layers of flattened superficial epithelial cells lying on an altered basement membrane, Bowman's membrane, or directly on the anterior stroma[17, 18] (Fig. 4–11).

Early in the course of the disorder there are multiple areas of fragmentation of the basement membrane, and later

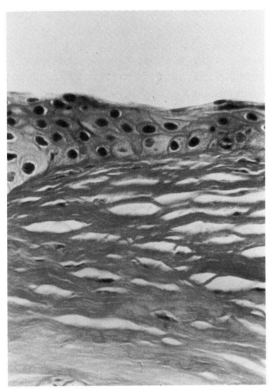

Figure 4–11. Thinned, disordered epithelial cells lying directly on the anterior stroma. (Courtesy of Thomas F. Freddo, Ph.D.)

(Fig. 4–12). These gaps occur at the base of the cone as well as at its apex and are filled either with newly formed connective tissue, presumably of stromal origin, or with epithelium. It is thought that these filled-in gaps in the continuity of Bowman's membrane correspond to the linear superficial scars seen clinically.

Except for its circular rather than linear pattern, the pigment ring in keratoconus, Fleischer's ring, seems to be identical in all respects to the Hudson-Stähli line, the horizontal brown line frequently visible in the superficial cornea of normal eyes along the line of lid closure. The ring is often incomplete or shows sector variation in intensity of pigmentation. Histopathologically, the pigmentation is not seen in tissue sections stained with hematoxylin and eosin or other commonly used stains. However, iron stains, utilizing the Prussian blue reaction, demonstrate the presence of iron in the cytoplasm of the corneal epithelium just peripheral to the

multiple dehiscences occur in this structure. The abnormalities in the basement membrane correspond in location to changes in Bowman's membrane and the epithelium.

Initially there is swelling and fibrillar degeneration of Bowman's membrane. With the phase contrast microscope the structure appears to be composed of multiple, wavy, fine fibrils rather than presenting its normal homogeneous appearance. As the process of fibrillation continues, the fibrils become coarse and extend to the adjacent stroma. These morphological changes are accompanied by changes in the staining characteristics of Bowman's membrane; there is an increased intensity of staining with toluidine blue and periodic acid–Schiff.

In the more advanced stages of keratoconus, Bowman's membrane is gradually destroyed. A characteristic lesion of Bowman's membrane results wherein the structure shows multiple narrow gaps and takes on a wavy appearance

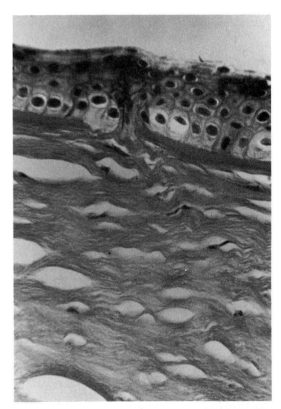

Figure 4–12. Break in Bowman's membrane filled with connective tissue. (Courtesy of Thomas F. Freddo, Ph.D.)

base of the cone in the region of normal corneal thickness. The iron tends to be most concentrated in the basal cells. However, the density of staining has been shown to vary from very faint staining of only the basal epithelium to very heavy staining of the entire epithelial layer. Iron also has been detected histopathologically in cases in which Fleischer's ring was not apparent clinically. Fleischer's ring is not necessarily related to fragmentation of the basement membrane or to breaks in or fibrillation of Bowman's membrane. Although cases have been documented in which there was degeneration of Bowman's membrane beneath Fleischer's ring, other published cases show an intact Bowman's membrane beneath the iron deposit and degeneration of Bowman's membrane central to the ring with no iron deposits in the overlying epithelium. Similarly, Fleischer's ring is not associated with neovascularization of the superficial corneal stroma. The origin of the iron in Fleischer's ring and the factors that lead to its deposition at the base of the cone are not known.[19, 20]

The most striking histological feature in the stroma, just as it is clinically, is the abnormal thinning and anterior protrusion of the central portion of the cornea. At the apex of the ectasia the stroma may be one third or less of its normal thickness. The lesions of Bowman's membrane seem to spread to the underlying stroma, which also shows areas of fibrillar degeneration. The superficial stroma eventually is destroyed and replaced with newly formed connective tissue that is irregularly arranged in a wavy pattern. In advanced cases the stromal lesion extends more widely and deeply.

Amyloid deposits have been demonstrated in corneal specimens (removed at the time of penetrating keratoplasty for keratoconus) using alkaline Congo red stains. The deposits were present in two forms. A large mass of amyloid was demonstrated lying immediately beneath the epithelium in an area normally occupied by Bowman's membrane and the superficial stroma. Amyloid deposits were also found intermittently along corneal lamellae at various depths of the corneal stroma. Occasional deposits were seen in stromal lamellae just above Descemet's membrane, in the central corneal parenchyma, and just below Bowman's membrane. In each instance these deposits stained well with alkaline Congo red and manifested a bright green birefringence when viewed with polarized light, properties that identify the deposits as amyloid.[20]

There may be folds in Descemet's membrane as well as in the overlying stroma in the early stages of keratoconus. However, no microscopic alterations are observed in Descemet's membrane itself until later stages of the disorder, when in some instances Descemet's membrane ruptures in the region of greatest ectasia. The break is evidenced by curling of the ruptured edges of Descemet's membrane anteriorly toward the stroma or by the formation of a hyaline nodule where the break had healed and Descemet's membrane had been replaced. The area is initially covered by endothelial cells, presumably adjacent cells that have enlarged to fill in the defect. Repair of the edematous, disrupted stroma is characterized by the formation of scar tissue.

The endothelium appears normal in the early stages of keratoconus. As the condition progresses, the endothelial cells flatten and their nuclei lie farther apart. Presumably this reflects a stretching of individual endothelial cells as they attempt to maintain their continuity over the progressively ectatic posterior corneal surface.

Thus, histopathologic changes in the early stages of keratoconus are confined chiefly to the anterior layers of the cornea, where the basal epithelium and its basement membrane, Bowman's membrane, and the anterior stroma are involved. Epithelial changes seem to be secondary, since they almost always occur concurrently with changes in the basement membrane and Bowman's membrane or with changes in the endothelium. The degenerative changes in basement membrane and Bowman's membrane are said to be the initial lesions because they have been observed when other layers of the cornea have been normal. However, most corneal specimens available for histopathologic study of keratoconus are removed at the time of penetrating keratoplasty, and the great majority of these patients previously have worn contact lenses. Buxton[4] raises the interesting question of whether pathologists differentiate between cases in which contact lenses have been worn and those in which they have not, implying that perhaps contact lenses contribute to the anterior corneal changes that have been described. Published reports give no indication that this point has been considered, and it merits investigation. In any event, fibrillation of Bowman's membrane occurs in keratoconus and the structure is greatly attenuated. There are gaps in its continuity, and these may be filled with newly formed connective tissue or with epithelium. The stroma is thinned, and there are folds in Descemet's membrane and the adjacent stroma. In a number of cases Descemet's membrane and the endothelium are stretched sufficiently to cause them to rupture. When this occurs, the gaps in these deeper structures permit aqueous humor to enter the stoma, causing marked edema of all layers.

CORNEAL HYDROPS

Acute ectasia of the cornea, or corneal hydrops, occurs as a complication of the existing keratoconus. Seemingly it results from an acute rupture of Descemet's membrane and the overlying endothelium.[21–23] Considerable aqueous humor enters the corneal stroma and produces immediate swelling and opacification of the cornea, often of frightening proportions (Fig. 4–13). A prominent, round, spongy-appearing, markedly elevated area is evident, and there is microcystic or bullous edema of the epithelium covering this area. Visual acuity is greatly reduced and the adjacent conjunctiva is red. Generally the patient is photophobic and tearing profusely. The cornea may appear as if perforation is imminent, but this complication has not been described. Hydrops appears to occur more frequently in keratoconus associated with Down's syndrome.[24–29]

In severe cases Bowman's membrane may rupture; these breaks are filled with fibrous tissue, a process that results in corneal scarring. In time the endothelial cells adjacent to the area of rupture apparently enlarge, fill in the defect, and ultimately effect regeneration of Descemet's membrane.[30] When this sequence of events occurs, the edema recedes (Fig. 4–14) and the cornea dehydrates spontaneously. Unfortunately, its occurrence is not invariable, and considerable edema may persist indefinitely in some cases of corneal hydrops (Fig. 4–15). In general, only symptomatic treatment need be undertaken, although there have been reports that topically administered corticosteroids exert a therapeutic effect on the condition.[22, 24, 31] Aquavella and

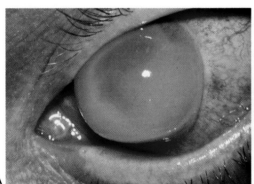 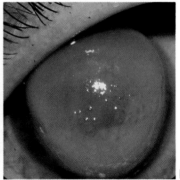

Figure 4–13. Acute corneal hydrops. *A,* Markedly swollen, elevated corneal stroma. *B,* Same as *A,* plus bullous edema of the epithelium.

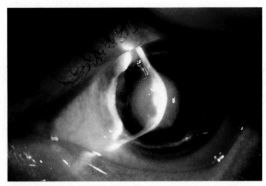

Figure 4–14. Acute corneal hydrops. Appearance of the cornea during spontaneous progressive recession of edema.

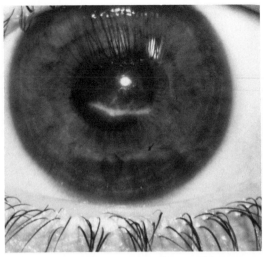

Figure 4–16. Flattening of cornea after episode of acute hydrops. Previously unable to wear a contact lens, patient is now able to wear the lens and achieve 20/40 vision (same cornea as shown in Figure 4–14).

colleagues have presented evidence that the local application of heat (thermokeratoplasty) may be useful in the treatment of chronic corneal hydrops.[32] Six cases treated by this method cleared within 3 weeks. These investigators found that the shrinkage of corneal collagen induced by the application of heat was effective in sealing small, full-thickness puncture wounds in rabbits. They believe that shrinkage of the deeper layers of the corneal stroma results in a reapproximation of the ruptured edges of Descemet's membrane, enabling the

adjacent endothelium to cover the break and seal the leak with a newly formed Descemet's membrane. If it is not axial, the subsequent stromal scarring induced by chronic edema and/or the thermokeratoplasty procedure may ultimately have a favorable effect. Sufficient flattening of the cornea may occur after resolution of the acute episode to improve vision or the ability to tolerate a contact lens (Fig. 4–16).

ASSOCIATED CONDITIONS

A number of entities are frequently associated with keratoconus. Many of these may be chance associations with no important pathogenic implications. The disorders associated with keratoconus include retinitis pigmentosa,[8, 33, 34] infantile tapetoretinal degeneration (Leber's congenital or infantile amaurosis),[35] and Down's syndrome.[24, 36, 37] Other ocular abnormalities documented to occur concurrently with keratoconus are blue sclera, microcornea, aniridia, corneal degeneration, congenital cataract, ectopia lentis, and lenticonus. There also appears to be a relationship between keratoconus and several entities thought to have an allergic etiology, e.g., vernal conjunctivitis,[38] atopic der-

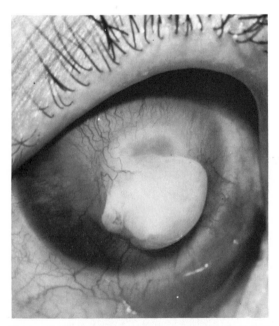

Figure 4–15. Persistent edema and elevated corneal scar following an episode of acute hydrops (same cornea as shown in Figure 4–13B).

matitis,[39–42] and other atopic conditions such as hay fever and asthma.[40, 43] Atopy often is associated with increased levels of IgE together with changes in other immunoglobulins.[44] In a study of 182 individuals with keratoconus,[45] a definite history of atopy was found in 35 per cent compared with 12 per cent of a matched control group. There was a male:female ratio of 2 to 1 among the atopic individuals with keratoconus. The commonest allergic disorder was hay fever, followed by asthma and eczema. The serum IgE level was significantly ($p < 0.001$) raised in keratoconus and markedly so in cases of keratoconus associated with atopic disease. Serum levels of IgG and IgM also were elevated, but, contrary to the findings of other observers, IgA levels were normal. The significance of these immunological changes in the pathogenesis and natural history of keratoconus is not known.

Many keratoconus patients rub their eyes excessively. This has been observed particularly among keratoconus patients with an associated atopic condition. The contribution of excessive rubbing of the eyes to the etiology of keratoconus is not clear, but at least one prominent authority concluded that it was the dominant causal factor in two thirds of patients with keratoconus who progress to contact lens wear.[46]

KERATOGLOBUS

When the entire cornea is involved in the ectatic process, the condition is called keratoglobus (Fig. 4–17). As the term indicates, the cornea assumes a globelike appearance characterized by a pronounced increase in curvature. Corneal diameter may be normal or it may be increased to 13 mm. or greater. The cornea generally remains clear and lustrous, but in all instances it is quite thin. In some cases of keratoglobus the thinning of the stromal parenchyma is generalized (Fig. 4–8); there is no significant difference between the central and peripheral portions of the cornea. In other cases, however, the pattern of thinning is just the reverse of that seen in keratoconus. The stromal tissue is thinnest in the periphery, in proximity to the limbus, rather than centrally. The corneal stroma in keratoglobus may be reduced in thickness to only one fifth that of the normal cornea, and it may be quite fragile. It is well documented that corneal perforation can occur in this disorder following minimal ocular trauma.[47–50]

Keratoglobus occurs much less frequently than keratoconus and is considered by many to represent simply an extreme form of keratoconus. This view is supported by the observation of cases in which one eye was found to have keratoglobus while the opposite eye of the individual harbored a typical case of keratoconus. There are also reports of families in which some members had keratoconus while others had keratoglobus.[51, 52] However, other authorities believe that keratoglobus is an independent condition and should not be considered an extreme form of kerato-

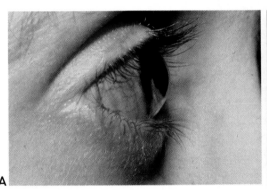
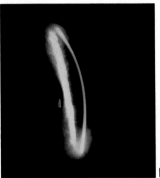

Figure 4–17. Keratoglobus. A, Profile of cornea. B, Slit-lamp view showing an enlarged, protruding, thin cornea. (Courtesy of J. H. Krachmer, M.D.)

conus. Support for this view is provided by the observation that in most instances keratoconus initially appears during the second decade; keratoglobus, on the other hand, generally occurs at or soon after birth and seemingly is a development anomaly. In some instances it appears to be part of a generalized connective tissue defect, and the occurrence of a distinct syndrome has been proposed by several authors.[47, 49, 52] Associated abnormalities include blue sclerae and one or more of the following: hyperextensibility of joints, abnormal teeth, reduced hearing, fractures, and spondylolisthesis.[47, 49, 52-54]

A case of keratoglobus seemingly acquired in adulthood fails to support the concept that the disorder is a developmental anomaly.[55] In this case keratoglobus was associated with thyroid ophthalmopathy, which interestingly preceded the onset of clinical symptoms of hyperthyroidism and the appearance of keratoglobus by almost 25 years. This patient's eyes were evaluated at age 33 because of bilateral exophthalmos. His visual acuity was 20/20 in each eye (the report does not state whether this was with or without correction), and no corneal abnormalities were described. Keratoglobus subsequently was noted.

Acute hydrops of the cornea occurs in cases of keratoglobus.[22, 47, 51, 56, 57] Its clinical characteristics are little different from those described when the phenomenon occurs in keratoconus (Fig. 4–18).

POSTERIOR KERATOCONUS

Posterior keratoconus is an entity characterized by an anterior conical protrusion of the posterior corneal surface

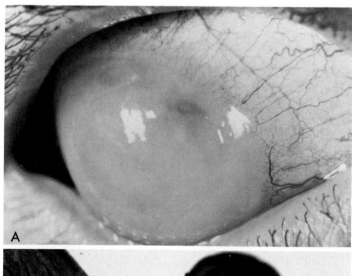

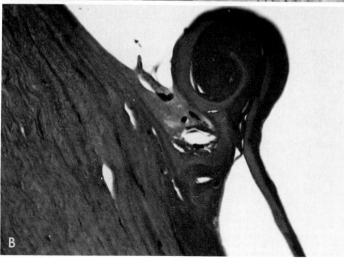

Figure 4–18. Acute hydrops of the cornea in a case of keratoglobus. *A,* Clinical appearance. *B,* Histopathologic appearance of the curled edge of Descemet's membrane at the site of the break in endothelium and Descemet's membrane responsible for the acute stromal edema. (Courtesy of J. V. Aquavella, M.D.)

along with a noninflammatory decrease in stromal thickness of the involved portion of the cornea. Although the name is anatomically descriptive, it implies that this entity has some relationship to true keratoconus, the condition described above. In fact, there is no evidence that the two abnormalities are related in any way. The entity is nonprogressive and generally is not associated with any significant alteration of curvature of the anterior corneal surface.

Two forms of posterior keratoconus have been described (Fig. 4–19). The first is characterized by a uniform, symmetrical increase in curvature of the posterior corneal surface, causing the central stroma to be much thinner than normal (keratoconus posticus totalis).[58, 59] The cornea generally is clear or almost so and generally is free of any clinically evident tears in Descemet's membrane, striae in the deep stromal lamellae, or other abnormalities that have been identified with the slit-lamp biomicroscope in cases of anterior keratoconus. Since the greatest part of corneal refraction occurs at the normal anterior corneal surface, these patients do not commonly have serious difficulty with vision.

The more common type of posterior keratoconus is characterized by a localized, dome-shaped excavation of the central portion of the posterior corneal surface with no alteration of the anterior corneal surface (keratoconus posticus circumscriptus).[60–64] Slit-lamp examination reveals an isolated crater, often half spherical in configuration, on the posterior corneal surface; most commonly only a single crater is encountered. The involved, thinned stroma often is opacified, and this, rather than the irregularity of the posterior corneal surface, accounts for the decrease in visual acuity that occurs in some of these patients. In addition to the localized loss of stromal substance, an increased density of the posterior corneal surface and opacities projecting into the aqueous humor have been reported.[65]

Posterior keratoconus may occur either unilaterally or bilaterally. It is

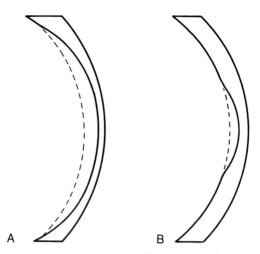

Figure 4–19. Posterior keratoconus. *A,* Generalized (keratoconus posticus totalis). *B,* Localized (keratoconus posticus circumscriptus).

generally considered to be a congenital defect, and evidence has been presented suggesting that it has its origin prior to the fifth or sixth month of gestation.[64] However, a traumatic etiology has also been reported.[66] Most cases are nonfamilial, but the condition has been described in more than one family member.[67–69]

A number of congenital anomalies have been described in association with posterior keratoconus.[59, 60, 65, 67, 69–72] The ocular abnormalities include corneal nebulae, endothelial precipitates and dystrophic changes, lens changes including anterior lenticonus, aniridia, iris atrophy, ectropion uveae, mesodermal tissue in the angle, and choroidal and/or retinal sclerosis. Nonocular abnormalities in patients with posterior keratoconus, although uncommon, include abnormal development of the bridge of the nose, hypertelorism, webbed neck, short stature, brachydactylia, and mental retardation.

Histologically, the involved stroma is markedly thinned in the posterior cornea and is covered by irregular epithelium varying from two to five cells in thickness. The epithelial basement membrane is partially absent and Bowman's membrane is replaced by fibrous tissue. There is an irregular arrangement of collagen in the thinned stroma. By light microscopy, the appearance of Descemet's membrane is variable. In one case[64] there were occasional excrescences, but Descemet's membrane appeared normal otherwise. In a second case there were many small breaks in Descemet's membrane.[73] Each of these breaks was sealed by a hyaline substance deposited on the posterior surface of Descemet's membrane by dense accumulations of endothelial cells. Most breaks showed excessive hyaline deposits, which formed large and sometimes bizarre-appearing excrescences extending into the anterior chamber. The breaks in Descemet's membrane appeared to be old, and the hyaline material stained much like Descemet's membrane itself. Longitudinal splitting or duplication of Descemet's membrane also was observed.[73] The electron microscope reveals striking changes in Descemet's membrane. The structure has a multilaminar appearance with areas of abnormal, widely spaced collagen.[64]

TREATMENT

There is no medical therapy that can ameliorate or otherwise favorably affect the course of keratoconus. Although suggestions to the contrary appear in earlier literature, neither corneal nor scleral contact lenses retard the progression of keratoconus. Indeed, it is possible that contact lens wear can infrequently cause sufficient corneal warping to produce a keratoconus-like picture. Apparently even well-fitted contact lenses can cause corneal warping, usually manifested as with-the-rule astigmatism. In some cases the cornea returns partially or completely to its original curvature after discontinuation of contact lens wear. In other cases, however, the alteration in corneal curvature is permanent; despite discontinuation of contact lens wear, there is no decrease in astigmatism. In the most marked of these cases the cornea becomes conical and the resultant irregular astigmatism no longer permits spectacle correction of vision to the pre–contact lens 20/20 level. Such cases demonstrate a positive Munson's sign,

distortion of the reflex of Placido's disk and keratometer mires, and the characteristic alterations of the red reflex seen with the retinoscope and the direct ophthalmoscope in primary keratoconus.[74–81] Seemingly, in certain instances a contact lens is able to exert sufficient pressure or interfere with corneal metabolism in a manner capable of inducing a secondary type of keratoconus. Hartstein has presented data that suggest that this type of keratoconus may be related to the long-term wearing of a contact lens on an eye that has low ocular rigidity,[76] but this thesis has not been proved. Another study failed to confirm that the coefficient of ocular rigidity is abnormally low in keratoconus.[82] Rather, the ocular rigidity coefficient, E, for all unoperated patients with keratoconus was not significantly different from that of the normal controls. Only if the conical cornea was thinned by 60 per cent or more was E significantly lower than that of normal eyes. However, in this latter group the ocular rigidity coefficient reverted to normal after penetrating keratoplasty. Replacement of the thinned cornea with one of normal thickness restored ocular rigidity to normal. These data do not support the generalization that most patients with keratoconus have an abnormally low ocular rigidity.

The milder forms of keratoconus often can be satisfactorily corrected with spectacles, and this is the treatment of choice for as long as it provides satisfactory visual acuity. Keratometric measurements will provide a rough estimate of the degree and the axis of astigmatism, but even in early stages of the disorder retinoscopy may be of limited value. A subjective refraction must be performed with painstaking care, during which the patient should be allowed to rotate the cylinder in the trial frame and to pick the axis that provides optimal vision. Patience and perseverance are required and surprisingly often are rewarded.

However, if keratoconus progresses and the ectatic process induces significant irregular corneal astigmatism, spectacles are at best of limited usefulness.

Contact lenses then become the treatment of choice. When a satisfactory fit can be obtained, contact lenses eliminate the irregular anterior cornea as a refracting surface and replace it with a spherical, regular optical element. Commonly this is accomplished with a hard or semirigid flexible lens that retains its shape. Although the literature contains sporadic reports of success with soft contact lenses fitted for keratoconus, my experience with these devices, particularly among more advanced cases, has been disappointing. Although soft contact lenses often are better tolerated than hard or flexible variants, they generally fail to improve vision adequately, presumably because some of the surface irregularities of the cornea are transmitted to the lens as the material conforms to the configuration of the globe. In some cases visual acuity can be improved by spectacle overrefraction, but in many instances this cannot be accomplished. Techniques for fitting a contact lens on a conical cornea are described in Chapter 31.

When a contact lens cannot be fitted satisfactorily, the patient is unable to tolerate a contact lens, or the contact lens fails to effect significant visual improvement because of stromal scarring or other pathological change, then the conical cornea must be replaced surgically. Penetrating keratoplasty is the procedure of choice. Among all corneal disorders for which transplantation surgery is undertaken, the greatest success is achieved in keratoconus (Fig. 4–20); virtually all authorities cite success rates of approximately 90 per cent. From time to time lamellar keratoplasty has been suggested as an alternative to penetrating keratoplasty for the treatment of advanced keratoconus.[83–85] Lamellar keratoplasty is an extraocular procedure, which presents less risk of intraoperative and postoperative complication. However, visual results are not, on the average, as good as those obtained by penetrating keratoplasty.[84, 85] Wrinkling of Descemet's membrane and scarring at the donor-recipient interface often reduce the optical clarity of lamellar

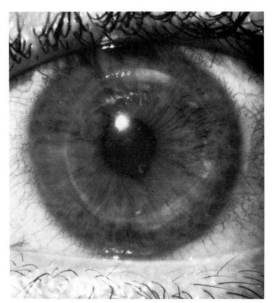

Figure 4–20. Successful penetrating keratoplasty performed for advanced keratoconus.

grafts. After successful penetrating keratoplasty it is common to encounter considerable astigmatism, so that visual rehabilitation of many keratoconus patients with clear corneal grafts requires contact lens wear postoperatively.

Following successful uncomplicated corneal transplantation for keratoconus, a fixed dilated pupil may be encountered postoperatively.[86–92] This phenomenon may be manifested fully within 24 hours of the operative procedure, or alternatively pupillary mydriasis may progressively develop during the first several postoperative days.[86, 90] In the complete form of the entity, dilatation of the pupil after surgery invariably is pronounced (the pupil may be 8.0 to 9.0 mm. in diameter) and the condition is permanent, although over a 1- to 2-year period the pupillary diameter may decrease slightly. However, cases have been reported wherein paresis of the pupil was transient and spontaneous recovery occurred over a period of weeks to months.[90] In such instances recovery of pupillary function may be partial or complete. Davies and Ruben[90] have also described cases with a partially dilated pupil, which they characterize as 1.5 mm. larger than that of the opposite unoperated eye. Although both pupils react to light and fixation at near, the partially dilated pupil does so incompletely, remaining larger than its fellow when a given stimulus is applied to both. Unlike the pupil in the complete form of the condition, the partially dilated pupil does constrict fully in response to topically administered miotics.

A permanently fixed dilated pupil is said to occur in 5 to 6 per cent of eyes undergoing penetrating keratoplasty for keratoconus.[90, 91] This problem rarely occurs after penetrating keratoplasty for corneal abnormalities other than keratoconus, and its cause is not known. It does not appear to be related to concurrent iris surgery; irreversible mydriasis has been reported in cases in which a peripheral iridectomy was performed at the time of penetrating keratoplasty as well as in cases in which no iridectomy was performed. The use of topically administered mydriatic-cycloplegic agents also has been cited as a contributory factor that, at the very least, increases the prevalence of a fixed, dilated pupil. However, it is well documented that the condition may appear in cases in which these drugs have not been used.[86, 90] The anterior chamber of affected eyes usually is deep, and mydriasis is not related to the presence of anterior or posterior synechiae. Glaucoma is no more a complication of keratoplasty for keratoconus than it is when the transplantation procedure is performed for other corneal disorders, and elevated intraocular pressure does not generally occur concomitantly with a postoperative paretic pupil in keratoconus.[90, 92] In the fully manifest form of this entity the pupil fails to respond either to parasympathomimetic (i.e., pilocarpine) or to anticholinesterase (i.e., echothiophate iodide) agents applied topically at the time abnormal mydriasis is first observed, nor does it respond to acetylcholine injected into the anterior chamber 3 to 4 weeks postoperatively.[86] This suggests an abnormality of the parasympathetic innervation of the iris sphincter, its neuromuscular junction, or the muscle fibers of the sphincter itself.

Abnormalities of the iris sphincter are not biomicroscopically evident, although transillumination of the iris reveals a high incidence of iris atrophy in keratoconus cases that have undergone penetrating keratoplasty. Two very different types, focal atrophy and sector atrophy, have been described.[90] Focal iris atrophy is more common and has been observed in eyes with fixed dilated pupils as well as in eyes with partially dilated pupils after keratoplasty. The abnormality consists of multiple focal areas in which the posterior pigmented epithelium of the iris is absent but the overlying stroma appears normal to examination with the slit-lamp biomicroscope. These areas of focal iris atrophy lie just beneath the host-donor junction of the corneal graft and are apparent shortly after surgery. Davies and Ruben[90] feel that this is not true iris atrophy but simply the result of surgical trauma disturbing the pigmented layer of the iris. Focal iris atrophy is not present in many cases of true and partial paretic pupil, and, conversely, it has been observed in many keratoconus cases in which the postoperative pupillary responses are normal. It is very much more common after keratoplasty for keratoconus than after keratoplasty for other corneal disorders,[90] suggesting that the iris in keratoconus is abnormal. The presence of focal iris atrophy in eyes with both normal and paretic pupils supports the conclusion that it is not a direct cause of the paretic pupil.

Sector iris atrophy, although much less common than the focal variety, was observed in all seven eyes with permanently dilated pupils reported by Davies and Ruben.[90] It is characterized by large areas of atrophy involving all layers of the iris. Often these extend to the margin of the pupil, and additional scattered areas of atrophy may be visible throughout the region of the sphincter pupillae. Interestingly, this type of iris atrophy occurred between 2 and 5 months postoperatively while in all cases the dilated pupils were noted within a few days after surgery.

It is not known whether sector iris atrophy is a cause or a consequence of mydriasis. Davies and Ruben suggest that the mydriasis results from ischemic injury to the sphincter pupillae during surgery. They have observed that during surgery the iris vessels are dilated peripheral to the cut edge of the host cornea and constricted central to it. They attribute this appearance to a vascular strangulation phenomenon caused by the intraocular contents pushing the lens-iris diaphragm against the posterior surface and cut edge of the host cornea. Ischemia paralyzes the sphincter and mydriasis results. The degree of ischemic atrophy of the pupillary sphincter determines whether mydriasis is permanent or the pupil recovers. However, this author has observed a definitely positive, albeit transient, miotic response of a fixed dilated pupil (which first appeared after a successful corneal graft had been performed for keratoconus) to the topical application of thymoxamine hydrochloride 0.5 per cent. This compound is an α-adrenergic blocking agent that can cause miosis and widen the angle without affecting either the intraocular pressure or the facility of outflow in normal patients and those with open-angle glaucoma.[93, 94] The iris dilator is sympathetically innervated and its receptors are α-adrenergic in nature. Thymoxamine hydrochloride paralyzes the dilator muscle selectively; thus, the miotic response we observed must be attributed to a functioning, parasympathetically innervated pupillary sphincter. However, the pupil in this case was not responsive either to pilocarpine hydrochloride 4 per cent or to echothiophate iodide 0.25 per cent, a seemingly contradictory observation that serves to emphasize that the etiology of this phenomenon is still to be elucidated.

The presence of a postoperative fixed dilated pupil is not synonymous with failure of the corneal graft. In most cases the intraocular pressure is within normal limits, the graft remains dehydrated and transparent, and corrected visual acuity is excellent. The patient unfortunately is left with the problem of photophobia, which is directly related to the size of the pupil and its lack of responsiveness. Tinted spectacles and/or contact lenses constitute the initial therapeutic modality for this problem. In severe cases a contact lens that provides a small pupillary aperture and upon which an iris has been painted has proven successful.

Several ophthalmologists have reported that a procedure known as thermokeratoplasty may be useful in keratoconus.[95–98] Thermokeratoplasty is simply the controlled application of heat to the cornea. At certain temperatures mammalian collagen fibers shrink appreciably when they are heated in water or other polar substances. This provides the rationale for the use of this technique. The temperature elevation causes stabilizing cross-linkages to rupture and the collagen fibers to shrink and increase in thickness. In keratoconus this hydrothermal shrinkage of collagen may result in a significant flattening of the cornea with a concomitant decrease in myopia and corneal astigmatism. The alteration in corneal curvature may permit contact lens wear that had previously been precluded by a steep cone. Thus, in successful cases thermokeratoplasty offers the possibility of visual rehabilitation without the need to resort to corneal transplantation surgery.

Despite this formidable attraction, the present role of thermokeratoplasty in the treatment of keratoconus is limited. The specific indications for the procedure are not clear, and the criteria for patient selection vary substantially among its advocates. Published reports indicate that the technique has not been standardized. The optimal temperature is not known; the optimal size and configuration of the probe have not been established; and precise guidelines relating to the optimal method, location, and duration for each thermal application are not available. Unfortunately, there is at present no adequate clinical technique for monitoring changes in corneal curvature, a factor that represents a major impediment to the timely resolution of these shortcomings.

Although it was initially thought that

the alteration of corneal curvature could be accomplished with minimal corneal trauma, frequent complications and therapeutic failures have been reported.[99-101] There is a substantial incidence of delayed epithelial regeneration, injury of the basement membrane and Bowman's membrane, recurrent erosion syndrome, and irreversible stromal scarring. Aseptic necrosis of the corneal stroma, a persistent, sterile, central stromal inflammatory infiltrate, and central neovascularization also have been reported. In many cases the apex of the cone is not significantly flattened by the application of heat. When substantial alterations in corneal curvature are obtained initially, subsequent steepening of the cone has been observed in many instances, indicating that some of the changes produced by thermokeratoplasty are transient.

Overall, the reported results of thermokeratoplasty indicate a measure of therapeutic success. For patients who are poor surgical risks, for those who are unwilling to undergo surgery, and for the mentally retarded, whose visual requirements may be limited and in whom the risk of postoperative complications is substantial, the procedure seemingly offers an alternative to keratoplasty. In a patient unable to wear a contact lens, in whom restoration of vision requires a corneal transplantation procedure, a limited initial trial of thermokeratoplasty is not unreasonable. Results are said to be better when the apex of the cone is below the corneal center and when there is little or no apical thinning or scarring. However, the procedure is unpredictable, and caution should be exercised in its use. Successful penetrating keratoplasty can be performed for keratoconus after unsuccessful thermokeratoplasty. There are, however, no controlled data on whether or not the hydrothermal shrinkage of collagen has any detrimental effect on the potential for success of a subsequent corneal graft.

REFERENCES

1. Barth, J.: Statistik über 300 Keratoconusfälle mit 557 befallenen Augen. Thesis. Zurich, 1948.
2. Thomas, C. I.: *The Cornea.* Springfield, Ill., Charles C Thomas, 1955, pp. 233–244.
3. Amsler, M.: Quelques Donées du problème du kératocône. Bull Soc Belge Ophtalmol 129:331, 1961.
4. Buxton, J. N.: Keratoconus. In *Symposium on Contact Lenses.* Transactions of the New Orleans Academy of Ophthalmology. St. Louis, C. V. Mosby Co., 1973, pp. 88–100.
5. Kim, J. O., and Hassard, D. T. R.: On the enzymology of the cornea: A new enzyme deficiency in keratoconus. Canad J Ophthalmol 7:176, 1972.
6. Robert, L., Schillinger, G., Moczar, M., Jungua, S., and Moczar, E.: Biochemical study of keratoconus. Arch Ophtalmol (Paris) 30:590, 1970.
7. Cannon, D. J., and Foster, C. S.: Collagen cross-linking in keratoconus. Invest Ophthalmol 17:63, 1978.
8. Franceschetti, A., and Klein, D.: Keratoconus. In Waardenburg, P. J., Franceschetti, A., and Klein D. (eds.): *Genetics in Ophthalmology.* Vol. 1. Assen, Netherlands, Van Gorcum, 1961, pp. 452–456.
9. Amsler, M.: Le Kératocône fruste. Bull Mem Soc Fr Ophtalmol 50:100, 1937.
10. Amsler, M.: Le Kératocône fruste au Javal. Ophthalmologica 96:77, 1938.
11. Amsler, M.: Kératocône classique et kératocône fruste: arguments unitaires. Ophthalmologica 111:96, 1946.
12. Amsler, M.: La Notion du kératocône. Bull Mem Soc Fr Ophtalmol 64:272, 1951.
13. Shaw, E. L., Sewell, J., and Gasset, A. R.: Photodiagnosis of keratoconus. Ann Ophthalmol 5:297, 1973.
14. Jonkers, G. H.: Keratoconus. Ophthalmologica 120:181, 1950.
15. Bron, A. J.: Superficial fibrillary lines. A feature of the normal cornea. Brit J Ophthalmol 59:133, 1975.
16. Bron, A. J., Lobascher, D. J., Dixon, W. S., Das, S. N., and Ruben, M.: Fibrillary lines of the cornea. A clinical sign in keratoconus. Brit J Ophthalmol 59:136, 1975.
17. Chi, H. H., Katzin, H. M., and Teng, C. C.: Histopathology of keratoconus. Amer J Ophthalmol 42:847, 1956.
18. Teng, C. C.: Electron microscopic study of the pathology of keratoconus. Amer J Ophthalmol 55:18, 1963.
19. Gass, J. D. M.: The iron lines of the superficial cornea: Hudson-Stähli line, Stocker's line and Fleischer's ring. Arch Ophthalmol 71:348, 1964.
20. McPherson, S. D., Jr., and Kiffney, G. T., Jr.: Some histologic findings in keratoconus. Arch Ophthalmol 79:669, 1968.
21. Rychener, R. O., and Kirby, D. B.: Acute hydrops of the cornea complicating keratoconus. Arch Ophthalmol 24:326, 1940.
22. Grayson, M.: Acute keratoglobus. Amer J Ophthalmol 56:300, 1963.

23. Wolter, J. R., Henderson, J. W., and Clahassey, E. G.: Ruptures of Descemet's membrane in keratoconus. Amer J Ophthalmol 63:1689, 1967.

24. Appelmans, M., Michiels, J., Nelis, J., and Massa, J. M.: Kératocône aigu chez le mongoloide. Bull Soc Belge Ophtalmol 128:249, 1961.

25. Heinmuller, G.: Akuter Keratoconus. Klin Monatsbl Augenheilk 134:410, 1959.

26. Hofmann, H.: Akuter Keratoconus bei mongoloider Idiotie. Klin Monatsbl Augenheilk 129:756, 1956.

27. Lefertatra, L. J.: Acute keratoconus in the presence of mongoloid idiocy. Ophthalmologica 137:432, 1959.

28. Slusher, M. M., Laibson, P. R., and Mulberger, R. D.: Acute keratoconus in Down's syndrome. Amer J Ophthalmol 66:1137, 1968.

29. Pierse, D., and Eustace, P.: Acute keratoconus in mongols. Brit J Ophthalmol 55:50, 1971.

30. Laing, R. A., Sandstrom, M. M., Berrospi, A. R., and Leibowitz, H. M.: The human corneal endothelium in keratoconus: A specular microscopic study. Arch Ophthalmol 97:1867, 1979.

31. Wilde, S.: Akuter Keratoconus bei mongoloider Idiotie. Ztschr Kinderheilk 81:550, 1958.

32. Aquavella, J. V., Buxton, J. N., and Shaw, E. L.: Thermokeratoplasty in the treatment of persistent corneal hydrops. Arch Ophthalmol 95:81, 1977.

33. Franceschetti, A., Francois, J., and Babel, J.: Dégénérescences tapéto-rétiniennes et kératocône dans les hérédo-dégénérescences chorio-rétiniennes. Rapp Soc Fr Ophtalmol 2:1110, 1963.

34. Streiff, E. B.: Kératocône et rétinite pigmentaire. Bull Mem Soc Fr Ophtalmol. 65:323, 1952.

35. Alstrom, C. H., and Olson, O.: Heredo-retinopathia congenitalis monohybrida recessiva autosomalis, a genetical-statistical study. Hereditas 43:1, 1957.

36. Wilde, S.: Akuter Keratoconus bei mongoloider Idiotie. Ztschr Kinderheilk 81:550, 1958.

37. Rados, A.: Conical cornea and mongolism. Arch Ophthalmol 40:454, 1948.

38. Bietti, G. B., and Ferraboschi, C.: L'Association du catarrhe printanier et du kératocône et son évidence statistique. Bull Mem Soc Fr Ophtalmol 71:185, 1958.

39. Brunsting, L., Reed, H. B., and Bavi, H. L.: Occurrence of cataracts and keratoconus with atopic dermatitis. Ann Derm Syph 72:237, 1955.

40. Galin, M. A., and Berger, E.: Atopy and keratoconus. Amer J Ophthalmol 45:904, 1958.

41. Spencer, W. H., and Fisher, J. J.: The association of keratoconus with atopic dermatitis. Amer J Ophthalmol 47:332, 1959.

42. Copeman, P. W. M.: Eczema and keratoconus. Brit Med J 2:977, 1965.

43. Stucchi, C. A., and Streiff, E. B.: Cheratocono e atopia atti. Soc Oftal Ital 18:477, 1960.

44. Taylor, B., Norman, A. P., Orgel, H. A., Stokes, C. R., Turner, M. W., and Soothill, J. F.: Transient IgA deficiency and pathogenesis of infantile atopy. Lancet 2:111, 1973.

45. Rahi, A., Davies, P., Ruben, M., Lobascher, D., and Menon, J.: Keratoconus and coexisting atopic disease. Brit J Ophthalmol 61:761, 1977.

46. Karseras, A. G., and Ruben, M.: Etiology of keratoconus. Brit J Ophthalmol 60:522, 1976.

47. Biglan, A. W., Brown, S. I., and Johnson, B. L.: Keratoglobus and blue sclera. Amer J Ophthalmol 83:225, 1977.

48. Stein, R., Lazar, M., and Adam, A.: Brittle cornea: A familial trait associated with blue sclera. Amer J Ophthalmol 66:67, 1968.

49. Hyams, S., Dar, H., and Neumann, E.: Blue sclerae and keratoglobus. Ocular signs of a systemic connective tissue disorder. Brit J Ophthalmol 53:53, 1969.

50. Gregoratos, N., Bartosocas, C., and Papas, K.: Blue sclerae with keratoglobus and brittle cornea. Brit J Ophthalmol 55:424, 1971.

51. Cavara, V.: Keratoglobus and keratoconus. Brit J Ophthalmol 34:621, 1950.

52. Greenfield, G., Romano, A., Stein, R., and Goodman, R.: Blue sclerae and keratoconus. Key features of a distinct heritable disorder of connective tissue. Clin Genet 4:8, 1973.

53. Tucker, D.: Blue sclerotics syndrome simulating buphthalmos. Amer J Ophthalmol 47:345, 1959.

54. Arkin, W.: Blue scleras with keratoglobus. Amer J Ophthalmol 58:678, 1964.

55. Jacobs, D. S., Green, W. R., and Maumenee, A. E.: Acquired keratoglobus. Amer J Ophthalmol 77:393, 1974.

56. Silva, D., and Quiroz, R.: Clinical report of a case of acute keratoglobus. An Soc Mex Oftal Oto-rino-lar 26:197, 1953.

57. Verrey, F.: Keratoglobe aigu. Schweiz Med Wschr 77:859, 1947.

58. Butler, T. H.: Keratoconus posticus. Trans Ophthalmol Soc UK 50:551, 1930.

59. Ross, J. V. M.: Keratoconus posticus generalis. Amer J Ophthalmol 33:801, 1950.

60. Greene, P. B.: Keratoconus posticus circumscriptus: Report of a case. Arch Ophthalmol 34:432, 1945.

61. Goldsmith, A. J. B.: Bilateral circumscribed posterior conical cornea. Trans Ophthalmol Soc UK 63:180, 1944.

62. Leopold, I. H.: Keratoconus posticus circumscriptus. Arch Ophthalmol 34:432, 1945.

63. Schacket, S. S., Phelps, W. L., and Petit, T. H.: Bilateral posterior circumscribed keratoconus. Amer J Ophthalmol 57:840, 1964.

64. Krachmer, J. H., and Rodrigues, M. M.: Posterior keratoconus. Arch Ophthalmol 96:1867, 1978.

65. Karline, D. B., and Wise, G. N.: Keratoconus posticus. Amer J Ophthalmol 52:119, 1961.

66. Jacobs, H. B.: Traumatic keratoconus posticus. Brit J Ophthalmol 41:40, 1957.

67. Haney, W. P., and Falls, H. F.: The occurrence of congenital keratoconus posticus circumscriptus (in 2 siblings presenting a previously unrecognized syndrome). Amer J Ophthalmol 52:53, 1961.

68. Jacobs, H. B.: Posterior conical cornea. Brit J Ophthalmol 41:31, 1957.

69. Collier, M.: Le Kératocône postérieur. Arch Ophtalmol (Paris) 22:376, 1962.

70. Hagedoorn, A., and Velzeboer, C. M. J.: Postnatal partial spontaneous correction of a severe congenital anomaly of the anterior segment of an eye. Arch Ophthalmol 62:685, 1959.

71. Charan, H.: Keratoconus posticus circumscriptus with indentation of the lens. Brit J Ophthalmol 51:486, 1967.

72. DeRosa, C.: Su di un caso di cheratocono posteriore. Arch Ottalmol 63:445, 1959.

73. Wolter, J. R., and Haney, W. P.: Histopathology of keratoconus posticus circumscriptus. Arch Ophthalmol 69:357, 1963.

74. Hartstein, J.: Corneal warping due to contact lenses. Amer J Ophthalmol 60:1103, 1965.

75. Hartstein, J.: Keratoconus that developed in patients wearing corneal contact lenses. Arch Ophthalmol 80:345, 1968.

76. Hartstein, J.: Research into the pathogenesis of keratoconus. Arch Ophthalmol 84:728, 1970.

77. Rubin, M. L.: The tale of the warped cornea: A real-life melodrama. Arch Ophthalmol 77:711, 1967.

78. Hardie, B.: Keratoconus and contact lenses. JAMA 208:539, 1969.

79. Nauheim, J. S.: Corneal curvature changes simulating keratoconus occurring in patients wearing contact lenses. Contact Lens Med Bull 2:7, 1969.

80. Gasset, A. R., Houde, W. L., Garcia-Bengochea, M.: Hard contact lens wear as an environmental risk in keratoconus. Amer J Ophthalmol 85:339, 1978.

81. Hartstein, J.: Keratoconus and contact lenses: A reappraisal. South Med J 64:151, 1971.

82. Foster, C. S., and Yamamoto, G. K.: Ocular rigidity in keratoconus. Amer J Ophthalmol 86:802, 1978.

83. Polack, F. M.: Lamellar keratoplasty. Arch Ophthalmol 86:293, 1971.

84. Wood, T. O.: Lamellar transplants in keratoconus. Amer J Ophthalmol 83:543, 1977.

85. Richard, J. M., Paton, D., and Gasset, A. R.: A comparison of penetrating keratoplasty and lamellar keratoplasty in the surgical management of keratoconus. Amer J Ophthalmol 86:807, 1978.

86. Uribe, L. E.: Fixed pupil following keratoplasty. Amer J Ophthalmol 63:1682, 1967.

87. Castroviejo, R.: *Atlas of Keratectomy and Keratoplasty.* Philadelphia, W. B. Saunders Co., 1966, pp. 336–337.

88. Ruedemann, A. D., Jr.: Keratoplasty. South Med J 57:1075, 1964.

89. Urrets-Zavalia, A., Jr.: Fixed, dilated pupil, iris atrophy and secondary glaucoma. Distinct clinical entity following penetrating keratoplasty in keratoconus. Amer J Ophthalmol 56:257, 1963.

90. Davies, D., and Ruben, M.: The paretic pupil: Its incidence and etiology after keratoplasty in keratoconus. Brit J Ophthalmol 59:223, 1975.

91. Gasset, A. R.: Fixed dilated pupil following penetrating keratoplasty in keratoconus (Castroviejo syndrome). Ann Ophthalmol 9:623, 1977.

92. Alberth, B., and Schnitzler, A.: Irreversible Mydriase nach Keratoplastik bei Keratokonus. Klin Monatsbl Augenheilk 159:330, 1971.

93. Wand, M., and Grant, W. M.: Thymoxamine hydrochloride. Effects on the facility of outflow and intraocular pressure. Invest Ophthalmol 15:400, 1976.

94. Wand, M., and Grant, W. M.: Thymoxamine test: Differentiating angle closure glaucoma from open angle glaucoma with narrow angles. Arch Ophthalmol 96:1009, 1978.

95. Gasset, A. R., Shaw, E. L., Kaufman, H. E., Itoi, M., Sakimoto, T., and Ishii, Y.: Thermokeratoplasty. Trans Amer Acad Ophthalmol Otolaryngol 77:OP441, 1973.

96. Gasset, A. R., and Kaufman H. E.: Thermokeratoplasty in the treatment of keratoconus. Amer J Ophthalmol 79:226, 1975.

97. Aquavella, J. V.: Thermokeratoplasty. Ophthal Surg 5:39, 1974.

98. Arentsen, J. J., and Laibson, P. R.: Thermokeratoplasty for keratoconus. Amer J Ophthalmol 82:447, 1976.

99. Keates, R. H., and Dingle, J.: Thermokeratoplasty for keratoconus. Ophthal Surg 6:89, 1975.

100. Fogle, J. A., Kenyon, K. R., and Stark, W. J.: Damage to epithelial basement membrane by thermokeratoplasty. Amer J Ophthalmol 83:392, 1977.

101. Aquavella, J. V., Smith, R. S., and Shaw, E. L.: Alterations in corneal morphology following thermokeratoplasty. Arch Ophthalmol 94:2082, 1976.

III

SWELLING OF THE CORNEA

Specular Microscopy | 5

HOWARD M. LEIBOWITZ, M.D.
RONALD A. LAING, Ph.D.

The corneal specular microscope is a reflected-light microscope. It projects a slit of light onto the cornea and utilizes the light reflected from an optical interface of the tissue for image formation (rather than light transmitted through the tissue sample, as in the case of the standard bright-field biological microscope). To date, the instrument has been used primarily to study the corneal endothelium, although other structures (e.g., the corneal epithelium and both the anterior and posterior surfaces of the crystalline lens) can also be visualized (Fig. 5–1).

HISTORICAL NOTES

In 1968 David Maurice, using an epi-illumination microscope that focused a slit of light onto the posterior corneal surface of an enucleated eye, published endothelial photographs of the rabbit.[1] Since the specular image of the endothelium was photographed, Maurice suggested the name specular microscope for the instrument he used. It required contact between the objective of the instrument and the corneal epithelium, but this instrument produced photographs of the endothelium at magnifications up to 400 × in the intact, enucleated eye. In 1970 Brown constructed a clinical photomicroscope that could be used in the specular mode to obtain endothelial photographs.[2] Contact with the epithelial surface was not necessary with this

instrument, but its useful magnification was limited to 10 ×. Bron and Brown used this instrument for clinical study of grafted corneas,[3] and although the photographs they obtained were considerably better than earlier drawings, they were not of sufficient quality or magnification for study of endothelial morphology. Hoefle and coworkers[4] demonstrated the usefulness of Maurice's specular microscope for evaluating the corneal endothelium of human eyes being considered as donor material for keratoplasty. These workers also showed that the instrument could be used to measure corneal thickness by ascertaining the distance traversed by the objective lens after alternatively focusing on the anterior and posterior corneal surfaces. Laing and coworkers[5] made several modifications of Maurice's instrument that resulted in photomicrographs of improved quality. A single field of cells could be photographed at 100 × to 200 × with sufficient resolution to clearly demonstrate individual cell boundaries and to distinguish numerous intracellular structures.

To this point, the development of instrumentation for corneal specular microscopy limited the procedure to stationary corneas, either excised and mounted in a perfusion chamber or in the intact enucleated globe. Laing and coworkers developed the first specular microscope suitable for in vivo use and published the first in vivo high-magnification endothelial photographs in

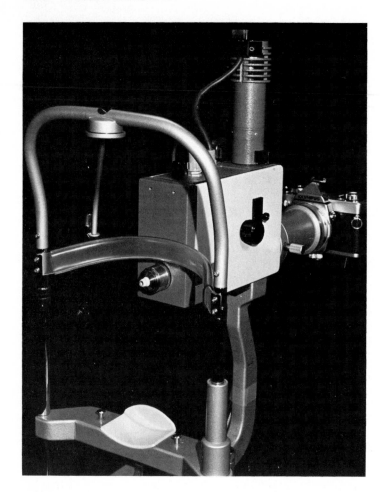

Figure 5–1. A typical clinical specular microscope.

1975.[6] Photomicrographs were obtained in rabbits, cats, monkeys, and humans by stabilizing the eye relative to the objective lens. An improved specular microscope, which contained a suction type corneal stabilizer and used a variable working distance objective lens (Nikon 77803, W20X), was constructed for this purpose. When the lens was fitted with the suction type corneal stabilizer, the cornea could be completely immobilized to facilitate focusing. For in vivo studies, the lens was used in a contacting and applanating mode. The first clinical specular microscope also was reported by Laing and coworkers.[6–8] The instrument provided a suitable head holder and horizontal mounting arrangement and produced endothelial photomicrographs at magnifications of 100 × or greater. The original unit operated by pulsating an incandescent lamp to a higher-than-normal brightness when the camera shutter opened, but this soon was replaced by a rapid-recycle flash-lamp power supply as a light source. The original instrument was crude in design and unwieldy in use, but it did produce high-magnification endothelial photomicrographs of sufficient quality to have clinical utility.

A variety of improvements and modifications of the corneal specular microscope have followed. Methodology using the ring setting on the objective lens to measure corneal thickness has been devised.[7, 9] The optical system has been redesigned to provide a wider field of view, more even illumination, and greater resolution. Some current objectives have a curved front surface, which "cushions" the cornea rather than applanating it, providing greater comfort and safety to the patient. A clinical scanning–slit specular microscope has been developed.[10] The major advantage of this instrument is its wider field. Alternative methods for obtaining a wide field of view utilize a calcium fluoride (fluorite) element affixed to the objective[11] or a fluid-filled adapter cap placed on the end of the objective.[12]

Further development of the noncontact macrophotography approach originated by Brown also has proceeded, although it must be emphasized that most "contact" specular microscopes can also function as noncontact microscopes by using a long working distance objective and, if desired, a slit illuminator. Some instruments designed as early as 1976 allow such additions to be made. Most noncontact methods employ a standard slit lamp to project a long vertical slit of light onto the endothelium; the specular reflection from the endothelium is photographed with a macro camera. With suitable lenses, viewing can be performed at 25 × to 60 × and photography at 13 × to 20 ×. A slit beam of large height can be used at these low magnifications, resulting in a larger number of cells per photograph than one obtains in the contact mode. However, the photographic resolution of these instruments, particularly in the periphery of the field, is less than that of contact mode instruments. Nonetheless, the image quality of medium power, noncontact specular microscopes, though less than that of the higher-power contact specular microscopes, is sufficient for many types of clinical observations. The noncontact feature of these instruments makes them especially useful for photographing children, overly apprehensive patients, and early postoperative cases.

Bigar and coworkers have developed a clinical instrument that uses two objectives mounted at a 45-degree angle, one for illumination, the other for observation.[13] Between the two objectives and the patient's cornea there is a special glass coupling element that applanates the cornea and provides the proper optical pathway for the dual lens system. The field is large and suitable for clinical screening, but the large angle between illuminating and viewing lenses may cause optical artifacts. Interpretation of some of the structures observed with the instrument is open to question.

Davidovits and Egger have reported still another technique for obtaining endothelial photomicrographs.[14] A small spot of laser light is scanned across the endothelial surface, and the reflected light is collected with a photomultiplier tube. Electronic circuits process the photomultiplier tube signal and form an image of the endothelium on an oscilloscope screen for photographic reproduction. This method should be capable of providing high-quality images of large fields of cells, but to date it has not been applied clinically.

OPTICAL PRINCIPLES OF SPECULAR MICROSCOPY

An understanding of the fundamental optical principles concerned with image formation by the specular microscope is useful in interpreting the endothelial photomicrographs obtained clinically.[15] Light striking a surface can be reflected, transmitted, or absorbed. Generally, some combination of the three effects occur, the relative proportions depending on such conditions as the wavelength of the light, the relative transparency of the medium below its surface, and the relative refractive indices on each side of the surface. Of primary importance in clinical specular microscopy is the reflected light. Light can be reflected from a surface in two ways, specular and diffuse (Fig. 5–2). Specular reflection is the type commonly associated with mirrors and other smooth surfaces, wherein the angle of reflection is equal to the angle of incidence. Diffuse reflection commonly is associated with rough surfaces (e.g., ground glass or fabric), and the reflected light is spread out over many angles. For most surfaces, reflection is a combination of specular and diffuse reflection; a majority of the reflected light is specularly reflected, although some light is also reflected at nonspecular angles.

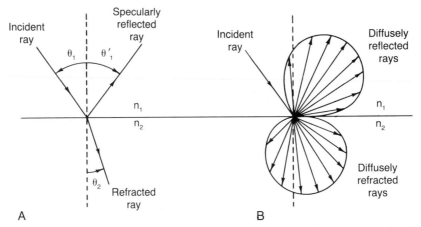

Figure 5–2. Reflection at a surface between two transparent media. *A,* Specular reflection. *B,* Diffuse reflection. θ_1 is the angle of incidence, θ_1' is the angle of reflection, θ_2 is the angle of refraction, n_1 is the index of refraction of medium 1, and n_2 is the index of refraction of medium 2.

For the normal, transparent cornea, most of the visible light incident on the epithelial surface is transmitted. Virtually no light is absorbed, but since an index of refraction gradient is present at the epithelial surface, some light is reflected (though the fraction of reflected light is small). As light passes into corneal tissue, three things can happen. The light can be transmitted through the tissue, it can be absorbed by the tissue, or it can be scattered. Scattering is a phenomenon that is similar to but more general than reflection; scattering encompasses light rays deviated through any angle, whereas reflection refers only to rays that are deviated "backwards" toward the incident light source. In the stroma of the normal cornea, most of the incident light is transmitted through the tissue, while a small, usually negligible portion is absorbed by cellular organelles, and another small amount is scattered. In edematous corneas, the fraction of scattered light increases and can become the dominant element.

As light strikes the posterior corneal surface, most of it is transmitted into the aqueous humor. Essentially no light is absorbed here, but because there is a change in index of refraction at the endothelium–aqueous humor interface, some light is reflected back into the cornea. For a smooth, posterior corneal surface, this has been calculated to be 0.022 per cent of the total incident light.

In pathologic corneas with a roughened or irregular posterior surface, there may be a substantial, diffuse component to the reflected light, decreasing the relative intensity of the specularly reflected light.

Hence, as the illumination beam of the specular photomicroscope passes through the cornea, it encounters a series of interfaces between optically distinct regions. At each of these interfaces, some light is reflected back toward the photomicroscope and some is transmitted farther into the cornea. The greater the difference in index of refraction between the two regions, the greater will be the amount of reflected light and the more intense the reflected light. The more edematous the tissue, the greater will be the intensity of scattered light. A portion of the reflected and backscattered light is collected by the objective lens of the specular microscope and an image of the plane at which the instrument is focused is formed at the film plane of the photomicroscope (Fig. 5–3).

Figure 5–4*A* shows a narrow slit of light from a specular microscope that is focused onto the posterior corneal surface. The incident light illuminates, in turn, the precorneal tear film or a coupling medium (e.g., saline, artificial tears, or Gonio-gel) between the objective lens and the cornea, the epithelium, Bowman's membrane, the stroma, Des-

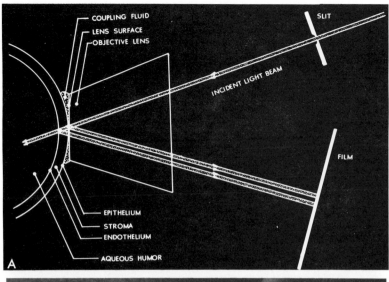

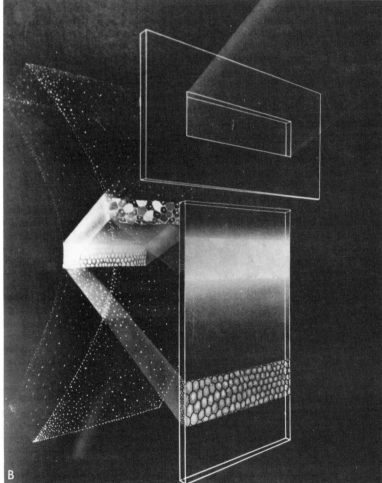

Figure 5–3. Pathway of light from its source in the clinical specular microscope, back to the film plane of the same instrument. *A,* Cross-sectional diagram. *B,* Graphic representation. Although both epithelium and endothelium are shown in focus on the film plane of the graphic representation, in practice only one layer is in focus at any one time because of the restricted depth of field of the instrument.

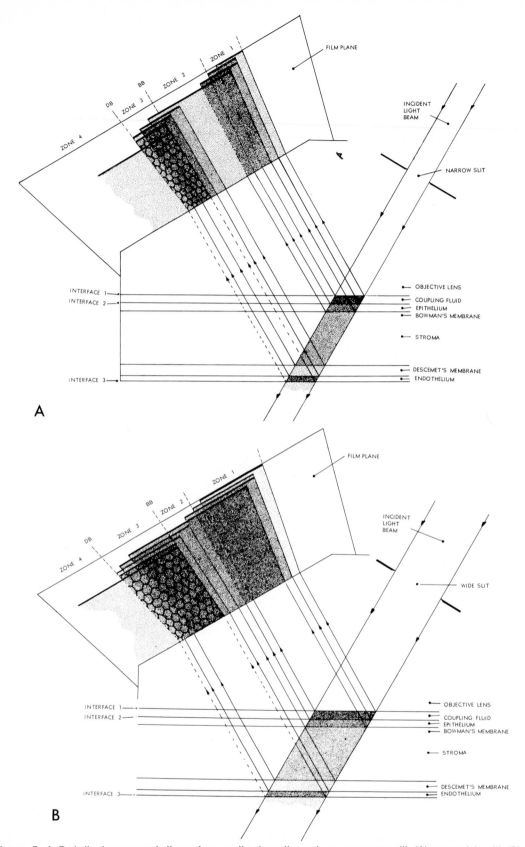

Figure 5–4. Detailed representation of an optical section when a narrow slit *(A)* or a wide slit *(B)* of light passes through various corneal layers and is focused on the posterior corneal surface. As drawn, the film plane is positioned at right angles to the plane of the paper. The zones shown are defined in the text. BB = bright boundary; DB = dark boundary.

128

cemet's membrane, the endothelium, and the aqueous humor. Within each of these regions some light is scattered back towards the film, and at the major optical interfaces (labeled 1, 2, and 3) considerable light is specularly reflected back toward the film. The fraction of light reflected from each of these interfaces has been calculated; it is 0.36 per cent from the objective lens–saline interface, 0.025 per cent from the saline–corneal epithelium interface, and 0.022 per cent from the corneal endothelium–aqueous humor interface using indexes of refraction of the objective lens, saline, cornea, and aqueous humor of 1.517, 1.333, 1.376, and 1.336, respectively. Intracorneal optical interfaces (e.g., between epithelium and Bowman's membrane or between stroma and Descemet's membrane) also reflect light, but the fraction of reflected light cannot be calculated because the index of refraction of the separate layers of the cornea has never been measured. These differences are undoubtedly small, and for our present purposes we will ignore intracorneal reflections. Anatomically distinct regions in the cornea also scatter light back to the specular microscope, and various parts of the cornea can behave differently in different types of corneal disorders. For example, in entities characterized by microcystic edema of the epithelium or by a roughened, irregular epithelial surface, the epithelium will scatter more light back to the film plane of the specular microscope than the stroma. Conversely, when stromal edema is the prominent abnormality, the opposite is true.

At the film plane of the specular microscope, light from various corneal regions and interfaces overlaps. Whenever a bright region and a dark region overlap, the dark region is not seen. If a sufficiently narrow slit of incident light is used, one can generally appreciate part of the aqueous humor (Zone 4), the endothelial region (Zone 3), part of the stromal region (Zone 2), and a bright region (Zone 1). The latter is formed by light reflected from the lens–coupling fluid or the coupling fluid–epithelial in-terfaces or both, depending on the index of refraction of the coupling fluid used.

The interface between Zone 3 and Zone 4 is called the dark boundary (Fig. 5–4).[15] This landmark separates the illuminated cornea from the nonilluminated structures located more posteriorly. One side of the boundary is dark because neglible light is scattered from the aqueous humor. In contrast, the interface between Zone 2 and Zone 3 is called the bright boundary. This landmark separates the endothelial reflection from the overlying illuminated corneal stroma. Since substantial amounts of light are scattered from this tissue, neither side of the boundary is dark. The light scattered from Descemet's membrane and stroma causes the bright boundary to be less distinct than the dark boundary and accounts for the progressively lower contrast as one approaches the bright boundary.

Of importance clinically is the width of the slit of light projected onto the cornea by the specular microscope. If the angle of incidence of the illuminating source is increased, a wider slit can be used and a larger field of endothelial cells can be seen (Figs. 5–4B, 5–5). However, the wider slit beam also illuminates more of the corneal tissue anterior to the endothelium, so that the volume of "interfering stroma" increases and more light is scattered back to the film plane of the specular microscope. The net result is a decrease in contrast of the endothelial image and a loss of cellular definition; a greater number of cells can be seen when a wider illuminating slit is used, but only at the expense of contrast and definition required for optimal visualization of intracellular structures and cell boundaries. This trade-off between the contrast of the photograph and the number of cells within a single frame is not due to an optical limitation of the instrument but rather to light scattering in the tissue overlying the endothelium. Moreover, use of a wider slit width requires that the angle of incidence of the illuminating source be increased. At a large angle of incidence (and a correspondingly large angle of

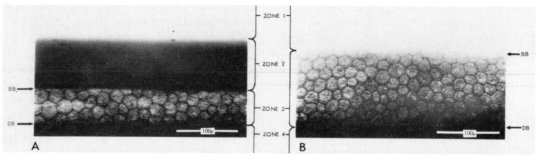

Figure 5–5. Specular photomicrograph of a normal human corneal endothelium using a narrow slit beam *(A)* and a wide slit beam *(B)*. Four zones are seen when the narrow slit beam is used: a bright zone originating from the objective lens–coupling fluid–epithelial interface (Zone 1), a gray zone originating in the stroma (Zone 2), the endothelial zone (Zone 3), and a dark zone originating in the aqueous humor (Zone 4). Zone 2 disappears and Zone 3 becomes larger when a wide slit beam is used. BB = bright boundary, DB = dark boundary.

reflection and observation) normal endothelial cells appear shortened in one direction. Thus, a wider illuminating slit beam results in a distorted endothelial cell pattern, making assessment of morphological details more difficult. A wide slit width with a large angle of incidence is used in most noncontacting types of specular microscopes.

When a narrow illuminating slit is used, the photographic image contains a region produced by scattered light exclusively of stromal origin (Zone 2). As we have indicated, this region progressively disappears as the slit is progressively widened. The intensity of light scattered solely from the stroma (when a narrow slit of incident light is employed) can be quantitatively determined by measuring the film density in this area of the specular photomicrograph. The resultant value is an objective measure of stromal edema. Though not in routine clinical use at present, specular microscopy offers the potential for more accurate measurement of stromal edema than any method currently in use.

Figure 5–5 shows an endothelial photomicrograph of a normal human cornea taken with a wide slit setting. It illustrates the various phenomena described above.[15] With a narrow slit four distinct zones are seen; with a wide slit only three zones are apparent. A bright zone, Zone 1, arises from the reflection at the objective lens–epithelial cell interface.

Zone 2 arises from light diffusely scattered from corneal stroma and is present only in narrow slit photographs. This zone is darker in clear corneas and brighter in edematous corneas, a phenomenon that can be used to grade the degree of stromal edema quantitatively. Zone 3 shows the endothelial cell pattern produced by light specularly reflected from the posterior corneal surface, while Zone 4, the dark zone, is the product of light scattered from the aqueous humor. Since little light is scattered in the aqueous humor and virtually no light from the region normally returns to the collection optics of the microscope, Zone 4 is generally dark. In eyes with considerable debris in the anterior chamber this zone occasionally can be brighter and show some structure, but in most instances it is uniformly dark. Two distinct boundaries are seen in Figure 5–5: the dark boundary (DB) between Zones 3 and 4, and the bright boundary (BB) between Zones 1 and 2. The average intensity is nearly constant along the length of the slit but varies linearly along its width. Abnormalities such as epithelial or stromal edema, stromal infiltration, and scarring will increase the amount of light scattered back to the instrument and obscure the image of the underlying endothelial cell pattern.

The degree of irregularity and/or roughness of the posterior corneal surface can be determined by evaluation of the dark boundary in the endothelial photomicrograph.[15] Regardless of the type of surface, a ray of light incident upon the cell boundary (CB) at the junction of an intercellular space and the anterior chamber is reflected in a manner that prevents its collection by the viewing optics. As a result the cell boundaries are not exposed on the film, and they appear dark on the prints. Figure 5–6 shows four different types of posterior corneal surfaces: smooth, rough, wavy, and a surface containing an excrescence. In the case of a smooth surface, all other light rays incident upon the surface are directed to the collection optics of the specular microscope. This manifests itself in the photograph in two ways: the illumination within each cell boundary is essentially uniform (except for the reflection of light from cellular organelles), and the dark boundary is straight and smooth. A rough posterior corneal surface pro-

duces a rough dark boundary with linear irregularities that correspond to the surface irregularities of the posterior corneal surface. To appear irregular in the photograph, the distance between adjacent high (or low) points of a given irregularity must be more than the wavelength of the illuminating light (approximately 0.5 μm). Otherwise the surface is optically smooth and the dark boundary appears straight. A rough posterior corneal surface also produces a pattern that contains dark regions within cell boundaries. The size and configuration of these intracellular dark regions depend upon the nature and the degree of the surface irregularities.

If the distance between irregularities of the posterior corneal surface is of the order of magnitude of the normal endothelial cell diameter, the posterior corneal surface has an undulating or wavy configuration. The dark boundary in an endothelial photomicrograph will ap-

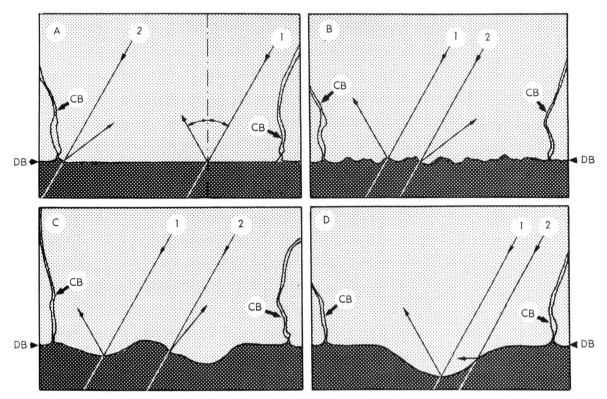

Figure 5–6. The nature of specular reflection from various types of posterior endothelial surfaces. *A,* Smooth. *B,* Rough. *C,* Wavy. *D,* A posterior endothelial surface containing an excrescence. In each instance, the ray labeled "1" is collected by the objective lens of the specular microscope, resulting in a bright area on the film. The ray labeled "2" is not collected by the objective lens of the specular microscope, resulting in a dark area on the film. CB = cell boundary, DB = dark boundary.

pear wavy, and illumination within individual cell boundaries will not be uniform. If the amplitude of the undulations is sufficiently large, the lack of uniformity in illumination will be visually apparent in the endothelial cell pattern of the photomicrograph. In the case of a posterior corneal surface containing an excrescence, the dark boundary also will contain an irregularity. However, the excrescence will be even more readily apparent in the endothelial cell pattern. The sides of the excrescence appear dark, whereas its apex specularly reflects incident light into the collection optics of the specular microscope and appears bright.[16, 17]

ANALYTICAL MEASUREMENTS WITH THE SPECULAR MICROSCOPE

Qualitative Analysis of the Corneal Endothelium

At present the clinical specular microscope is used primarily to evaluate the corneal endothelium. Both qualitative and quantitative assessments of this layer can be made. In making a qualitative cellular analysis, one looks for the presence of abnormal endothelial structures and grades the endothelium either according to the number or size of the abnormal structures present or on the basis of an overall visual assessment of endothelial appearance. The goal is not to assign a precise numerical value to the photograph (although a rough value such as 1+ or 2+ may be given) but rather to provide a subjective evaluation of the endothelium. This type of analysis is useful in providing a rapid clinical evaluation of the endothelium to assess the risks of intraocular surgery, to establish a diagnosis, or to decide upon treatment. However, one must be careful to eliminate optical artifacts from consideration when performing this type of evaluation.

A complete qualitative analysis requires that several parameters be evaluated.[16] These include (1) cell conformation, (2) cell boundaries and their intersections, (3) configuration of the dark boundary, and (4) presence of acellular structures.

Cell Conformation

The specular microscope resolves the endothelial pattern of the normal cornea into a quasi-regular and quasi-hexagonal pattern of contiguous cells having well defined cell boundaries. The central endothelial cells of young people with normal eyes are approximately the same size and the distribution of cell area is approximately normal (gaussian). With age the average cell area increases, the cellular pattern becomes distinctly pleomorphic, and the cell size distribution becomes skewed toward larger cell areas (Fig. 5–7). In young people with normal eyes the cell side lengths are all roughly equal. In older individuals, the side lengths lose this regularity and one sees an increasing variation. The angles of intersection between the cell sides are roughly 120 degrees at all ages, although in older individuals and in patients who have suffered cell loss considerable variation in intersection angles is seen.

Several distinct variations in endothelial cell conformation have been observed. For example, cell size can vary over a wide range in a number of disorders (Fig. 5–8). To date neither cellular pleomorphism nor uniform cellular enlargement, to at least a factor of five, has been shown to be related to a loss in the ability of the endothelium to maintain corneal deturgescence. However, we believe that pleomorphism and cellular enlargement reflect a loss in the reserve capacity of the endothelium, that is, in the ability of this cellular layer to recover from a subsequent insult.

In addition to changes in size, endothelial cells may assume a shape that is substantially different from the usual quasi-hexagonal configuration. Figure 5–9A shows endothelial cells that are both enlarged and elongated. These cells were encountered near the corneal apex in a case of keratoconus. They appear to be aligned in the same direction and to follow lines of stress as if they have been

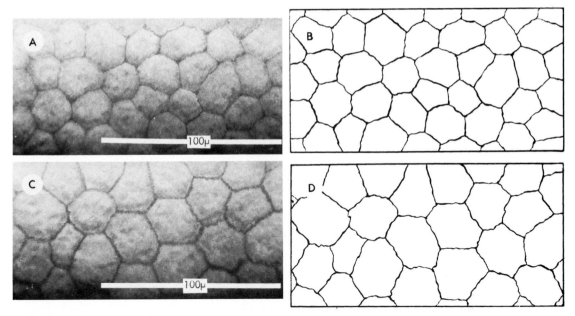

Figure 5–7. Cell pattern configurations photographed with the clinical specular microscope. *A,* 18-year-old normal endothelium. *B,* Tracing of cell boundaries in *A. C,* 69-year-old normal endothelium. *D,* Tracing of *C.*

stretched by gross deformation of the cornea. Cells with scalloped rather than conventional straight sides are occasionally seen (Fig. 5–9B). So, too, are round cells (Fig. 5–9C and D), square cells (Fig. 5–9E), and triangular cells (Fig. 5–9F). As in the case with changes in endothelial cell size, alterations in shape have not been directly related to changes in the physiologic function of the affected cells.

Cell Boundaries and Intersections

Normal cell boundaries most commonly appear as dark, straight, narrow lines (Fig. 5–10A).[16] However, several additional types of cell boundaries, collectively referred to as doubled boundaries, have been observed. The most common type of doubled boundary exhibits a less distinct secondary dark line within the cell, running adjacent and parallel to the

Figure 5–8. Variations in the configuration of the corneal endothelium. *A,* Cellular pleomorphism—great variation in the size of the cells.*B,* Relatively uniform enlargement of the cells.

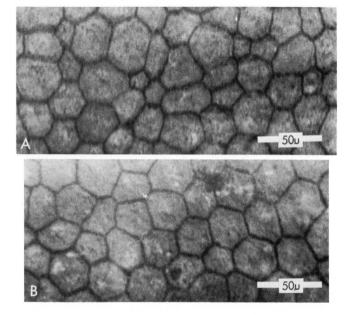

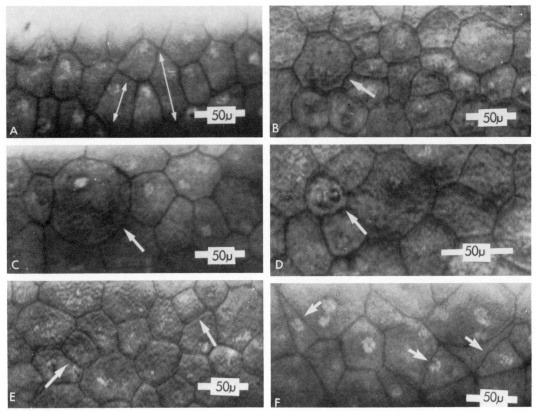

Figure 5–9. Variations in the configuration of the corneal endothelium. *A*, Elongated cells. *B*, Cell with scalloped edges. *C* and *D*, Round cell. *E*, Square cell. *F*, Triangular cell.

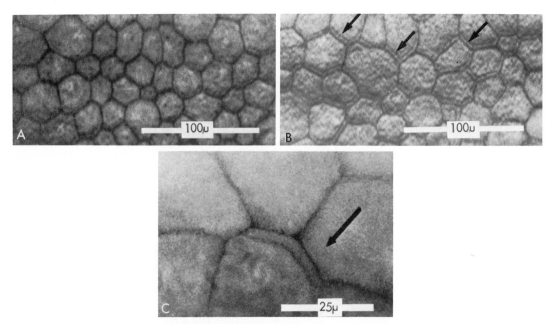

Figure 5–10. Variations in the morphology of endothelial cell boundaries. *A*, Single (the most commonly encountered type). *B* and *C*, Doubled cell boundaries (arrows).

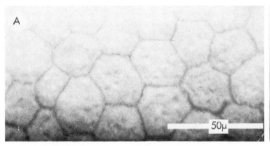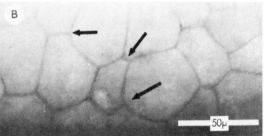

Figure 5–11. Variations in the pattern of cell boundary intersections. *A*, Normal cell pattern with normal intersections. *B*, Abnormal intersections (arrows).

usual primary boundary (Fig. 5–10B). It usually involves one or two cell sides, occurs in many cells in a given field, and always is seen on the same sides of the cells. This suggests that the formation of such boundaries may be a shadowing phenomenon. A less common variety of doubled boundary affects only occasional cells (Fig. 5–10C). Here the secondary boundary line lies within the cell. It is visually as dark as the primary boundary and it runs adjacent and parallel to two or more cell sides. These two types of doubled cell boundaries are seen in corneas that appear normal by slit-lamp biomicroscopy. Their significance is not clear, and we have no information indicating that endothelial cells containing such boundaries are physiologically abnormal.

In the normal endothelium, cell boundaries intersect in a manner that results in three angles of intersection that are each approximately 120 degrees.[16] Cell boundary intersections also are seen wherein the angles of intersection vary considerably from 120 degrees (Fig. 5–11). Such intersections are thermodynamically unstable, suggesting that they are formed by abnormal cells or by cells undergoing a transition in shape that has been brought about by endothelial cell loss or movement of nearby cells.

The Posterior Corneal Surface

As we have stated above, information about the posterior surface of the endothelium can be obtained by examining the appearance of the dark boundary, the interface between the endothelial cell pattern and the adjacent dark zone produced by the aqueous humor. If the endothelial surface is smooth, the resulting dark boundary will be straight, whereas an irregular endothelial surface produces an irregular dark boundary. Four different basic configurations of the dark boundary are possible (Figs. 5–5, 5–12). Clinically one not only encounters these four basic types of dark boundary but also may encounter combinations of the four types. Specific relationships between these abnormal variations in the posterior surface configuration of the endothelium and in the physiologic function of the cells have not been established.

Miscellaneous Structures

A number of inter- and intra-endothelial cell structures, which may be either dark or bright in appearance, are seen in endothelial photographs.[16] One type of dark structure disrupts the endothelial cell pattern and can range in size from a structure smaller than to one larger than an individual endothelial cell. Each such structure generally has dark sides and a central bright spot (Fig. 5–13A). Such structures represent a smooth excrescence of Descemet's membrane (i.e., cornea guttata) and often are surrounded by a ring of abnormally shaped cells. Cornea guttata can be seen at a much earlier stage with the specular microscope than with the conventional slit-lamp biomicroscope.[17] When these excrescences are abundant, they begin to touch one another and to coalesce. One

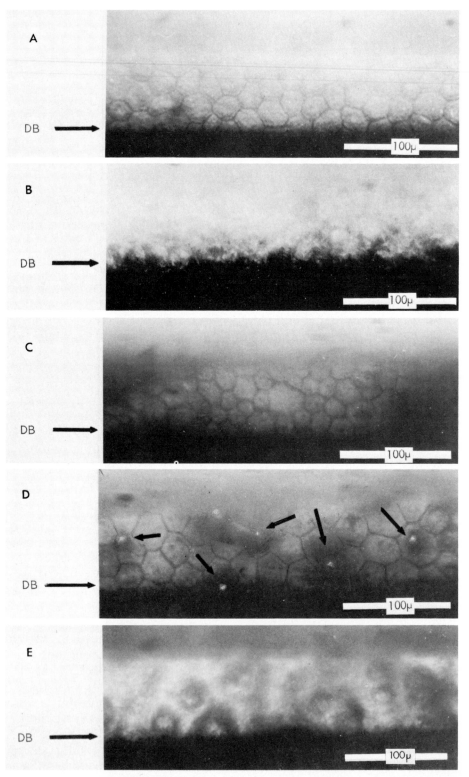

Figure 5–12. Variations in the appearance of the posterior corneal surface, the dark boundary (DB). *A,* Normal endothelium, smooth dark boundary. *B,* Rough dark boundary. *C,* Smooth, uneven dark boundary (wavy). *D,* Multiple excrescences (cornea guttata) (arrows). *E,* Combined type of dark boundary abnormality (wavy-rough).

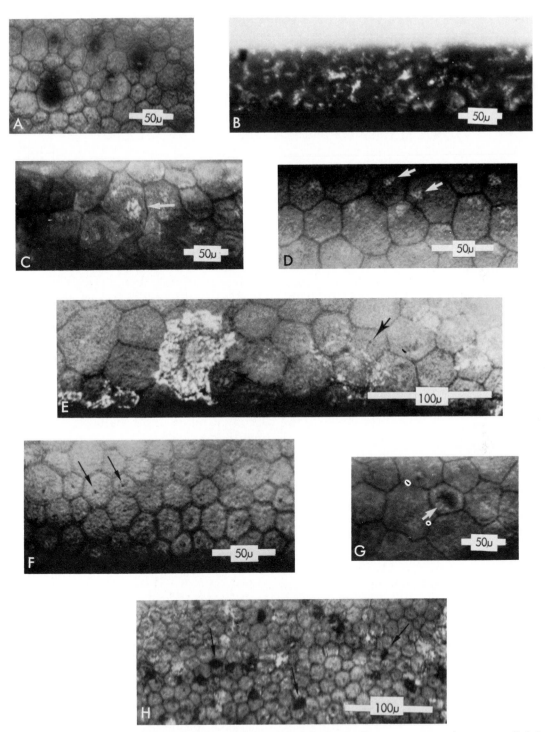

Figure 5–13. Miscellaneous endothelial structures. *A,* Isolated smooth excrescences (cornea guttata). *B,* Multiple coalesced excrescences. *C* and *D,* Intracellular bright structures. *E,* Pigmented endothelial deposits. *F* and *G,* intracellular dark structures. *H,* intercellular dark structures, believed to be invading inflammatory cells. (*D, E,* and *F* courtesy of L. Neubauer, M.D.)

sees the pattern illustrated in Fig. 5–13B, and, although the endothelial cell pattern is not visible, the bright reflection from the apex of each excrescence is clearly seen. (See the discussion of Fuchs' dystrophy later in this chapter.)

Intracellular bright structures, some of which may be only the cell nucleus, have been seen in endothelial photomicrographs.[16] They are variable in size and typically are contained completely within a single endothelial cell (Fig. 5–13C and D). Occasional exceptions do occur, however, wherein the bright structure seems to cross a cell boundary. We believe that these intracellular bright structures are found in stressed cells, explaining why they commonly are seen within enlarged cells such as those encountered in successful corneal transplants. Their size or number (multiple bright structures may occur within a single greatly enlarged cell) seems to be proportional to the size of the cell. That is, the larger the endothelial cell, the larger the intracellular bright structure.

A second type of bright structure spans several endothelial cells (Fig. 5–13E) and is positioned at random on the endothelial cell pattern of the specular photomicrographs. When viewed directly, these structures appear to sparkle; some are orange, while others are white. Slit-lamp biomicroscopy of these corneas reveals numerous pigment deposits on the endothelium. The bright structures seen with the clinical specular photomicroscope appear to correspond to the pigmented endothelial deposits seen with the slit-lamp biomicroscope, and presumably they are the same abnormality.

Two additional types of dark bodies, both intracellular in location, have been observed. The first type is small, generally located in the central or paracentral portion of the cell, and has sharp, well-defined edges showing that it is located on the posterior surface of the cell (Fig. 5–13F). This structure has been seen in clinically normal corneas, and, when present, it occurs in many but not all cells. It presumably represents the base of an endothelial cilia, although histo-logic verification of this has not yet been obtained. The second type of dark body is considerably larger and has indistinct edges, suggesting that it is located within the cell (Fig. 5–13G). It may represent an intracellular vacuole or bleb.

Intercellular dark structures, lying predominantly at endothelial cell intersections, have been observed (Fig. 5–13H).[16] They tend to be uniform in size, and within a given frame they are randomly positioned across the endothelial cell pattern. These structures occur in patients with anterior uveitis, and it is believed they represent invading inflammatory cells.

A variety of endothelial structures that are not visible with the slit-lamp biomicroscope can be seen with the clinical specular microscope. Morphologic variations in endothelial cell configuration, cell surface properties, and intercellular boundaries, as well as the presence of numerous intracellular structures, can be identified. Although the nature and significance of many of these abnormalities are not presently known, their recognition represents an initial step in the elucidation of their pathophysiological significance.

QUANTITATIVE CELL ANALYSIS

Although a qualitative description of the corneal specular photograph suffices for many applications, more quantitative information is desirable for others. The aim of quantitative analysis is to assign a number (or set of numbers) to the specular photomicrograph that can provide a measure of the endothelial status.

There are a variety of morphological parameters that can be quantitated. These include cell size (cell area or cell density), cell perimeter, average cell side length, cell shape, and so forth. Histograms or frequency distributions of these quantities can also be determined. To date only cell size and several variables related to it have been shown to be measurably changed and to be useful in determining endothelial status. As more precise and sophisticated methods of analysis are developed, we anticipate that additional morphologic parameters may be found to be of clinical value.

Two equivalent parameters have been used to quantitate endothelial cell size. They are mean cell area and cell density (or cell count). Cell area has most often been expressed in units of μm.^{2} per cell and cell density in units of cells per mm.^{2} These two quantities are related by the following equations:

Mean cell area (μm.^{2}/cell)
$$= 10^6/\text{cell density (cells/mm.}^2)$$

Cell density (cell/mm.^{2})
$$= 10^6/\text{mean cell area } (\mu\text{m.}^2/\text{cell})$$

Two different methods, fixed frame analysis and variable frame analysis, exist for measuring either of these two parameters of cell size.

Fixed Frame Analysis of Cell Size

In fixed frame analysis one counts the number of cells within a frame or window of constant área. All cells lying completely within the frame are counted as whole cells. However, along the boundary of the frame there are many cells that lie only partly in the frame, and for these cells it is usually impossible to determine the fraction of the cellular area that lies within the borders of the frame. Each cell that is only partially within the frame is counted as one half cell regardless of the fractional area of that cell located within the frame. The total number of cells (the cell count) is then taken as the sum of the number of whole and half cells within the frame. To speed up the counting process one commonly invokes a symmetry principle and counts only the cells cut by two of the boundaries as whole cells. (Those cells cut by the other two boundaries are not counted.) As long as the number of boundary cells is small compared to the total number of whole cells within the frame, and cellular pleomorphism is not too great, this method can give reasonably accurate values for mean cell size.

The size is usually obtained by dividing the cell count by the area of the frame and expressed as cell density in cells per mm.^{2} The area of the frame must be referred to the endothelium. This is accomplished by dividing the actual area of the frame by the square of the linear magnification of the specular microscope and, if the cells were counted from an enlargement of the negative, by the square of the linear magnification of the enlargement. One could also divide the area by the cell count and report mean cell area as well.

Variable Frame Analysis of Cell Size

In variable frame analysis one measures the variable area occupied by an integral number of cells. The variable frame area is obtained by using either a planimeter or a digitizer. The stylus of the instrument is used to trace around the boundary of the group of cells being analyzed, and when the stylus returns to the starting point, the area is read directly from the instrument. The cell density is then calculated by dividing the number of cells that have been traced by the area of the frame. An equivalent value, the mean cell area, can be obtained by dividing the frame area by the number of cells that have been circumscribed. Since this method eliminates the problem of counting fractional cells along the boundary, it provides a more accurate determination of mean cell size, again assuming that cellular pleomorphism is not too great and that the cell sample is representative of the area under study.

In the event that extensive cellular pleomorphism is present, the number of cells within a frame, either fixed or variable, may not be representative of the entire population of endothelial cells, and the cell density or the mean cell area calculated may not be representative of the endothelium. For present endothelial cameras, which all photograph more than 100 normal cells per field, this is seldom a problem except in cases of greatly reduced cell density.

Individual Cell Analysis

In fixed frame analysis only average cell size can be determined. The same holds true for variable frame analysis if only a group of cells is circumscribed. However, using the variable frame technique, only a single cell can be traced with the stylus of the planimeter or digitizer, and this then permits individual cell analysis.[7] Such an analysis provides much more information about the endothelial cell pattern than can be obtained with methods that determine only cell density or average cell area. Individual cell analysis can be performed either manually or automatically. The more sophisticated, automatic analyses are accomplished with a digitizer. The cell boundaries are traced with a special pen or a cross-hair cursor. As this is being done, the x and y coordinates of the boundary points are automatically entered into a computer. The computer determines when the cell has been completely circumscribed and calculates the area (or other programmed morphologic parameter) of that cell. It then instructs the operator to trace another cell. The cell density or mean cell area can be obtained by averaging the data on a group of cells. In addition, a frequency

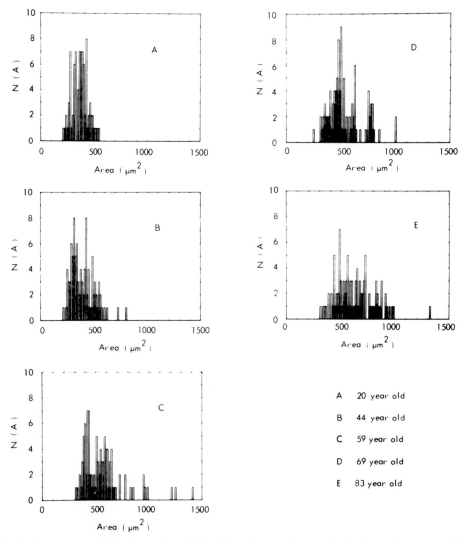

Figure 5–14. Frequency distribution of endothelial cell areas for subjects of varying ages. N(A) is the number of endothelial cells having an area between A and A + 0.125 mm.[2] (on film) or, approximately, between A and A + 12.5 μm[2] (on endothelium).

distribution (or histogram) of cell size can be obtained as shown in Figure 5–14. Although such frequency distributions provide considerable information about the endothelium, the procedure is extremely tedious and few studies using this method have been reported. Fortunately, automated methods of individual cell analysis in which the tedious task of manual digitization is replaced by an automated method of digitization or scanning of the endothelial photograph are being developed. Because of the complexity of an endothelial photograph, automated methods, at least for the foreseeable future, will not be able to function without operator input and will require interaction and decision-making by a human operator.

IN VIVO FINDINGS OF SPECULAR MICROSCOPY

Aging

Most studies with the specular microscope to date have evaluated the central corneal endothelium. Several investigators concur that the central endothelium changes as a function of age.[7,18–22] In most individuals the cell density decreases (or mean cell area increases) from birth to death. These changes seem to occur in several steps. From birth to adolescence the cell density decreases rapidly, though it is not known whether this represents true cell loss or is simply a reflection of the normal enlargement of the globe that occurs during this period. From age 20 through approximately age 50 endothelial cell density seems to be relatively stable. After the age of 60 cell density decreases significantly in most people, although there is a great deal of individual variability. Since at this age the globe does not change in size, this observation seems to represent a true loss of endothelial cells. Generally there is no significant difference in endothelial cell density between the two eyes of an individual. However, in some people a significant difference may appear as the individual becomes older, and

this difference may increase with age. The reason for this phenomenon is not known. No changes in pleomorphism (variability of cell size), cell shape, or other non–size related parameters have yet been found to correlate with age.

It is not known why endothelial cells are lost with age. Shaw and coworkers[23] divided the population they studied into those who exhibited cell size variability (polymegathism or pleomorphism) and those who did not. These investigators proposed that their data suggest that individuals with polymegathism or pleomorphism at an early age show more cell loss with increasing age than those who do not. Unfortunately, the distinction between normal individuals with endothelial cells that are of uniform size and those with endothelial cells that are variable in size is relatively subjective. Current technology does not allow a large percentage of people to be classified unambiguously into one group or the other.

Fuchs' Dystrophy

Cornea guttata are focal accumulations of collagen on the posterior surface of Descemet's membrane. They apparently are formed by stressed or abnormal endothelial cells and appear as warts or excrescences of Descemet's membrane. These structures characterize Fuchs' endothelial dystrophy but are not pathognomonic for this disorder. Cornea guttata also occur as a result of aging[24, 25] and corneal inflammation.[26]

Fuchs' endothelial dystrophy is a progressive disorder. Initially, central guttate endothelial changes are observed in the absence of biomicroscopically apparent alterations of the other corneal layers or visual symptoms. Over an interval that may span many years, the central cornea guttata become more numerous and prominent and begin to spread toward the corneal periphery. Edema of the corneal epithelium and stroma then appears, causing blurred vision. The progressive morphologic changes of cornea guttata in Fuchs'

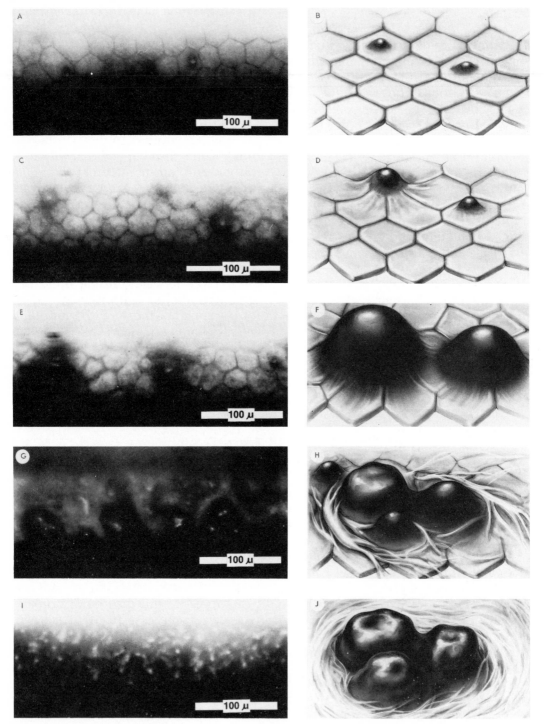

Figure 5–15. Specular photomicrographs and diagrammatic representations of various stages of cornea guttata in Fuchs' dystrophy (× 100). *A* and *B*, Stage 1: Earliest form of cornea guttata seen by specular microscopy. Excrescences are smaller than individual endothelial cells. Dark areas are the sides of the excrescence. Bright spots are each a reflex from the apex of the excrescence. *C* and *D*, Stage 2: Cornea guttata approximate the average endothelial cell in size. *E* and *F*, Stage 3: Cornea guttata are considerably larger than the average endothelial cell. Adjacent endothelial cells are abnormal in appearance. *G* and *H*, Stage 4: Individual cornea guttata have coalesced and contain more than one apical bright spot. Boundaries of adjacent endothelial cells are absent or difficult to identify. *I* and *J*, Stage 5: Coalesced excrescences and nearly complete disorganization of adjacent endothelial mosaic. Numerous bright structures presumably are collagenous material deposited at the level of Descemet's membrane or on the posterior corneal surface.

endothelial dystrophy have been characterized by clinical specular photomicroscopy.[17] Five specific stages in the development of excrescences can be discerned during the early evolution of Fuchs' dystrophy (Fig. 5–15). Indeed, all five stages of cornea guttata can occur in a cornea clinically free of edema. Several stages can be observed in the same cornea at a given time, although in most cases the majority of cornea guttata seem to have progressed to the same stage of development.

Specular microscopic findings strongly suggest that the individual excrescence begins as a minute structure, substantially smaller in size than an individual endothelial cell, and that it gradually and progressively grows larger, presumably as a result of the deposition and incorporation of additional collagen. Initially the endothelial cell lying behind the excrescence as well as neighboring endothelial cells all appear normal, and the specular microscopic studies contribute no information about the basic processes involved in the formation of the excrescence. As the excrescence grows larger, it obscures the view of the endothelial cell lying directly behind it, but the neighboring endothelial cells begin to appear distinctly abnormal. Clearly, there are definite endothelial abnormalities in the absence of clinically evident corneal edema in patients with Fuchs' dystrophy. Whether the enlarged excrescence damages the endothelium or the abnormal endothelium manufactures a larger excrescence is not clear.

Two types of cornea guttata can be identified in vivo with the specular microscope (Fig. 5–16).[17] One has a smooth, regular posterior surface, whereas the posterior contour of the second is irregular. Ultrastructural studies similarly have identified rounded excrescences and excrescences with a flat, broad posterior surface containing a central depression.[27, 28] The latter, umbilicated excrescences tend to be large, perhaps on the average larger than the rounded excrescences, suggesting that the irregular posterior surface may represent a maturation change and that that particular excrescence is long lived. However, one cannot differentiate·between the endothelial changes adjacent

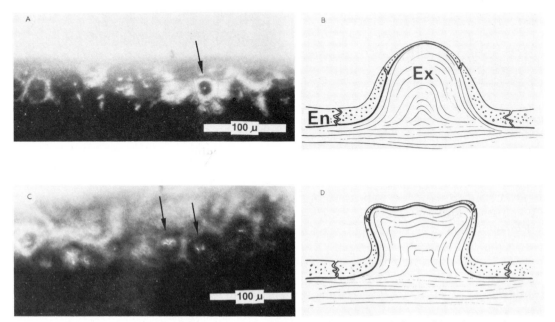

Figure 5–16. Specular photomicrographs and diagrammatic representation of two types of cornea guttata (× 100). A and B, Smooth excrescence (Ex) characterized by a roughly circular dark area containing a regular, circular bright apical spot. En = endothelial cell. C and D, Rough excrescence characterized by a dark area containing an irregular, bright spot in which there are random variations of brightness. Ratio of bright to dark area is greater than that encountered with smooth excrescences.

to the two types of cornea guttata, nor is one able to identify either type of excrescence as a specific contributor to endothelial decompensation.

Specular microscopy provides no information that directly relates the morphologic characteristics of cornea guttata and the physiologic status of the adjacent endothelium. We are able to say little more than that there is an association of cornea guttata and corneal edema, but we cannot specifically link the functional status of the endothelium to any particular aspect of the associated excrescences. Specular microscopic studies suggest that the more advanced stages of development of excrescences correlate with clinically prominent cornea guttata seen with the slit-lamp biomicroscope and with early endothelial decompensation and edema. Unfortunately, exceptions to this rule have been observed and we are unable to pronounce such a correlation with certainty. To date patients with predominantly stage 4 and/or stage 5 changes invariably exhibit biomicroscopic evidence of Fuchs' dystrophy, though not necessarily edema.

Iridocorneal Endothelial Syndrome

The iridocorneal endothelial syndrome includes progressive essential iris atrophy, Chandler's syndrome, and the iris nevus (Cogan-Reese) syndrome. This spectrum of diseases is characterized by abnormalities of the cornea, anterior chamber angle, and iris.[29] Corneal edema occurs in some cases and growth of a membrane onto the iris is encountered in others. Contraction of the membrane may cause peripheral anterior synechiae with secondary glaucoma and various iris abnormalities.

It has been suggested that a defect of the corneal endothelium may be the fundamental change in these disorders.[30] The endothelium often has a fine, beaten-silver appearance when examined with the slit-lamp biomicroscope, but this is not diagnostic and can be readily confused with cornea guttata.

However, the unilateral tendency of these diseases and the maintenance of excellent vision in most of those affected, even in the face of substantial endothelial abnormalities, suggests a different pathophysiology from that of Fuchs' dystrophy. Ultrastructural studies of cases with advanced corneal edema reveal a decreased endothelial cell population of abnormal cells covering a thickened, multilayered Descemet's membrane.[31, 32]

Although in many patients with iridocorneal endothelial syndrome the cornea is clear and normal in thickness, most of the anterior chamber angle is closed by peripheral anterior synechiae and substantial endothelial abnormalities are present. However, in other eyes afflicted with this disorder synechial attachments involve less than 25 per cent of the angle despite the presence of severe central endothelial abnormalities,[33] supporting the thesis that the endothelial changes are primary and that the peripheral anterior synechiae, iris atrophy, and iris nodule or nevus formation occur secondarily to endothelial migration onto the anterior iris surface. This theory, most recently espoused by Campbell and coworkers[30] holds that essential iris atrophy begins as an abnormality of the corneal endothelium. This abnormality results in corneal edema in some cases and leads to the production of a cuticular membrane composed of a single layer of endothelial cells and a Descemet's membrane–like structure. The membrane grows over the open anterior chamber angle and onto the anterior surface of the iris. Subsequent contraction of the membrane leads to the formation of peripheral anterior synechiae, to distortion of the pupil, and to iris atrophy. Peripheral anterior synechiae are not a prerequisite for growth of a membrane across the anterior chamber angle; histopathologic studies show the membrane growing across an open angle.[29, 32, 34, 35]

An early report of the specular microscopic appearance of the corneal endothelium in Chandler's syndrome described grossly abnormal cells and suggested that the changes could be confused with cornea guttata.[36] However, a subsequent study indicated that this similarity in specular microscopic findings might be problematic only in advanced cases of the iridocorneal endothelial syndrome and Fuchs' dystrophy, and that the abnormalities observed in the former entity were rather distinctive. In minimally affected corneas the clinical specular microscopic appearance of the endothelium was characterized as a "rounding-up" of the endothelial cells. There was a loss of cellular definition and hexagonal shape, and many pentagonal cells were evident. There was also an increased granularity of the intracellular details, and small, eccentric dark areas appeared in individual cells. These changes seemed to affect virtually all cells.[37]

Moderately affected corneas were characterized by an increased pleomorphism of the endothelial cells and an enlargement of the intracellular dark areas. In some instances these structures extended to the cell margin but they did not appear to cross cell boundaries. In markedly affected corneas a true endothelial mosaic was no longer recognizable, but the dark areas seemingly remained confined within individual cells and did not cross cell boundaries. Surprisingly, corneas with this degree of morphologic endothelial abnormality remained clear and dehydrated, permitting excellent visualization and specular photomicroscopy. It is perhaps important to note that specular microscopy of apparently uninvolved opposite eyes of these patients often revealed a degree of endothelial cell pleomorphism that was inconsistent with the patient's age.[37] The significance of this observation is not known.

Keratoconus

Histologic studies of the cornea in keratoconus suggest that the disorder affects the anterior part of the cornea primarily and the posterior part of the cornea only secondarily. In the early stages of keratoconus reported microscopic changes include fragmentation of the basement membrane of the corneal epithelium along with fibrillar degeneration of Bowman's membrane and the anterior stroma. As the disorder progresses, this is followed by folds and buckles in Descemet's membrane and in the overlying deep stroma.[38, 39]

In cases of keratoconus examined with the clinical specular microscope, the endothelial cells are not radically different from normal.[40] The usual quasi-hexagonal pattern is intact and the dark boundary is smooth. There are no excrescences, pigment deposits, or bright bodies. Overall, the mean cell area is not significantly different from that of a group of age-matched, normal subjects. These observations are perhaps not surprising since, in the great majority of cases of keratoconus, the cornea remains transparent and clinically free of edema and inflammation. However, the endothelium cannot satisfactorily be visualized and photographed with the specular microscope in all cases of keratoconus. The more pronounced the ectasia, the more difficult it becomes to obtain satisfactory specular photomicrographs, so that the relatively benign state of the endothelium in reported series may to some degree reflect an absence of the most severe cases.

While specular microscopy has not uncovered any evidence that incriminates the endothelium as a primary site in the pathogenesis of keratoconus, it has demonstrated the presence of endothelial abnormalities.[40] There appears to be an increase in cellular pleomorphism, a finding that is particularly unusual in view of the relative youth of the population studied. Many cells considerably smaller than normal are distributed throughout the endothelial population. Indeed, after clinically scanning the photomicrographs the examiners were left with the distinct impression that there were two populations of cells, one larger than normal, the other considerably smaller than normal. Unfortunately, the latter observation could not be substantiated by centroid analysis of individual cells.

The most striking abnormality in keratoconus is a directional enlargement of many endothelial cells (Fig. 5–9A).[40] The long axis of these cells seems oriented toward the apex of the cone, and the cells themselves appear to have been stretched by the ectatic process. This observation is consistent with the current concept of acute corneal hydrops, wherein stretching of the endothelium and Descemet's membrane is presumed to result ultimately in the rupture of both structures, allowing considerable aqueous humor to enter the corneal stroma.

In most cases of acute ectasia of the cornea (or corneal hydrops) dehydration of the cornea ultimately occurs. It is presumed that with time the endothelial cells adjacent to the area of rupture enlarge, fill in the defect, and ultimately effect regeneration of Descemet's membrane. The single cornea with a history of acute hydrops in our published series contained a localized area of endothelium in which the cells were seven to ten times larger than normal Fig. 5–17.[40] In other areas of this cornea the endothelial cells were normal both in size and in morphologic appearance. This suggests that the endothelium and Descemet's membrane ruptured in the area of enlarged cells and that the dramatic increase in the size of these cells reflects the changes necessary to repair the affected site, an interpretation that is consistent with our understanding of acute corneal hydrops and its resolution.

The specular photomicrographs also revealed that many endothelial cells contained a dark structure (Fig. 5–18), which in all instances was completely contained within the cell. Invariably there was a normal-appearing area between the dark structure and the cell boundary, and the latter was normal. These intracellular dark structures seemed to occur less frequently in larger endothelial cells. They are consistent in appearance with blebs or vacuoles seen with the electron microscope,[41] but their role in the pathogenesis of keratoconus is completely open to speculation.

Glaucoma

Persistently elevated intraocular pressure produces endothelial trauma, which may result in a gradual diminution of the total endothelial cell population.[42] This detrimental effect upon the site of the mechanisms involved in corneal deturgescence is manifested physiologically by an inverse relationship between the intraocular pressure and the ability of the hydrated cornea to excrete water.[43, 44] Clinically, the deterioration of individual cells and the decrease in the total endothelial cell population are

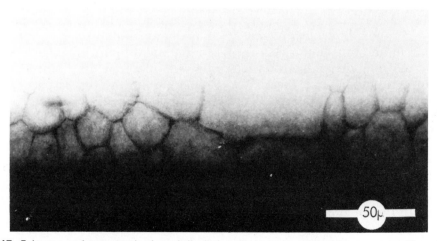

Figure 5–17. Extreme enlargement of endothelial cells in a keratoconic cornea with a history of acute hydrops. Cells in this area are seven to ten times larger than normal.

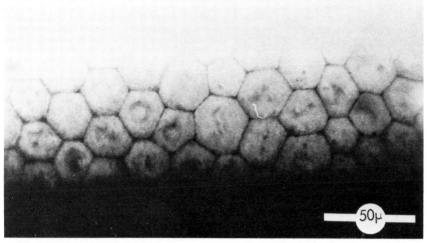

Figure 5–18. Intracellular structures, presumably blebs or vacuoles, in the endothelial cells of a keratoconic cornea.

reflected in the decreasing levels of intraocular pressure at which the cornea becomes edematous in many glaucoma patients as their disease progresses. Irvine reported such a case.[42] At one point in the course of the disease there was no evidence of corneal edema at intraocular pressure levels of 40 to 50 mm. Hg. Two years later, however, the cornea was noted to be edematous when the intraocular pressure exceeded 25 mm. Hg. Specular microscopic studies in patients with unilateral glaucoma or with a history of unilateral attacks of glaucomatocyclitic crisis often show a lower endothelial cell density in the eye afflicted with glaucoma.[45, 46]

Intraocular Inflammation

Experimental studies in rabbits have demonstrated that in the course of an acute anterior uveitis mononuclear inflammatory cells penetrate the apical junctional complexes of corneal endothelial cells and insinuate themselves between endothelial cells as well as between endothelial cells and Descemet's membrane. Endothelial cells seem to suffer little intracellular damage as a result of the inflammatory cell invasion, but in the most advanced cases the inflammatory cells dislodge individual endothelial cells and cause them to float free in the aqueous humor.[47] In his study of the role of the endothelium in bullous keratopathy, Irvine cites intraocular inflammation as a cause of endothelial degeneration and demonstrates histologically the relationship of keratic precipitates to areas of defective endothelium.[48] A clinical specular microscopic study of patients with unilateral iridocyclitis yielded results consistent with animal experiments and histopathologic examination of human tissue. Chronic severe iridocyclitis with mutton-fat keratic precipitates was associated with a decrease in the central endothelial cell count (in comparison with the opposite unaffected eye). In contrast, patients with recurrent attacks of unilateral, nongranulomatous uveitis did not show interocular differences in endothelial cell densities between healthy and affected eyes. In the latter instance, characterized by less severe inflammatory disease, neither the inflammatory process itself nor the accompanying small, round keratic precipitates had a deleterious effect on the central corneal endothelium.[49]

Cataract Extraction

Following conventional cataract extraction (not using phacoemulsification) some degree of endothelial cell loss generally occurs. Numerous investigators have reported their findings,[50–58] and the data show a degree of variability. In uncomplicated cases mean cell loss varies from approximately 6 per cent to 17 per cent, but individual cases range from virtually no cell loss to levels that exceed 40 per cent. Even the latter degree of endothelial cell loss is consistent with corneal transparency during the period of observation, at least in some cases. Intraoperative and postoperative complications are generally associated with a greater mean cell loss than that encountered in uncomplicated cases.[51, 57] We are unaware of any prospective studies comparing the relative endothelial trauma of intracapsular and extracapsular techniques, and we do not know of any data that define the relative trauma to the endothelium of cryoextraction and forceps delivery. Since in many cases of uncomplicated cataract extraction endothelial cell loss is relatively small, the answers to these questions will require large samples and carefully controlled conditions, requirements that are difficult to satisfy clinically. Most studies to date do not show a progressive decrease in endothelial cell density 1 year after cataract extraction.

Phacoemulsification or similar procedures in which the cataract is fragmented by an ultrasonic probe and in which the lens fragments are then irrigated and aspirated from the eye can damage the endothelium. This has been documented in experimental animals, and the endothelial damage has variously been attributed to mechanical injury caused by anterior chamber instrumentation and/or anterior chamber manipulation of a hard lens nucleus, to the ultrasonic vibration, to heat generated by the ultrasonic tip, and to prolonged intraocular irrigation.[59–61] The same type of damage can occur when the procedure is performed clinically in the human eye, and it is more likely to injure the endothelium if Fuchs' dystrophy or similar dystrophic changes are present.[62] Cataract extraction performed by phacoemulsification or a similar method generally results in greater endothelial cell loss than more conventional forms of extraction.[58, 63, 64] Cell loss ranging from 14 per cent to 34 per cent has been reported.

There is specular microscopic evidence that, following cataract extraction, endothelial damage is greatest in the superior part of the cornea in the area of maximal manipulation adjacent to the incision.[65, 66] The inferior portion of the cornea is least affected and shows the least endothelial cell loss. Central endothelial cell counts are intermediate between the other two and may be more a mathematical average of endothelial cell density than an indicator of overall, uniform density. This vertical disparity in endothelial cell density occurs following cataract extraction by conventional techniques or by phacoemulsification, and it has been observed in cases both with and without implantation of an intraocular lens. No such regional differences in endothelial density have been documented in cataractous eyes prior to lens extraction, and time does not appear to alter the vertical cell disparity caused by surgical trauma.

Intraocular Lens Implantation

Although a rare mitotic figure has been observed in the human corneal endothelium,[67] spontaneous division of endothelial cells does not appear to occur to any significant degree in the adult cornea.[68–70] Any type of damage to the endothelium is followed by a decrease in density and an increase in size of the corneal endothelial cells of the injured eye.[71, 72] This is presumed to reflect a process wherein the remaining viable cells enlarge and spread (or slide) to cover the posterior corneal surface left bare by the injured cells. To a surprising degree, these enlarged endothelial cells seem able to compensate physiologically for the cell loss sustained at the time of injury and to maintain corneal deturgescence.

These phenomena are observed following intraocular lens implantation.[50, 51] Even momentary contact between an intraocular lens and the corneal endothelium produces significant endothelial damage and cell loss.[73–75] Available evidence suggests that upon contact, the methacrylate surface of the intraocular lens adheres to the corneal endothelium. Subsequent separation of the two surfaces causes the cell membrane to be torn from endothelial cells, irreversibly damaging most cells. Scanning electron microscopy of the surface of an intraocular lens after contact with the endothelium demonstrates cell membrane material adherent to the lens surface. Other substances such as glass and stainless steel also produce endothelial damage on contact, but the natural crystalline lens of the eye appears to cause little or no damage when it is touched to the endothelium for short periods. Similarly, contact between the corneal endothelium and hydrophilic contact lens material (hydroxyethyl methacrylate) produces minimal endothelial cell damage.[74]

This type of damage to the endothelium can be lessened (and perhaps even eliminated) by two approaches. The first is to coat the hydrophobic surface of the typical intraocular lens with a hydrophilic material.[75, 76] The effectiveness of this approach has been demonstrated experimentally. Immersion of an intraocular lens in either a 40 per cent solution of polyvinyl pyrrolidone or a 1 per cent solution of methylcellulose substantially decreases the amount of endothelial cell damage resulting from subsequent contact of the intraocular lens with the endothelium (in comparison to the degree of damage resulting from contact with an uncoated, acrylic lens). Similarly, coating of the intraocular lens with salt-poor human albumin or serum sharply reduces the damage resulting from contact between the device and the corneal endothelium. Surprisingly, commercial suppliers of intraocular lenses have not utilized this approach to date, but hyaluronic acid (Healon) placed on the surface of the implant prior to its insertion seems to provide a measure of protection for the endothelium.

Alternatively, endothelial damage can be averted by preventing contact between the intraocular lens and the corneal endothelium. Maintenance of a deep anterior chamber at all times during the surgical procedure minimizes the potential for contact. The introduction of hyaluronic acid or an air bubble into the anterior chamber seems to be the most practical and effective way of attaining this result.[77] Contact of the air bubble itself with the endothelium can cause damage to the endothelium.[5, 78, 79] Nonetheless, the degree of reduction in intraocular lens–related endothelial cell damage seems to more than compensate for the inherent toxicity of the air bubble.

Available data provided by specular microscopic studies of the cornea following intraocular lens implantation firmly support the conclusion that the lens implantation procedure is more traumatic to the endothelium than is an uneventful, conventional cataract extraction.[50–56, 58, 66, 80, 81] There is a wide range of reported values of endothelial cell loss after intraocular lens implantation, 7 per cent to 62 per cent, but most are significantly greater than the level of cell loss observed after uncomplicated cataract extraction. This tends to be especially true when results of both procedures performed by the same surgeon are compared. The variability in findings presumably reflects, at least in part, differing degrees of surgical trauma to the corneal endothelium resulting from different lens designs, from different surgical techniques, and from differing levels of surgical skill, as well as methodological limitations of clinical specular microscopy and analysis of the resultant data.

Some investigators have found that a significant number of endothelial cells continue to be lost for many months, and perhaps years, after intraocular lens implantation but not after conventional cataract extraction.[52, 81–83] During the initial postoperative period the central region of the corneal endothelium may not show substantial alterations, but abnormalities invariably are noted in the endothelium of the superior peripheral cornea, presumably the result of surgical trauma. Later in the postoperative period, however, the endothelium covering the central region of the cornea undergoes an increase in cell size, sugesting that these cells have contributed to the repopulation of the traumatized peripheral cornea. Still later, however, there appears to be a progressive, continuing decline in endothelial cell density of eyes containing an intraocular lens implant. Persistent intraocular inflammation is a likely cause of the progressive endothelial cell loss, and Doane has shown that iris plane implants can physically traumatize the corneal endothelium during normal ocular movements.[84] Undoubtedly, however, not all of the etiologic mechanisms have been identified with certainty. Moreover, neither the interval during which these changes take place nor the ultimate degree of endothelial cell damage is known. Indeed, other investigators have not confirmed these findings.[54, 66]

Nonetheless, the weight of current evidence indicates a progressive endothelial cell loss after intraocular lens implantation. This phenomenon appears to occur relatively slowly, so that years may elapse before the critical cell density value below which corneal deturgescence cannot be maintained is reached. If true, this observation suggests the alarming possibility that the relatively advanced average age of patients undergoing intraocular lens implantation tends statistically to favor their death before the critical amount of endothelial cell loss is reached, and merely this fortuitous circumstance explains why the incidence of postoperative edema is not higher. In any event caution should be the byword, particularly when one contemplates an implantation procedure in a younger patient.

Penetrating Keratoplasty

Several investigators have used specular microscopy to observe and evaluate the endothelium of donor corneas prior to their use for penetrating keratoplasty.[58, 85–90] Special chambers that permit evaluation of the endothelium of an excised cornea stored in McCarey-Kaufman medium and that allow inspection of donor endothelium in the intact globe have been constructed. These techniques provide for more detailed and more accurate evaluation of the suitability of donor material for keratoplasty than does observation with the slit-lamp biomicroscope, but as yet they do not appear to be in routine use.

Endothelial changes resulting from or occurring after penetrating keratoplasty also have been studied,[3, 8, 20, 58, 91–95] although it is apparent that such studies are limited to successful, transparent corneal grafts. Giant endothelial cells, indicating extensive cell loss, have been observed (Fig. 5–19). Current theory holds that the relatively uninjured central endothelium compensates for the peripheral cellular damage sustained at the time of surgery.[96] The central endothelial cells enlarge to replace the damaged peripheral cells, providing a functional, limiting, posterior cellular layer for the cornea. There is great variability in endothelial cell loss. In some instances a grafted cornea can remain transparent and support 20/20 vision with less than 20 per cent of its normal endothelial cell complement.[8, 92] On the other hand, little or no endothelial cell loss is observed in other corneal grafts, and one cannot distinguish clinically between a successful corneal transplant with extensive cell loss and one with virtually no cell loss.

In a prospective study in which the endothelial cells were counted preoperatively in the donor eye and in the recipient eye after the transplantation procedure, a 21 per cent cell loss was reported.[58] In a second prospective study the endothelial cell density of the donor tissue was first measured preoperatively in vitro while the tissue was being stored in McCarey-Kaufman medium and then again in the early postoperative period following penetrating keratoplasty. A 23 per cent loss of endothelial cells was reported.[94] There is also an unusual case report in the literature of a donor cornea from a 13-month-old transplanted to an

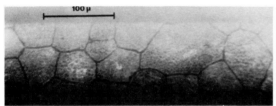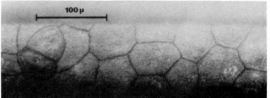

Figure 5–19. Marked enlargement of corneal endothelial cells, indicating extensive cell loss, in successful penetrating corneal transplants. (Courtesy of L. Neubauer, M.D.)

81-year-old recipient with Fuchs' dystrophy and frank bullous keratopathy. In this instance no endothelial cell loss was documented during the 9-month observation period.[97]

Endothelial cell loss occurs much faster in a transplanted cornea than in an innate cornea after intraocular surgery, suggesting a greater vulnerability of the grafted endothelium. There is also evidence that the endothelium of a corneal graft remains in a state of transition for a considerable length of time postoperatively, seemingly reflecting a prolonged healing process. Cell density may decrease and mean cell area increases with time.[20, 95, 98] These changes are progressive and may continue for months and perhaps for years after surgery. Their end point is not known, but presumably this finding explains the sudden decompensation of a grafted cornea years after successful corneal transplantation surgery.

No correlation has been demonstrated between endothelial cell loss (i.e., increased endothelial cell size) and cell shape, donor age, recipient age, time between death and enucleation (within the conventionally accepted limits), or time between enucleation and surgery (again within the conventionally accepted limits). Evidence has been presented that fewer endothelial cells are lost when the corneal grafting procedure is performed in an aphakic eye than when the procedure is performed in a phakic eye.[94] This finding was attributed to the deeper anterior chamber and the absence of endothelial trauma from the lens-iris diaphragm in the aphakic eye. However, it has not been confirmed by subsequent studies.[58, 95]

Sato's study confirmed that there is considerable endothelial cell loss following successful keratoplasty.[20] He found that mean endothelial cell size in a corneal graft was about three times that of endothelial cells of normal individuals in their seventh decade of life and concluded that cell loss was due to surgical trauma and postoperative inflammation and that recovery took place largely by expansion of the surviving cells. Sato also demonstrated in transparent grafts that, although the transplanted cornea recovered excellent deturgescence capabilities, a small but statistically significant increase in corneal thickness (in comparison with normal corneas) persisted. The correlation between graft thickness and endothelial cell size or endothelial cell pleomorphism was not significant. However, the transfer coefficient of fluorescein from the aqueous humor to the cornea was significantly greater in cases of uneventful keratoplasty than in normal corneas, indicating a persistent increase in the endothelial permeability of successful corneal grafts. Thus, endothelial function of the clear graft is not completely normal. The correlation between graft thickness and endothelial permeability (as measured by the transfer coefficient of fluorescein) is statistically significant,[20, 99] suggesting that endothelial permeability, rather than the size or pleomorphism of endothelial cells, is the major factor that determines the thickness of a clear corneal graft.

The specular microscopic data on successful corneal grafts indicate that substantial endothelial cell loss occurs at or slightly after surgery. In many instances there also may be a progressive and sustained cell loss for a considerable period thereafter. There undoubtedly is a critical endothelial cell density below which corneal deturgescence cannot be maintained and irreversible edema occurs. What has been revealed by the specular microscope is the surprisingly low endothelial cell density that can at times maintain the cornea in a dehydrated, transparent state.

Intraocular Irrigating Solutions

Closed intraocular surgery (e.g., phacoemulsification, vitrectomy) requires the introduction into the eye of a large volume of an irrigating solution over a relatively prolonged time period. Several corneal perfusion studies have demonstrated that endothelial structure and function is best maintained when solutions that resemble aqueous humor in composition are used.[100–102] Optimal physiologic function of the endothelium requires that the solution bathing the endothelium have a pH of 7.4, an osmolarity of about 306 milliosmoles, an energy source such as glucose, and appropriate amounts of such ions as Na^+, Ca^{++}, Mg^{++} and HCO_3^-. A bicarbonate buffer system seems to be preferable, reflecting the fact that HCO_3^- is the normal aqueous humor buffer. The addition of adenosine and reduced glutathione to an irrigating solution help maintain endothelial function. These substances improve the performance of the endothelial pump mechanism and prevent ultrastructural changes among the endothelial cells. While glucose is a necessary substrate for cellular aerobic metabolism, adenosine apparently drives the pentose shunt, which increases the rate of adenosine triphosphate (ATP) production and may account for the improvement in the endothelial pump mechanism.[103] Glutathione may prevent the depletion of endothelial ATP levels[104] and may play a role in maintaining cell membrane integrity and endothelial cell junctional complexes.[105–109] Irrigating solutions not satisfying these requirements can rapidly produce adverse endothelial changes and corneal edema. In vitro perfusion experiments demonstrate that these endothelial changes and the resultant corneal swelling are caused by many commercially available intraocular irrigating solutions that are deficient in some essential component. Edelhauser and associates[102] have shown that the intraocular irrigating solution that best maintains endothelial structure and function during in vitro perfusion is glutathione bicarbonate Ringer's (GBR), followed by balanced salt solution, lactated Ringer's, Plasmalyte 148 in water, and 0.9 per cent saline. Although GBR contains all essential ingredients needed to maintain the corneal endothelium, it is not chemically stable once it is formulated. The pH becomes more alkaline with time, and reduced glutathione apparently becomes oxidized within 2 hours.[110] Among commercially available products, BSS Plus maintains human endothelial cell function and ultrastructure throughout a 3- to 4-hour period. BSS Plus is similar to GBR without the adenosine and with the addition of $NaHPO_4$ and oxidized glutathione. It contains the essential ingredients necessary for continued endothelial cell function and is able to maintain its pH stability at 7.4 throughout a 24-hour period. This has been achieved through the addition of $NaHPO_4$ while maintaining a 28-mM. concentration of sodium bicarbonate. Since BSS Plus is able to maintain pH throughout a 24-hour period and since it contains the essential ions and substrates, it meets the current need of ocular surgery.

The adverse effect of various intraocular irrigating solutions on the corneal endothelium has primarily been documented by in vitro perfusion experiments and by measurement of the mean rate of corneal swelling. Increases in the corneal swelling rate can be correlated with degenerative changes in endothelial cells, and the latter have been clearly demonstrated by transmission and scanning electron microscopy.[100–102] There is a paucity of comparable published material describing the effect on the endothelium of intraocular irrigating solutions in vivo using the specular microscope. The few clinical data we have encountered appear to confirm the experimental findings.

Vitreocorneal Contact

Persistent corneal edema, resulting from contact of formed vitreous humor with the corneal endothelium, can occur months to years after uneventful intracapsular cataract extraction, but the precise mechanism of corneal decompensation is not known.[111-114] Since corneal dehydration is controlled primarily by the endothelium, it is assumed that vitreous contact mechanically injures the endothelium and interferes with its physiologic function. Experimental evidence suggests that contact of solid, collagenous elements of the vitreous humor with the endothelium interferes with transport of fluid out of the cornea,[115] and most clinicians agree that liquid or loosely formed vitreous humor is better tolerated and less apt to cause corneal edema than well-formed vitreous humor, particularly if the latter has an intact anterior hyaloid face. However, exceptions certainly occur. Mere contact between formed vitreous humor and the corneal endothelium is not invariably followed by corneal edema, and in those cases in which the phenomenon is encountered the cornea may tolerate vitreous contact and remain clear and dehydrated for extended periods before edema is observed. Factors that appear to contribute significantly to this process include the duration of contact, the density of contact, and the location of contact. Also highly important is the condition of the endothelium at the time of contact; a partially compromised endothelium, such as that encountered in Fuchs' dystrophy, is more apt to succumb to the adverse effects of vitreous contact than is a normal endothelium.[111, 114]

Specular microscopic studies tend to support these clinical concepts.[116, 117] Several types of morphologic abnormalities are observed in the endothelium of corneas in the early stages of decompensation as a result of vitreous contact (Fig. 5–20). Some endothelial cells are markedly enlarged and grossly abnormal in shape. Others contain abnormal bright or dark structures within their cell boundaries. Abnormal cell intersections and side length distributions are encountered, and the central guttate excrescences of Fuchs' dystrophy are not uncommon. However, no structure consistent with the retrocorneal fibrous membrane described by Snip and co-workers[118] has been identified with the specular microscope in the early stages of corneal decompensation due to vitreous touch. These abnormalities have not been seen in an endothelium in contact with formed vitreous humor in the absence of clinical evidence of corneal decompensation, leading to the presumption that they are related to the production of corneal edema. Unfortunately, we have little other objective information about the mechanisms through which vitreous contact causes corneal edema.

Removal of vitreous humor from the anterior chamber by closed vitrectomy, with the elimination of vitreous contact, may result in substantial improvement in the state of corneal hydration and in some cases in the elimination of clinically significant corneal edema.[116, 117, 119] Surprisingly, those endothelial changes seen in edematous corneas prior to vitrectomy appear to persist following vitrectomy and corneal deturgescence (Fig. 5–20C). Despite the seeming irreversibility of the endothelial changes, clinical reversal of corneal edema at times may occur in cases of moderately prolonged vitreous contact. Cases in which closed vitrectomy does not produce complete reversal of corneal edema are those with Fuchs' dystrophy and those with the most bizarre endothelium. Apparently the endothelial changes wrought by vitreous contact progress and can reach a stage of functional irreversibility. In this instance surgical intervention will not result in a visually significant improvement of the corneal edema.

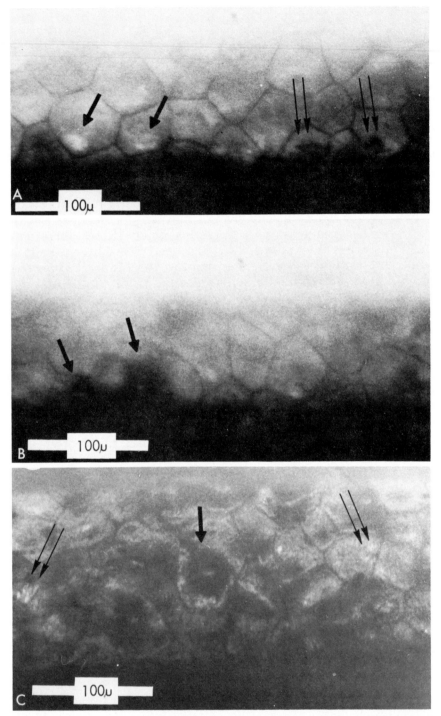

Figure 5–20. Endothelial changes associated with vitreocorneal contact (× 100). *A*, Cells are larger than normal with abnormal shapes and intersections. Intracellular bright (arrows) and dark (double arrows) structures are present. *B*, Extremely large endothelial cells and cornea guttata (arrows). *C*, After vitrectomy (same patient as *B*): Greatly enlarged and misshapen cells containing cornea guttata (arrow) and brightly colored pigment deposits (double arrows) persist despite resolution of corneal edema.

Overall, available data indicate that closed vitrectomy can be a useful procedure for the treatment of corneal decompensation secondary to vitreous contact, particularly if specular photomicroscopy shows that endothelial cell abnormalities are not pronounced. Corneal edema may be reversed and useful vision may be recovered in a substantial percentage of patients despite relatively prolonged periods of vitreous contact and corneal decompensation. On the other hand, vitreous contact does not invariably lead to endothelial destruction and corneal edema, and edema, even of relatively long duration, may be reversible. This would appear to contraindicate the use of closed vitrectomy for vitreous contact in the absence of corneal edema.

Epithelialization of the Anterior Chamber

The endothelial surface of the cornea has been photographed in vivo with the specular microscope during varying stages of epithelialization of the anterior chamber in an effort to define clinical signs that would permit a definite diagnosis to be made in the absence of histopathologic verification. The findings vary somewhat, which is not surprising since evaluation of the corneal endothelium in this entity by specular microscopy is laborious and demanding. Even in the most cooperative of patients, cellular structures may be difficult to detect and, when seen, they often cannot be distinctly focused. Smith and Parrett reported a sharply defined border between normal corneal endothelial cells and the area of epithelial downgrowth.[120] In contrast, in the region occupied by the clinically observed endothelial demarcation line, Laing and coworkers observed enlarged, abnormally shaped endothelial cells inferiorly, blending into an acellular, structureless area superiorly (Fig. 5–21).[121] By focusing more deeply in the seemingly structureless area superiorly, these investigators were able to visualize poorly defined structures that they suggested represented multilayered epithelial cells. However, neither epithelial nor endothelial cells could be identified with certainty in the region above the demarcation line seen with the slit-lamp biomicroscope.

In the four patients examined by Laing and coworkers[121] because of an apparent clinical diagnosis of epithelialization of the anterior chamber, the diagnosis was later verified histopathologically. When the endothelium was successfully visualized with the specular microscope, it usually appeared to be abnormal. Considerable cell loss seemed to have occurred, as evidenced by the large size of the remaining cells. Whether this cell loss results from a traumatic insult during the prior surgery and contributes to the subsequent epithelial invasion of the anterior chamber or, alternatively, whether it is produced by the advancing layer of epithelium is not clear. The specular photomicrographs show only that endothelial cells are present but are large and abnormal-appearing when the clinically visible demarcation line is well above the region photographed. Experimentally it has been shown that the epithelium will migrate and cover a stromal surface as well as Descemet's membrane if the latter is devoid of endothelium. However, epithelial advancement is inhibited if the epithelium makes contact with the endothelium.[122] These experimental observations suggest that normally functioning endothelial cells are necessary to inhibit epithelial invasion of the anterior chamber. Presumably damage or destruction of the corneal endothelium contributes to epithelial invasion of the anterior chamber. This concept is supported by the in vivo demonstration with the specular microscope of abnormal endothelial cells well below the site of clinically evident epithelialization in eyes in which the invading epithelium subsequently advanced.

When epithelialization was moderately advanced, cellular structures were seen that did not have the morphologic appearance of endothelial cells. Presumably these were epithelial cells, but this

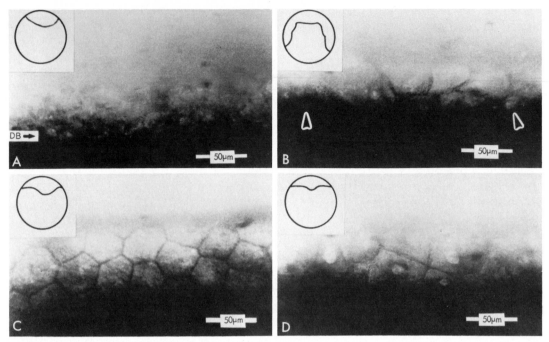

Figure 5–21. Endothelial changes associated with epithelialization of anterior chamber (× 100). Inset accompanying each specular photomicrograph shows the clinical appearance of the endothelial demarcation line. In each instance the specular photomicrograph was taken below the demarcation line. DB = dark boundary. *A,* Only well-focused amorphous structures are seen. *B,* Visible cells are substantially enlarged and morphologically abnormal. Arrows point to amorphous structures. *C,* Cells are 2.5 times larger than those seen in normal subject of same age. *D,* Poorly delineated cells are approximately six times larger than those seen in normal subjects of same age. Bright structures are present within many cells.

is not certain. In the most advanced cases no distinct cell boundaries at all could be seen. Only a disorganized, amorphous, membranous layer containing some formed structures was visualized. Again, the presumption is that this is a thickened, multilayered epithelial membrane whose structure does not permit satisfactory resolution by the specular microscope. This presumption is supported by the fact that the problem of endothelial resolution was encountered in corneas that were optically clear on examination with the slit-lamp biomicroscope and free of significant edema as measured with the corneal pachymeter. In the absence of corneal edema, the inability to see endothelial structures distinctly with the specular microscope suggests either that the endothelium is disorganized or that more than a single layer of cells is·present. The invading epithelium also produces an irregular layer of fibrillar material along the epi-

thelial–Descemet's membrane interface[123] that may contribute to the gray appearance of the involved cornea and to the difficulty encountered in obtaining a clear image of the structures in the zone of specular reflection.

We have pointed out above that information about the posterior surface of the endothelium (i.e., the surface in contact with the aqueous humor) can be obtained by evaluating the appearance of the dark boundary, the interface between the endothelial cell pattern and the adjacent dark zone produced by the aqueous humor. If, as in the normal eye, the posterior endothelial surface is smooth, the resulting dark boundary will be straight and smooth; an irregular endothelial surface produces an irregular dark boundary. In the specular photomicrographs of patients with epithelialization of the anterior chamber following cataract extraction, the dark boundary varies from ragged to smooth

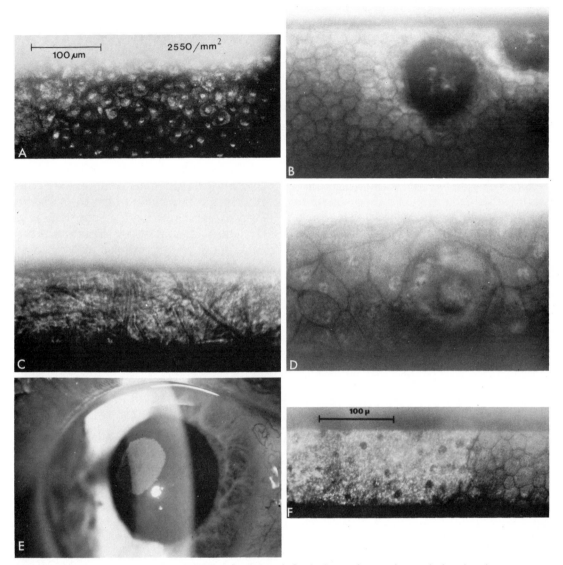

Figure 5–22. Miscellaneous endothelial findings. *A,* Posterior polymorphous dystrophy: Appearance of endothelium in area of deep dystrophic change. *B,* Posterior polymorphous dystrophy: endothelium in area of deep dystrophic change is obscured. Immediately surrounding endothelial cells are elongated or irregular in shape, or both. Endothelium at a distance from the dystrophic change appears normal. *C,* Specular photomicrograph of a thickened, irregular Descemet's membrane. The endothelium is not seen in this photograph but can be visualized by focusing at a deeper plane. *D,* Unusual endothelial structure and enlarged cells with bright bodies in a corneal transplant following successful therapy of a rejection reaction. *E,* Clinical photograph of iris pigment epithelial cells, presumably dislocated during cataract surgery, on the corneal endothelium. This abnormality was observed to enlarge progressively before it stabilized at this size about 8 months postoperatively. *F,* Specular photomicrograph of this structure including its border with the adjacent normal endothelium. Note the circular dark spots, which we believe represent the nuclei of iris pigment epithelial cells. (*A, C, E,* and *F* courtesy of L. Neubauer, M.D.)

and uneven, indicating the presence of irregularities in the contour of the posterior corneal surface, even in the absence of a recognizable endothelial pattern (Fig. 5–21).

Blunt Trauma

Blunt trauma to the cornea can damage the endothelium. Bourne and coworkers[124] have reported their findings on a 16-year-old boy who had suffered a BB injury of the right eye 2 years previously. Clinically, both corneas were clear and free of edema; evidence of prior endothelial damage was revealed only by clinical specular microscopy. The endothelial cells on the right were enlarged and central endothelial cell density was only 47 per cent of that of the opposite, normal left eye. Although it is suspected that in instances such as this the residual endothelial cells might be more sus-

ceptible to subsequent trauma than normal cells, no additional cell loss was documented following cataract extraction by phacoemulsification in this particular case.

The impact of small, nonpenetrating foreign bodies on the cornea may give rise to clinically apparent gray rings on the corneal endothelium.[125, 126] Reproduction of these rings in experimental animals reveals that they consist of swollen or disrupted endothelial cells. The center of each ring corresponds to the epithelial impact site of the foreign body, with the least disruption of the endothelium occurring here. Specular microscopic studies confirm that posterior annular keratopathy occurring after blunt corneal trauma in humans represents a contusion injury and consists of disrupted and swollen endothelial cells.[127] The damaged cells may still be evident many days after the clinically visible endothelial rings disappear and,

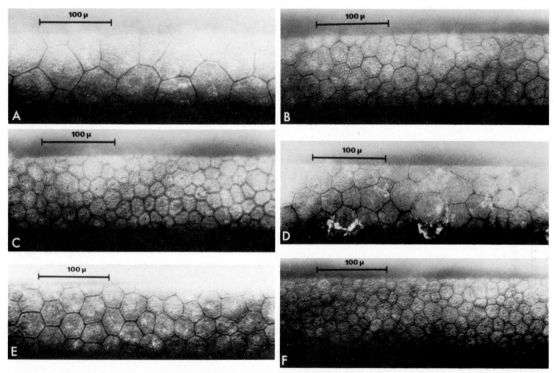

Figure 5–23. Miscellaneous endothelial findings: *A–C,* Vertical disparity after cataract extraction and insertion of Binkhorst iris clip intraocular lens implant. *A,* Superior cornea (cell count = 339/mm²). *B,* Inferior cornea (cell count = 1436/mm²). *C,* Opposite unoperated eye of same patient (cell count = 2766/mm²). *D,* Vitreocorneal contact—pigment on the anterior vitreous face in contact with endothelium. *E,* Eye of a patient treated for buphthalmos for 19 years. Intraocular pressure regulated with medication—no history of surgery (cell count = 1170/mm²). *F,* Opposite normal eye of same patient (cell count = 3325/mm²). (Courtesy of L. Neubauer, M.D.)

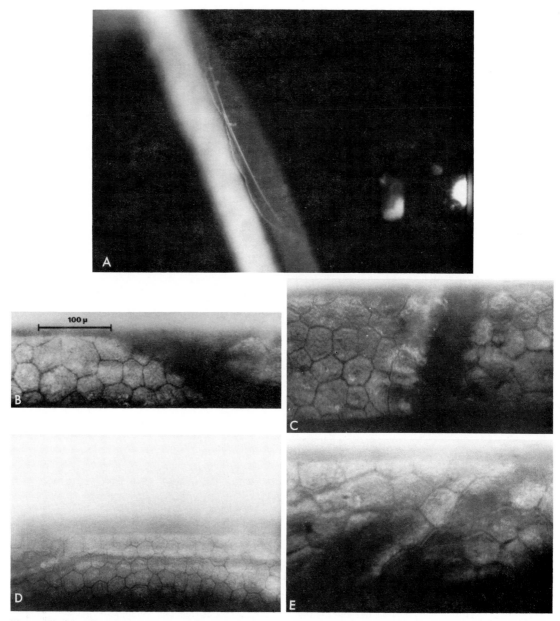

Figure 5–24. Miscellaneous endothelial findings: *A*, Slit lamp photograph of rupture of Descemet's membrane. *B*, Specular photomicrography of cornea pictured in *A*. *C*, Specular photomicrograph of a second patient with rupture of Descemet's membrane induced by forceps delivery. *D* and *E*, Linear structure representing an artifact caused by applanation of the objective lens cone of the contact specular microscope. (*A, B,* and *D* courtesy of L. Neubauer, M.D.)

indeed, permanent cell loss may occur. As might be expected, the degree of endothelial cell loss appears to be related to the severity of the injury; a measurable decrease in cell density occurs only in the more severely injured corneas.

most such cases our knowledge of the nature and significance of these findings is limited, and for the present we can do little better than describe what we see and speculate. However, continuing studies with improved instrumentation are certain to uncover many of the mysteries of the corneal endothelium.

Miscellaneous Endothelial Findings

A number of other interesting and unusual findings can be observed and documented in or adjacent to the corneal endothelium using the clinical specular photomicroscope. Examples are illustrated in Figures 5–22 through 5–24. In

Acknowledgment

The authors are indebted to Setsuko S. Oak and to Lorenz Neubauer, M.D., for their assistance with the final preparation of this chapter.

REFERENCES

1. Maurice, D. M.: Cellular membrane activity in the corneal endothelium of the intact eye. Experientia 24:1094, 1968.
2. Brown, N.: Macrophotography of the anterior segment of the eye. Brit J Ophthalmol 54:697, 1970.
3. Bron, A. J., and Brown, N.: Endothelium of the corneal graft. Trans Ophthalmol Soc UK 94:863, 1974.
4. Hoefle, F. B., Maurice, D. M., and Sibley, R.: Human corneal donor material. A method of examination before keratoplasty. Arch Ophthalmol 84:741, 1970.
5. Leibowitz, H. M., Laing, R. A., and Sandstrom, M.M.: Corneal endothelium. The effect of air in the anterior chamber. Arch Ophthalmol 92:227, 1974.
6. Laing, R. A., Sandstrom, M. M., and Leibowitz, H. M.: In vivo photomicrography of the corneal endothelium. Arch Ophthalmol 93:143, 1975.
7. Laing, R. A., Sandstrom, M. M., Berrospi, A. R., and Leibowitz, H. M.: Changes in the corneal endothelium as a function of age. Exp Eye Res 22:587, 1976.
8. Laing, R. A., Sandstrom, M. M., Berrospi, A. R., and Leibowitz, H. M.: Morphological changes in corneal endothelial cells after penetrating keratoplasty. Amer J Ophthalmol 82:459, 1976.
9. Bourne, W. M., and Enoch, J. M.: Some optical principles of the clinical specular microscope. Invest Ophthalmol 15:29, 1976.
10. Koester, C. J.: Scanning mirror microscope with optical sectioning characteristics: Applications in ophthalmology. Appl Optics 19:1749, 1980.
11. Sherrard, E. S., and Buckley, R. J.: Contact clinical specular microscopy of the corneal endothelium: Optical modifications to the applanation objective cone. Invest Ophthalmol Vis Sci 20:816, 1981.
12. Laing, R. A., Neubauer, L., and Oak, S. S.: Personal communication, 1982.
13. Bigar, F., Witmer, R., and Thaer, A.: Die Spiegelmikroskopie des Hornhautendothels. Klin Monatsbl Augenheilk 173:742, 1978.
14. Davidovits, P., and Egger, M. D.: Photomicrography of corneal endothelial cells in vivo. Nature 244:366, 1973.
15. Laing, R. A., Sandstrom, M. M., and Leibowitz, H. M.: Clinical specular microscopy. I. Optical principles. Arch Ophthalmol 97:1714, 1979.
16. Laing, R. A., Sandstrom, M. M., and Leibowitz, H. M.: Clinical specular microscopy. II. Qualitative evaluation of corneal endothelial photomicrographs. Arch Ophthalmol 97:1720, 1979.
17. Laing, R. A., Leibowitz, H. M., Chang, R. C., Theodore, J., and Oak, S. S.: The endothelial mosaic in Fuchs' dystrophy. A qualitative evaluation with the specular microscope. Arch Ophthalmol 99:80, 1981.
18. Bourne, W. M., and Kaufman, H. E.: Specular microscopy of the human corneal endothelium in vivo. Amer J Ophthalmol 81:319, 1976.
19. McCarey, B. E.: Noncontact specular microscopy. A macrophotography technique and some endothelial cell findings. Ophthalmology 86:1848, 1979.
20. Sato, T.: Studies on the endothelium of the corneal graft. Jpn J Ophthalmol 22:114, 1978.
21. Blatt, H. L., Rao, G. N., and Aquavella, J. V.: Endothelial cell density in relation to morphology. Invest Ophthalmol 18:856, 1979.
22. Laule, A., Cable, M. K., Hoffman, C. E., and Hanna, C.: Endothelial cell population changes of human cornea during life. Arch Ophthalmol 96:2031, 1978.
23. Shaw, E. L., Rao, G.N., Arthur, E. J., and Aquavella, J. V.: The functional reserve of corneal endothelium. Ophthalmology 86:640, 1978.
24. Goar, E. L.: Dystrophy of the corneal endothelium (cornea guttata), with a report of a histological examination. Amer J Ophthalmol 17:215, 1934.
25. Lorenzetti, D. W. C., Uotila, M. H., Parikh, N., and Kaufman, H. E.: Central cornea guttata. Incidence in the general population. Amer J Ophthalmol 64:115, 1967.
26. Waring, G. O., Font, R. L., Rodrigues, M. M., and

Mulberger, R. D.: Alterations of Descemet's membrane in interstitial keratitis. Amer J Ophthalmol 81:773, 1976.

27. Polack, F. M.: The posterior corneal surface in Fuchs' dystrophy: Scanning electron microscopic study. Invest Ophthalmol 13:913, 1974.

28. Waring, G. O., Rodrigues, M. M., and Laibson, P. R.: Corneal dystrophies. II. Endothelial dystrophies. Surv Ophthalmol 23:147, 1978.

29. Shields, M. B.: Progressive essential iris atrophy, Chandler's syndrome and the iris nevus (Cogan-Reese) syndrome. A spectrum of diseases. Surv Ophthalmol 24:3, 1979.

30. Campbell, D. G., Shields, M. B., and Smith, T. R.: The corneal endothelium in the spectrum of essential iris atrophy. Amer J Ophthalmol 86:317, 1978.

31. Quigley, H. A., and Forster, R. F.: Histopathology of cornea and iris in Chandler's syndrome. Arch Ophthalmol 96:1878, 1978.

32. Shields, M. B., McCracken, J. S., Klintworth, G. K., and Campbell, D. G.: Corneal edema in essential iris atrophy. Ophthalmology 86:1533, 1979.

33. Hirst, L. W., Quigley, H. A., Stark, W. J., and Shields, M. B.: Specular microscopy of iridocorneal endothelial syndrome. Amer J Ophthalmol 89:11, 1980.

34. Rodrigues, M. M., Streeten, B. W., Spaeth, G. L.: Chandler's syndrome as a variant of essential iris atrophy. A clinicopathologic study. Arch Ophthalmol 96:646, 1978.

35. Scheie, H. G., Yanoff, M., and Kellogg, W. T.: Essential iris atrophy. Report of a case. Arch Ophthalmol 94:1315, 1976.

36. Hetherington, J., Jr.: The spectrum of Chandler's syndrome. Ophthalmology 85:240, 1978.

37. Hirst, L. W., Quigley, H. A., Stark, W. J., and Shields, M. B.: Specular microscopy of iridocorneal endothelial syndrome. Amer J Ophthalmol 89:11, 1980.

38. Chi, H. H., Katzin, H. M., and Teng, C. C.: Histopathology of keratoconus. Amer J Ophthalmol 42:847, 1956.

39. Teng, C. C.: Electron microscopic study of the pathology of keratoconus. Amer J Ophthalmol 55:18, 1963.

40. Laing, R. A., Sandstrom M. M., Berrospi, A. R., and Leibowitz, H. M.: The human corneal endothelium in keratoconus. A specular microscopic study. Arch Ophthalmol 97:1867, 1979.

41. Jakus, M. A.: Further observations on the fine structure of the cornea. Invest Ophthalmol 1:202, 1962.

42. Irvine, A. R.: The role of the endothelium in bullous keratopathy. Arch Ophthalmol 56:338, 1956.

43. Harris, J. E., Gehrsitz, L., and Gruber, L.: The hydration of the cornea. II. The effect of the intraocular pressure. Amer J Ophthalmol 42:325, 1956.

44. Ytteborg, J., and Dohlman, C. H.: Corneal edema and intraocular pressure. II. Clinical results. Arch Ophthalmol 74:477, 1965.

45. Vannas, A., Setala, K., and Ruusuvaara, P.: Endothelial cells in capsular glaucoma. Acta Ophthalmol 55:951, 1977.

46. Setala, K., and Vannas, A.: Endothelial cells in glaucomato-cyclitic crisis. Adv Ophthalmol 36:218, 1978.

47. Inomata, H., and Smelser, G.: Fine structural alterations of corneal endothelium during experimental uveitis. Invest Ophthalmol 9:272, 1970.

48. Irvine, A. R., Jr.: The role of the endothelium in bullous keratopathy. Arch Ophthalmol 56:338, 1956.

49. Setala, K.: Corneal endothelial cell density in iridocyclitis. Acta Ophthalmol 57:277, 1979.

50. Bourne, W. M., and Kaufman, H. E.: Endothelial damage associated with intraocular lenses. Amer J Ophthalmol 81:482, 1976.

51. Forstot, S. L., Blackwell, W. L., Jaffe, N. S., and Kaufman, H. E.: The effect of intraocular lens implantation on the corneal endothelium. Trans Amer Acad Ophthalmol Otolaryngol 83:195, 1977.

52. Hirst, L. W., Snip, R. C., Stark, W. J., and Maumenee, A. E.: Qualitative corneal endothelial evaluation in intraocular lens implantation and cataract surgery. Amer J Ophthalmol 84:775, 1977.

53. Cheng, H., Sturrock, G. D., Rubinstein, B., and Bulpitt, C. J.: Endothelial cell loss and corneal thickness after intracapsular extraction and iris clip lens implantation: A randomized controlled trial (interim report). Brit J Ophthalmol 61:785, 1977.

54. Sugar, A., Fetherolf, E. C., Lin, L. L. K., Ostbaum, S.A., and Galin, M.A.: Endothelial cell loss from intraocular lens insertion. Ophthalmology 85:394, 1978.

55. Sugar, J., Mitchelson, J., and Kraff, M.: Endothelial trauma and cell loss from intraocular lens insertion. Arch Ophthalmol 96:449, 1978.

56. Drews, R. C., and Waltman, S. R.: Endothelial cell loss in intraocular lens placement. Amer Intraoc Implant Soc J 4:14, 1978.

57. Bourne, W. M., and Kaufman, H. E.: Cataract extraction and the corneal endothelium. Amer J Ophthalmol 82:44, 1976.

58. Abbott, R. L., and Forster, R. K.: Clinical specular microscopy and intraocular surgery. Arch Ophthalmol 97:1476, 1979.

59. Binder, P. S., Sternberg, H., Wickman, M. G., and Worthen, D. M.: Corneal endothelial damage associated with phacoemulsification. Amer J Ophthalmol 82:48, 1976.

60. Polack, F. M., and Sugar, A.: The phacoemulsification procedure. II. Corneal endothelial changes. Invest Ophthalmol 15:458, 1976.

61. McCarey, B. E., Polack, F. M., and Marshall, E.: The phacoemulsification procedure. I. The effect of intraocular irrigating solutions on the corneal endothelium. Invest Ophthalmol 15:449, 1976.

62. Polack, F. M., and Sugar, A.: The phacoemulsification procedure. III. Corneal complications. Invest Ophthalmol Vis Sci 16:39, 1977.

63. Irvine, A. R., Kratz, R. P., and O'Donnell, J. J.: Endothelial damage with phacoemulsification and intraocular lens implantation. Arch Ophthalmol 96:1023, 1978.

64. Sugar, J., Mitchelson, J., and Kraff, M.: The effect of phacoemulsification on corneal endothelial cell density. Arch Ophthalmol 96:446, 1978.

65. Hoffer, K. J.: Vertical endothelial cell disparity. Amer J Ophthalmol 87:344, 1979.

66. Galin, M. A., Lin, L. L., Fetherolf, E., Ostbaum, S. A., and Sugar, A.: Time analysis of corneal endothelial cell density after cataract extraction. Amer J Ophthalmol 88:93, 1979.

67. Kaufman, H. E., Capella, J. A., and Robbins, J. E.: The human corneal endothelium. Amer J Ophthalmol 61:835, 1966.

68. Smelser, G. K., and Ozanics, V.: New concepts in the anatomy and histology of the cornea. In King, J. H., and McTigue, J. W. (eds): The Cornea: First World Congress. London, Butterworth & Co., 1964, pp. 1–20.

69. Van Horn, D. L., Sendels, D. D., Seideman, S. S.,

and Buco, D. J.: Regenerative capacity of the corneal endothelium in rabbit and cat. Invest Ophthalmol Vis Sci 16:597, 1977.

70. Van Horn, D. L., and Hyndiuk, R. A.: Endothelial wound repair in primate cornea. Exp Eye Res 21:113, 1975.

71. Kaufman, H. E., and Katz, J.: Pathology of the corneal endothelium. Invest Ophthalmol Vis Sci 16:265, 1977.

72. Bourne, W. M., McCarey, B. E., and Kaufman, H. E.: Clinical specular microscopy. Trans Amer Acad Ophthalmol Otolaryngol 81:743, 1976.

73. Kaufman, H. E., Katz, J., Valenti, J., Sheets, J. W., and Goldberg, E. P.: Corneal endothelium damage with intraocular lenses: Contact adhesion between surgical materials and tissue. Science 198:525, 1977.

74. Kaufman, H. E., and Katz, J. I.: Endothelial damage from intraocular lens insertion. Invest Ophthalmol 15:996, 1976.

75. Kirk, S., Burde, R. M., and Waltman, S. R.: Minimizing corneal endothelial damage due to intraocular lens contact. Invest Ophthalmol Vis Sci 16:1053, 1977.

76. Katz, J., Kaufman, H. E., Goldberg, E. P., and Sheets, J. W.: Prevention of endothelial damage from intraocular lens insertion. Trans Amer Acad Ophthalmol Otolaryngol 83:204, 1977.

77. Bourne, W. M., Brubaker, R. F., and O'Fallon, W. M.: Use of air to decrease endothelial cell loss during intraocular lens implantation. Arch Ophthalmol 97:1473, 1979.

78. Van Horn, D. L., Edelhauser, H. F., Aaberg, T. M., and Pederson, H. J.: In vivo effects of air and sulfur hexafluoride gas on rabbit corneal endothelium. Invest Ophthalmol 11:1028, 1972.

79. Olsen, R. J.: Air and the corneal endothelium. An in-vivo specular microscopic study in cats. Arch Ophthalmol 98:1283, 1980.

80. Binkhorst, C. D., Nygaard, P., and Loones, L. H.: Specular microscopy of the corneal endothelium and lens implant surgery. Amer J Ophthalmol 85:597, 1978.

81. Rao, G. N., Stevens, R. E., Harris, J. K., and Aquavella, J. V.: Long term changes in corneal endothelium following intraocular lens implantation. Ophthalmology 88:386, 1981.

82. Rao, G. N., Shaw, E. L., Arthur, E., and Aquavella, J. V.: Morphological appearance of the healing corneal endothelium. Arch Ophthalmol 96:2027, 1978.

83. Hoffer, K. J.: Corneal decompensation after corneal endothelium cell count. Amer J Ophthalmol 87:252, 1979.

84. Doane, M. G., Miller, D., and Korb, D.: Applications of high-speed cinematography in the evaluation of intraocular and contact lenses. Invest Ophthal Vis Sci 22(Suppl.):164, 1982.

85. Hoefle, F. B., Maurice, D. M., and Sibley, R. C.: Human corneal donor material: A method for examination before keratoplasty. Arch Ophthalmol 84:741, 1970.

86. Bigar, F., Schimmelpfennig, B., and Giesler, R.: Routine evaluation of endothelium in human donor corneas. Albrecht von Graefes Arch Klin Exp Ophthalmol 200:195, 1976.

87. Schimmelpfennig, B., Bigar, F., Witmer, R., and Hürzeler, R.: Endothelial changes in human donor corneas. Albrecht von Graefes Arch Klin Exp Ophthalmol 200:201, 1976.

88. Bigar, F., Schimmelpfennig, B., and Hürzeler, R.: Cornea guttata in donor material. Arch Ophthalmol 96:653, 1978.

89. Bourne, W. M.: Examination and photography of donor corneal endothelium. Arch Ophthalmol 94:1799, 1976.

90. McCarey, B. E., and McNeil, J. I.: Specular microscopic evaluation of donor corneal endothelium. Ann Ophthalmol 9:1279, 1977.

91. Ruben, M., Colebrook, E., and Guillon, M.: Keratoconus, keratoplasty thickness, and endothelial morphology. Brit J Ophthalmol 63:790, 1979.

92. Bourne, W. M., and Kaufman, H. E.: The endothelium of clear corneal transplants. Arch Ophthalmol 94:1730, 1976.

93. Rao, G. N., Shaw, E. L., Arthur, E. J., and Aquavella, J.V.: Morphological appearance of the healing corneal endothelium. Arch Ophthalmol 96:2027, 1978.

94. Bourne, W. M., and O'Fallon, W. M.: Endothelial cell loss during penetrating keratoplasty. Amer J Ophthalmol 85:760, 1978.

95. Rao, G. N., Stevens, R. E., Mandelberg, A. I., and Aquavella, J. V.: Morphologic variations in graft endothelium. Arch Ophthalmol 98:1403, 1980.

96. Doughman, D. J., Van Horn, D. L., Rodman, W. P., Byrnes, P., and Lindstrom, R. L.: Human corneal endothelial layer repair during organ culture. Arch Ophthalmol 94:1791, 1976.

97. Rao, G. N., Waldron, W. R., and Aquavella, J. V.: Fate of endothelium in a corneal graft. Ann Ophthalmol 16:645, 1978.

98. Bourne, W. M.: One-year observation of transplanted human corneal endothelium. Ophthalmology 87:673, 1980.

99. Ota, Y.: Endothelial permeability of fluorescein in corneal grafts and bullous keratopathy. Jpn J Ophthalmol 19:286, 1975.

100. Edelhauser, H. F., Van Horn, D. L., Hyndiuk, R. A., and Schultz, R. O.: Intraocular irrigating solutions. Their effect on the corneal endothelium. Arch Ophthalmol 93:648, 1975.

101. Edelhauser, H. F., Van Horn, D. L., Schultz, R. O., and Hyndiuk, R. A.: Comparative toxicity of intraocular irrigating solutions on the corneal endothelium. Amer J Ophthalmol 81:473, 1976.

102. Edelhauser, H. F., Gonnering, R., and Van Horn, D. L.: Intraocular irrigating solutions. A comparative study of BSS Plus and lactated Ringer's solution. Arch Ophthalmol 96:516, 1978.

103. McCarey, B. E., Edelhauser, H. F., and Van Horn, D. L.: Functional and structural changes in the corneal endothelium during in vitro perfusion. Invest Ophthalmol 12:410, 1973.

104. Fischbarg, J.: Active and passive properties of the rabbit corneal endothelium. Exp Eye Res 15:615, 1973.

105. Dikstein, S., and Maurice, D. M.: The metabolic basis to the fluid pump in the cornea. J Physiol 221:29, 1972.

106. Dikstein, S.: Efficiency and survival of the corneal endothelial pump. Exp Eye Res 15:639, 1973.

107. Kosower, E. M., and Kosower, N. W.: Lest I forget thee, glutathione. Nature 224:117, 1969.

108. Epstein, D. L., and Kinoshita, J. H.: The effect of diamide on lens glutathione and lens membrane function. Invest Ophthalmol 9:629, 1970.

109. Edelhauser, H. F., Van Horn, D. L., Miller, M. P., and Pederson, H. J.: The effect of thiol-oxidation of glutathione with diamide on corneal endo-

thelial function, junctional complexes, and microfilaments. J Cell Biol 68:567, 1976.

110. Anderson, E. I., Fischbarg, J., and Spector, A.: Disulfide stimulation of fluid transport and effect on ATP level in rabbit corneal endothelium. Exp Eye Res 19:1, 1974.

111. Leahy, B. D.: Bullous keratitis from vitreous contact. Arch Ophthalmol 46:22, 1951.

112. Chandler, P. A.: Complications after cataract extraction: Clinical aspects. Trans Amer Acad Ophthalmol Otolaryngol 58:382, 1954.

113. Goar, E. L.: Postoperative hyaloid adhesions to the cornea. Amer J Ophthalmol 45:99, 1958.

114. Jaffe, N. S.: Cataract surgery and its complications. 2nd ed. St. Louis, C. V. Mosby Co., 1976, pp. 256–271.

115. Fischbarg, J., and Stuart, J.: The effect of vitreous humor on fluid transport by rabbit corneal endothelium. Invest Ophthalmol 14:497, 1975.

116. Leibowitz, H. M., Laing, R. A., Chang, R., Theodore, J., and Oak, S. S.: Corneal edema secondary to vitreocorneal touch. Arch Ophthalmol 99:417, 1981.

117. Homer, P. I., Peyman, G.A., and Sugar, J.: Automated vitrectomy in eyes with vitreocorneal touch associated with corneal dysfunction. Amer J Ophthalmol 89:500, 1980.

118. Snip, R. C., Kenyon, K. R., and Green, W. R.: Retrocorneal fibrous membrane in the vitreous touch syndrome. Amer J Ophthalmol 79:233, 1975.

119. Wilkinson, C. P., and Rowsey, J. J.: Closed vitrectomy for the vitreous touch syndrome. Amer J Ophthalmol 90:304, 1980.

120. Smith, R. E., and Parrett, C.: Specular microscopy of epithelial downgrowth. Arch Ophthalmol 96:1222, 1978.

121. Laing, R. A., Sandstrom, M. M., Leibowitz, H. M., and Berrospi, A. R.: Epithelialization of the anterior chamber. Clinical investigation with the specular microscope. Arch Ophthalmol 97:1870, 1979.

122. Cameron, J. D., Flaxman, B. A., and Yanoff, M.: In vitro studies of corneal wound healing: Epithelial-endothelial interactions. Invest Ophthalmol 13:575, 1974.

123. Jensen, P., Minckler, D., and Chandler, J. W.: Epithelial ingrowth. Arch Ophthalmol 95:837, 1977.

124. Bourne, W. M., McCarey, B. E., and Kaufman, H. E.: Clinical specular microscopy. Trans Amer Acad Ophthalmol Otolaryngol 81:OP743, 1976.

125. Cibis, G. W., Weingeist, T. A., and Krachmer, J. H.: Traumatic corneal endothelial rings. Arch Ophthalmol 96:485, 1978.

126. Forstot, S. L., and Gasset, A. R.: Transient traumatic posterior annular keratopathy of Payrau. Arch Ophthalmol 92:527, 1974.

127. Maloney, W. F., Colvard, D. M., Bourne, W. M., and Gordon, R.: Specular microscopy of traumatic posterior annular keratopathy. Arch Ophthalmol 97:1647, 1979.

6 Corneal Edema

JAMES V. AQUAVELLA, M.D.

To perform its primary function, the refraction of light, the cornea must be relatively thin and dehydrated and it must retain a smooth anterior refracting surface. In a normal cornea optical transparency is directly related to the state of hydration of the tissue. If the cornea swells, it increases in thickness and its surface becomes irregular. Both changes downgrade its optical properties and interfere with vision.

The maintenance of normal hydration is achieved by several mechanisms acting in concert. The epithelium and endothelium act as semipermeable membranes, creating a barrier to the flow of water into the cornea from tears and aqueous humor.[1] Evaporation from the corneal surface osmotically extracts water from the cornea, although this plays a minor role in corneal dehydration in man.[2] Finally, there is a continuous, physiologic transport of water from the cornea. Metabolic energy is required for this function, which occurs in the endothelium.[3-5]

Current concepts relating to the functional capacity of the cornea to remain dehydrated attribute primary responsibility for the state of corneal deturgescence to an active metabolic pump in the endothelium. Clinical attention is focused on the dynamic reserve of the endothelium, since a variety of intrinsic and extrinsic insults may compromise the corneal endothelium. In some instances the damage results in latent morphologic changes that are unrecognized because they are not associated with immediate clinical signs of decompensation. In other instances there is overt decompensation with clinical edema. Such episodes may be of sufficient magnitude to preclude a return to the normal state of deturgescence, or they may be of a transient or reversible nature, allowing for ultimate return of normal corneal thickness, transparency, and normal corneal function. However, even in instances of complete clinical recovery the capacity of the endothelium to sustain future trauma may have been permanently compromised, leaving the cornea more vulnerable to a future insult.

Thus, at any given moment the functional capacity of the corneal endothelium, and therefore the ability of the cornea to remain in its normal state of deturgescence, is a measure of the sum total of limitations imposed by a variety of factors. These factors may be inherited, presenting as a congenital abnormality, or they may be correlated with aging. They may act alone or in concert with traumatic, toxic, or inflammatory stimuli to influence endothelial function. Manifestations of corneal disease may be morphologic or functional or both. The resultant defects may be latent or they may be clinically manifest in a variety of objective and subjective sequelae.

The classical morphologic response of a compromised endothelial cell is the elaboration of Descemet's membrane, which may differ qualitatively and quantitatively from that observed in the young healthy cornea (cornea guttata). A second set of morphologic characteristics is associated with the altered appearance of the endothelial cells themselves. As a result, cell density, size, and architecture are becoming increasingly viewed as valid parameters of endothelial cell function.

THE NATURE OF THE INSULT

A number of classifications have been proposed to differentiate various types of corneal dysfunction on an etiologic basis. Because the term "dystrophy" is firmly entrenched in the literature, Stocker[5] elected to retain the term while broadening its definition to include defective nourishment, abnormal development, and degeneration. Therefore, the primary endothelial dystrophies are considered to occur as a result of intrinsic factors such as constitution, heredity, and aging. The secondary endothelial dystrophies encompass those entities in which degeneration occurs as a result of an extrinsic condition. Bearing in mind the concept of a dynamic endothelium, one can easily conceive of a cornea whose functional capacity is limited by hereditary factors (primary dystrophy) but ultimately succumbs to the added burden imposed by elevated intraocular pressure, chronic inflammation, or surgical trauma (secondary dystrophy).

Primary Endothelial Dystrophies

The primary endothelial dystrophies include congenital dystrophies (malformations) as well as those developing in later life. Several specific types of congenital endothelial dystrophy have been described in the literature and are reported by Stocker[5] and Duke-Elder.[6] They may be differentiated on the basis of history, biomicroscopic appearance, or clinical course, and occasionally on the basis of light and electron microscopy in cases that have been treated by corneal transplantation.

The condition known as congenital hereditary endothelial dystrophy (Fig. 6–1) has been described in detail, and the abnormalities in the endothelium and Descemet's membrane have been documented by electron microscopy.[7, 8] Autosomal dominant and recessive forms have been distinguished.[9] Both corneas are symmetrically involved by marked stromal edema, which usually is gradually progressive over a period of years. Microcystic epithelial edema generally is present, but bullae are uncommon. These corneas are of normal diameter and are free of vascularization. Intraocular pressure in involved eyes is normal. The corneas of asymptomatic family members may have lesions resembling those of posterior polymorphous dystrophy,[10] which may itself be a rare cause of corneal edema.[11]

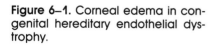

Figure 6–1. Corneal edema in congenital hereditary endothelial dystrophy.

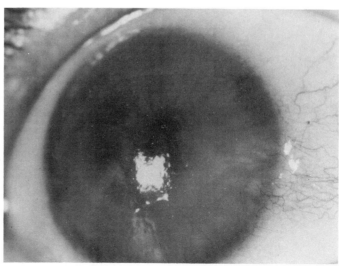

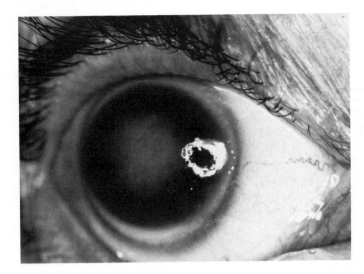

Figure 6–2. Primary chronic edema.

Primary endothelial dystrophies that develop in later life are Fuchs' dystrophy and the entity known as primary chronic edema (Fig. 6–2). The latter entity is characterized by edema that occurs despite normal endothelial appearance, normal intraocular pressure, and the absence of a history or other evidence of previous trauma or disease. The earliest changes of Fuchs' dystrophy are limited to the posterior portion of the cornea and present as central cornea guttata (Fig. 6–3), which are excrescences on Descemet's membrane elaborated by endothelial cells. Although guttate changes, known as Hassall-Henle warts, are frequently observed in the corneal periphery, where they represent an aging change of little consequence,[12] those associated with Fuchs' dystrophy

have a predilection for the central portion of the corneal endothelium. This finding alone does not warrant a diagnosis of Fuchs' dystrophy. A substantial portion of the population has isolated central cornea guttata,[13] and only a relatively small number of cases with demonstrable excrescences go on to develop epithelial and stromal edema consistent with a diagnosis of Fuchs' dystrophy. The incidence and the severity of the central guttate changes increase with the age of the patient, just as do the peripheral excrescences.[14] In overt Fuchs' dystrophy increasing numbers of excrescences also appear in the corneal midperiphery as the disorder progresses.

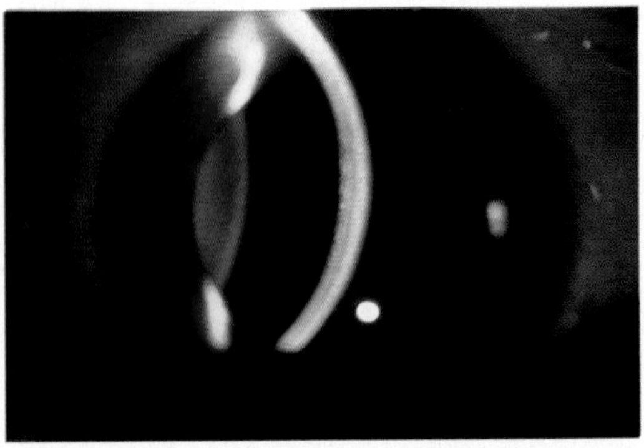

This initial phase of Fuchs' dystrophy, characterized by central cornea guttata and varying amounts of a brownish pigment that appears to have been dusted onto the endothelium, is not generally accompanied by symptoms. There may be a small increase in stromal thickness that can be measured by pachymetry, but vision usually is not affected. Invariably many years pass before the slowly progressive endothelial embarrassment results in clinical decompensation characterized by an increase in corneal thickness. Fluid now penetrates the endothelial barrier in a quantity that exceeds the capacity of the damaged endothelial pump. Coincident with fluid infiltration into the stroma, a grayish zone of in-

Figure 6–3. Central cornea guttata of Fuchs' dystrophy. (Courtesy of Howard M. Leibowitz, M.D.)

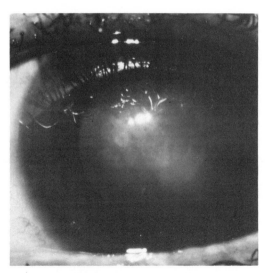

Figure 6–4. Central stromal edema producing corneal turbidity in Fuchs' dystrophy. (Courtesy of Howard M. Leibowitz, M.D.)

creased turbidity can be observed on slit-lamp examination (Fig. 6–4) and folds appear in Descemet's membrane (Fig. 6–5). Descemet's folds form because the anterior limiting membrane of the cornea largely maintains its original curvature despite the stromal edema. This results in the posterior displacement of Descemet's membrane, causing it, in effect, to become too long and therefore less taut.[15] As a consequence, accordion-like folds become visible.

Fluid in the cornea ultimately permeates the epithelial layers, and the small droplets characteristic of micro-

cystic epithelial edema can be seen in retroillumination with the slit-lamp biomicroscope. This represents intracellular edema of the basal epithelial cells. As the disease progresses, individual cells burst, intercellular edema occurs, and typical blisters or bullae form (Fig. 6–6). These changes are almost invariably confined to the central portions of the cornea; only in late stages of the disorder is the corneal periphery involved. However, an unusual sector or pie-shaped form of Fuchs' dystrophy, in which the decompensation is noted to start at the periphery and to progress towards the pupillary area, has been reported. Corneal sensitivity may be markedly reduced in Fuchs' dystrophy, and, as long as the bullae remain intact, there is only slight discomfort. With the rupture of a bulla, however, severe pain may occur. Late stages of Fuchs' dystrophy are characterized by the addition of subepithelial connective tissue, vascularization, and scarring.

When stromal thickness increases by approximately 70 per cent, a visual deficit ensues.[16] Even small amounts of epithelial edema cause a more marked decrease in vision, and the late pannus formation, neovascularization, and stromal scarring reduce vision even further. These late changes do, however, result in some benefit; they enhance the adhesion of the epithelium to the underlying tissue, reducing the formation of bullae and ameliorating the pain.

Figure 6–5. Folds in Descemet's membrane in chronic stromal edema of Fuchs' dystrophy.

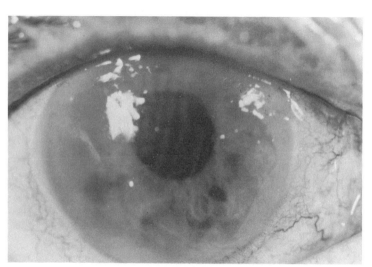

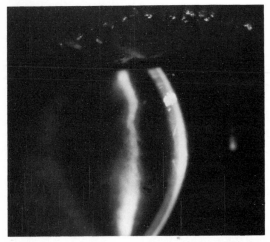

Figure 6-6. Slit-lamp photograph showing corneal edema, folds in Descemet's membrane, and bullae. (Courtesy of Howard M. Leibowitz, M.D.)

Secondary Endothelial Dystrophies

The paramount role of the endothelium in maintaining the normal state of corneal hydration leads us to the concept of what we shall call secondary endothelial dystrophy. This is based on the knowledge that endothelial dysfunction can be initiated by a number of factors that constitute the classic causes of secondary corneal edema. They include glaucoma, blunt and penetrating trauma, and intraocular inflammation and hemorrhage. Indeed, almost any noxious insult (depending on its severity and/or chronicity) has at least the potential for inciting the degenerative processes.

Whether these deleterious effects are related to the products of inflammation (keratic precipitates, altered composition of the aqueous) or whether they represent a more direct toxic effect is not clearly understood. Noxious elements have the capacity to compromise both the barrier function of the endothelium and its pump mechanism; the relative extent to which each is involved is variable, depending on the nature of the insult. With increased use of specular microscopy, the precise mechanisms underlying various entities will come under closer scrutiny.

Glaucoma

Experimental studies have demonstrated the relationship between intraocular pressure and corneal hydration,[17, 18] and every experienced ophthalmologist is aware that at any given level of endothelial function there is a point at which a further elevation of the intraocular pressure will result in overt corneal edema. Even if the corneal endothelium is normal, an acute rise in intraocular pressure that exceeds the swelling pressure of the corneal stroma will result in epithelial edema and the associated symptoms of halos around lights, photophobia, and reduced vision. The level of intraocular pressure also will affect the clinical appearance of

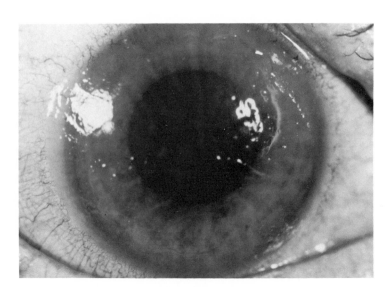

Figure 6-7. Corneal edema secondary to chronic glaucoma.

corneal decompensation in an eye with a compromised corneal endothelium. In such an eye the state of corneal hydration often will be an exquisite measure of the intraocular pressure level. Corneal edema may occur at a relatively low intraocular pressure but largely clear when the pressure is lowered further.[19] Chronic elevation of intraocular pressure will permanently damage the endothelium (Fig. 6–7); the degree of damage is directly related to the level of pressure elevation and its duration.

Trauma

This category encompasses accidental (and purposeful) injury to the eye as well as the unavoidable trauma of surgery. Blunt, nonpenetrating trauma can damage the endothelium and cause corneal edema.[20] Most often the injury is reversible and the edema clears, but irreversible endothelial damage can result from nonpenetrating blunt trauma (e.g., BB injury). Perforating ocular injuries can, of course, damage the endothelium either directly, if the injury involves the cornea (Fig. 6–8), or secondarily through the adverse effects of the resulting glaucoma, inflammation, hemorrhage, or synechiae. Whether or not the cornea recovers normal hydration and transparency depends upon the nature of the injury, its severity, and the status of the endothelium prior to the injury. A tiny, unobtrusive foreign body that gains entrance to the anterior chamber during a perforating injury and lodges in the anterior chamber angle can be the cause of progressive corneal edema.[21] Most often the edema caused by this mechanism begins in the inferior periphery because the foreign body settles inferiorly (Fig. 6–9). The corneal edema responds favorably to removal of the foreign body.

A number of other sources of trauma deserve mention because they produce well-characterized clinical entities. Forceps applied to the head of an infant in the birth canal during delivery can cause sufficient pressure on the globe to rupture Descemet's membrane (Fig. 6–10). Corneal edema often results but slowly clears over a period of weeks to months as the endothelium regenerates. Typical double-contoured striae are visible once the cornea clears (Fig. 6–11), but the irrevocable nature of the injury is reflected in the observation that the cornea may again decompensate several decades later (Fig. 6–12).[22] Congenital glaucoma can similarly rupture Descemet's membrane (Fig. 6–13), and so-called corneal hydrops seen in keratoconus (Fig. 6–14) is also the result of a break in Descemet's membrane. Both can cause a striking degree of corneal edema. In addition to these mechanical injuries, noxious chemicals, especially alkali, which

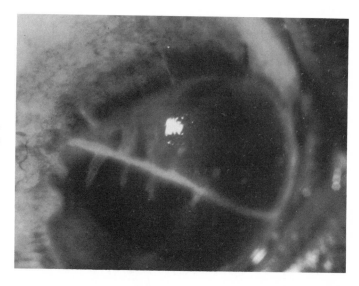

Figure 6–8. Corneal edema resulting from the trauma of a perforating laceration.

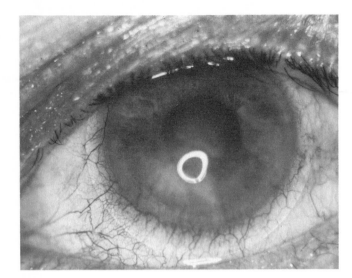

Figure 6–9. Edema of the inferior cornea due to a foreign body in the inferior angle. A hydrophilic contact lens has been fitted to alleviate the patient's discomfort.

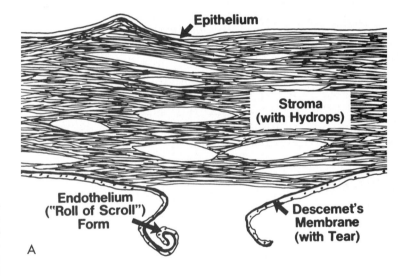

Figure 6–10. Rupture of Descemet's membrane. *A*, Schematic illustration showing the break in Descemet's membrane and endothelium (which results in stromal edema) and the typical "curling up" of the free end of Descemet's membrane. *B*, Histopathologic section showing the curled end of Descemet's membrane.

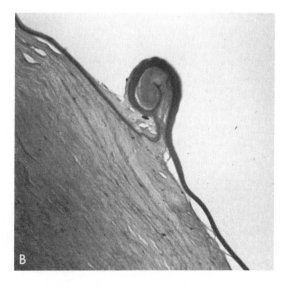

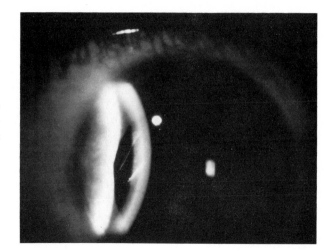

Figure 6–11. Double-contoured striae reflecting a rupture in Descemet's membrane. (Courtesy of Howard M. Leibowitz, M.D.)

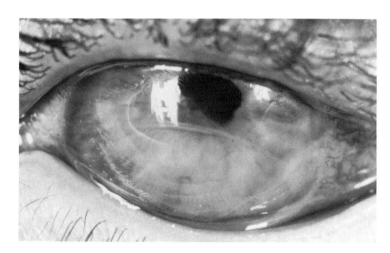

Figure 6–12. Corneal edema due to rupture of Descemet's membrane.

Figure 6–13. Corneal edema secondary to congential glaucoma.

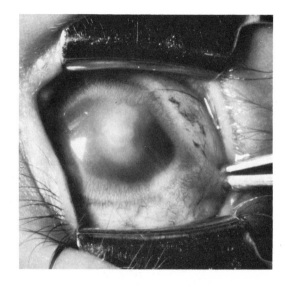

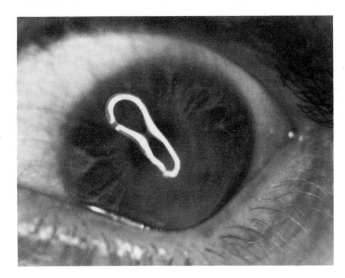

Figure 6–14. Chronic hydrops in keratoconus due to rupture of Descemet's membrane.

is capable of rapid corneal penetration, can destroy the endothelium.

More commonly, however, corneal edema results from the trauma of intraocular surgery. Since cataract extraction is the intraocular procedure performed most frequently, so-called aphakic bullous keratopathy (Fig. 6–15) forms the largest category within this group of secondary endothelial dystrophies. Even the most successful of cataract surgical procedures is a traumatic event to the corneal endothelium; virtually all corneas are edematous during the early postoperative period. Although the vast majority clinically recover, a significant increase in stromal thickness can be demonstrated by pachymetry months

later,[23] and a definite loss of endothelial cells can be documented with the specular microscope.[24, 25] The opportunities for insult to the corneal endothelium during a "routine" cataract extraction are numerous. The incision into the anterior chamber can strip away portions of Descemet's membrane or even the endothelium itself (Fig. 6–16). Excessive handling and bending of the cornea, various manipulations in the anterior chamber, faulty instrumentation or other errors in surgical technique, and hemorrhage into the anterior chamber (Fig. 6–17) can all take their toll on the endothelium.

The preoperative existence of an abnormal endothelium is an important fac-

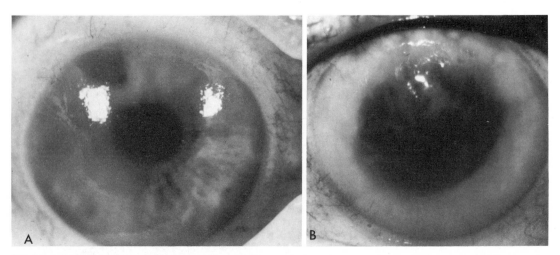

Figure 6–15. Aphakic bullous keratopathy. *A,* Following round pupil intracapsular extraction. *B,* Following intracapsular extraction wih sector iridectomy.

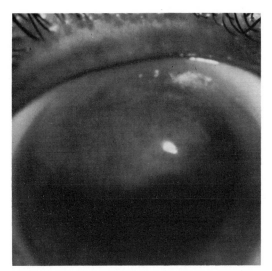

Figure 6–16. Edema of the superior cornea, the result of traumatic stripping of Descemet's membrane during cataract extraction.

the absence of any discernible morphologic alteration. Although current diagnostic techniques are greatly improved over those available even a decade ago, they remain insufficient to identify all corneas that will succumb to the trauma of cataract extraction.

A number of drugs and solutions used intraocularly during surgery have the potential to adversely influence endothelial function and to potentiate, or perhaps directly cause, secondary endothelial dystrophy. Epinephrine and even normal saline can be toxic to the endothelium.[26, 27] Experimental evidence indicates that a balanced salt solution containing glutathione is the least toxic substitute for aqueous humor, particularly when prolonged intraocular irrigation is required.

Additional hazards are present in the postoperative period. Contact of vitreous humor with the endothelium can cause irreversible corneal edema, particularly if the anterior hyaloid face of the vitreous is intact (Fig. 6–18).[28, 29] This is especially apt to occur if Fuchs' dystrophy is present or the endothelium is otherwise compromised. A flat anterior chamber allowing the iris to come into prolonged contact with the corneal endothelium can similarly result in endothelial decompensation; this complication is particularly devastating if a lens implant is in place and comes into contact with the central endothelium (Fig. 6–19).[30] Pronounced irreversible

tor in the subsequent development of secondary corneal edema. A careful preoperative examination with the slit-lamp biomicroscope and preoperative evaluation with the specular microscope will often allow the ophthalmic surgeon to identify eyes at increased risk of corneal decompensation. Unfortunately, recognition of dense cornea guttata, substantial morphologic abnormalities in the endothelial mosaic, or a significant reduction in the endothelial cell population may be of little more than prognostic value when a dense cataract limits vision and must be removed. Moreover, a predisposition of the endothelium to surgical trauma may exist in

Figure 6–17. Corneal edema following cataract extraction complicated by anterior chamber hemorrhage.

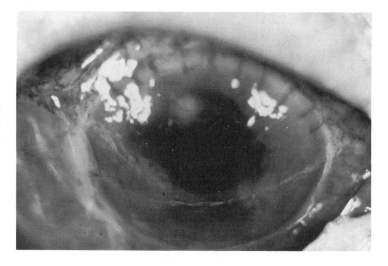

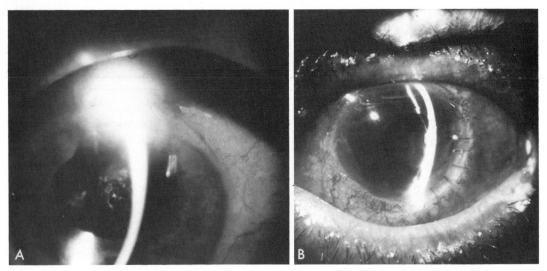

Figure 6–18. Corneal edema resulting from vitreocorneal contact. *A,* Onset 2 years after successful cataract surgery. *B,* Onset 3 days after removal of lens through inferotemporal wound from a glaucomatous eye with a successful superonasal filtering sclerectomy. (Courtesy of Howard M. Leibowitz, M.D.)

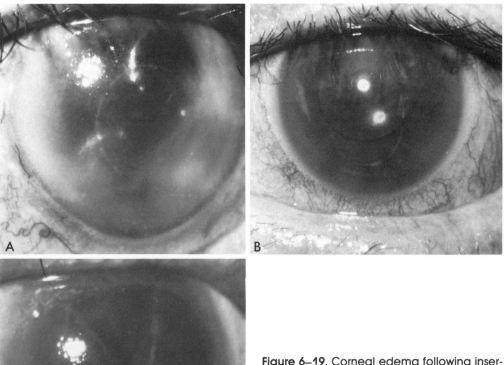

Figure 6–19. Corneal edema following insertion of intraocular lens implant. *A,* Dislocated iris plane lens. *B,* Well-placed iris plane lens. *C,* Anterior chamber lens.

edema is the invariable consequence, resulting from severe mechanical damage to the endothelial cells. Uveitis, secondary glaucoma, endophthalmitis, and epithelialization of the anterior chamber can also contribute to postoperative corneal edema. While cataract extraction is the single largest cause of the iatrogenic secondary corneal dystrophies, other surgical procedures (e.g., glaucoma surgery, retinal detachment surgery, vitrectomy, and penetrating keratoplasty) are frequently associated with secondary bullous keratopathy.

Contact Lenses

Contact lenses are perhaps the most common cause of corneal edema. Most often this presents as microcystic epithelial edema near the center of the resting position of the contact lens, best seen with sclerotic scatter illumination of the slit lamp, and is referred to as Sattler's veil. It is caused by an insufficient supply of oxygen to the corneal epithelium, which results in the depletion of glycogen and the accumulation of lactic acid within the epithelial cells.[31] If allowed to continue, stromal edema and folds in Descemet's membrane are observed. This type of edema is readily reversible by removing the contact lens or altering its fit to allow sufficient circulation of freshly oxygenated tears beneath the contact lens to supply the epithelium adequately with its oxygen requirements.

Iridocorneal Endothelial Syndrome

Yanoff has proposed the name iridocorneal endothelial syndrome to describe the spectrum of disorders that includes essential iris atrophy, Chandler's syndrome, and the iris-nevus (Cogan-Reese) syndrome.[32] The corneal changes in each of these disorders are variable, but each may present with guttate changes and frank corneal edema. Clinically, essential iris atrophy is characterized by distortion of the pupil, peripheral anterior synechiae, and iris atrophy with prominent full-thickness holes in the iris. This entity occurs most often in Caucasian women in their fourth and fifth decades. It is generally unilateral, and glaucoma commonly is present in the involved eye.

Chandler's syndrome is used to describe cases whose clinical characteristics differ somewhat from essential iris atrophy. The guttate endothelial changes and/or corneal edema tend to be more prominent, but the intraocular pressure is normal or only slightly elevated and iris atrophy is minimal. In early descriptions,[33] true holes were said not to form in the iris, nor was the pupil grossly distorted. The iris-nevus (Cogan-Reese) syndrome[34] is characterized by pigmented iris nodules which histopathologically are benign nevi, along with peripheral anterior synechiae, heterochromia, sector iris atrophy, and glaucoma.

The corneal endothelium may be abnormal in each of these three entities, and in each the peripheral endothelium along with Descemet's membrane—like material may proliferate over the anterior chamber angle onto the anterior surface of the iris. Campbell and colleagues[35] have advanced the so-called membrane theory, proposing that contraction of this membrane, resulting from the proliferation of abnormal corneal endothelium and consisting of a single layer of endothelial cells and a basement membrane, produces the peripheral anterior synechiae and pupillary distortion with subsequent iris thinning. Certainly the degree and type of corneal and iris changes in each of these entities vary over a wide spectrum (Fig. 6–20). Cases have been reported that do not fit into any of the three typical categories, and the features of these three entities clearly overlap; some patients with Chandler's syndrome progress to hole formation in the iris, and many with essential iris atrophy show signs of endothelial disease.[35] Indeed, iris nodules have been observed in eyes with the typical features of essential iris atrophy, including the formation of holes in

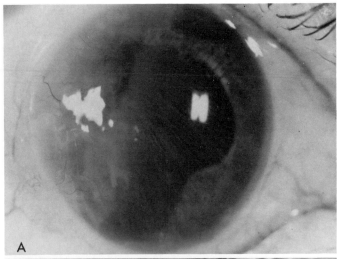

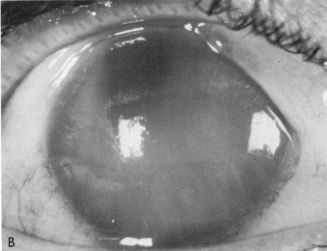

Figure 6–20. Iridocorneal endothelial (ICE) syndrome. *A,* Distortion of pupil, peripheral anterior synechiae, iris atrophy with full-thickness holes in iris, and corneal edema. *B,* More pronounced corneal edema, slight elevation of intraocular pressure, and pupillary distortion.

the iris.[35, 36] Mounting evidence appears to support the thesis that these three entities represent a continuum of findings of a single disorder[37] and supports the use of the term iridocorneal endothelial syndrome to describe that disorder. However, Campbell and coworkers believe that these disorders are primarily abnormalities of the cornea and involve the iris only secondarily. They propose a new designation for the spectrum of abnormalities, primary proliferative endothelial degeneration.[38]

MANIFESTATIONS OF CORNEAL EDEMA

Regardless of the nature of the insult, the important manifestations of corneal edema are reduced visual acuity, pain, and alterations in the normal corneal structure.

Altered Visual Acuity

When endothelial function can no longer maintain deturgescence, stromal edema ensues and is followed by epithelial edema. Although a 70 per cent increase in the stromal thickness per se may be compatible with relatively normal acuity,[16] a small amount of epithelial edema can result in a great reduction in acuity. Epithelial edema may be intracellular, intercellular, or a combination of the two types.

In the presence of a compromised endothelium, corneal deturgescence becomes directly related to extrinsic factors such as temperature, humidity, and air flow; such a cornea is at the mercy of its environment. Typically, epithelial edema and the accompanying reduced acuity are more severe in the early morning. During sleep, with the lids closed, there is no opportunity for evaporation of tears, and as the day progresses, increased evaporation can result in a diminution of the epithelial edema. Consequently, vision may improve as the day progresses. Visual acuity also will fluctuate in response to variations in intraocular pressure. Patients maintained on ocular hypotensive therapy may recognize a pattern of variations in vision that are related to the time at which their medication is administered.

In more advanced cases of edema gross surface irregularities and stromal opacification present further obstacles to the normal refractive processes. Posterior irregular astigmatism associated with Descemet's membrane folds and irregularities may be an additional barrier to vision. Associated iritis, cataract, glaucoma, retinopathy, and optic nerve changes in an eye with corneal edema can be responsible for some of the reduced acuity. A careful evaluation of these factors is necessary before an accurate prognosis can be given to the patient and a rational therapeutic approach established.

A few drops of glycerine may clear the cornea sufficiently for observation of the anterior chamber and posterior segment.[15] An exhaustive examination is often necessary to determine the extent of visual reduction due to the corneal edema. Refraction over a hydrophilic lens in marginal cases can often indicate the functional capacity of the posterior segment. Ultrasonography, electroretinography, and tests of macular function also may be of value.

Pain and Discomfort

Pain and discomfort associated with corneal edema result from disruption of the abundant sensory innervation of the ep-

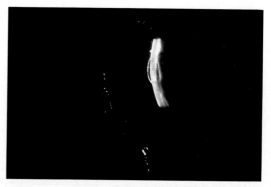

Figure 6–21. Slit-lamp view of the elevation of a large area of epithelium from the underlying basement membrane to form a bulla. (Courtesy of Howard M. Leibowitz, M.D.)

ithelium. As the edema progresses, large areas of epithelium are detached from the underlying basement membrane to form bullae (Figs. 6–21, 6–22). The rupture of a bulla causes severe pain. Typically, secondary corneal edema is associated with a greater degree of discomfort. Acute episodes of pain generally are accompanied by significant photophobia and epiphora, and charac-

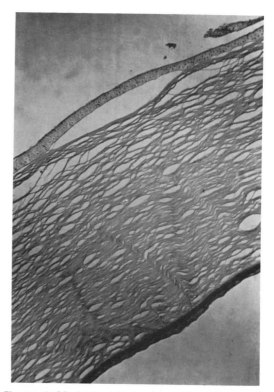

Figure 6–22. Histopathologic section of an epithelial bulla.

teristically there is a narrowing of the palpebral aperture. However, the degree of discomfort is extremely variable among individuals.

In moderate to advanced cases the discomfort is enhanced by the presence of chronic anterior uveitis. All too often, however, the degree of corneal opacification precludes an accurate diagnosis of anterior chamber inflammation. This is particularly true in cases of iatrogenic bullous keratopathy. In such cases initial therapy might well include mydriatics and topical steroids.

Photophobia, resulting from light scattering in the edematous cornea as well as from inflammation, increases discomfort. Reflex stimulation of tears by both pain and photophobia often results in epiphora, and the pain and tearing can in turn cause blepharospasm. Given this environment of lid and tear film dysfunction, chronic blepharitis may develop. Secondary infection of the cornea is a potential hazard, but, surprisingly, it is uncommon and is not an important factor in the management of these patients.

Altered Corneal Morphology

Slit-lamp examination will often reveal cornea guttata as well as the presence of a dense, brownish reflex originating from the posterior aspects of the stroma and indicative of a thickened Descemet's membrane. When decompensation occurs, corneal edema is recognized by increased density in the stroma and an overall increase in corneal thickness. This can be measured with a pachymeter; corneal thickness measurements are usually in excess of 0.60 mm. in the central corneal area.

In cases in which edema involves the epithelium a wide variation of patterns may be noted. These range from minute bedewing of the corneal epithelium to gross swelling and irregularity of the edematous epithelial cells. Formation of bullae is easily observed with the slit-lamp biomicroscope. The areas occupied by ruptured bullae readily stain with fluorescein dye. In cases of chronic corneal edema, such as late Fuchs' dystrophy or aphakic bullous keratopathy, neovascularization, pannus formation, and corneal leukomata are visible (Fig. 6–23).

Cornea guttata and alteration of endothelial mosaic patterns can be seen with the aid of specular illumination. Scanning and transmission electron microscopy provide evidence of specific morphologic changes in the endothelium. Using specular microscopy, one sees a characteristic endothelial appearance[38] in which individual cornea guttata and the endothelial cells are enlarged with an increased perimeter and a reduced density. Pleomorphism can be widespread. Evidence of an alteration of the cell membranes and interspaces has

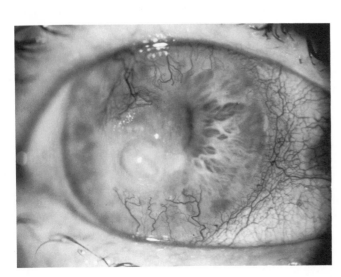

Figure 6–23. Chronic edema showing multiple structural alterations of the cornea including bulla formation, stromal edema, stromal scarring, and neovascularization. (Courtesy of Howard M. Leibowitz, M.D.)

been associated with a decrease in the endothelial barrier function and with clinical edema.

CLINICAL MANAGEMENT

A number of therapeutic modalities have been advocated for the treatment of corneal edema. All are aimed at improving vision and/or alleviating pain.

An often overlooked aspect in the treatment of chronic corneal edema is the control of intraocular pressure. Traditional diagnostic methods, such as Schiøtz or applanation tonometry, often are not reliable indicators of the intraocular pressure in the presence of an edematous cornea with an irregular surface; a MacKay-Marg electronic tonometer or an electronic pneumotonometer will provide a far more reliable estimation of the intraocular pressure. In all cases of corneal edema, when elevation of intraocular pressure is documented, its control with systemic carbonic anhydrase inhibitors and/or topical antiglaucoma medications is of paramount concern. Even if the intraocular pressure is only moderately elevated, its control may result in a significant reduction of epithelial edema and in some cases in complete corneal deturgescence and recovery. The effect tends to be most dramatic in early cases of Fuchs' dystrophy. Regrettably, because of the progressive nature of Fuchs' dystrophy, the improvement may be short-lived; ultimately corneal edema may recur despite the lower intraocular pressure.

When the intraocular pressure remains elevated despite maximum systemic and topical medical therapy, surgical intervention must be considered, even in the presence of a compromised corneal endothelium. In aphakic eyes cyclocryotherapy may be helpful. Should a filtering operation be necessary, a trabeculectomy is undoubtedly the safest form of this procedure. It carries with it the lowest incidence of loss of the anterior chamber, an important factor in the face of a compromised corneal endothelium.

The goal of topical therapy is the removal of fluid from the edematous cornea either through evaporation or through the establishment of an osmotic gradient. Patients who find their visual acuity most reduced after they sleep may be helped by exposure of their eyes to a moving stream of warm air. A few minutes spent in front of a hair dryer shortly after arising may initiate evaporation and a reduction in the degree of early morning corneal edema, resulting in an improvement in vision.

Topical application of hyperosmotic agents can remove a small amount of fluid from the edematous cornea. For this treatment to be effective, the epithelium must be intact and capable of functioning as a semipermeable membrane. Nonetheless, this approach is limited because most highly hypertonic agents cause too much discomfort to be of practical value. Five per cent sodium chloride in solution or ointment is the most commonly used clinical agent;[39, 40] despite its instillation at hourly or even more frequent intervals, it is effective only in mild forms of edema.

If inflammation is a contributory cause of corneal edema, topically applied corticosteroids can be very helpful. Treatment of any coexisting iritis or blepharitis, as well as inflammation within the cornea itself, is essential. If the etiology of the corneal edema is not apparent, an aggressive 10-day course of topical corticosteroids can serve a diagnostic as well as a therapeutic purpose. Amelioration of the edema establishes the causal contribution of an inflammatory process. Relatively long-term use of topical corticosteroids may be required to control and reverse the edema. The potential hazards of long-term corticosteroid use must be borne in mind.

In patients with early corneal decompensation and mild degrees of corneal edema a careful refraction may improve vision. However, when all treatment modalities discussed thus far (i.e., control of intraocular pressure, application of warm air and topical hyperosmotic agents, and a careful refraction) fail to improve the visual acuity, a therapeutic hydrophilic contact lens should be considered. Particularly in monocular cases, an attempt should be made to fit the involved cornea with a thin hydrophilic lens that is fitted flat to allow for maximum contact between the lens and the irregular epithelium. Topical hyperosmolar agents (e.g., 5 per cent sodium chloride solution) may be instilled while the lens is in place, and an adequate trial (up to several weeks) should be carried out. If this trial is unsuccessful, a variety of lens fitting combinations should be tried before this approach is abandoned. Ideally, the lens should be inserted and removed daily, but continuous contact lens wear may be successful, particularly in cases of Fuchs' dystrophy.[41] Overrefraction and a change of spectacles, if necessary, should be attempted prior to final evaluation of the efficacy of this mode of therapy.

In cases of painful bullous keratopathy visual improvement with a hydrophilic contact lens may be limited. Although the irregular epithelial surface can easily be eliminated by the contact lens, advanced stromal edema, scarring, and neovascularization often are present and prevent substantial visual improvement. Nevertheless, a trial with a hydrophilic contact lens is indicated, primarily to relieve discomfort. In the presence of optic nerve damage, maculopathy, or other causes of a poor visual prognosis, relief of pain should be the predominant therapeutic objective. This goal can be accomplished in a very high percentage of cases of painful bullous keratopathy by the fitting of a hydrophilic contact lens.[42, 43] If pain is not successfully alleviated by application of a hydrophilic contact lens, several surgical procedures are available to accomplish this goal. They include the application of radiodiathermy or other forms of electrocautery to Bowman's membrane.[44] This produces a fibrous adhesion between the stroma and the epithelium, preventing the formation of bullae. Alternatively, a Gundersen type of conjunctival flap with or without an accompanying la-

mellar keratectomy can be performed.[45] Both procedures are highly effective in relieving pain but substantially diminish corneal transparency and so limit the ability to visualize intraocular structures. In a blind, painful eye with absolute glaucoma, enucleation may represent the optimal procedure; discomfort secondary to chronic uveitis and/or absolute glaucoma may persist despite a conjunctival flap.

In the absence of pain or discomfort, if there is a possibility of restoring vision, surgical intervention in the form of penetrating keratoplasty should be considered whenever acuity is inadequate for the patient's requirements. Penetrating keratoplasty is equally successful in painful eyes and should be undertaken instead of cauterization of Bowman's membrane or a conjunctival flap if the potential for visual recovery exists. Although a detailed fundus examination and fluorescein angiography may not be possible, every attempt should be made to rule out overt macular disease before advising this form of surgery. Topical application of glycerine to temporarily dehydrate the cornea may afford a view of the posterior segment. The prognosis for penetrating keratoplasty, even when combined with cataract extraction, is very good (80 per cent or better) when employed for most types of corneal edema (Fig. 6–24). Glaucoma must be satisfactorily controlled before

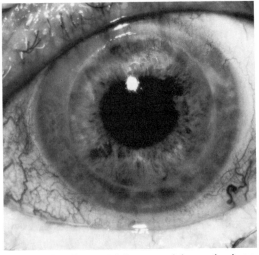

Figure 6–24. Successful corneal transplant performed for aphakic bullous keratopathy.

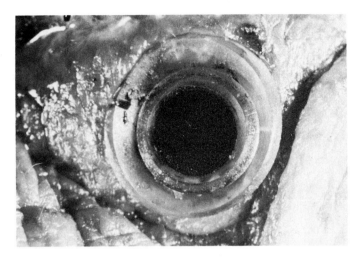

Figure 6–25. Use of a keratoprosthesis, a "last ditch" effort to visually rehabilitate an eye with severe corneal edema and multiple graft failures.

corneal transplantation is attempted. However, even in secondary aphakic bullous keratopathy penetrating keratoplasty combined with vitrectomy and iridoplasty carries a relatively good prognosis.

In cases of multiple graft failures, especially if corneal thickness exceeds 1.5 mm., use of a keratoprosthesis has been advocated (Fig. 6–25). This procedure carries with it a high potential for complication and failure,[46] and it is viewed by most authorities as a "last ditch" effort to visually rehabilitate an eye. It should be undertaken only when there is a reasonable prospect for improving vision; preoperative ultrasonography and electroretinography may be helpful in making this determination. In cases of severe bilateral corneal edema meeting the criteria cited above, placement of a keratoprosthesis in the worst eye may preserve vision and make the decision to attempt another standard keratoplasty in the fellow eye a reasonable one. Although a nut-and-bolt keratoprosthesis has been advocated by some as a primary procedure in corneal edema,[47] at the current state of development the vast majority of corneal surgeons considers this an operation of desperation, to be used only when there is little or no hope for conventional keratoplasty.

REFERENCES

1. Mishima, S.: Corneal thickness. Surv Ophthalmol 13:57, 1968.
2. Mishima, S., and Maurice, D. M.: The effect of normal evaporation on the eye. Exp Eye Res 1:46, 1961.
3. Harris, J. E., and Nordquist, L. T.: The hydration of the cornea: I. Transport of water from the cornea. Amer J Ophthalmol 40:100, 1955.
4. Harris, J. E.: The physiologic control of corneal hydration. Amer J Ophthalmol 44:262, 1957.
5. Stocker, F. W.: *The Endothelium of the Cornea and Its Implications.* 2nd ed. Springfield, Ill., Charles C Thomas, 1971.
6. Duke-Elder, S., and Leigh, A. G.: *Diseases of the Outer Eye.* In Duke-Elder, S. (ed.): *System of Ophthalmology.* Vol. 8. Part 2. St. Louis, C. V. Mosby Co., 1965, pp. 863–992.
7. Kenyon, K. R., and Antine, B.: The pathogenesis of congenital hereditary endothelial dystrophy of the cornea. Amer J Ophthalmol 72:787, 1971.
8. Kenyon, K. R., and Maumenee, A. E.: Further stud-

ies of congenital hereditary endothelial dystrophy of the cornea. Amer J Ophthalmol 76:419, 1973.
9. Judisch, G. F., and Maumenee, I. H.: Clinical differentiation of recessive congenital hereditary endothelial dystrophy and dominant hereditary dystrophy. Amer J Ophthalmol 85:606, 1978.
10. Levenson, J. E., Chandler, J. W., and Kaufman, H. E.: Affected asymptomatic relatives in congenital hereditary endothelial dystrophy. Amer J Ophthalmol 76:467, 1973.
11. Cibis, G. W., Krachmer, J. A., Phelps, C. D., and Weingeist, T. A.: The clinical spectrum of posterior polymorphous dystrophy. Arch Ophthalmol 95:1529, 1977.
12. Hogan, M. J., and Zimmerman, L. E. (eds.): *Ophthalmic Pathology.* 2nd ed. Philadelphia, W. B. Saunders Co., 1962, pp. 288–290.
13. Waring, G. O., III, Rodrigues, M. M., and Laibson, P. R.: Corneal dystrophies: II. Endothelial dystrophies. Surv Ophthalmol 23:147, 1978.
14. Lorenzetti, D. W., Uotila, M. H., Pariker, N., and

Kaufman, H. E.: Central cornea guttata. Amer J Ophthalmol 64:1155, 1967.

15. Cogan, D. G.: Clearing of edematous corneas by glycerine. Amer J Ophthalmol 26:551, 1943.

16. Zucker, B. B.: Hydration and transparency of corneal stroma. Arch Ophthalmol 75:228, 1966.

17. Ytteborg, J., and Dohlman, C. H.: Corneal edema and intraocular pressure: I. Animal experiments. Arch Ophthalmol 74:375, 1965.

18. Ytteborg, J., and Dohlman, C. H.: Corneal edema and intraocular pressure: II. Clinical results. Arch Ophthalmol 74:477, 1965.

19. Irvine, A. R., Jr.: The role of the endothelium in bullous keratopathy. Arch Ophthalmol 56:338, 1956.

20. Bourne, W. M., McCarey, B. E., and Kaufman, H. E.: Clinical specular microscopy. Trans Amer Acad Ophthalmol Otolaryngol 81:743, 1976.

21. Laibson, P. R.: Inferior bullous keratopathy. Arch Ophthalmol 74:191, 1965.

22. Spencer, W. H., Ferguson, W. J., Jr., Shaffer, R. N., and Fine, M.: Late degenerative changes in the cornea following breaks in Descemet's membrane. Trans Amer Acad Ophthalmol Otolaryngol 70:973, 1966.

23. Miller, D., and Dohlman, C. H.: Effect of cataract surgery on the cornea. Trans Amer Acad Ophthalmol Otolaryngol 74:369, 1970.

24. Rao, G. N., Stevens, R. E., Harris, J. K., and Aquavella, J. V.: Long term changes in corneal endothelium following intraocular lens implantation. Ophthalmology 88:386, 1981.

25. Abbott, R. L., and Forster, R. K.: Clinical specular microscopy and intraocular surgery. Arch Ophthalmol 97:1476, 1979.

26. Hull, D. S., Chenotti, T., Edelhauser, H. F., Van Horn, D. L., and Hyndiuk, R. A.: Effect of epinephrine on the corneal endothelium. Amer J Ophthalmol 79:245, 1978.

27. Edelhauser, H. F., Van Horn, D. L., Schultz, R. O., and Hyndiuk, R. A.: Comparative study of intraocular irrigating solutions on the corneal endothelium. Amer J Ophthalmol 81:473, 1976.

28. Leahy, B. D.: Bullous keratitis from vitreous contact. Arch Ophthalmol 46:22, 1951.

29. Leibowitz, H. M., Laing, R. A., Chang, R., Theodore, J., and Oak, S. S.: Corneal edema secondary to vitreocorneal touch. Arch Ophthalmol 88:1013, 1979.

30. Kaufman, H. E., and Katz, J. I.: Endothelial damage from intraocular lens insertion. Invest Ophthalmol 15:996, 1976.

31. Friend, J.: Biochemistry of ocular surface epithelium. Int Ophthalmol Clin 19:73, 1979.

32. Yanoff, M.: Iridocorneal endothelial syndrome. Unification of a disease spectrum. Surv Ophthalmol 24:1, 1979.

33. Chandler, P. A.: Atrophy of the stroma of the iris, endothelial dystrophy, corneal edema and glaucoma. Amer J Ophthalmol 41:607, 1956.

34. Cogan, D. G., and Reese, A. B.: A syndrome of iris nodules, ectopic Descemet's membrane and unilateral glaucoma. Doc Ophthalmol 26:424, 1969.

35. Campbell, D. G., Shields, M. B., and Smith, T. R.: The corneal endothelium and the spectrum of essential iris atrophy. Amer J Ophthalmol 86:317, 1978.

36. Shields, M. B., Campbell, D. G., and Simmons, R. J.: The essential iris atrophies. Amer J Ophthalmol 85:749, 1978.

37. Shields, M. B.: Progressive essential iris atrophy, Chandler's syndrome, and the iris-nevus (Cogan-Reese) syndrome: A spectrum of disease. Surv Ophthalmol 24:3, 1979.

38. Laing, R. H., Leibowitz, H. M., Oak, S. S., Chang, R., Berrospi, A. R., and Theodore, J.: The endothelial mosaic in Fuchs' dystrophy: A qualitative evaluation with the specular microscope. Arch Ophthalmol 99:80, 1981.

39. Marisi, A., and Aquavella, J. V.: Hypertonic saline solution in corneal edema. Ann Ophthalmol 7:229, 1975.

40. Luxenberg, M. N., and Green, K.: Reduction of corneal edema with topical hypertonic agents. Amer J Ophthalmol 71:847, 1971.

41. Takahashi, G. H., and Leibowitz, H. M.: Hydrophilic contact lenses in corneal disease. III. Topical hypertonic saline therapy in bullous keratopathy. Arch Ophthalmol 86:133, 1971.

42. Aquavella, J. V.: Chronic corneal edema. Amer J Ophthalmol 76:201, 1973.

43. Leibowitz, H. M., and Rosenthal, P. R.: Hydrophilic contact lenses in corneal disease: II. Bullous keratopathy. Arch Ophthalmol 85:283, 1971.

44. DeVoe, A. G.: Electrocautery of Bowman's membrane. Arch Ophthalmol 76:768, 1966.

45. Gundersen, T.: Conjunctival flaps in the treatment of corneal disease with reference to a new technique of application. Arch Ophthalmol 60:880, 1958.

46. DeVoe, A. G.: Symposium: Keratoprosthesis—summary. Trans Amer Acad Ophthalmol Otolaryngol 83:282, 1977.

47. Donn, A.: Additional follow-up of 34 cases of prosthokeratoplasty. Trans Amer Acad Ophthalmol Otolaryngol 83:281, 1977.

IV

DISORDERS OF THE LIMBAL REGION

The Corneal Limbus | 7

ROBERT H. POIRIER, M.D.

The limbus is the zone of transition between the transparent cornea and the opaque sclera. This blue-gray zone, which includes the marginal cornea, is readily identifiable, and it is the classic area for the placement of a surgical incision for cataract extraction. A host of disease processes have a predilection for the limbus, and it is to these entities that this chapter will direct its attention. The discussion of the disorders that affect the corneal limbus will proceed as outlined in Table 7–1.

LIMBAL AND MARGINAL CORNEAL MANIFESTATIONS OF METABOLIC DISEASES

Superior Limbic Keratoconjunctivitis of Theodore (SLK)

In 1963 Theodore first described an unusual inflammation of the limbal conjunctiva and marginal cornea that was bilateral in the majority of cases and was associated with filaments of the superior cornea in about one third of the cases. Its etiology remains undetermined. The superior bulbar conjunctiva is usually markedly injected in a distribution that resembles an inverted trapezoid (Fig. 7–1) and often appears lusterless, probably because of keratinization of the epithelial cells. Conjunctival scrapings from the area show markedly keratinized epithelial cells. In addition to the superior corneal filaments, superficial punctate epithelial erosions often are observed (Fig. 7–2). This finding seems to be more common in eyes with redundant folds of the superior bulbar conjunctiva.[1-3]

Tenzel first pointed out the possible relationship between thyroid disease and SLK.[4] A variety of thyroid disorders may occur in association with SLK, but in my clinical experience the most common has been goiter. However, simple chemical hyperthyroidism (i.e., elevated serum protein–bound iodine) may be the only abnormal metabolic finding, so that it is my practice to evaluate all patients with superior limbic keratoconjunctivitis for thyroid disease, including referral to an internist or endocrinologist.

Patients with SLK commonly present with burning and irritated eyes and occasionally complain of mild tearing. Photophobia has not been a significant symptom in my experience. The use of conjunctival cytology as an adjunct for establishing the diagnosis of SLK inadvertently led to the observation that the technique also has significant therapeutic value. Although topical application of 0.5 per cent silver nitrate to the superior bulbar and tarsal conjunctiva is

Table 7–1. DISORDERS OF THE CORNEAL LIMBUS

1. Limbal and marginal corneal manifestations of metabolic diseases
2. Limbal corneal findings secondary to the deposition of substances
3. Infections of the limbal area
4. Hypersensitivity reactions at the corneal limbus
5. Limbal corneal manifestations of collagen vascular diseases
6. Limbal ulcerations due to autoimmunity
7. Dysplastic and neoplastic limbal lesions
8. Degenerations of the corneal limbus

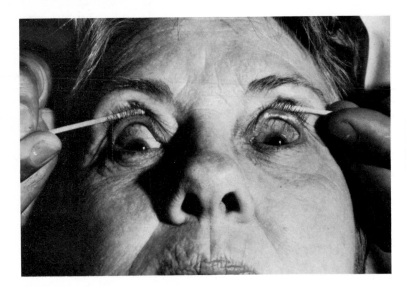

Figure 7–1. Superior limbic keratoconjunctivitis with injected keratinized bulbar conjunctiva.

commonly recommended as treatment for this disorder, I have found simple scraping of the bulbar and tarsal conjunctiva after instillation of an anesthetic to be just as effective. This technique relieves both symptoms and signs of external ocular inflammation. Following conjunctival scraping, the eye is not patched, nor are local antibiotics or corticosteroids administered. Should this procedure not be effective, particularly in cases in which the conjunctiva is excessively redundant, simple excision of the excess conjunctiva has been recommended.

Arcus Juvenilis and Arcus Senilis

Annular infiltration of the peripheral corneal stroma by lipids is known as arcus senilis. Usually there is a relatively clear zone between the lipoidal deposits and the sclera (Fig. 7–3). The deposits consist of neutral fats and phospholipids[5, 6] and appear to develop much earlier in life in black individuals than in Caucasians.

Peripheral corneal lipid deposits are common in elderly patients, and in this instance the finding has no clinical significance. However, the presence of

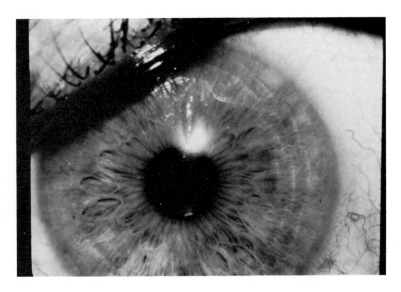

Figure 7–2. Corneal filament near the superior limbus in a patient with SLK.

these lipoidal deposits in young people (where they are called arcus juvenilis), particularly if found in conjunction with xanthelasma, strongly suggests the possibility of a serious metabolic lipid disorder. Blood vessels may be seen within the lipoidal infiltrate when it is associated with a disorder of lipid metabolism. Any patient under 40 years of age with a significant arcus senilis merits a complete evaluation for hyperlipidemia. This is particularly important in individuals with a family history of hypercholesterolemia;[7] clinical studies show a significant association between fatal heart disease and familial hypercholesterolemia.[8]

Patients heterozygous for familial hypercholesterolemia tend to develop arcus juvenilis and tendon xanthomas by the second decade, and by the third decade these findings are present in approximately 50 per cent of such individuals. The mean age of coronary artery disease in patients with familial hypercholesterolemia is 43 years of age in males and 53 years of age in females. The risk of a myocardial infarction in males with this entity is 5 per cent by age 30, 51 per cent by age 50, and 85 per cent by age 60; in women it is 0 per cent, 12 per cent, and 58 per cent respectively. Perhaps a more meaningful comparison is that the incidence of coronary artery disease is 25 times greater in persons with familial hypercholesterolemia than it is in individuals who are unaffected and do not carry this particular gene. Homozygotes have hypercholesterolemia at birth and develop cutaneous xanthomas in early childhood; their mean age at death is 21 years.[8] Arcus juvenilis is an important clinical sign for the detection of both forms of this disease.

Wilson's Disease (Hepatolenticular Degeneration)

This rare disorder of copper metabolism may have as one of its earliest manifestations the deposition of copper deep within the limbal cornea at the level of Descemet's membrane. It may be seen initially in the vertical meridians and may be found later in the horizontal meridians, ultimately forming the classic Kayser-Fleischer ring (Fig. 7–4). Commonly the early findings are not visible with the unaided eye, but they can be readily detected with the slit-lamp biomicroscope. Occasionally the early deposition of copper deep within the peripheral cornea is best seen by gonioscopy. An additional ocular manifestation of this disease is the occasional presence of a typical sunflower cataract not unlike that seen in association with

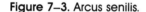
Figure 7–3. Arcus senilis.

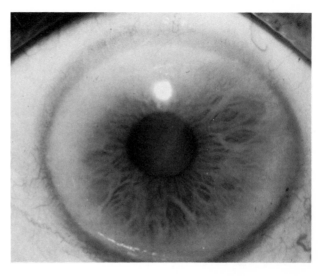

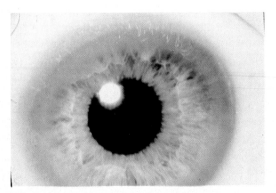

Figure 7–4. Advanced Kayser-Fleischer Ring. (Courtesy of Howard M. Leibowitz, M.D.)

intraocular copper foreign bodies and secondary chalcosis.

Patients with Wilson's disease have elevated tissue and urinary copper levels, whereas the blue, copper-carrying protein, ceruloplasmin, and its related oxidase activity is reduced rather consistently in the serum. The disease is characterized by a continued output of amino acids and copper in the urine. There is an increased absorption of copper from the gastrointestinal tract and an increased deposition of copper in all tissues, but particularly within the basal ganglia and the liver. Clinically the patient may present with a mild tremor that can progress to a full-blown cerebellar type of abnormality along with pill-rolling movements of the fingers similar to that seen with Parkinson's disease. If the disorder is untreated, death usually occurs in 1 to 3 years. The liver frequently is affected with a form of nodular cirrhosis, and the patient may succumb to this aspect of the disease with terminal hepatic coma.[9] The treatment of Wilson's disease has included BAL (2,3-dimercaptopropanol) and DL-penicillamine.[10]

Gout

Gout may affect the eye. Its most common manifestation is a conjunctivoepiscleritis located adjacent to the limbus (Fig. 7–5); true involvement of the sclera occurs but is rare. Uric acid crystals occasionally can be seen deposited in the limbal area adjacent to episcleral vessels, and limbal masses of ureates that mimic pinguecula have been described.[11] Clinical gout is present in 7 per cent of patients with episcleritis and in 2 per cent of those with scleritis.[12]

A classic attack of gout, i.e., a male awakening in the early morning with extreme pain in the metatarsal joint of the big toe, is usually easy to diagnose. Unfortunately, the classic picture is not always present; only three attacks in four affect the big toe, and one attack in ten can affect more than one joint. Gout typically affects postpubertal males and postmenopausal females, and the attack of arthritis usually subsides within a couple of weeks. In addition to classic

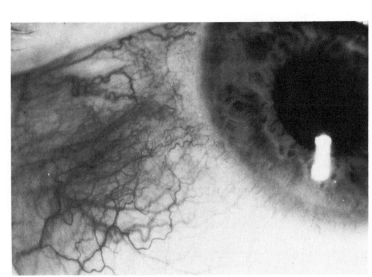

Figure 7–5. Conjunctivoepiscleritis in a patient with gout.

primary gout, there are secondary forms associated with failure of the renal uric acid excretory mechanism, so that there is a decrease in the urinary excretion of uric acid. Compounds that block uric acid excretion, such as the thiazide diuretics, can cause this disorder. Another form of secondary gout occurs when there is a pathologic increase in uric acid production. This is encountered in occasional patients with leukemia and in patients receiving chemotherapy for carcinoma.[13, 14] The chances of a clinical attack of gout increase proportionately to the level of serum uric acid. Treatment of hyperuricemic patients with recurrent episcleritis is directed at reduction of the serum uric acid level.

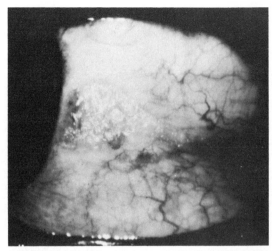

Figure 7–6. Bitot's spot in a patient with severe nutritional deficiency.

Vitamin A Deficiency

In its primary form vitamin A deficiency is a disease of dietary insufficiency, not a true metabolic disease. However, this disorder also can occur secondarily, the result of a metabolic disease such as cystic fibrosis. In the latter instance infants and children are particularly susceptible.[15] Vitamin A deficiency is not commonly encountered in the United States, but it may be seen in dietary fanatics who exclude foods containing vitamin A.

The classic ocular sign of vitamin A deficiency is a Bitot spot (Fig. 7–6), although this finding occurs with nutritional deficiency states in general and is not pathognomonic of vitamin A deficiency. Bitot spots are small, gray or white, generally round or oval, sharply outlined areas located near the limbus. They commonly have a frothy or foamy appearance, but the more well-developed lesions are perhaps best described as cheeselike patches. Bitot spots are not wetted normally by tears, and they reform rapidly after removal by mechanical debridement. They can form on both the nasal and temporal sides of the limbus, but the latter location is more common. Histopathologically, the conjunctival epithelium becomes epidermoid in character, goblet cells disappear, and hyaline degeneration of the epithelial cells is observed. The foamlike appearance is said to be due to vesicular formation and irregularity of the superficial layers of the keratinized epithelium. Scrapings show meibomian secretions, epithelial debris, fatty globules, and large numbers of *Corynebacterium xerosis* and other bacterial organisms.

Xerophthalmia or epithelial xerosis, an excessive keratinization of the conjunctival and corneal epithelium, results from vitamin A deficiency, and some of its earliest ocular manifestations occur at the limbus. There may be folds in the limbal conjunctiva along with keratinized, heaped-up corneal epithelium and marginal corneal infiltrates. In advanced cases the entire cornea becomes necrotic and vascularized.

Peripheral Corneal Opacification with Skeletal Deformities

In 1970 Brown and Kuwabara described an unusual case of peripheral thinning of the cornea in a patient suffering from arthritis that was similar to rheumatoid arthritis. There was annular limbal opacification along with pannus formation. It may be related to a form of mucopolysaccharidoses.[16]

Gaucher's Disease (Cerebroside Lipidosis)

In Gaucher's disease there is a deficiency of glucocerebroside-cleaving enzyme, and excess glucocerebroside accumulates in the reticuloendothelial cells of the spleen, liver, lymph nodes, and bone marrow. Decreased activity of this enzyme can be demonstrated in the peripheral blood by testing the leukocytes.[17] There are at least two forms of the disease, an infantile and an adult form. The infantile form is panethnic (not more prevalent among Jews) and is invariably fatal; its most common ocular manifestation is strabismus. The adult form is more prevalent among Ashkenazi Jews and is characterized by onset late in childhood or in the adult and by a prolonged course free of neurologic involvement. Limbal pingueculae may be found in this form of the disease.[18, 19] Although pingueculae adjacent to the limbus are common among older individuals, those seen in association with Gaucher's disease appear to be more deeply pigmented (yellow-brown) and are vascularized.[18] Histologically, these pingueculae contain large epithelioid cells with foamy cytoplasm.[20]

Juvenile Xanthogranuloma (JXG)

Although not properly a disease of lipid metabolism per se, JXG is included in this section because its histologic picture resembles histiocytosis X. Seemingly this disorder is an inflammatory response of an undetermined nature. It usually affects youngsters between the ages of 4 months and 10 years and will remit spontaneously. It is characterized by the presence of small (0.5 to 2.0 cm.) yellow granulomas that can be found on the skin, conjunctiva, sclera, orbit, and limbus.[21, 22] The most important ocular lesions of JXG, however, are the granulomas that involve the iris and ciliary body.[23] They can cause a spontaneous hyphema or secondary glaucoma and may require biopsy for microscopic confirmation of the diagnosis. Histopathologically, the lesions consist of fat deposits in the histiocytes of granulomas.

Alkaptonuria (Ochronosis)

This metabolic disease is an autosomal recessive characterized by dark pigmentation of the skin, sclera, and cartilage. It is caused by the absence of the enzyme homogentisic acid oxidase, which converts homogentisic acid to maleylacetoacetic acid during the degradation of tyrosine. The urine will turn a dark color upon oxidation. The clinical disease, ochronosis, results from the deposition of homogentisic acid in connective tissue, particularly sclera and cartilage. The presence of homogentisic acid in the urine occurs at an early age, whereas the ocular manifestations do not usually become manifest until middle age. The interpalpebral region of the sclera and the upper sclera appear to be particularly prone to pigmentation. In addition, there may be deeply pigmented areas anterior to the insertion of the medial and lateral recti, and these occasionally involve the peripheral sclera and limbal area.[24, 25] The pigmentation is extracellular and there is little inflammation associated with it. Systemically, patients may have trouble walking because of serious back problems, including complete spinal rigidity due to narrowed intervertebral discs and calcification.

Amyloidosis

Amyloidosis is a disorder characterized by the extracellular deposition in various tissues of a protein substance called amyloid. The protein contains sulfated mucopolysaccharides, including heparan sulfate. When deposited on the ocular surface, the material forms pink to yellow nodular masses that histopathologically have characteristic staining properties. Amyloid is amorphous, exhibiting metachromasia when stained with crystal violet and showing dichroism under polarized light when stained with Congo red. Two major types of protein are deposited; they may be found singly or they may coexist. One group of proteins, first identified by Glenner, often is the sole type found in primary amyloidosis. This group does not have the amino acid sequence of immunoglobulin and is called the A.L. (amyloid-L-chain) protein. The other group of proteins in amyloid fibrils have an amino acid sequence that closely resembles that of the light chains of immunoglobulins.[26]

The usual clinical classification divides amyloidosis into systemic and localized disease, and each is further subdivided into primary and secondary categories. Considerable overlap may occur. Primary forms of the disorder are not associated with chronic infection or inflammation, and their origin remains obscure. In contrast, secondary forms are associated with chronic infection or inflammation (e.g., osteomyelitis, rheumatoid arthritis). The eye and surrounding tissues may be involved in all but the secondary systemic form of the disease.

Amyloid can be deposited as fleshy, tumorlike masses in the tarsal or bulbar conjunctiva, or the deposits can be located deep within the fornices. Fleshy, nodular lesions also may be encountered at the limbus, where the tumor may be large enough to masquerade as a lipodermoid. Corneal manifestations of amyloidosis include a fan-shaped keratopathy and nodular masses resembling those of Salzmann's nodular corneal degeneration. Evidence has been presented that lattice dystrophy is a localized or isolated form of primary, familial amyloidosis.[27, 28] The skin of the lids may be involved, and other ocular variants include a chronic uveitis, orbital involvement with proptosis, and the formation of vitreous opacities.[29–32] Visual acuity in the latter group may be improved by pars plana vitrectomy.

Porphyrias

The porphyrias are characterized by abnormal porphyrin metabolism; porphyrin and its precursors are produced in excess and can be demonstrated in blood, urine, and feces. Patients with porphyria exhibit a wide range of symptoms and signs. The two most common clinical forms are severe, acute, intermittent porphyria, which has no ocular manifestations, and the chronic cutaneous form, which may be associated with ocular manifestations and porphyria variegata.[33] In the second or third decade patients with the chronic variety may develop conjunctival scarring and symblepharon formation similar to mucous membrane pemphigoid. Yellow-brown thickening of the episclera and conjunctiva may be present and may extend onto the limbus. These areas have been described as appearing like "milk curds" in ultraviolet light. In addition, patients with this form of porphyria may suffer spontaneous limbal perforation secondary to scleromalacia perforans.[34]

Cryoglobulinemia

A group of serum proteins known as cryoglobulins precipitate when exposed to cold and dissolve when returned to body temperature. Multiple myeloma has been found in 50 per cent of patients with a marked elevation in the concentration of cold precipitable serum proteins. These proteins may even precipitate at 37° C if their concentration increases sufficiently. In addition to the mechanical problems they create, it has been suggested that precipitating cryoglobulins also may be antigenic and provoke autoimmunization. The only treatment for essential cryoglobulinemia is the avoidance of cold temperatures. Treatment of cryoglobulinemia secondary to diseases such as multiple myeloma and chronic lymphatic leukemia is directed at the underlying disease.

The ocular manifestations of cryoglobulinemia include the occasional limbal deposition of curious, deep, maplike, whitish-gray deposits. The maplike lesions may change as the ambient temperature changes, suggesting that they may be precipitated cryoglobulins deposited at the limbus (Fig. 7–7).

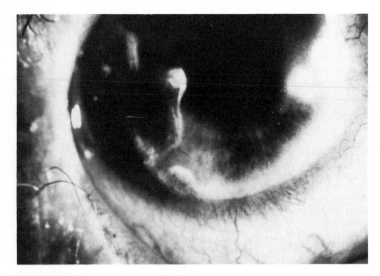

Figure 7–7. Peculiar deposits in a patient with cryoglobulinemia.

Monoclonal Gammopathy

In addition to the unusual findings occasionally associated with cryoglobulinemia, crystalline corneal opacities have been found in patients with so-called benign monoclonal gammopathy.[35, 36] Although these tend to be most dense in the deep stroma at the midperiphery of the cornea rather than at the limbus, the entity is mentioned here for sake of completeness.

LIMBAL CORNEAL FINDINGS SECONDARY TO THE DEPOSITION OF SUBSTANCES

Limbal Deposits of Gold (Chrysiasis)

Gold deposits will occasionally be observed in the corneas of patients who receive gold injections for the treatment of rheumatoid arthritis. The earliest deposition of gold may be in the midstroma near the limbus (Fig. 7–8). When gold is deposited in the central cornea, it tends to become more superficial. Gold should not be confused with copper, which is a darker yellow in color.[37]

Copper Deposits (Chalcosis)

In Wilson's disease copper is deposited in the peripheral cornea at the level of Descemet's membrane and forms the Kayser-Fleischer Ring. Wilson's disease is discussed more fully earlier in this chapter.

Iron Deposits

Iron lines in the cornea are associated with many conditions, but the iron deposits closest to the limbus are those at the base of a glaucoma filtering bleb, i.e., the Ferry line, and those at the advancing edge of a pterygium, i.e., the Stocker line. In each instance the iron is deposited within the corneal epithelium.[38, 39]

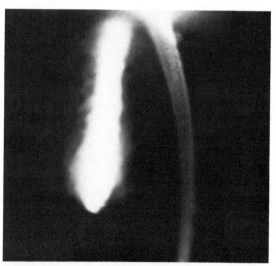

Figure 7–8. Corneal deposits of gold in a patient with severe rheumatoid arthritis.

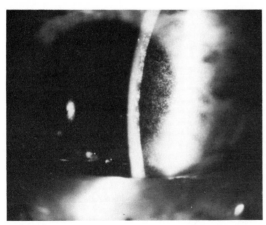

Figure 7–9. Deep corneal deposits found in a patient taking phenothiazines for years.

Phenothiazines

Long-term administration of phenothiazine compounds to individuals with psychiatric disturbances may be accompanied by the deposition of this material deep within the corneal stroma at the level of Descemet's membrane. These deposits initially may be found at the limbus, but eventually the entire cornea may become involved (Fig. 7–9). There may be an associated pigmentary retinopathy in many of these patients.[40]

INFECTIONS OF THE LIMBAL AREA

Bacterial Limbal Ring Ulcers and Infiltrates

The presence of a limbal ring ulcer is one of the most serious corneal conditions that the ophthalmologist encounters. Most frequently it is due to infection of the peripheral cornea by *Streptococcus pneumoniae* or *Pseudomonas aeruginosa* and is characterized by a dense cellular infiltrate. Generally there is significant pain associated with these peripheral corneal ulcers, and the bulbar conjunctiva is markedly hyperemic. Limbal ring ulcers can quickly progress to complete coalescence and can deteriorate to perforation with 24 to 48 hours (Fig. 7–10). Usually there is an accompanying severe uveitis with dense flare and cells in the aqueous humor, and frequently a hypopyon is present. Many patients with corneal ring ulcers are debilitated; they have serious systemic diseases, often a malignancy, and there also seems to be an increased prevalence of this type of lesion in patients with Sjögren's syndrome. It is imperative to establish the microbiologic etiology of a limbal ring infiltrate or an ulcer as soon as possible. The limulus lysate assay is a rapid and reliable method for the detection of minute amounts of Gram-negative endotoxin. It is a useful adjunct to the traditional methods of diagnosis (i.e., Gram stain and culture), permitting the swift detection of Gram-negative infection and the prompt selection of appropriate antimicrobial agents.[41, 42]

Treatment follows the usual guidelines for bacterial keratitis. In general, if the agent is Gram positive, antibiotic therapy must be effective against the penicillinase producing staphylococci and *Streptococcus pneumoniae.* Recommended drugs include the semisynthetic penicillins, the cephalosporins, bacitracin, and vancomycin. If a Gram-negative organism is seen in the Gram stain or if the limulus lysate test is positive, antimicrobial therapy must cover *Pseudomonas aeruginosa.* Drugs commonly used for *Pseudomonas* keratitis include gentamicin, tobramycin, carbenicillin, colistin, and polymyxin B. Antibiotics are administered as "fortified" topical formulations and by periocular injection. Corticosteroids are not used primarily for peripheral bacterial ulcers. Mydriatic-cycloplegic agents are instilled to prevent synechia formation as a result of the accompanying severe uveitis. Anticollagenase compounds often are administered to reduce the likelihood of peripheral corneal melting associated with the production of proteases and collagenases by *Pseudomonas* organisms,[43, 44] but their clinical effectiveness has not been established. The treatment of bacterial infections of the cornea is discussed in detail in Chapter 15.

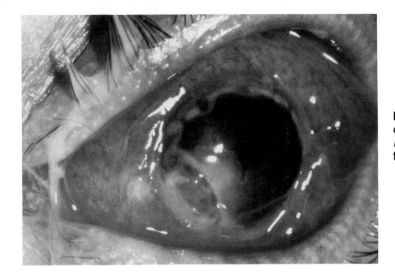

Figure 7–10. Limbal ring ulcer due to *Streptococcus pneumoniae* in a patient with keratoconjunctivitis sicca.

Limbal Corneal Infections Due to Viruses

Herpes Simplex Infections (Limbal Herpes)

Herpes simplex virus classically produces dendrites that tend to involve the central cornea. However, it may occasionally produce peripheral corneal lesions that are difficult to diagnose and that tend to have a somewhat more protracted natural history than central dendrites.[45, 46] In patients with a history of herpetic disease who present with hypesthetic epithelial lesions at the limbus, the suspicion of recurrent herpetic infection should be very high (Fig. 7–11). Small areolar areas of keratitis or even microdendrites are not uncommonly seen in children with primary herpes infection (Fig. 7–12). Recurrent limbal herpetic epithelial disease will eventually be characterized by a moderate amount of concomitant stromal edema and often by sector neovascularization of the limbus. The importance of rose bengal as a diagnostic stain in these patients cannot be overemphasized, and the presence of multinucleated giant cells (demonstrated by Giemsa staining) and/or the presence of intranuclear inclusions from scrapings (best demonstrated by the Papanicolaou technique) tend to support the clinical suspicion of herpes simplex.[47]

The management of limbal herpes follows the guidelines of central epithelial herpes simplex keratitis with only minor exceptions. Most of these patients are not threatened with visual loss from stromal keratitis or neovascularization, but the disease does tend to be more protracted and more difficult to manage with available antiviral compounds. The use of debridement, advocated for the treatment of herpetic dendritic keratitis,[48] is an excellent choice for treatment of lesions located at the limbus. Recurrent epithelial herpes simplex keratitis at the limbus increases the likelihood of severe stromal reactions. These stromal infiltrates may occasionally be confused

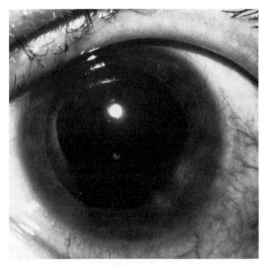

Figure 7–11. Recurrent herpetic keratitis involving the peripheral cornea. (Courtesy of Howard M. Leibowitz, M.D.)

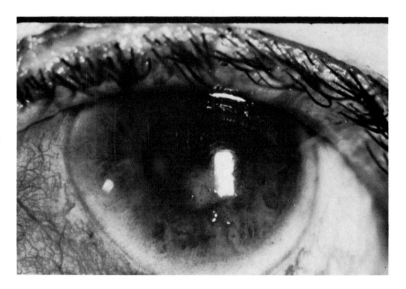

Figure 7–12. *Areolar keratitis due to herpes simplex.*

with the marginal corneal infiltrates caused by staphylococci, but it is important to differentiate clinically between the two entities. Topically applied corticosteroids often are very helpful in treating the bacterial problem but frequently are contraindicated as treatment for the marginal herpetic keratitis.

Varicella-Zoster

A limbal lesion occasionally will occur in children with chickenpox (Fig. 7–13). These lesions are actually small areas of raised punctate epithelial keratitis (PEK). Very small, shallow, limbal ul-

cers and associated areas of limbal infiltration also may occur, and a very mild episcleritis is encountered on rare occasions. The limbal lesions of chickenpox are self-limited and tend to fade with the skin lesions. They rarely require antiviral treatment.[49]

Zoster infections of the eye rank among the most serious.[50] In this chapter their discussion could also be placed in the hypersensitivity section. Patients with herpes zoster ophthalmicus will occasionally show, either in conjunction with the acute attack or at a later date, a dense inflammation of the peripheral cornea and adjacent sclera (Fig. 7–14). This sclerokeratitis responds to topical corticosteroids. Less frequently zoster

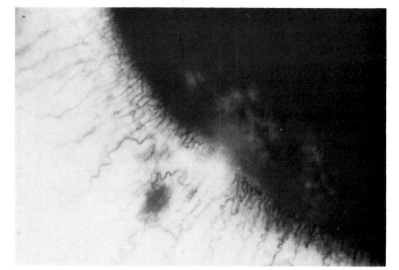

Figure 7–13. *Varicella lesion at the limbus.*

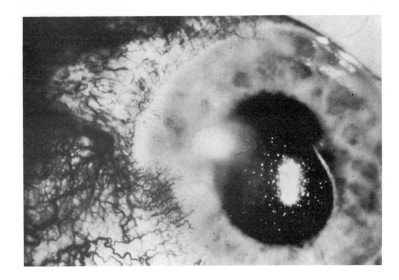

Figure 7–14. Marked sclerokeratitis in a patient with herpes zoster ophthalmicus.

immune rings, or arcs, and shallow limbal ulcers also occur (Fig. 7–15).

Vaccinia

Since the reduction in mass immunization programs for smallpox, blepharoconjunctivitis caused by autoinoculation of the lids with live vaccinia virus has decreased (Fig. 7–16). However, when recently vaccinated children or their siblings present with an acute ulcerative blepharoconjunctivitis and cellulitis, the possibility of autoinoculation with vaccinia must be kept in mind.[51]

These patients may have limbal edema and peripheral corneal dendrites (Fig. 7–17). The central cornea can also be involved by the epithelial lesions, and to a certain extent they resemble primary herpes simplex reactions. It is important to keep in mind, however, that the follicular reaction of primary herpes simplex is absent in these children. Vaccinia virus can be recovered from the lesions, and the characteristic brick-shaped virus can be identified by electron microscopy.

Antiviral compounds are effective in the management of patients with ocular vaccinia.[52, 53] In addition, systemic vaccine immune globulin (VIG) has been used in serious cases, but there is a possibility that VIG may worsen the stromal keratitis. Vaccinial stromal keratitis responds to topical corticosteroids,

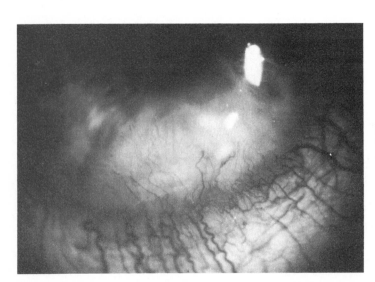

Figure 7–15. Herpes zoster immune ring 4 months after skin eruption.

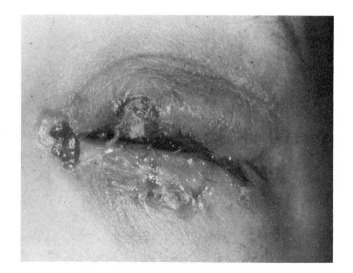

Figure 7–16. Marked vaccinial reaction.

but they should be used with caution along with topical antiviral agents as an umbrella cover.[54]

HYPERSENSITIVITY REACTIONS AT THE CORNEAL LIMBUS

Phlyctenular Keratitis

Phlyctenular keratitis classically has been associated with endemic tuberculosis. It is extremely common where untreated cases of tuberculosis are widespread. In the continental United States pulmonary tuberculosis is largely controlled, and chronic staphylococcal blepharitis appears to be the entity most commonly associated with phlyctenular keratitis. Other causes of phlyctenular reactions of the cornea include candida and coccidioidomycosis.[55, 56]

The limbal phlyctenule is a microabscess that typically appears as a raised, inflamed nodule near the limbus (Fig. 7–18). A small central ulceration often develops and the lesion then eventually regresses. Repeated attacks may occur; occasionally this is evident because of the presence of triangular-based limbal scars.

There is a spectrum of phlyctenular reactions that differ from the classic limbal phlyctenule. A wandering phlyctenule, which along with a leash of vessels progresses over the surface of the cornea,

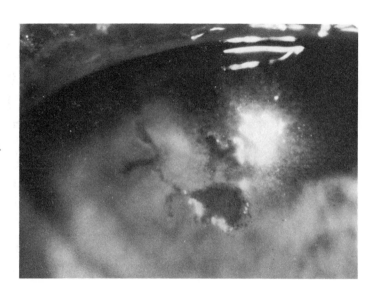

Figure 7–17. Vaccinial dendrite.

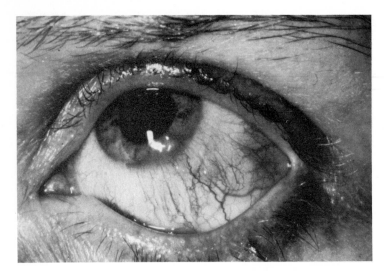

Figure 7–18. Limbal phlyctenule.

occurs rarely. Perforations due to phlyctenular disease are extremely unusual in this country but may be encountered in areas where tuberculosis is severe. In children presentation of the disease includes an inferior pannus and even a circumferential pannus. Anterior stromal opacification and small areas of epithelial and subepithelial infiltration commonly accompany the superficial vascularization (Fig. 7–19).

Management of phlyctenular disease due to endemic tuberculosis requires control of the tuberculosis. Management of phlyctenular reactions accompanying bacterial blepharitis, on the other hand, calls for lid hygiene and the application of antimicrobial ointments to the lid margins with cotton-tipped applicators. Patients will also usually require topical corticosteroids to control the inflammatory reactions.[57]

Vernal Disease

Vernal disease may be characterized as itching keratitis.[58] The characteristic compound papillae (cobblestone papillae) of the tarsal conjunctiva are well known. The corneal manifestations include the presence of punctate epithelial erosions (PEE) and punctate epithelial keratitis (PEK) located near the superior marginal cornea. In addition, there may be limbal vegetations (Fig. 7–20), which

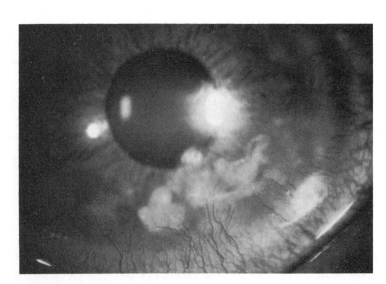

Figure 7–19. Areas of epithelial and subepithelial keratitis in a young child with staphylococcal blepharitis.

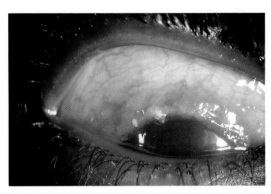

Figure 7–20. Limbal vegetations in vernal disease. (Courtesy of Howard M. Leibowitz, M.D.)

can be effective. Some children have chronic staphylococcal lid disease that requires the application of antimicrobial ointments to the lid margins. The introduction of disodium cromoglycate has been a significant advance in the management of patients with severe vernal disease. Topical administration of cromolyn sodium 4 per cent may be effective in reducing symptoms and in improving both the conjunctival and the corneal manifestations of the disease. It may permit a significant reduction of the amount of corticosteroids being used.[59]

can occur without the classic compound papillary reaction of the tarsal conjunctiva. Trantas' dots are associated with this disorder and are merely collections of eosinophils that appear at the limbus. Hooded edema of the limbal conjunctiva in the form of a pseudogerontoxon may be seen, and in severe cases there may be a superior pannus. Superior horizontal, oval vernal corneal ulcers may occasionally be observed.

The management of patients with vernal disease is difficult and prolonged. Most affected children have other atopic problems. They commonly require topical corticosteroids to relieve their ocular symptoms and to lessen the conjunctival response. In addition, these children produce an abnormal mucus that may require control with a topical mucolytic compound. Topically applied acetylcysteine 10 per cent (Mucomyst)

Rosacea

Patients with acne rosacea often have chronic staphylococcal blepharitis that may produce recurrent marginal corneal infiltrates and ulcers. These infiltrates are commonly midstromal and may be a dense yellow in color, appearing similar to a limbal corneal abscess. Recurrent bouts of these limbal corneal infiltrates often leave the patient with deep marginal corneal neovascularization and eventual thinning and opacification.[60]

Limbal Marginal Infiltrates and Ulcers Due to Staphylococcal Hypersensitivity

Marginal ulceration of the cornea in association with chronic staphylococcal blepharokeratoconjunctivitis has al-

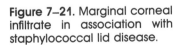

Figure 7–21. Marginal corneal infiltrate in association with staphylococcal lid disease.

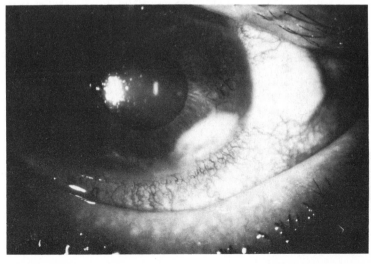

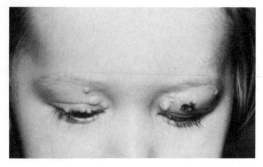

Figure 7–22. Molluscum contagiosum.

nodule may be hidden on the lid margin, or it may be found near the lateral canthus. On the other hand, the diagnosis may be readily apparent in young children who present with a large crop of molluscum nodules on the skin of the lids, face, and forehead (Fig. 7–22). A significant superior limbal pannus may be present and lead the examiner to falsely suspect trachoma. The reaction will subside completely after the excision of the molluscum nodule.

ready been mentioned. These patients may present with conjunctival papillary injection and with limbal corneal infiltrates or ulcers of sudden onset (Fig. 7–21). The lesions may be ulcerated, and typically the infiltrates have their long axis in parallel with the limbus. Generally there is a clear zone between the infiltrate and the limbus. The infiltrates respond to the reduction of staphylococcal antigenic load by the application of antimicrobial ointments to the lid margins. It may be necessary to use dilute topical corticosteroid preparations to eliminate them completely.[61]

Molluscum Contagiosum

Molluscum contagiosum may be associated with a chronic unilateral conjunctivitis whose cause frequently has eluded practitioners. The molluscum

LIMBAL CORNEAL MANIFESTATIONS OF COLLAGEN VASCULAR DISEASES

Patients with disorders characterized as collagen vascular diseases will occasionally present with limbal manifestations of their systemic disorder. Most commonly the problem is encountered in patients with rheumatoid arthritis, and characteristically the lesion is a marginal corneal furrow (Fig. 7–23)[62] capable of spontaneous perforation. The ulcer occasionally will respond to the institution of systemic corticosteroids or to increasing the level of corticosteroid that the patient may already be taking. Often, however, the lesion continues relentlessly to progress and deepen. In my experience the use of topical corticosteroids has been fraught with hazard and may cause the ulcer to perforate rapidly (Fig. 7–24).

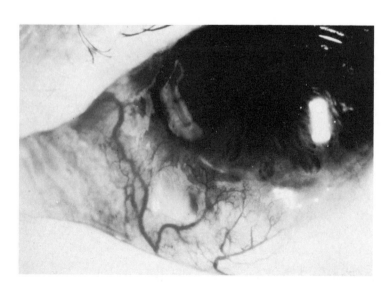

Figure 7–23. Rheumatoid marginal corneal furrow after perforation.

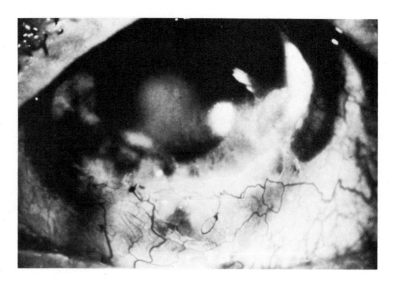

Figure 7–24. Tectonic lamellar graft for perforated marginal corneal furrow following treatment with topical corticosteroids.

In addition to rheumatoid marginal corneal furrows, the peripheral cornea may be affected in patients with other collagen vascular diseases. There is a characteristic marginal keratolysis in patients with polyarteritis nodosa; the marginal cornea appears to melt away, leaving a deep limbal gutter. Severe peripheral corneal melting also occurs in patients with midline granuloma, Wegener's granulomatosis and, less commonly, in patients with systemic lupus erythematosus. Occasionally this phenomenon is encountered in patients with ulcerative colitis and colitic arthropathy along with deep stromal vascularization of interstitial keratitis (Fig. 7–25). In many instances the ulcerative process in the peripheral cornea is accompanied by surprisingly few signs of external ocular inflammation.

LIMBAL ULCERATIONS DUE TO AUTOIMMUNITY (MOOREN'S ULCER)

Progressive furrow ulceration of the peripheral cornea in the absence of a collagen vascular disorder is called Mooren's ulcer. It generally occurs in older individuals but may be encountered in young blacks, and evidence has been presented attributing the disorder to autoimmune phenomena.[63–65] The condition is characterized by circumferential melting of the peripheral cornea that

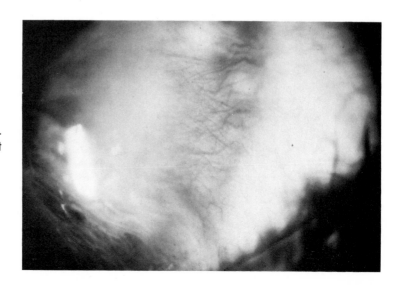

Figure 7–25. Deep limbal interstitial keratitis in a patient with colitic arthropathy.

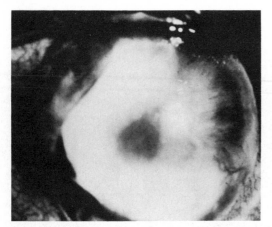

Figure 7–26. Mooren's corneal ulcer.

may eventually destroy the entire peripheral corneal substance, leaving only a central corneal cap (Fig. 7–26). The management of patients with Mooren's corneal ulcers is an extremely difficult problem. Many of these patients are elderly, and they may be confined to a wheelchair or be bedridden. They usually have extreme pain. Conjunctival excision has been beneficial as has the use of systemic immunosuppression.[66–69]

DYSPLASTIC AND NEOPLASTIC LIMBAL LESIONS

Hereditary Benign Dyskeratosis

Hereditary benign dyskeratosis of the limbus is dominantly transmitted and the ocular sequelae usually are minor. In these individuals there may be a dense hyaline-like plaque of dyskeratotic epithelium heaped up in the limbal area.

Intraepithelial Epithelioma

In addition to intraepithelial epithelioma, the ophthalmic literature refers to this disorder as limbal dysplasia, carcinoma in situ, and Bowen's disease. It tends to occur in older individuals (though this is not invariable), particularly among those who have lived in zones of intense ultraviolet radiation. At

times intraepithelial epithelioma presents as a lumpy, gray, elevated epithelial lesion extending from the limbus onto the central cornea (Fig. 7–27). There may be an associated fine pannus, and in some cases the opacified epithelium assumes a characteristic "caput medusae" configuration. More typically, however, the intraepithelial epithelioma is located at the limbus; it is elevated and vascularized and appears very much like a small strawberry (Fig. 7–28). Histologically the lesion consists of atypical, haphazardly arranged epithelial cells containing bizarre mitotic figures. Although these changes are considered to be malignant, the basal epithelial layer is intact and the stroma is not invaded; these lesions can be removed by simple excision.[70]

Squamous Cell Carcinoma

Squamous cell carcinoma of the bulbar conjunctiva and limbal area is unusual. The lesions tend to be raised and elevated to a greater degree than benign lesions (Fig. 7–29). Limbal squamous cell carcinomas may remain superficial and do not invariably invade the ocular tissues deeply (Fig. 7–30). Superficial excision in these cases may be satisfactory, resulting in a cure for the patient. At times, however, a limbal squamous cell carcinoma can invade the intraocular structures.[71]

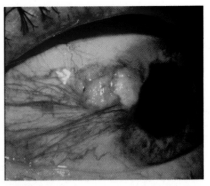

Figure 7–27. Carcinoma in situ (Bowen's disease). (Courtesy of Howard M. Leibowitz, M.D.)

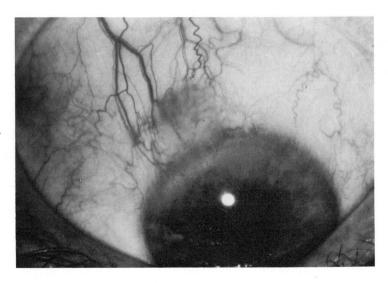

Figure 7–28. Intraepithelial epithelioma (Bowen's disease).

Limbal Melanoma

Melanomas may occur at the limbus (Fig. 7–31), and they should be surgically managed, as are melanomas elsewhere, with a wide surgical resection. Enucleation, radiation, and chemotherapy may also be indicated. They should not be confused with cystic nevi that commonly occur at the limbus and may show activity at or around the time of puberty (Figs. 7–32 and 7–33). If there is any doubt concerning a pigmented lesion of the limbal area, an excisional biopsy of the lesion should be done for histopathologic confirmation.[72]

Limbal Epibulbar Dermoid

These lesions (choristomas) represent normal tissue found in an abnormal location. They vary from small limbal lesions to large ones that may extend over the cornea in association with a scleral staphyloma (Fig. 7–34).[73] The presence of epibulbar dermoids in association with auricular and vertebral abnormalities is known as Goldenhar's syndrome. Patients with this disorder should have a complete physical evaluation and should be referred to an otorhinolaryngologist for the prevention of hearing loss. The surgical management of all of

these superficial disorders has been previously summarized by the author.[74]

DEGENERATIONS OF THE CORNEAL LIMBUS

Pinguecula

It is very common to see fleshy, elastoid pingueculae near the limbus (Fig. 7–35). They have no clinical significance, although it has been postulated that these raised lesions may under certain circumstances lead to localized dried areas that may eventually contribute to the formation of a pterygium. In any event, pin-

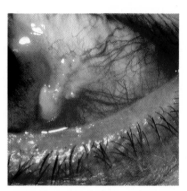

Figure 7–29. Limbal lesion, clinically thought to be Bowen's disease, proved histopathologically to be a squamous cell carcinoma. (Courtesy of Howard M. Leibowitz, M.D.)

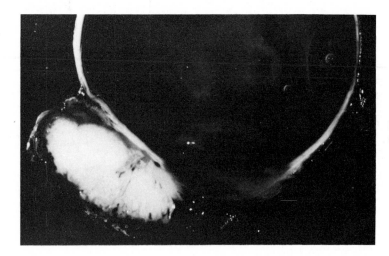

Figure 7–30. Squamous cell carcinoma of the limbus.

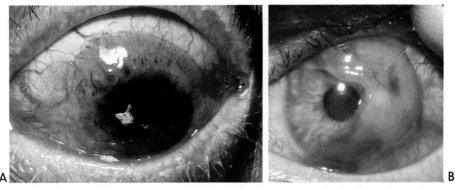

A   B

Figure 7–31. Limbal melanoma. *A*, Moderately advanced lesion. *B*, More advanced lesion with extensive corneal invasion. Both cases were successfully treated by a wide, deep local excision, application of cryotherapy, and a segmental lamellar keratoplasty. Excellent retention of vision with no recurrence of tumor after 5 years in both cases. (Courtesy of Howard M. Leibowitz, M.D.)

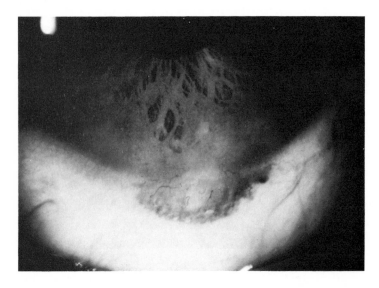

Figure 7–32. Cystic limbal nevus.

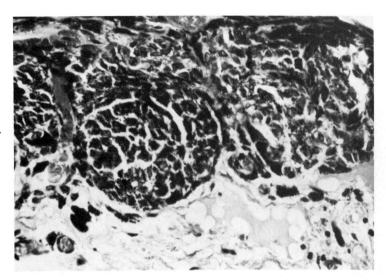

Figure 7–33. Nests of limbal nevus cells.

gueculae in general are of no consequence, should be recognized as such, and should be left undisturbed.

White Limbic Girdle of Vogt

The white limbic girdle of Vogt is a common marginal corneal finding. It is a degenerative change located in the superficial cornea and is usually confined to the interpalpebral fissure (Fig. 7–36). It is of no clinical consequence.

Band Keratopathy

Band keratopathy usually begins with the subepithelial deposition of calcium at the 3 and 9 o'clock meridians adjacent to the limbus (Fig. 7–37). It is often associated with elevation of serum calcium and, in addition, it occurs in eyes with chronic uveitis. It is commonly found in patients with juvenile rheumatoid arthritis (JRA, Still's disease) who have uveitis. Band keratopathy also may be seen in patients suffering from longstanding open-angle glaucoma requiring long-term miotic therapy and in patients with blind, painful eyes. The removal of band keratopathy is accomplished after the epithelium is removed from the cornea; the calcium is chelated with topically applied 0.02 molar disodium EDTA.[75]

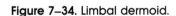

Figure 7–34. Limbal dermoid.

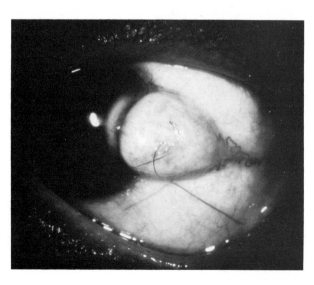

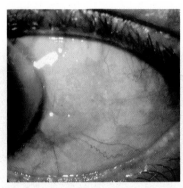

Figure 7–35. Pinguecula.

Pterygium

There are probably as many explanations for the pathogenesis of pterygium as there are differences in the behavior of these conjunctival limbal degenerations (Fig. 7–38). The incidence of pterygia is higher in tropical than in temperate regions. Tropical areas of the earth receive the most intense ultraviolet radiation, and it seems likely that ultraviolet radiation is involved in the pathogenesis of pterygium. As discussed previously, it also is possible that in some individuals pinguecula and an associated localized drying phenomenon produce pterygia.[76]

In any event patients affected with pterygia fall generally into two broad categories: (1) those with a small atrophic pterygium that shows little or no evidence of progression over a long period of time, and (2) those in whom the pterygium behaves in a much more aggressive fashion. In the latter case there tends to be deep hyperemia within the lesion and an associated advancing area of grayish opacification preceded by an epithelial iron line. The pterygium invades the superficial peripheral cornea and moves relentlessly toward the visual axis, causing distortion of the cornea, irregular astigmatism, and visual loss. The surgical management includes simple excision with lamellar keratectomy, free conjunctival or buccal mucosal grafts, and lamellar keratoplasty for severe recurrent lesions.[77]

Post-Irradiation Scleromalacia

In patients who have received excessive beta radiation subsequent to the excision of a pterygium or other limbal lesion, there may be sudden melting in the area of the original excision some years later. Patients who experience diffuse scleromalacia and corneal melting subsequent to irradiation may have a concomitant debilitating systemic disease. This is not meant to detract from the potentially worthwhile effects of judiciously applied beta radiation as an adjunct to the treatment of pterygia. However, I

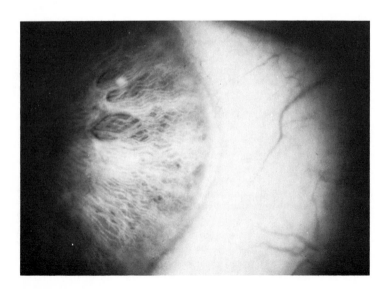

Figure 7–36. White limbic girdle of Vogt.

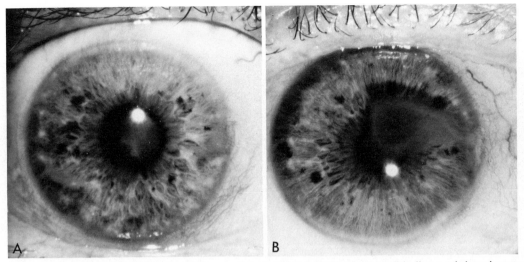

Figure 7–37. Band keratopathy. *A,* Right eye. Subepithelial calcium deposit in the peripheral cornea at three o'clock and a second faint deposit at eight o'clock. *B,* Left eye of same patient. Subepithelial calcium deposition has progressed to involve the central, interpalpebral portion of the cornea.

have abandoned the *routine* use of beta radiation following pterygium excision.

Droplet Keratopathy

The presence of fine, oily-appearing droplets at the limbal area has been described in detail.[78] This characteristic corneal change was originally reported in Labrador, but it is also very common in agricultural workers of the southern United States and has been seen in large scale trachoma field trials in southern Iran. The cause of Labrador keratopathy is controversial and ill-defined, but it is thought by many to be related to environmental trauma, e.g., exposure to ultraviolet rays, fine dust, and heat.

Dellen

Sudden marginal corneal stromal thinning without tendency to perforate may occur after surgical procedures at or near the limbus that alter the tear film and leave dry spots (Fig. 7–39). The nature of these benign lesions has been well described.[79, 80]

Figure 7–38. Pterygium in a patient from San Antonio, Texas.

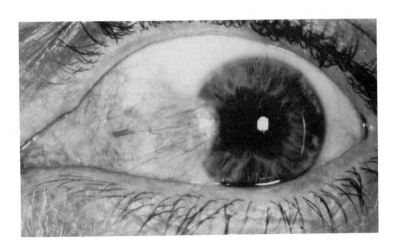

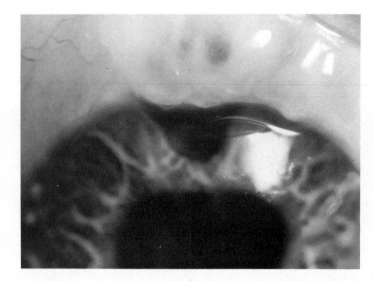

Figure 7–39. Dellen adjacent to an elevated conjunctival filtering bleb. (Courtesy of Howard M. Leibowitz, M.D.)

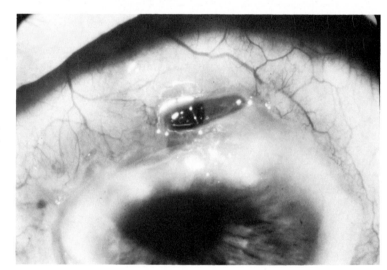

Figure 7–40. Marginal degeneration following cataract surgery.

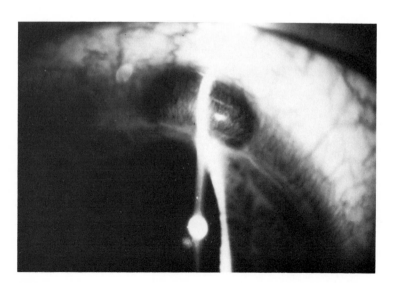

Figure 7–41. Terrien's marginal degeneration with perforation in a 4-year-old male.

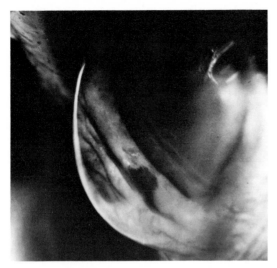

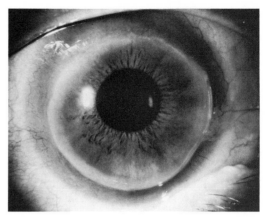

Figure 7–43. Asymptomatic marginal thinning in an elderly patient.

Figure 7–42. Normal thickness cornea, located just above an area of thinned inferior peripheral stroma, protruding anteriorly and downward in a case of pellucid marginal degeneration. (Courtesy of Howard M. Leibowitz, M.D.)

Marginal Degeneration After Cataract Surgery

A rare complication following cataract surgery is chronic melting and progressive thinning of the marginal cornea and sclera (Fig. 7–40).[81] This disorder is thought by some authors to represent ischemic necrosis of the peripheral cornea; periocular injection of heparin has been advocated as treatment for presumed ischemia of the peripheral cornea.[82] However, I have recently managed two cases successfully using the technique of conjunctival excision, and others recommend short-term systemic immunosuppression.[68, 69]

Terrien's Marginal Corneal Degeneration

This entity is a noninflammatory peripheral corneal thinning of unknown etiology. It initially affects the superior cornea and is found most commonly in adult males. However, I have treated a 4-year-old Latin American male be-

lieved to be the youngest patient with this condition; he presented after spontaneous perforation and required lamellar keratoplasty (Fig. 7–41).[74] Others have used this technique with good results for tectonic structural reinforcement.[83]

Pellucid Marginal Degeneration

Pellucid marginal degeneration of the cornea[84] is a bilateral disorder of unknown etiology characterized by an arcuate area of thinning in the inferior peripheral cornea. Typically, the area of thinning is 1 to 2 mm in width, is concentric to the inferior limbus and separated from it by 1 to 2 mm of normal thickness cornea, and is clear; there is no scarring, infiltration, lipid deposition, or neovascularization. The cornea above the thinned area is normal in thickness but protrudes anteriorly and downward (Fig. 7–42), generally resulting in a high degree of irregular astigmatism. This condition seemingly differs from keratoconus and keratoglobus, is not associated with inflammation, and does not appear to be related to the asymptomatic marginal thinning that occurs in the cornea of elderly patients (Fig. 7–43).

REFERENCES

1. Theodore, F. H.: Superior limbic keratoconjunctivitis. Eye Ear Nose Throat Monthly 42:25, 1963.
2. Theodore, F. H.: Further observations on superior limbic keratoconjunctivitis. Trans Amer Acad Ophthalmol Otolaryng 71:341, 1967.
3. Theodore, F. H., and Ferry, A. P.: Superior limbic keratoconjunctivitis. Clinical and pathological correlations. Arch Ophthalmol 84:481, 1970.
4. Tenzel, R. R.: Comments on superior limbic filamentous keratitis: II. Arch Ophthalmol 79:508, 1968.
5. Cogan, D. G., and Kuwabara, T.: Ocular changes in experimental hypercholesteremia. Arch Ophthalmol 61:219, 1959.
6. Hogan, M. J., and Zimmerman, L. E.: *Ophthalmic Pathology*. 2nd ed. Philadelphia, W. B. Saunders Co., 1962, p. 334.
7. Blodi, F. C., and Yarbrough, J. C.: Ocular manifestations of familial hypercholesterolemia. Trans Am Ophthalmol Soc 60:304, 1962.
8. Feldman, E. B.: Familial hypercholesterolemia— Predecessor of coronary heart disease. Res Staff Physician 24(6):70, 1978.
9. Chalmers, T. C., Iber, F. L., and Uzman, L. L.: Hepatolenticular degeneration (Wilson's disease) as a form of idiopathic cirrhosis. N Engl J Med 256:235, 1957.
10. Harrison, T. R. (ed.): *Principles of Internal Medicine*. New York, McGraw-Hill, 8th ed., 1977, p. 664.
11. Heinz, K., Schbel, F., and Gunther, R.: Augenbefunde bei Gicht und Hyperurikämie. Wien Klin Wochenschr 83:42, 1971.
12. Watson, P. G., and Hazleman, B. L.: *The Sclera and Systemic Disorders*. Philadelphia, W. B. Saunders Co., 1976, pp. 327–331.
13. Yu, T. F., and Gutman, A. B.: A study of the paradoxical effects of salicylates in low, intermediate and high dosage on the renal mechanisms for excretion of ureate in man. J Clin Invest 38:1298, 1959.
14. Watts, R. W.: Allopurinol in the therapy of neoplasia and blood diseases. Metabolic aspects. Ann Rheum Dis. 25:657, 1966.
15. Poppell, S., and Poirier, R.: Xerophthalmia in an infant with cystic fibrosis. Metab Ophthal 2(1):41, 1978.
16. Brown, S. I., and Kuwabara, T.: Peripheral corneal opacification and skeletal deformities. Arch Ophthalmol 83:667, 1970.
17. Kampine, J. P., Brady, R. O., Kanfer, J. N., Feld, M., and Shapiro, D.: Diagnosis of Gaucher's disease and Niemann-Pick disease with small samples of venous blood. Science 155:86, 1967.
18. Spaeth, G. L.: Ocular manifestations of the lipidoses. In Tasman, W. (ed.): *Retinal Disease in Children*. New York, Harper & Row, 1971, p. 148.
19. Groen, J. J.: Gaucher's disease: Hereditary transmission and racial distribution. Arch Intern Med 113:543, 1964.
20. East, T., and Savin, L. H.: A case of Gaucher's disease with biopsy of the typical pingueculae. Brit J Ophthalmol 24:611, 1940.
21. Nordentoft, B., and Andersen, S. R.: Juvenile xanthogranuloma of the cornea and conjunctiva. Acta Ophthalmol 45:720, 1967.
22. Grayson, M., and Pieroni, D.: Solitary xanthoma of the limbus. Brit J Ophthalmol 54:562, 1970.
23. Blank, H., Eglick, P. G., and Beerman, H.: Nevoxanthoendothelioma with ocular involvement. Pediatrics 4:349, 1949.
24. Allen, R. A., O'Malley, C., and Straatsma, B. R.: Ocular findings in hereditary ochronosis. Arch Ophthalmol 65:657, 1961.
25. Seitz, R.: Über die ochronosischen Pigmentierungen am Auge. Klin Monatsbl Augenheilk 125:432, 1954.
26. Glenner, G. G., Ein, D., and Terry, W. D.: The immunoglobulin origin of amyloid. Amer J Med 52:141, 1972.
27. Klintworth, G. K.: Lattice corneal dystrophy: An inherited variety of amyloidosis restricted to the cornea. Amer J Pathol 50:371, 1967.
28. Bowen, R. A., Hassard, T. R., Wong, V. G., DeLellis, R. A., and Glenner, G. G.: Lattice dystrophy of the cornea as a variety of amyloidosis. Amer J Ophthalmol 70:822, 1970.
29. Brownstein, M., Elliott, R., and Helwig, E.: Ophthalmologic aspects of amyloidosis. Amer J Ophthalmol 69:423, 1970.
30. Knowles, D., Jacobiec, F., Rosen, M., and Howard, G. M.: Amyloidosis of the orbit and adnexae. Surv Ophthalmol 19:367, 1975.
31. Doughman, D.: Ocular amyloidosis. Surv Ophthalmol 13:133, 1968.
32. Paton, D., and Duke, J. R.: Primary familial amyloidosis: Ocular manifestations with histopathologic observations. Amer J Ophthalmol 61:736, 1966.
33. Douglas, W. H.: Congenital porphyria: General and ocular manifestations. Trans Ophthalmol Soc UK 92:541, 1972.
34. Watson, P. G., and Hazleman, B. L.: *The Sclera and Systemic Disorders*. Philadelphia, W. B. Saunders Co., 1976, pp. 332–335.
35. Rodrigues, M. M., Kratchmer, J. H., Miller, S. D., and Newsome, D. A.: Posterior corneal crystalline deposits in benign monoclonal gammopathy. Arch Ophthalmol 97:124, 1979.
36. Eiferman, R. A., and Rodrigues, M. M.: Unusual superficial stromal corneal deposits in IgG K monoclonal gammopathy. Arch Ophthalmol 98:78, 1980.
37. Roberts, W. H., and Wolter, J. R.: Ocular chrysiasis. Arch Ophthalmol 56:48, 1956.
38. Ferry, A. P.: A "new" iron line of the superficial cornea. Arch Ophthalmol 79:142, 1968.
39. Gass, J. D.: The iron lines of the superficial cornea. Arch Ophthalmol 71:348, 1964.
40. Meredith, T. A., Aaberg, T. M., and Willerson, D.: Progressive chorioretinopathy after receiving thioridazine. Arch Ophthalmol 96:1172, 1978.
41. Poirier, R. H., and Jorgensen, J.: Endotoxin assay for rapid diagnosis of *Pseudomonas* corneal ulcer. Lancet 2:85, 1977.
42. Wolters, R. W., Jorgensen, J. H., Calzada, E., and Poirier, R. H.: Limulus lysate assay for early detection of certain gram-negative corneal infections. Arch Ophthalmol 97:875, 1979.
43. Brown, S. I.: Symposium on corneal infection and immunity. Collagenase and corneal ulcers. Invest Ophthalmol 10:203, 1971.
44. Berman, M.: Regulation of collagenase. Trans Ophthalmol Soc UK 98:397, 1978.
45. O'Day D. M., and Jones, B. R.: Herpes simplex keratitis. In Duane, T. D. (ed.): *Clinical Ophthal-*

mology. Vol. 4. Hagerstown, Md., Harper & Row, 1976.

46. Lanier, J. D.: Marginal herpes simplex keratitis. Ophthalmol. Dig., Mar. 15, 1976.

47. Plotkin, J., Reynaud, A., and Okumoto, M.: Cytologic study of herpetic keratitis. Preparation of corneal scrapings. Arch Ophthalmol 85:597, 1971.

48. Coster, D. J., Jones, B. R., and Falcon, M. G.: Role of debridement in the treatment of herpetic keratitis. Trans Ophthalmol Soc UK 97:314, 1977.

49. Cairnes, J. E.: Varicella of the cornea treated with 5-iodo-2'-deoxyuridine. Brit J Ophthalmol 48:288, 1964.

50. Jones, D. B.: Herpes zoster ophthalmicus. In Golden, B. (ed.): *Ocular Inflammatory Disease.* Springfield, Ill., Charles C Thomas, 1974, pp. 198–209.

51. Jones, B. R., and Al-Hussaini, M. K.: Therapeutic considerations in ocular vaccinia. Trans Ophthalmol Soc UK 83:613, 1963.

52. Fulginiti, V. A., Winograd, L. A., Jackson, M., and Ellis, P.: Therapy of experimental vaccinial keratitis. Effect of idoxuridine and VIG. Arch Ophthalmol 74:539, 1965.

53. Hyndiuk, R. A., Okumoto, M., Damiano, R. A., Valenton, M., and Smolin, F.: Treatment of vaccinial keratitis with vidarabine. Arch Ophthalmol 94:1363, 1976.

54. Thygeson, P.: Etiology and treatment of phlyctenular keratoconjunctivitis. Amer J Ophthalmol 34:1217, 1951.

55. Thygeson, P.: Nontuberculous phlyctenular keratoconjunctivitis. In Golden, B. (ed.): *Ocular Inflammatory Disease.* Springfield, Ill., Charles C Thomas, 1974, p. 50.

56. Thygeson, P.: Microbic allergy in ocular tissues. In Golden, B. (ed.): *Ocular Inflammatory Disease.* Springfield, Ill., Charles C Thomas, 1974, p. 54.

57. Thygeson, P., and Fritz, M. H.: Cortisone in treatment of phlyctenular keratoconjunctivitis. Amer J Ophthalmol 34:357, 1951.

58. Jones, B. R.: Vernal keratitis. Trans Ophthalmol Soc UK 81:2115, 1961.

59. Easty, D., Rice, N. S. C., and Jones, B. R.: Disodium cromoglycate (Intal) in the treatment of vernal kerato-conjunctivitis. Trans Ophthalmol Soc UK 91:491, 1971.

60. Borrie, P.: Rosacea with special reference to its ocular manifestations. Brit J Dermatol 65:458, 1953.

61. Chignell, A. H., Easty, D. L., Chesterton, J. R., and Thompsitt, J.: Marginal ulceration of the cornea. Brit J Ophthalmol 54:433, 1970.

62. Brown, S. I., and Grayson, M.: Marginal furrows. A characteristic corneal lesion of rheumatoid arthritis. Arch Ophthalmol 79:563, 1968.

63. Foster, C. S., Kenyon, K. R., Greiner, J., Greineder, D. K., Friedland, B., and Allansmith, M. R.: The immunopathology of Mooren's ulcer. Amer J Ophthalmol 88:149, 1979.

64. Mondino, B. J., Brown, S. I., and Rabin, B. S.: Cellular immunity in Mooren's ulcer. Amer J Ophthalmol 85:788, 1978.

65. Brown, S. I., Mondino, B. J., and Robin, B. S.: Autoimmune phenomenon in Mooren's ulcer. Amer J Ophthalmol 82:835, 1976.

66. Brown, S. I.: Mooren's ulcer. Treatment by conjunctival excision. Brit J Ophthalmol 59:675, 1975.

67. Aviel, E.: Combined cryoapplications and peritomy in Mooren's ulcer. Brit J Ophthalmol 56:48, 1972.

68. Easty, D. L., Madden, P., Jayson, M. I. V., Carter, C., and Noble, B. A.: Systemic immunosuppression in marginal keratolysis. Trans Ophthalmol Soc UK 98:410, 1978.

69. Foster, C. S.: Immunosuppressive therapy in external ocular inflammatory disease. Ophthalmology 87:140, 1980.

70. Linwong, M., Herman, S. J., and Rabb, M. F.: Carcinoma in situ of the corneal limbus in an adolescent girl. Arch Ophthalmol 87:48, 1972.

71. Rasteiro, A., and Cunha-Vaz, J. G.: Squamous cell carcinoma of the limbus with intraocular invasion. Ophthalmologica 172:332, 1976.

72. Cassady, J. V.: Malignant melanoma of the corneal limbus. Trans Amer Ophthalmol Soc 66:379, 1968.

73. Hutchison, D. S., Green, W. R., and Iliff, C. E.: Ectopic brain tissue in a limbal dermoid associated with a scleral staphyloma. Amer J Ophthalmol 76:984, 1973.

74. Poirier, R. H.: Role of corneal surgery in destructive corneal disease. Trans Ophthalmol Soc UK 98:418, 1978.

75. Kennedy, R. E., Roca, P. D., and Landers, P. H.: Atypical band keratopathy in glaucomatous patients. Amer J Ophthalmol 72:917, 1971.

76. Paton, D.: Pterygium management based upon a theory of pathogenesis. Trans Amer Acad Ophthalmol Otolaryngol 79:603, 1975.

77. Poirier, R. H., and Fish, J. R.: Lamellar keratoplasty for recurrent pterygium. Ophthalmic Surg 7(4):38, 1976.

78. Freedman, A.: Labrador keratopathy. Arch Ophthalmol 74:198, 1965.

79. Baum, J. L., Mishima, S., and Boruchoff, S. A.: On the nature of dellen. Arch Ophthalmol 79:657, 1968.

80. Tessler, H. H., and Urist, M. J.: Corneal dellen in the limbal approach to rectus muscle surgery. Brit J Ophthalmol 59:377, 1975.

81. Artentsen, J. J., Christiansen, J. M., and Maumenee, A. E.: Marginal ulceration after intracapsular cataract extraction. Amer J Ophthalmol 81:194, 1976.

82. Elliot, J. H., Aronson, S. B., Moore, T. E., and WIlliams, F. C.: Heparin therapy of peripheral corneal ischemic syndrome. In *Symposium on the Cornea.* Transactions of the New Orleans Academy of Ophthalmology. St Louis, C. V. Mosby Co., 1972, p. 78.

83. Fine, M: Lamellar corneal transplants. In *Symposium on the Cornea.* Transactions of the New Orleans Academy of Ophthalmology. St. Louis, C. V. Mosby Co., 1972, p. 204.

84. Krachmer, J. H.: Pellucid marginal corneal degeneration. Arch Ophthalmol 96:1217, 1978.

V

SUPERFICIAL CORNEAL DISORDERS

Anterior Corneal Dystrophies and Corneal Erosions

8

PETER R. LAIBSON, M.D.

Dystrophies are primary diseases of the cornea unassociated with prior inflammation or systemic disease. This definition distinguishes them from corneal degenerations, which can sometimes resemble a dystrophy but are either a reflection of the aging process or occur secondary to another corneal disorder. Anterior corneal dystrophies generally affect the epithelium, its basement membrane, and/or Bowman's membrane.

ANTERIOR CORNEAL DYSTROPHIES

Epithelial Basement Membrane Dystrophy

By far the most common anterior corneal dystrophy is epithelial basement membrane dystrophy. Its prevalence exceeds the combined prevalence of all other entities in this group. The literature also refers to this disorder as Cogan's microcystic dystrophy,[1] map-dot-fingerprint dystrophy,[2] and microcystic corneal dystrophy.[3] Cogan and coworkers[1] first identified this entity as a specific disorder in 1964, describing five cases that they classified as a dystrophy because of the spontaneous and symmetrical appearance of the corneal findings. They observed grayish-white, discrete corneal epithelial changes that were usually small and variable in size; some were pinpoint, while others were comma-shaped and irregularly oval (Fig. 8–1). Commonly the epithelial changes were located in the central cornea and were capable of causing some reduction in vis-

ual acuity. The predominant anatomic findings were intraepithelial cysts containing pyknotic nuclei with debris and anomalous basement membrane within the epithelium. No uniform cause was uncovered.

In 1965 Guerry[4] reviewed nine additional cases. He observed the microcysts reported by Cogan but also described irregular, faintly gray, linear patterns of varying length with clear zones lying between the gray zones. Guerry called the latter changes "maplike areas" (Fig. 8–2). A third finding, fingerprint lines in the cornea, was first described by Vogt in 1930,[5] and others subsequently have mentioned fingerprint lines in the cornea as representing areas of anomalous membrane in parallel lines (Fig. 8–3). It is recognized that fingerprint lines are similar to the maplike changes and that any combination of fingerprint lines, microcysts, and maplike changes may appear in the epithelium of the same cornea. The three types of alterations simply represent variations of the same basic dystrophy, resulting in the colloquial name of map-dot-fingerprint dystrophy.[2] However, the name epithelial basement membrane dystrophy[3] is more appropriate anatomically and will be used here.

Epithelial basement membrane dystrophy has been reported to occur as early as age 5 and increases in prevalence after age 30.[6] It is bilateral, shows equal predilection for both sexes, and appears to be dominantly inherited.[7] The pattern of maps, dots, and fingerprint lines changes with time, although

215

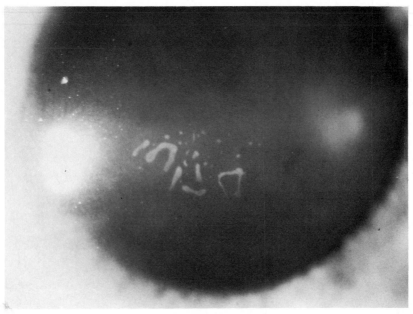

Figure 8–1. Cogan's microcystic dystrophy. Intraepithelial cysts containing cytoplasmic and nuclear debris. They appear somewhat milky in color, are variable in size, and change their position and configuration as they empty their contents onto the epithelial surface.

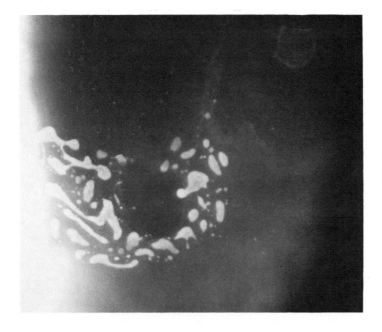

Figure 8–2. Epithelial basement membrane dystrophy. Epithelial microcysts, as described by Cogan, and maplike areas of Guerry.

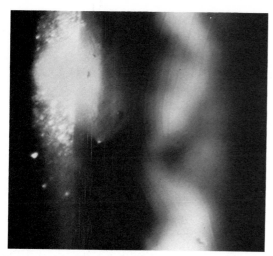

Figure 8–3. Epithelial basement membrane dystrophy. Fingerprint lines in the corneal epithelium.

pupil or with high magnification in the retroilluminating light of a narrow slit beam reflected from the iris (Fig. 8–5). Increased breakup time of the precorneal tear film may occur over areas of pathology. About 50 per cent of affected patients show more than one type of corneal change.[2, 9]

Maps appear as diffuse gray areas that contain oval clear lacunae and are separated by clear zones. The gray sheets become gradually less visible as one moves away from the discrete, sharp, geographically shaped edge that blends with the more normal cornea. They may be small and discrete or cover several square millimeters of cornea. Discrete white microcysts often appear within the maplike change but rarely in the clear zones (Fig. 8–6). Two distinct types of dots or microcysts occur. So-called putty-gray cysts are discrete, milky dots that are round, ameboid, or comma-shaped and are commonly located in the central cornea (Fig. 8–7). The majority are 0.05 to 0.5 mm. in diameter, but larger confluent cysts may be 1.0 mm. In contrast, blebs are considerably smaller (15 to 100 μm.). They present as fine, closely clustered, clear round dots seen only in retroillumination. Alternatively, they may present as refractile lines or rows of blebs that follow the polygonal outline of the anterior corneal mosaic, forming a pattern called nets. Neither disrupts the overlying tear film.

this phenomenon often is not readily apparent unless careful drawings or photographic records are maintained. Neither systemic nor ocular disease is associated with this corneal disorder, and no consistently associated abnormality of the precorneal tear film or of tear function has been demonstrated.[8]

Because the lesions are small, intraepithelial, and translucent, they are difficult to detect. Map changes are seen best in a broad slit-lamp beam directed tangentially over the corneal surface, where they appear as irregular gray patches (Fig. 8–4). Microcysts and fingerprint lines are best visualized against the red fundus reflection of a dilated

Figure 8–4. Epithelial basement membrane dystrophy. Maplike changes in the corneal epithelium seen in a broad slit-lamp beam directed tangentially over the corneal surface.

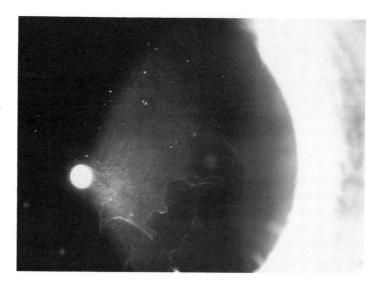

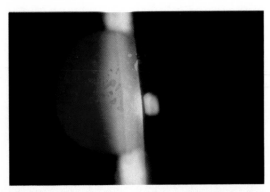

Figure 8–5. Epithelial basement membrane dystrophy. Microcysts seen in retroillumination against the red fundus reflection.

Superficial corneal lines are the most frequent form of presentation of epithelial basement membrane dystrophy. Fingerprint lines, a less common pattern, are roughly parallel refractile lines with an elongated or whorl pattern seen only in retroillumination. The tear film pattern may break up rapidly over a cluster of fingerprint lines.

Histopathologically, there are three basic elements present in epithelial basement membrane dystrophy: (1) thickened basement membrane with extension into the epithelium, (2) abnormal epithelial cells and intraepithelial microcysts, and (3) fibrillar material between the epithelial basement membrane and Bowman's layer.[6] Maps are composed primarily of a very thick epithelial basement membrane that extends into the epithelium as multilaminar sheets 2 to 6 μm. thick. Putty-gray dots are intraepithelial pseudocysts that contain cytoplasmic and nuclear debris.

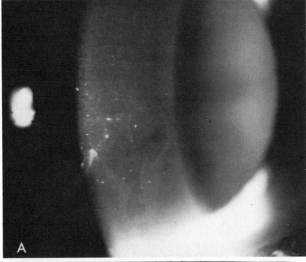

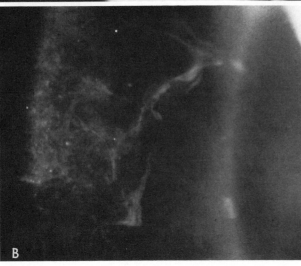

Figure 8–6. Epithelial basement membrane dystrophy. *A*, Discrete white microcysts within maplike changes. *B*, Higher magnification of microcysts within maplike epithelial alterations.

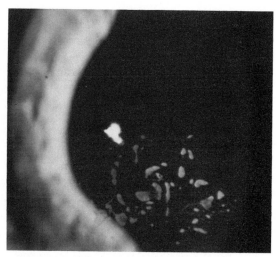

Figure 8–7. Epithelial basement membrane dystrophy. Discrete, milky, round, ameboid, or comma-shaped dots. (Same changes originally referred to as Cogan's microcystic dystrophy.)

These cysts, whose walls are formed by the corrugated normal border of the intact adjacent epithelial cells, form beneath the aberrant intraepithelial sheets of basement membrane and later surface to discharge their contents. Blebs are formed by an accumulation of a continuous layer of fibrillogranular material between the basement membrane of the epithelium and Bowman's membrane. The anterior surface of this material forms discrete mounds, which indent the overlying basal epithelial cells. The fingerprint lines also appear to be formed by the combination of sheets of subepithelial and intraepithelial basement membrane material and a fine fibrillogranular substance. Presumably, focal thickenings or undulations of this material form the fingerprint lines seen clinically.

The maps, dots, and fingerprint lines of epithelial basement membrane dystrophy often do not cause symptoms. However, when prominent and located in the axial cornea, they can produce sufficient irregular astigmatism to reduce visual acuity (Fig. 8–8). Surface irregularity can be documented with a keratoscope or keratometer and tends to be aggravated by a dry, hot environment and by exposure to wind. Visual loss, as measured with the Snellen chart, generally is not great (rarely to less than 20/50 in the absence of other defects), but the quality of the visual image is reduced. Halos around lights, blurred second images, and wavy lights are frequent associated complaints.

The dystrophic corneal changes can result in faulty adhesion of the epithelium to basement membrane,[10] predisposing the patient to or actually causing recurrent erosion. (It must be emphasized that although an anterior corneal dystrophy may be an underlying cause of recurrent corneal erosion, this problem also occurs in an eye with a normal cornea that has suffered an oblique superficial abrasion.) Recurrent erosion will be discussed in detail later in this chapter.

Blurred vision resulting from map,

Figure 8–8. Epithelial basement membrane dystrophy. Microcysts in the pupillary zone causing slight epithelial irregularity, which reduces the quality of the visual image and decreases visual acuity somewhat.

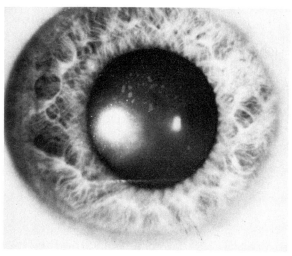

dot, or fingerprint abnormalities in the central cornea is managed by mechanical removal of the involved offending epithelium. This can be done under topical proparacaine anesthesia, and the use of an operating microscope is recommended. Following the procedure a pressure dressing is applied to promote re-epithelialization. In many instances epithelial regeneration is curative, at least for a time, and results in a clear, smooth, normal-appearing epithelium that permits normal vision. Unfortunately, recurrences are common and the procedure may have to be repeated at intervals. Management of recurrent erosion associated with epithelial basement membrane dystrophy is more complex and is discussed in the section on recurrent erosion.

Meesmann's Juvenile Epithelial Dystrophy

Meesmann described a corneal dystrophy affecting the epithelium that appears in the first few months of life.[10] The entity is bilaterally symmetrical and gradually progressive, with autosomal dominant inheritance.[11] It is manifested as fine epithelial cystlike changes best viewed by retroillumination with the broad beam of the slit lamp (Fig. 8–9). In the usual case the patient remains asymptomatic until middle age. The vesicles may then involve the entire epithelium, and in more severe cases they may produce sufficient irregular astigmatism to blur vision. At times vesicles may break through the epithelial surface and cause intermittent irritation and photophobia. In my experience recurrent erosion has not been a problem in cases of Meesmann's dystrophy.

The hallmark of this disorder is the presence of myriads of tiny round or oval, closely spaced, bubblelike blebs in the corneal epithelium. The individual lesions are well circumscribed, and the cornea between lesions is transparent. On examination with the slit-lamp biomicroscope the lesions appear as discrete gray dots in direct focal illumination and as transparent vesicles in retroillumination. They tend to aggregate in the palpebral fissure but affect the entire epithelium out to the limbus. Over a period of time the pattern changes, reflecting the migration of vesicles to the surface. In advanced stages of this dystrophy fine sinuous lines within the epithelium and small, subepithelial, amorphous gray opacities are observed along with the vesicles.

Microscopic examination of the tissue shows a thickened epithelium with poor maturation of cells from the basal layer to the surface. Intraepithelial cysts are found most prominently in the anterior epithelium, and at times their cavities, which contain cellular debris, are open to the epithelial surface. Presumably these cysts correspond to the vesicles seen clinically. The multilaminar epithelial basement membrane is thickened and more fibrillar than normal and sends projections into the basal epithelium. So-called peculiar substance accumulates within the cytoplasm of some of the corneal epithelial cells. It appears as a focal collection of fibrillogranular material surrounded by tangles of cytoplasmic filaments.[11, 12] The chemical composition of "peculiar substance" is unknown, but it is a characteristic ultrastructural finding in Meesmann's dystrophy. Although it does not accumulate in all epithelial cells, its presence allows diagnosis on histopathologic grounds alone.

The great majority of individuals with Meesmann's juvenile epithelial dystrophy have few symptoms and require no treatment. Removal of the affected epithelium is followed by rapid re-epithelialization, but vesicles reappear within the new epithelium in a short time. In contrast, epithelial regeneration after superficial keratectomy is said to proceed normally without recurrence of vesicles.[1] Apparently in conflict with this observation is the report that after lamellar and penetrating keratoplasties the epithelium often develops the abnormalities of Meesmann's dystrophy.[13]

Stocker and Holt described a rare hereditary anterior corneal dystrophy that

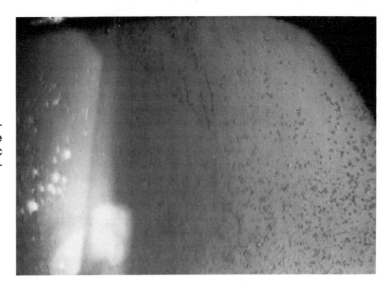

Figure 8–9. Meesmann's juvenile epithelial dystrophy. Fine corneal epithelial cystic changes seen in retroillumination.

occurred only in members of one family descended from Moravian settlers.[13] In a discussion of the paper by Cogan and coworkers on microcystic dystrophy, Stocker stated that the two dystrophies were definitely different.[14] Corneal changes were seen in all age groups examined by Stocker, and it was felt that patients had the disease to some degree from birth or early childhood. In most cases there were small white dots and wavy lines in the superficial cornea. Application of fluorescein revealed superficial punctate staining of the corneal surface. Corneal sensitivity was reduced. A thickened amorphous layer of dark, red-staining material, thought to be a product of the epithelial cells, was present between Bowman's membrane and the basal epithelium. Vision was reduced in the more severely involved cases. This entity is most likely a variant of Meesmann's juvenile epithelial dystrophy.[6]

BOWMAN'S MEMBRANE DYSTROPHIES

Reis-Bücklers Ring-Shaped Dystrophy

Reis in 1917[15] and Bücklers in 1949[16] described a bilateral, symmetrical, central corneal dystrophy with autosomal dominant inheritance. It appears in the first few years of life as a reticular superficial corneal opacification. The disorder initially is asymptomatic, but spontaneous epithelial erosions invariably occur, causing acute episodes of pain, photophobia, ocular redness, and blurred vision. These episodes tend to occur several times each year and usually involve only one eye at a time. In the second and third decades of life the central opacities extend into the midperiphery of the cornea and take on the appearance of irregular rings arranged in a fishnet pattern at the level of Bowman's membrane (Fig. 8–10). There is an associated superficial stromal haze and a decrease in corneal sensation. After the age of 30 the erosions tend to become infrequent, but visual acuity continues to decline as a result of increased superficial corneal opacification and surface irregularity.

Histopathologic examination reveals the epithelium to be irregular in thickness with considerable abnormality of individual cells and epithelial architecture. The basement membrane is focally absent, and the residual portions of basement membrane, though not thickened, are separated from the overlying basal epithelium by amorphous or fibrillar material.[17] This severe disruption of the basal epithelial cells and their stromal attachments accounts for the frequent epithelial erosions and the finding at surgery that the epithelium is very loosely attached.[17, 18] Much of Bowman's membrane is replaced by fibrocellular

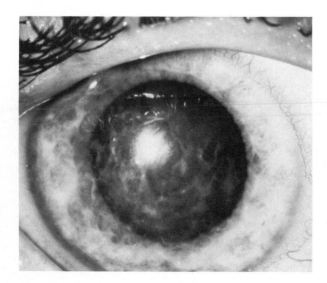

Figure 8–10. Reis-Bücklers ring-shaped dystrophy. Marked irregularity of the anterior corneal surface caused by edema of the superficial cornea and replacement of Bowman's membrane by scar tissue.

connective tissue, and fingers of fibrillar tissue indent the basal epithelium. The fibrocellular tissue also interdigitates with the anterior stroma and may correspond to the gray stromal opacity seen clinically.

Management of the epithelial erosions in Reis-Bücklers dystrophy is similar to that of epithelial erosions from other causes, as discussed in the section on recurrent erosion. When superficial opacification becomes severe enough to impair vision, superficial keratectomy may improve visual acuity.[17, 19, 20] In more severe cases lamellar or penetrating keratoplasty is necessary; the latter generally produces a superior visual result. However, the superficial ring-shaped opacification may recur in the graft.[21–23]

Grayson and Wilbrandt[24] described a family with corneal changes resembling Reis-Bücklers dystrophy. Their patients had a PAS staining material between Bowman's membrane and the corneal epithelium, a finding that was not present in typical Reis-Bücklers dystrophy. Bowman's membrane was destroyed in some areas, but corneal sensitivity was not decreased as it is in Reis-Bücklers dystrophy. It has been suggested that the anterior membrane dystrophy of Grayson and Wilbrandt as well as the honeycomb dystrophy of Thiel and Behnke[25] represent clinical variants of Reis-Bücklers dystrophy. The epithelium tends to remain smoother in both of these entities than in typical Reis-Bücklers dystrophy, with the result that visual acuity generally is not as severely affected.

RECURRENT EROSION OF THE CORNEA

Recurrent erosion of the cornea may occur in eyes that previously have suffered trauma to the corneal epithelium,[26] or the initial episode seemingly may be spontaneous with up to 40 per cent of all patients unable to recall any prior ocular trauma.[27] In eyes with documented trauma a sudden, sharp, glancing, abrading injury appears to predispose to recurrent erosion. A scratch by a fingernail seems to be the most common identifiable cause. Glancing abrasions caused by the edge of a piece of paper or a tree branch may also be followed by recurrent erosion. In contrast, injuries produced by small, partially penetrating foreign bodies that strike the cornea directly and become imbedded in the superficial stroma rarely predispose to recurrent corneal erosion. The superficial injury generally results in a true epithelial abrasion, which heals rapidly, leaving neither clinical evidence of residual damage nor a visual deficit. After an interval varying from days to years, symptoms suddenly recur in the absence of any obvious cause. In most instances they again subside promptly and spontaneously, only to recur periodically in similar fashion at varying intervals.

Classically, recurrent attacks have their onset at about the time of awakening. Many patients begin to experience symptoms immediately after they first open their eyes in the morning, and others are awakened by ocular pain. Each acute episode generally is characterized by ocular pain, photophobia, lacrimation, and blepharospasm. Objective corneal signs vary from a localized, grayish roughening or clouding of the epithelium to an epithelial bulla or a true abrasion. Therefore, frank epithelial loss is not required to establish the diagnosis when objective findings are associated with the typical clinical history. Indeed, the less severe corneal signs resolve quite rapidly, and often when the patient is examined within hours of an acute recurrence, no clinically evident abnormality is discernible.

Bilateral recurrent erosion is uncommon, although Brown and Bron[27] reported it in 10 per cent of their cases. The frequency of recurrences is quite variable as is the interval required for healing (1 hour to more than a week). The degree of visual impairment also varies and is directly related to the extent of epithelial disruption and to whether or not the axial cornea is involved. Recurrent erosion of the cornea usually occurs sporadically, but a familial occurrence has been documented in a few instances.[28, 29]

Chandler classified recurrent erosion into macroform and microform types.[26] In the macroform variety a large area of epithelium is separated from the stroma (Fig. 8–11). This is the more readily recognizable form, but it is the less common. As a rule, there is a history of a traumatic epithelial abrasion. During a recurrence the involved area is usually similar in location and extent to that of the original injury, but this is not invariably the case. Microform recurrent erosion is characterized by intraepithelial microcysts, which may or may not be accompanied by a minor break in the epithelium (Fig. 8–12). There is less likely to be a history of injury to the corneal epithelium, and when present, the injury is more likely to be a slight one. Recurrent attacks are milder and of shorter duration than those of the macroform variety. While the division into macroform and microform types is useful for descriptive purposes, the distinction is not a sharp one. Both forms may occur in the same individual at different times.[27]

It has long been recognized that the corneal epithelium is loosely attached to Bowman's membrane, both at the time of a recurrent attack[30] and between attacks, when the cornea is entirely healed and the patient is symptom-free.[31] More recently a relationship between various

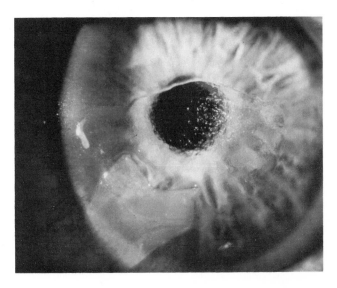

Figure 8–11. Recurrent erosion of the cornea. Macroform type characterized by spontaneous separation of a large area of epithelium from the underlying stroma. The involved epithelium is lying loose on the corneal surface, still attached at one area only, and the underlying stroma is clear.

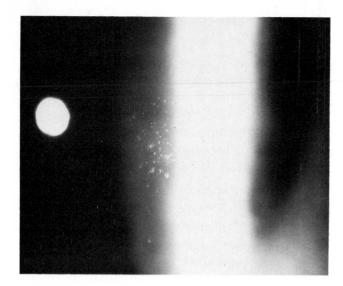

Figure 8–12. Recurrent erosion of the cornea. Microform type characterized by fine, relatively uniform intraepithelial microcysts.

superficial corneal dystrophies and recurrent erosion has been reported.[2, 27, 32–34] Most corneal abrasions heal satisfactorily and are not followed by recurrent erosion,[35, 36] suggesting that recurrent erosion occurs in a cornea that is already abnormal. Brown and Bron[27] found a much higher prevalence of superficial corneal dystrophies in the affected and unaffected eyes of patients with recurrent erosion than in controls and concluded that the superficial dystrophies were precursors of the erosion rather than the result of it. They also pointed out that the recurrent erosion appears to erase the dystrophic changes, and as a result they may be absent or only minimally present in the healed cornea.

Evidence has been presented that there is anomalous production of basement membrane material within and beneath the corneal epithelium in the superficial corneal dystrophies.[4, 33, 37–40] Normally healing of a corneal abrasion occurs in two stages. First, epithelial integrity is restored by lateral sliding of adjacent epithelial cells into the defect; mitotic proliferation of these cells subsequently restores the epithelial layer in the involved area to normal thickness. Then the healing mechanism must reestablish tight adhesion of the regenerated epithelium to the underlying tissue. The basement membrane and the hemidesmosomes of the basal epithelium are important to epithelial adherence.[41] In

the rabbit, epithelial scraping with a scalpel blade leaves remnants of the basement membrane that are utilized by regenerating epithelial cells to establish effective adherence within days. In contrast, if a superficial keratectomy is performed, no residual basement membrane is available. Regenerating basal epithelial cells must develop entirely new basement membrane complexes to effect their secure adhesion to the underlying tissue—a process that requires up to 2 months for completion. During this interval recurrent erosion can occur, the result of inadequate epithelial adhesion. Ultrastructural studies of a developing adhesion system in the rabbit reveal obvious gaps and redundancies in basement membrane complexes between basal cells and stroma.

The observations in the experimental model are remarkably similar to those of recurrent erosion of apparently varying etiology in the human. A defective basement membrane has been demonstrated in traumatic recurrent erosion[42] as well as in spontaneous recurrent erosion.[43] In the latter instance there is also an absence of hemidesmosomes in relation to the affected basal cells. Hemidesmosome–basement membrane discontinuities have been shown in Reis-Bücklers dystrophy,[17, 44, 45] an entity in which recurrent erosion is common. Seemingly, recurrent erosion is related, at least in part, to the presence of abnormal basement membrane complexes and to the presence of anomalous intraepithelial and subepithelial connective tissue, resulting in a disturbance of the basic epithelial adhesion mechanism.

The treatment of recurrent corneal erosion is frustrating, both for the patient and for the ophthalmologist. There is no definitive therapy for this disorder, but various approaches to re-epithelization and prevention of recurrent erosion may be attempted. Acute episodes are treated prophylactically with a topically applied antibiotic whenever there is a break in the epithelium. A short-acting mydriatic also is instilled and a pressure dressing is applied to such eyes. Some authorities advise that sheets of loose epithelium be carefully debrided with a scalpel blade prior to application of the pressure dressing (Fig. 8–13).[27] This appears to increase the healing rate of that episode but does not alter the incidence of recurrence. Once healing is complete, 5 per cent sodium chloride ointment is prescribed for instillation at bedtime. During sleep tears are hypotonic, and presumably this causes fluid to accumulate in the epithelium. Moreover, drying resulting from the physiologic decrease in tear secretion during sleep may promote sufficient adhesion between the corneal epithelium and the palpebral conjunctiva to cause that portion of the epithelium with abnormal basement membrane complexes to lift off when the eyes are first opened. Hypertonic saline ointment provides lubrication, and it is theorized that it also may transiently produce an osmotic gradient, drawing fluid from the epithelium and promoting the adherence of the epithelial cells to the underlying tissue. These functions may be accomplished more effectively by additional instillation of 5 per cent sodium chloride drops four or more times during the day. For patients unable to tolerate the hypertonic saline formulations a bland ophthalmic ointment (Dura Tears, Lacrilube) can be substituted at bedtime and an artificial tear preparation during the day. If therapeutic success is achieved, these medications should continue to be administered for as long as a year while normal basement membrane complexes are formed.

If, despite the administration of topical medications, recurrences persist, the use of a therapeutic hydrophilic contact lens is recommended. I prefer the 04 ultrathin lenses manufactured by Bausch and Lomb or comparable ultrathin lenses made by CooperVision. The soft contact lens is worn continuously 24 hours a day, usually for several months. Antibiotic drops and 5 per cent sodium chloride drops may be instilled concurrently with contact lens wear at the discretion of the ophthalmologist. (There are no reliable data indicating whether or not these medications have

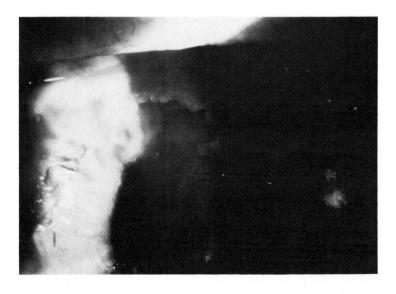

Figure 8–13. Recurrent erosion of the cornea. Appearance of acute lesion of the macroform type after debridement of the loose epithelium.

any positive effect in this situation.) The lens presumably protects the corneal epithelium from trauma of the lid margins during blinking and prevents the epithelium from adhering to the tarsal conjunctiva and being lifted off. Clinical experience suggests that this mode of therapy decreases the incidence of recurrent erosion, but it is not a panacea. Erosions can occur beneath the lens.

When corneal erosion recurs beneath a contact lens, debridement of the abnormal epithelium may encourage regeneration of epithelial cells more capable of developing a normal basement membrane. Particularly when a dystrophic epithelium is apparent on biomicroscopic examination, mechanical removal of the involved epithelium often is followed by regrowth of more normal-appearing epithelium. Should repeated debridement fail to limit recurrences, light cauterization of Bowman's membrane may result in satisfactory adherence of the epithelium. Cauterization is best controlled by the application of radiodiathermy. A broad, nonpenetrating diathermy probe is used. The energy setting of the apparatus and the length of each application should be just sufficient to produce a light gray surface haze on observation through the operating microscope. The procedure generally leaves a faint scar; therefore, except in desperate cases, it should not be used in the axial cornea. Long-term instillation of a hypertonic saline formulation is recommended following epithelial regeneration after debridement and/or cauterization.

In the most severe cases of recurrent erosion many episodes may occur before the problem resolves. Nonetheless, patients can be reassured that in the absence of a severe anterior corneal dystrophy (e.g., Reis-Bücklers dystrophy) episodes of recurrent erosion ultimately cease and the cornea remains transparent. I have rarely encountered a patient with severe recurrent erosion in whom the problem did not eventually resolve with maintenance of good vision.

REFERENCES

1. Cogan, D. G., Donaldson, D. D., Kuwabara, T., and Marshall, D.: Microcystic dystrophy of the corneal epithelium. Trans Amer Ophthalmol Soc 62:213, 1964.
2. Trobe, J. D., and Laibson, P. R.: Dystrophic changes in the anterior cornea. Arch Ophthalmol 87:378, 1972.
3. Laibson, P. R.: Microcystic corneal dystrophy. Trans Amer Ophthalmol Soc 74:488, 1976.
4. Guerry, D.: Observations on Cogan's microcystic dystrophy of the corneal epithelium. Trans Amer Ophthalmol Soc 62:320, 1965.
5. Vogt, A.: Lehrbuch und Atlas Spaltlampenmikroskopie des lebenden Auges. Berlin, Julius Springer, 1930.
6. Waring, G. O., Rodrigues, M. M., and Laibson, P. R.: Corneal dystrophies. I. Dystrophies of the epithelium, Bowman's layer and stroma. Surv Ophthalmol 23:71, 1978.
7. Laibson, P., and Krachmer, J. H.: Familial occurrence of dot (microcystic), map, fingerprint dystrophy of the cornea. Invest Ophthalmol 14:397, 1975.
8. Luxenberg, M. N., and Friedland, B. R.: Superficial microcystic corneal dystrophy. Arch Ophthalmol 93:107, 1975.
9. Bron, A. J., and Brown, N. A.: Some superficial corneal disorders. Trans Ophthalmol Soc UK 91:13, 1971.
10. Meesmann, A., and Wilke, F.: Klinische und anatomische Untersuchungen über eine bisher unbekannte, dominant vererbte Epitheldystrophie der Hornhaut. Klin Monatsbl Augenheilk 103:361, 1939.
11. Burns, R. P.: Meesmann's corneal dystrophy. Trans Amer Ophthalmol Soc 66:530, 1968.
12. Fine, B. S., Yanoff, M., Pitts, E., and Slaughter, F. D.: Messmann's epithelial dystrophy of the cornea. Amer J Ophthalmol 83:633, 1977.
13. Stocker, F. W., and Holt, L. B.: Rare form of hereditary epithelial dystrophy; Genetic, clinical and pathologic study. Arch Ophthalmol 53:536, 1955.
14. Stocker, F. W.: Discussion of Cogan, D. G., Donaldson, D. D., Kuwabara, T., and Marshall, D.: Microcystic dystrophy of the corneal epithelium. Trans Amer Ophthalmol Soc 62:223, 1964.
15. Reis, W.: Familiäre, fleckige Hornhautentartung. Dtsch Med Wschr 43:575, 1917.
16. Bücklers, M.: Ueber eine weitere familiäre Hornhautdystrophie (Reis). Klin Monatsbl Augenheilk 114:386, 1949.
17. Rice, N. S. C., Ashton, N., Jay, B., and Blach, R. K.: Reis-Bücklers' dystrophy. A clinico-pathological study. Brit J Ophthalmol 52:577, 1968.
18. Fogle, J. A., Green, W. R., and Kenyon, K. R.: Anterior corneal dystrophy. Amer J Ophthalmol 77:529, 1974.
19. Hall, P.: Reis-Bücklers dystrophy. Arch Ophthalmol 91:170, 1974.
20. Jones, S. T., and Stouffer, L. K.: Reis-Bücklers corneal dystrophy. A clinicopathologic study.

Trans Amer Acad Ophthalmol Otolaryngol 74:417, 1970.

21. Caldwell, D. R.: Postoperative recurrence of Reis-Bücklers dystrophy. Amer J Ophthalmol 35:567, 1978.

22. Olson, R. J., and Kaufman, H. E.: Recurrence of Reis-Bücklers corneal dystrophy in a graft. Amer J Ophthalmol 85:349, 1978.

23. Winkelman, J. E., and Delleman, J. W.: Reis-Bücklers Hornhautdystrophie und die Rolle der Bowmanschen Membran. Klin Monatsbl Augenheilk 155:380, 1969.

24. Grayson, M., and Wilbrandt, H.: Dystrophy of the anterior limiting membrane of the cornea (Reis-Bücklers Type). Amer J Ophthalmol 61:345, 1966.

25. Thiel, H. J., and Behnke, H.: Eine bisher unbekannte subepitheliale hereditäre Hornhautdystrophie. Klin Monatsbl Augenheilk 150:862, 1967.

26. Chandler, P. A.: Recurrent erosion of the cornea. Amer J Ophthalmol 28:355, 1945.

27. Brown, N., and Bron, A.: Recurrent erosion of the cornea. Brit J Ophthalmol 60:84, 1976.

28. Francheschetti, A.: Hereditäre rezidivierende Erosion der Hornhaut. Zscht Augenheilk 66:309, 1928.

29. Wales, J. H.: A family history of corneal erosions. Trans Ophthalmol Soc NZ 8:77, 1955.

30. Haab, J.: Über einige seltenere Hornhauterkrankungen. Inaug Diss, Zurich 1890.

31. von Szily, A.: Ueber Disjunction des Hornhautepithels. Arch f Ophth, 51:486, 1900.

32. Kaufman, H. E., and Clower, J. W.: Irregularities of Bowman's membrane. Amer J Ophthalmol 61:227, 1966.

33. Broderick, J. D., Dark, A. J., and Peace, W.: Fingerprint dystrophy of the cornea. Arch Ophthalmol 92:483, 1974.

34. Brown, N. A., and Bron, A. J.: Superficial lines and associated disorders of the cornea. Amer J Ophthalmol 81:34, 1976.

35. Jackson, H.: Effect of eye-pads on healing of simple corneal abrasions. Brit Med J 2:713, 1960.

36. Guyard, M., and Perdriel, G.: Apropos of the treatment of recurrent erosions of the cornea. Bull Soc Ophtal Franc 6:579, 1961.

37. King, R. G., Jr., and Geeraets, R.: Cogan-Guerry microcystic corneal epithelial dystrophy. A clinical and electron microscopic study. Med Coll Va Qrtly 8:241, 1972.

38. Tripathi, R. C., and Bron, A. J.: Cystic disorders of the corneal epithelium. Brit J Ophthalmol 57:376, 1973.

39. Rodrigues, M. M., Fine, B. S., Laibson, P. R., and Zimmerman, L. E.: Disorders of the corneal epithelium. A clinicopathologic study of dot, geographic and fingerprint patterns. Arch Ophthalmol 92:475, 1974.

40. Fogle, J. A., Kenyon, K. R., Stark, W. J., and Green, W. R.: Defective epithelial adhesion in anterior corneal dystrophies. Amer J Ophthalmol 79:925, 1975.

41. Khoudadoust, A. A., Silverstein, A. M., Kenyon, K. R., and Dowling, J. E.: Adhesion of regenerating corneal epithelium: The role of basement membrane. Amer J Ophthalmol 65:339, 1968.

42. Goldman, J. N., Dohlman, C. H., and Kravitz, J.: The basal membrane in recurrent epithelial erosion. Trans Amer Acad Ophthalmol Otolaryngol 73:471, 1969.

43. Tripathi, R. C., and Bron, A.: Ultrastructural study of non-traumatic recurrent corneal erosion. Brit J Ophthalmol 56:73, 1972.

44. Griffith, D. G., and Fine, B. S.: Light and electron microscopic observations in a superficial corneal dystrophy, probably early Reis-Bücklers type. Amer J Ophthalmol 63:1659, 1967.

45. Akiya, S., and Brown, S. I.: The ultrastructure of Reis-Bücklers' dystrophy. Amer J Ophthalmol 72:549, 1971.

9 Superficial Punctate Keratopathy

HOWARD M. LEIBOWITZ, M.D.
GLENN J. GREEN, M.D.

The conditions discussed in this chapter are grouped together here only because each can present as, or cause, minute changes in the corneal epithelium and at times in the subjacent Bowman's membrane and superficial stroma. At first glance this common pathologic alteration might seem a flimsy basis for associating a number of diverse entities. All too often, however, it is the predominant clinical sign confronting the ophthalmologist as he evaluates a patient and seeks to establish a diagnosis. Unfortunately, there is a great array of epithelial lesions, and many disorders are characterized by several different types, appearing simultaneously or in succession. All too frequently it is impossible to make a definitive etiologic diagnosis on the basis of the morphologic appearance of lesions in the corneal epithelium. Nonetheless, it is our hope that a discussion from this vantage point may bring a semblance of order to a vexing clinical problem. We will use the term superficial punctate keratopathy in a broad descriptive sense with no intent to imply etiologic specificity.

MORPHOLOGIC TYPES

Minute pathologic alterations in the corneal epithelium and subjacent tissues can be divided into three major types based on their morphologic characteristics when viewed with the slit-lamp biomicroscope.[1, 2] They are referred to as punctate epithelial erosions, punctate epithelial keratitis, and punctate subepithelial infiltrates.

Punctate Epithelial Erosions

Punctate epithelial erosions are true exfoliations of the corneal epithelium that appear as fine depressions or pits on examination at high magnification. The depressions may extend through all layers of the epithelium or involve only the more superficial epithelial layers. Generally there is no accompanying inflammatory infiltrate or loss of transparency; the cornea is clear and the epithelial pits are difficult or impossible to see in direct illumination. However, they are stained brilliantly by fluorescein dye (Fig. 9–1), and recognition of the defects, particularly the extent to which they are present, requires the use of this diagnostic aid. Following the application of fluorescein, it is not unusual to discover that a cornea appearing normal on slit-lamp examination with direct illumination is spattered with punctate epithelial erosions, revealed by the bright green fluorescent dye. Like all epithelial defects, they cause discomfort, generally characterized as irritation or a foreign body sensation, which may be accompanied by photophobia and lacrimation.

Punctate Epithelial Keratitis

The lesions of punctate epithelial keratitis provide a direct contrast to the

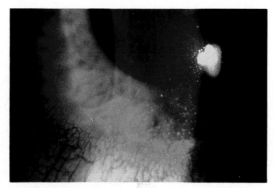

Figure 9–1. Punctate epithelial erosions.

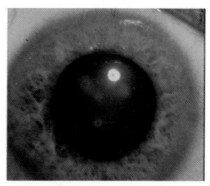

Figure 9–3. Punctate subepithelial infiltrates.

largely invisible punctate epithelial erosions. They are gray or white, well-circumscribed epithelial spots that may be slightly elevated and are easily visible in direct illumination at the magnification provided by the slit-lamp biomicroscope (Fig. 9–2). The involved opaque epithelial cells stain irregularly with fluorescein; usually the lesions do not appear as bright green as punctate epithelial erosions. Rose bengal, a vital dye with an affinity for degenerate but still viable cells, often stains this type of lesion more prominently than does fluorescein. Commonly punctate epithelial keratitis is accompanied by punctate epithelial erosions. Indeed, in some instances the spots of punctate epithelial keratopathy break down and give rise to punctate epithelial erosions.

Jones[1, 2] has classified the lesions of punctate epithelial keratitis according to their size and shape; categories include

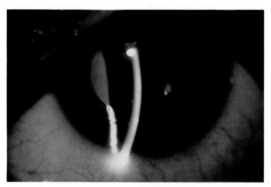

Figure 9–2. Punctate epithelial keratitis.

fine, coarse, areolar, and stellate. Although one type of lesion may predominate, the various types of lesions generally occur in combination. At times the larger, coarse lesions can be seen by the naked eye.

Punctate Subepithelial Infiltrates

Punctate subepithelial infiltrates are gray to white, well circumscribed spots located in the most superficial layers of the stroma (Fig. 9–3). Commonly these lesions accompany punctate epithelial keratitis or punctate epithelial erosions, and almost invariably the subepithelial spot lies beneath an epithelial lesion. The two types of changes (epithelial and subepithelial) may occur simultaneously or sequentially. Generally the subepithelial lesion follows a punctate epithelial keratitis, resulting in a combined epithelial-subepithelial punctate keratopathy. In most cases the epithelial lesions subsequently heal, while the subepithelial changes persist for varying lengths of time. When punctate subepithelial keratopathy persists, the epithelium generally reverts to a normal state and no longer stains with either fluorescein or rose bengal. Occasionally, however, the epithelium overlying subepithelial lesions may again become abnormal late in the course of the disease. The status of the overlying epithelium seems related to the severity of the focal subepithelial infiltrate.

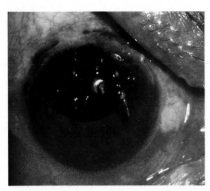

Figure 9–4. Filamentary keratopathy.

Filamentary Keratopathy

An entity that may accompany punctate changes in the superficial cornea is filamentary keratopathy. Corneal filaments (Fig. 9–4) apparently arise as a result of hypertrophy of a disordered epithelium. The hypertrophic epithelium desquamates but, for reasons that are unknown, remains attached at one point. All but the attached point of the filament moves freely, particularly on blinking, and the epithelium tends to elongate and coil. It may coil about a strand of mucus or, alternatively, mucus may adhere to the filament. One or many filaments may occur on a given cornea. They stain with both fluorescein and rose bengal and invariably are accompanied by ocular irritation or a foreign body sensation and by photophobia. After a short time they fall off, leaving an epithelial erosion at the point of attachment. Filaments have a tendency to recur, and new filaments tend to arise in different locations on the corneal surface.

MICROSCOPIC CHANGES

Information about the microscopic changes that occur in superficial punctate keratopathy is scanty. Although the epithelium can be removed with relative ease and little trauma, the required manipulations very often produce artifactual changes and generally are not justified clinically. Lamellar en bloc dissection of the involved epithelium and Bowman's membrane along with the un-

derlying superficial stroma occasionally is performed to establish a diagnosis. However, tissue excision must be confined to the corneal periphery; repair of the keratectomized area results in varying degrees of scarring and may produce more permanent tissue alterations than the original disorder. In general the superficial location of the entity, the relatively minor degree of tissue damage that it causes, and the regenerative capacity of the corneal epithelium (i.e., its ability not simply to heal but to replace itself with identical cells) combine to provide few specimens for study.

Published descriptions of punctate epithelial erosions say little more than that the entity is characterized microscopically by degeneration of the superficial epithelial cells in the involved area and by edema of the surrounding cells. Punctate epithelial keratitis, on the other hand, is characterized by discrete infiltrates in the epithelium. Microscopic examination of the infiltrates reveals edema and swelling of the epithelial cells, intercellular edema, and exudates beneath the epithelium. The infiltrate is said to contain primarily polymorphonuclear leukocytes in its initial stages and lymphocytes subsequently. Other histologic characteristics include prominent edema of the basal epithelial cells and absence of hemidesmosomes from the basement membrane.

Punctate subepithelial infiltrates are typified by discrete collections of white cells that lie in the stromal fibers just beneath Bowman's membrane and may also infiltrate this structure. In the type associated with adenoviral infection there is edema of these stromal fibers and perhaps also of Bowman's membrane initially, and several days later the area is invaded predominantly by lymphocytes. Splitting and degeneration of collagen fibers have been described, but these changes tend to be mild and permanent scarring is not severe. The peripheral marginal infiltrates associated with staphylococcal blepharoconjunctivitis also generally lie just beneath the epithelium. However, these infiltrates consist primarily of polymorphonuclear leukocytes, and microscopic examination shows more severe necrosis of the corneal tissue. Healing occurs by fibroblastic proliferation, and scarring tends to be more prominent.

DIFFERENTIAL DIAGNOSIS OF SUPERFICIAL PUNCTATE KERATOPATHY

Establishing an etiologic diagnosis in a given case of superficial punctate keratopathy can be both difficult and frustrating. Those entities capable of producing this abnormality are listed in Table 9–1. A brief discussion of each, stressing its salient characteristics, is presented.

Bacterial Infection of the Lids and Conjunctiva

Bacteria commonly infect the lid margins (with colonization of the lash follicles and the meibomian glands) and the conjunctiva. Often there is simultaneous involvement of both areas, producing the typical clinical picture of a blepharoconjunctivitis. Staphylococci are the most common etiologic organisms,[3] and both S. aureus and S. epidermidis are documented pathogens. A superficial punctate keratopathy is a frequent accompaniment of staphylococcal infection of the lid margins and/or the conjunctiva.[4] When they are secondary to a

Table 9–1. DIFFERENTIAL DIAGNOSIS OF SUPERFICIAL PUNCTATE KERATOPATHY

1. Bacterial infection of the lids and conjunctiva
2. Viral infection of the lids and conjunctiva
   A. Adenovirus
   B. Herpes simplex
   C. Herpes zoster
   D. Molluscum contagiosum and verrucae
   E. Vaccinia
   F. Other—myxoviruses, varicella, measles, rubella
3. Ocular chlamydial infections
4. Lacrimal insufficiency
5. Trauma: mechanical, chemical, radiational
6. Exposure keratopathy
7. Neurotrophic keratopathy
8. Thygeson's superficial punctate keratitis
9. Superior limbic keratoconjunctivitis
10. Allergy
11. Vernal keratoconjunctivitis
12. Rosacea
13. Reiter's disease

staphylococcal blepharitis, the lesions in the corneal epithelium tend to be located primarily in the inferior corneal periphery. Early in the course of a staphylococcal conjunctivitis, on the other hand, the punctate epithelial lesions are more apt to be diffusely and nonspecifically spattered over the entire cornea. Initially the corneal lesions are largely punctate epithelial erosions, but staphylococcal infections of the lid and conjunctiva often are persistent, and in this instance the punctate epithelial erosions are accompanied by punctate epithelial infiltrates. The more severe, chronic cases typically are also characterized by localized marginal infiltrates involving the anterior stroma (Fig. 9–5); these may

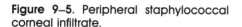
Figure 9–5. Peripheral staphylococcal corneal infiltrate.

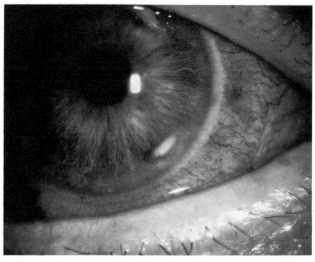

progress to ulceration. Organisms are not isolated from these lesions, which presumably are caused by staphylococcal exotoxins.[5]

While staphylococci are the most common causal organisms, several Gram-positive and Gram-negative bacteria are known to cause blepharitis and conjunctivitis. All such infections may be accompanied by superficial punctate keratopathy, which is characterized by punctate epithelial erosions, or in long-standing cases by coexisting punctate epithelial erosions and the infiltrates of punctate epithelial keratitis. The lesions in the corneal epithelium may be scattered over the entire corneal surface or they may be more dense in the corneal periphery. Neither the clinical appearance of individual lesions nor their location on the cornea provides a reliable clue to the species of bacteria causing the problem.

Superficial punctate keratopathy associated with an acute bacterial conjunctivitis is treated with topically applied antimicrobial agents. In a general ophthalmic practice cultures are not routinely obtained, so an agent providing broad-spectrum coverage is required. We prefer tobramycin 0.3%, but sulfacetamide in a 10 to 15 per cent concentration is also generally effective. Largely because ointments blur vision and cause aesthetic difficulties, we use aqueous formulations, but we know of no evidence that reliably documents the therapeutic superiority of either form. Drops are initially instilled at 2-hour intervals during waking hours, and after 48 hours of treatment they are tapered to four times daily. In less severe cases the latter regimen (i.e., four times a day) can be used from the outset. Seven to 10 days of treatment generally is adequate.

Bacterial cultures should be obtained whenever an acute conjunctivitis is resistant to therapy and in all chronic cases. Choice of an antimicrobial agent then is influenced by the in vitro sensitivities of the causal organism. In chronic cases in which scarring and other structural changes are present, we administer a corticosteroid, usually a 0.125 per cent suspension of prednisolone acetate, on a dose-for-dose basis with the antibiotic. Experiments in animals have shown that this does not enhance bacterial replication,[6] and clinical studies have demonstrated its effectiveness and safety.[7]

Superficial punctate keratopathy associated with a chronic bacterial blepharitis is infrequently eliminated solely by topical instillation of antibiotics. The organisms have colonized the lid margins and the glands of the lid, and in most instances they cannot be eradicated by topical (or systemic) medications. The ophthalmologist should aggressively remove all crusts from the lid margins. If there is a pronounced meibomitis, the lids should be compressed between two glass rods or similar implements and excess meibomian secretions should be expressed. This procedure can be repeated by the physician on subsequent visits as necessary. The patient must be instructed to cleanse his lid margins mechanically (Fig. 9–6). We recommend the use of a Q-tip and Johnson's Baby Shampoo or similar product that is said to cause minimal discomfort should it come in contact with the conjunctiva or cornea. The Q-tip is dipped into the shampoo, compressed against a second Q-tip to express any excess shampoo, and used to scrub the everted lid margin. If the patient is carrying out the procedure himself, it is generally done in front of a well-lighted mirror. Residual shampoo is removed from the lid margin using a Q-tip moistened with any sterile ophthalmic irrigating solution. Initially the patient is instructed to scrub his lid margins twice daily, on arising and before retiring; later the frequency is decreased to once daily at bedtime. A broad-spectrum antibiotic and a corticosteroid are instilled concurrently. We favor a neomycin-polymyxin B-dexamethasone combination preparation (Maxitrol) in aqueous form. Initially this is instilled four times daily, and after 10 to 14 days it is slowly but progressively tapered and discontinued. In many cases the nightly lid scrubs are maintained indefinitely.

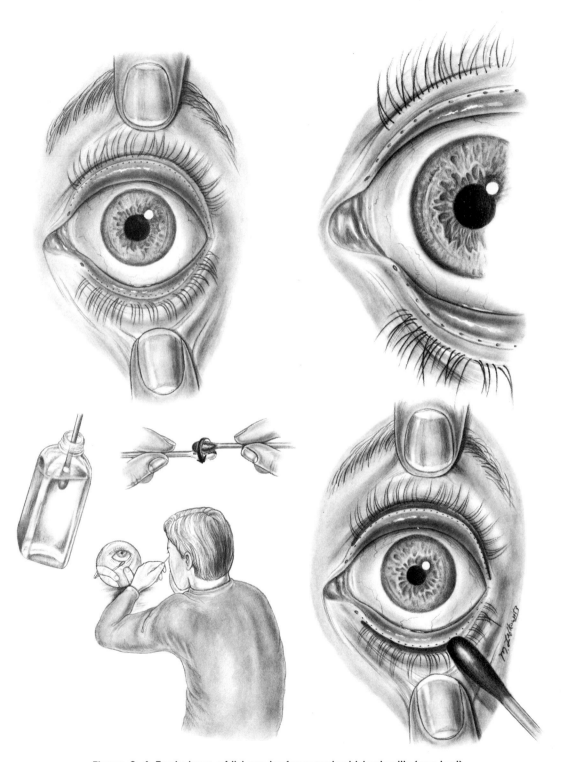

Figure 9–6. Technique of lid scrubs for marginal blepharitis (see text).

Viral Infection of the Lid and Conjunctiva

It is generally held that viral infections are a common cause of acute conjunctivitis in the United States, and a variety of viral agents have been incriminated. These include adenoviruses, vaccinia, herpes simplex, and herpes zoster. Each of these agents tends to affect the epithelium of both the conjunctiva and the cornea; as a result an epithelial keratitis is a frequent accompaniment of a viral conjunctivitis. Myxoviruses (influenza, mumps, and Newcastle disease) can also cause a minor punctate keratopathy in association with a conjunctivitis. In general a viral keratitis is characterized by punctate epithelial erosions that stain prominently with fluorescein and are often accompanied by punctate infiltrates in the epithelium. If the conjunctivitis persists or is severe, there may be a disturbance in the anterior stroma beneath the epithelial abnormalities. The stromal abnormalities may be ephemeral and resolve despite persistence of the epithelial keratitis or, as in the case of an adenovirus infection, they may persist for a period of years, long after the epithelial changes have resolved (Fig. 9–7). In the latter instance the subepithelial infiltrates are thought to be immunologic in origin, the result of an antigen-antibody reaction. While the persistence of such subepithelial infiltrates is sufficiently characteristic to enable a specific diagnosis to be made, the punctate epithelial changes rarely are sufficiently distinct morphologically to permit a specific type of virus to be identified as the etiologic agent.

Adenoviruses

Adenovirus infection of the outer eye is typified by the entity known as epidemic keratoconjunctivitis (EKC).[8–11] Types 8, 19, 1, 2, 3, 4, 5, 6, 7, 9, 10, 11, 13, 14, 15, 16, and 29 have all been documented to be causal agents,[8] and there are no clinical features that allow identification of the infecting adenovirus type. All ages and both sexes are affected. The average

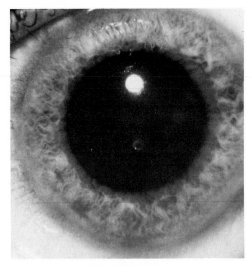

Figure 9–7. Subepithelial infiltrates present two years after an acute attack of adenoviral epidemic keratoconjunctivitis. The epithelium is intact and does not stain.

incubation period is 8 days, with a range of 2 to 16 days. The infection starts unilaterally and may remain so, but most cases are bilateral with an interval of up to 1 week between involvement of the first and second eye in most instances. The disorder is characterized by a red, irritated, lacrimating eye, and preauricular adenopathy is present in the great majority of cases. Both ocular involvement and preauricular adenopathy are more prominent on the side that is involved first. Systemic illness, including fever, malaise, a sore throat, and an upper respiratory infection sometimes complete the clinical picture, especially in children.

The conjunctivitis is characterized by hyperemia, chemosis, a follicular reaction, and at times pseudomembrane formation. Commonly this clears within 2 weeks, but it may persist for 6 weeks or longer. The virus generally can be isolated up to 2 weeks from the onset of the conjunctivitis. Corneal involvement is frequent and generally makes its appearance 7 to 10 days after the onset of the conjunctivitis. Initially this is a fine, diffuse punctate epithelial keratitis with sensation unaffected. It can last days to weeks and clear spontaneously, or it can persist with the formation of larger epithelial infiltrates and the appearance of focal areas of edema and infiltration in the anterior stroma beneath many of the epithelial infiltrates. The epithelial infiltrates generally resolve, but the subepithelial lesions (Figs. 9–3 and 9–7), most often located centrally, remain for varying periods, usually in the order of months. Frequently, however, the subepithelial opacities persist for a year or two. We have seen two cases in which the subepithelial infiltrates persisted for more than 10 years before clearing without residual scar formation. As its name indicates, the disease occurs in epidemic proportions; hand-to-eye transmission is common, and ophthalmic solutions and instruments are a frequent cause of contamination.

Although adenovirus is a DNA virus with some in vitro sensitivity to idoxuridine and trifluorothymidine, none of the available antiviral antimetabolites is effective clinically. A topical astringent, antibiotic, or sulfonamide commonly is instilled four times daily, largely as supportive therapy for symptomatic relief. (Bacterial superinfection is a very infrequent complication.) If anterior uveitis is present, a short-acting mydriatic (e.g., cyclopentolate) also is administered four times a day. A potent ophthalmic corticosteroid, such as 1.0 per cent prednisolone acetate, will dramatically suppress the conjunctival inflammatory signs, relieve symptoms, and cause the subepithelial infiltrates in the cornea to disappear.[12] However, adenovirus infections usually are self-limited and permanent visual loss is rare. Since corticosteroids are not innocuous agents, their use generally is limited to cases with symptoms and blurred vision of sufficient severity to be incapacitating.

Many authors stress that the subepithelial infiltrates in the cornea often reappear when corticosteroids are discontinued. Since the natural course of the disorder is characterized by subepithelial infiltrates that can persist for months or even years, this is not surprising. Corticosteroids in no way alter the basic pathogenetic mechanisms of the disease; they simply suppress the manifestation of its signs. There are no controlled data substantiating the conclusion that corticosteroids prolong the disease or the persistence of subepithelial infiltrates.

If corticosteroids are used, 1.0 per cent prednisolone acetate administered four times daily will eliminate subepithelial infiltrates in virtually all cases within a short period of time. The dosage is then progressively reduced to the least amount of drug that will maintain the patient's comfort and keep the cornea free of infiltrates. Prednisolone acetate 0.125 per cent, instilled twice daily or even less frequently, will accomplish this in most cases. Since the subepithelial infiltrates in untreated cases can persist for months or years, corticosteroid therapy may be required for prolonged periods. At a point that is chosen empirically, corticosteroid therapy is discontinued and the ocular response is observed. Subepithelial infiltrates may recur, but if their reappearance is not associated with significant symptoms, the disease can be allowed to run its course and corticosteroid therapy need not be reinstituted. Should incapacitating symptoms accompany the recurrent corneal infiltrates, corticosteroids are again administered in sufficient dosage to effect their suppression. Subsequently they are tapered to a minimum maintenance dose and ultimately the cycle is repeated.

Herpes Simplex

Primarily ocular herpes simplex infection[2, 13, 14] characteristically causes a follicular conjunctivitis that is often associated with an enlarged, somewhat tender, ipsilateral preauricular lymph node. The disorder occurs predominantly in infants and young children but can present in individuals of any age. Commonly only one eye is involved, and it is red and irritable with a watery discharge. Vesicles may be present on the eyelid or face (Fig. 9–8), the eyelids may be swollen, and there may be an ulcerative blepharitis. Rarely are these findings severe. Within 2 weeks after the onset of conjunctivitis, an epithelial ker-

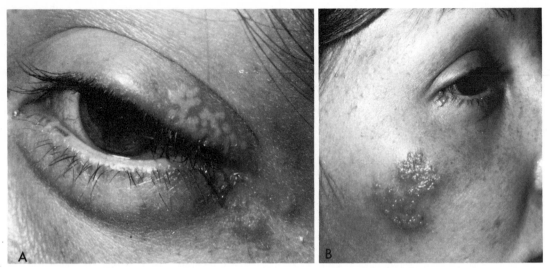

Figure 9–8. Herpes simplex vesicles on the skin of the eyelids *(A)* and the face *(B)*.

atitis may develop. Generally this is accompanied by a mild foreign body sensation and photophobia, and it frequently causes blurring of vision.

The corneal component is variable in appearance. It may manifest itself as a diffuse, fine, punctate epithelial keratitis. The epithelial infiltrates stain poorly with fluorescein (and often little better with rose bengal) and many desquamate to form punctate epithelial erosions. Conversely, corneal involvement may occur in the form of a coarse punctate epithelial keratitis with white plaques of opaque epithelial cells reaching 1.0 to 2.0 mm. in diameter.[2] These lesions may progress to form typical dendritic figures (Fig. 9–9). Rarely is there stromal involvement initially, but subsequently (generally within about 2 weeks) subepithelial infiltrates appear with frequency. These tend to be transient and to clear without significant residua, though they may persist for several weeks before gradually resolving and leaving light gray focal superficial scars.

Recurrent herpes simplex keratitis also can begin as a diffuse, coarse (areolar or stellate shaped lesions) punctate epithelial keratitis. This is not associated with a follicular conjunctivitis. The lesions contain replicating virus and stain brightly with rose bengal. Invariably within a day or two the coarsely punctate lesions assume a dendritic

shape, and shortly thereafter the involved epithelial cells desquamate to form the typical linear, branching, dendritic ulcer. Associated punctate epithelial erosions are common.

Punctate lesions in the corneal epithelium caused by herpes simplex virus are treated with topically applied antiviral antimetabolites. Details are presented in Chapters 13 and 16.

Herpes Zoster

Involvement of the trigeminal ganglion by varicella-zoster virus results in a striking and pathognomonic clinical picture referred to as herpes zoster ophthalmicus. Presumably the virus is widely

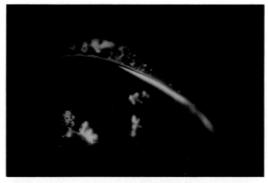

Figures 9–9. Multiple small dendritic epithelial lesions of herpes simplex keratitis. Twenty-four hours earlier a coarse, punctate epithelial keratopathy had been present.

disseminated in the body during an initial varicella illness and persists in an inactive form in certain tissues. Herpes zoster ophthalmicus is said to be caused by a reactivation of the latent varicella-zoster virus in the trigeminal ganglion. The virus appears to replicate within the ganglion and to migrate down the peripheral fibers of the fifth cranial nerve, particularly the ophthalmic branch.[15–17]

The patient experiences a systemic illness of relatively abrupt onset marked by fever, generalized malaise, nausea and vomiting, and neuralgic pain along the affected division of the trigeminal nerve. Shortly thereafter (within days) the skin supplied by the involved portion of the nerve becomes exquisitely sensitive, red, and edematous, and vesicles appear. Initially these are filled with clear fluid (from which virus can be cultured for approximately 3 days), but the fluid rapidly becomes turbid and yellow. Over the course of several days, the vesicles burst, forming eschars. This can be a necrotizing process involving the dermis, so that when the eschars are shed, permanent pitted scars remain. The ophthalmic division of the trigeminal nerve is affected most often, and when this includes its lacrimal and nasociliary branches, ocular involvement is common. The nasociliary branch provides sensory innervation for the anterior portion of the eye and the conjunctiva as well as for the skin around the medial canthus and the side and tip of the nose. This accounts for Hutchinson's rule that the eye is frequently involved if there are vesicles along the side and at the tip of the nose.

Conjunctival involvement frequently is manifested simply as hyperemia of the tissue. At times a follicular response, a mucopurulent discharge, and/or a regional adenopathy occur. Corneal involvement commonly presents as a coarse, punctate, epithelial keratitis with ragged, irregularly shaped aggregations of opaque epithelial cells (Fig. 9–10). These tend to desquamate spontaneously and to heal without ulceration. Alternatively, epithelial involvement may be characterized by the appearance of vesicles or dendritic lesions (see Chapter 17) resembling those of herpes simplex keratitis.[18, 19] In zoster keratitis the dendrite is said to be comprised of gray, swollen, elevated epithelial cells that stain irregularly with fluorescein, whereas the dendrite of herpes simplex keratitis is characterized by ulceration of the epithelium, causing it to stain brightly with fluorescein. Zoster virus has been isolated from the dendritic lesions,[18] which upon clearing often leave mild anterior stromal nebulae. The punctate epithelial keratopathy may resolve spontaneously within 2 to 3 weeks, or it may persist despite treatment for considerable periods. It sometimes progresses to a combined epithelial and subepithelial keratopathy, and the latter may further progress to a punctate subepithelial keratopathy. Here nummular opacities 1.0 to 2.0 mm. in size characteristically appear in the most superficial layers of the stroma. In more

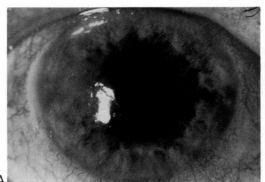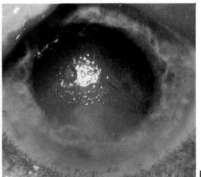

Figure 9–10. Herpes zoster keratitis. *A*, A coarse, punctate epithelial keratopathy. *B*, More severe involvement; epithelium is ragged and desquamating.

severe cases extensive stromal involvement may occur with neovascularization of the cornea, particularly when the involvement is peripheral. Corneal sensation commonly is depressed in herpes zoster ophthalmicus, but neurotrophic keratitis is not an invariable accompaniment. In many instances the cornea remains clear and there is a gradual recovery of sensation. Nonetheless, a severe neurotrophic keratitis can occur in cases marked by persistent hypesthesia or anesthesia. Here epithelial and stromal ulceration, stromal infiltration and necrosis, and neovascularization result, and the outcome is dense scarring or even perforation.

The virus of varicella (chickenpox) is identical with that of herpes zoster, and the most common clinical manifestation of the virus is chickenpox. Occasionally the lesions of chickenpox involve the eye. Commonly these are unilateral, small, papular lesions that erupt along the lid margin or at the limbus. They may resolve without sequelae or become pustular and form painful, reactive conjunctival ulcers. At times the cornea also is involved. Usually this presents as a relatively benign superficial punctate keratopathy, but stromal involvement also can occur.[20]

The superficial punctate keratopathy produced by varicella-zoster virus should be treated conservatively. A mild astringent (e.g., zinc sulfate 0.25 per cent) can be instilled four times a day, but commonly an antibiotic or sulfonamide preparation is used. These agents seem to afford a degree of symptomatic relief, perhaps through a placebo effect, but secondary bacterial infection is rare. A short-acting mydriatic-cycloplegic also may be helpful in restoring comfort; its use is mandatory if the keratopathy is accompanied by active inflammation in the anterior chamber. Antiviral antimetabolites are ineffective. We generally reserve topical corticosteroids for cases with epithelial and subepithelial infiltrates and/or anterior uveitis. The response, though not as dramatic as that obtained in adenovirus infection, is often favorable. Local corticosteroid

therapy of ocular involvement by varicella-zoster does not produce the enhancement of viral replication and worsening of corneal disease encountered with herpes simplex virus infection of the corneal epithelium.

Molluscum Contagiosum and Verrucae

The viruses of molluscum contagiosum and of verrucae can cause a tumorlike epithelial proliferation. Both can produce lesions on the eyelids, and in the presence of such lesions a conjunctivitis and a superficial punctate keratopathy may be encountered.[21] The typical lesion of molluscum contagiosum is a small, discrete, elevated globular tumor with a central umbilication (Fig. 9–11). The disorder is basically a benign dermatologic condition caused by a filterable virus, apparently a DNA virus of the pox group. As a result the disease is transmissible but the degree of contagion is quite low. The virus stimulates hyperplasia of the deeper epidermal cells to produce the tumor. Histologically, a fibrous capsule surrounds the tumor and fibrous septa divide it into lobules, each of which is formed by a mass of epithelial cells. Some of these epithelial cells become greatly enlarged. The nucleus within these cells is eccentrically displaced and ultimately is destroyed, and the cytoplasm is replaced by an enormous inclusion body. The huge intracytoplasmic inclusions within degenerated epithelial cells are shed into the central core of the tumor and presumably form the curdlike material that often can be expressed from the lesions. The surface indentation is filled with keratinized epithelial cells containing inclusion bodies.

Both the upper and lower lids can be involved, and the lesions occur singly or in groups. Generally the tumor is located at or near the lid margin and may be partially obscured by the lashes. Occasionally it presents in the conjunctiva, primarily in the lower palpebral conjunctiva, and a molluscum tumor has even been reported to evolve in the cor-

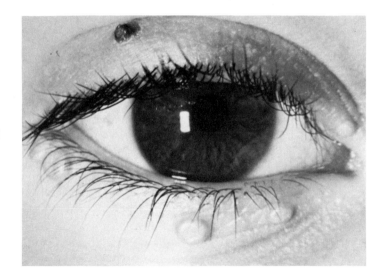

Figure 9–11. Typical lesion of molluscum contagiosum.

nea,[22] although the latter location is a rarity. The lesions growing on the lid margins (as well as those occasionally appearing in the conjunctiva) induce a secondary conjunctivitis. Most often this is a mild to moderate, chronic, follicular conjunctivitis affecting both the upper and lower fornices. Mononuclear cells predominate in smears of the exudate. The conjunctivitis is resistant to therapy as long as the lid lesions are present, and if allowed to persist, it is accompanied by corneal abnormalities. Initially the corneal disorder is a diffuse superficial punctate keratopathy characterized primarily by fine epithelial erosions. Subsequently, if the corneal abnormality is allowed to progress, a punctate epithelial keratitis as well as punctate subepithelial infiltrates appear. These inflammatory lesions tend to be most prevalent in the superior portion of the cornea. If the problem is not treated appropriately, peripheral neovascularization and scarring, a phlyctenular lesion, or ulceration of the cornea may occur. Replicating virus has not been isolated from conjunctival or corneal epithelium. The inflammatory changes in the cornea and conjunctiva are not helped by steroids or antibiotics but resolve following the removal of the tumors from the lid margin. This supports the conclusion that both the conjunctivitis and the keratitis are a response to toxic viral products released from the lid lesions.

Similarly, the verruca virus attacks epithelial cells and after a long incubation period (months to years) produces a papilliform proliferation in the form of a wart (Fig. 9–12). If these lesions are located at or near the lid margins, a mild, subacute catarrhal conjunctivitis may occur. This affects only the eye with the warts on the lid margin and remains confined to that eye. The conjunctivitis may be accompanied by a superficial punctate keratopathy characterized by multiple punctate epithelial erosions. Like molluscum contagiosum, the verrucose conjunctivitis and the keratitis

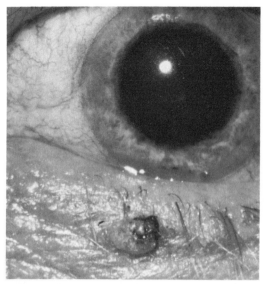

Figure 9–12. Papilliform lid lesion produced by the verruca virus. The associated chronic conjunctivitis and superficial punctate keratopathy cleared after excision of the lesion.

both are resistant to therapy with all forms of topically administered agents, but they respond promptly to simple removal of the wart. Presumably the conjunctivitis and the keratitis are an inflammatory response to a toxin released from the lid lesion.

Vaccinia

Ocular vaccinia[2, 23, 24] invariably presents in a patient who has been vaccinated within the prior 10 days or who has been in contact with someone successfully vaccinated during that period. The eye or adnexae are accidentally inoculated, usually as a result of viral transmission by the patient's hands. Ocular involvement usually is unilateral and often is accompanied by enlarged preauricular lymph nodes on the involved side. The severity of the resultant clinical disease tends to be directly proportional to the patient's immune status with regard to the virus. If the individual has been vaccinated previously and a good level of immunity is present, the disease is mild and generally is manifested by little more than an acute focal purulent blepharoconjunctivitis. In contrast, severe reactions may occur in unvaccinated or weakly immune individuals.

Typically the eyelids are swollen, and in most instances single or multiple vaccinial lesions are present (Fig. 9–13). These lesions may be located on the eyelid, at or near the lid margin, on the periocular skin, or on the conjunctiva. Characteristically the lesion is elevated and appears pustular. The center of the pustule is umbilicated and necrotic, and the surrounding skin generally is erythematous. The conjunctiva is hyperemic and chemotic, and mucopurulent exudate commonly is present. If a vaccinial lesion involves the conjunctiva, conjunctival ulceration may occur; the ulcers often are covered by an adherent, inflammatory membrane.

Vaccinial keratitis often is first manifested by a grayish, granular opacification of the epithelium. Sometimes these are focal, pinhead-sized lesions, but the

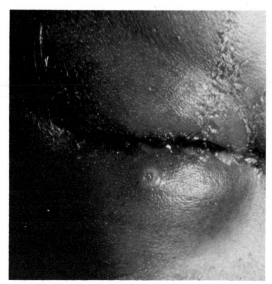

Figure 9–13. Vaccinial lesion on the eyelid. There is an associated blepharoconjunctivitis and a punctate epithelial keratopathy.

entire corneal epithelium may be affected. The involved epithelial cells contain virus and stain with rose bengal. Punctate epithelial erosions occur and yellow opacities may appear in the superficial stroma. The latter range from punctate subepithelial opacities that develop beneath disordered epithelial cells to large stromal abscesses. The small lesions evolve into a gray, punctate subepithelial keratitis reminiscent of epidemic keratoconjunctivitis and follow a course similar to that of an adenovirus infection. In the case of vaccinia, however, the subepithelial opacities may be central, peripheral, or form a ring in the corneal midperiphery. They persist for months to years, and an associated neovascularization with some degree of permanent scarring is not uncommon. Deeper, more severe vaccinial stromal involvement tends to follow a course like that of severe herpes simplex keratitis. The disease is protracted; stromal infiltration, necrosis, and ulceration occur; and corneal scarring and neovascularization, or even perforation, result.

Other Viruses

A number of other viruses, including the myxoviruses,[2, 25] picornavirus (Fig. 9–

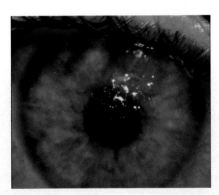

Figure 9–14. Punctate epithelial keratopathy caused by picornavirus in a case of acute hemorrhagic conjunctivitis.

14)[26,27] measles (rubeola),[28, 29] and postnatally acquired rubella,[30] have been documented to cause keratitis. In well-nourished individuals with normal immune systems, ocular involvement is relatively mild in degree and tends to resolve spontaneously without adverse sequelae. Typically, corneal involvement accompanies a nondescript, catarrhal conjunctivitis and takes the form of a minor superficial punctate keratopathy. Usually the keratitis has no distinguishing morphologic characteristics. When factors such as malnutrition are associated with the viral infection, serious corneal involvement and permanent blindness can occur.[31]

Ocular Chlamydial Infections

Chlamydia, the so-called TRIC agents that cause trachoma and inclusion conjunctivitis, can produce a punctate keratopathy.[1, 32, 33] In the early stages of trachoma, punctate keratopathy typically is associated with a chronic follicular conjunctivitis involving the upper tarsal conjunctiva primarily. Often, superficial capillaries extend across the superior limbus, invade the anterior corneal stroma, and form a pannus. Limbal lymphoid follicles may develop in this area (i.e., the superior limbus); Herbert's pits result when the follicles resolve by scarring. The corneal surface may appear generally gray and roughened, and there is a diffuse epithelial keratopathy characterized by relatively ragged punctate epithelial erosions that stain brightly with fluorescein. Subsequently, punctate yellow to gray subepithelial infiltrates may appear; they may persist for months, long after the epithelial erosions have healed, or they may resolve and be replaced by new infiltrates in different locations, much like an adenovirus infection. The corneal changes of trachoma primarily involve the upper half of the cornea. If untreated, the entity tends to be persistent, causing ocular irritation, photophobia, and lacrimation. Significant disability may result.

The exudate in trachoma contains both polymorphonuclear and mononuclear cells. Giemsa stained conjunctival scrapings also may demonstrate classic Halberstaedter–von Prowazek inclusion bodies in the cytoplasm of conjunctival epithelial cells. The organism is difficult to isolate in culture, and facilities for this purpose are not generally available. Topically administered tetracyclines are the mainstay of trachoma chemotherapy programs. If tetracycline cannot be used, erythromycin ophthalmic ointment is a suitable substitute.

The chlamydial agent that causes inclusion conjunctivitis is genitally transmitted. Therefore, the disease occurs in those who come into contact with genital tract secretions, i.e., newborns and sexually active adults. In the adult the infection usually presents as an acute follicular conjunctivitis predominantly involving the conjunctiva of the lower lid and fornix. Inclusion conjunctivitis does not commonly produce the conjunctival scarring and pannus formation seen with trachoma, but exceptions occur. It is also much less apt than trachoma to cause a punctate keratopathy but has been well documented to do so. The superficial corneal changes consist of a ragged, punctate epithelial keratitis or a combined epithelial-subepithelial punctate keratopathy. Discrete subepithelial infiltrates similar to those found in association with bacterial conjunctivitis have been described at the limbus and in the central cornea and have been said to occur in the absence of a preced-

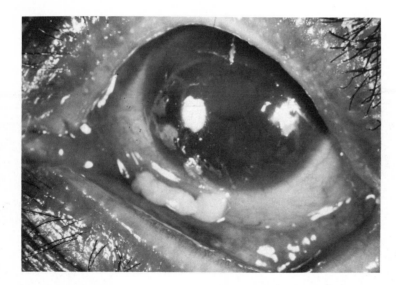

Figure 9–15. Excess mucus in a case of keratoconjunctivitis sicca.

ing epithelial keratitis. In general the superficial corneal lesions of inclusion conjunctivitis are little different from those of trachoma, except that they tend to involve primarily the central and/or inferior cornea.

The conjunctival exudate of inclusion conjunctivitis, like that of trachoma, contains polymorphonuclear and mononuclear cells. Giemsa stained conjunctival scrapings taken from affected infants contain many typical chlamydial intracytoplasmic inclusions, but these occur infrequently in adults. Adult inclusion conjunctivitis responds to oral tetracyclines. When undesirable side effects result from tetracycline therapy, erythromycin can be used.

Lacrimal Insufficiency

Keratoconjunctivitis sicca and other dry eye syndromes result from a diminution in the secretion of the main or accessory lacrimal glands and from localized disease of the conjunctiva. The insufficiency of tears causes a chronic conjunctivitis that tends to be nonspecific in its clinical appearance, although there may be concentric folds in the hyperemic bulbar conjunctiva, particularly in its lower half. The conjunctivitis may be mild in degree. It is frequently associated with considerable ocular irritation and photophobia, and it is not unusual

for the symptoms of the disorder to exceed the signs in severity. The precorneal tear film may be irregular in thickness, with an abnormally short breakup time, and the marginal tear strip may be scanty. Both often contain excessive debris. Characteristically, strands of mucus are present and are seen in the lower fornix or on the cornea (Fig. 9–15). Corneal involvement is encountered with regularity. The early or least severe form is a punctate epithelial keratopathy (Fig. 9–16) composed of epithelial erosions (which stain brightly with fluorescein and rose bengal dyes) and punctate epithelial infiltrates. These lesions occur most frequently in the interpalpebral portion of the cornea or in its lower half, but it is not unusual for them to be more widespread. With time dry areas of epithelium may keratinize (Fig. 9–17) and

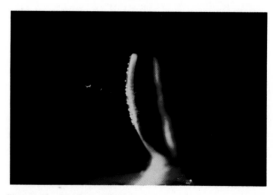

Figure 9–16. Superficial punctate keratopathy in a case of keratoconjunctivitis sicca.

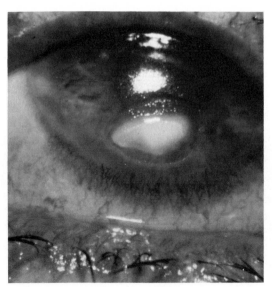

Figure 9–17. A plaque of keratinized epithelium in a case of keratoconjunctivitis sicca.

localized infiltrates may appear in Bowman's membrane and in the anterior stromal lamellae. Epithelial filaments (Fig. 9–4) commonly are encountered in keratitis sicca, although their occurrence is not pathognomic of this disorder. More serious corneal complications occur in the severe forms of this entity; these include corneal neovascularization and pannus formation, persistent stromal infiltrates, and indolent ulcers of varying size and depth (see Chapter 20).

Several tests of tear deficiency are available. They include the Schirmer test, tear breakup time, rose bengal staining, the fluorescein dilution test, and lysozyme assay. The last two, the fluorescein dilution test and lysozyme assay, require equipment or laboratory facilities that are not generally available in a clinical setting. The Schirmer test provides a gross measure of aqueous tear secretion, tear breakup time is useful in delineating an unstable tear film, and rose bengal staining colors and defines devitalized, desiccated epithelial cells and mucin. Unfortunately, none of these tests is sufficiently accurate, reproducible, or discriminatory to permit a diagnosis to be established with a high degree of confidence. In a seemingly normal individual it is not uncommon

to find an abnormality in a single tear function test, but this type of isolated finding generally is of little significance in establishing the diagnosis of dry eyes. To do so, one must consider the findings of the entire battery of clinical examinations and tear function tests, not just the results of a single test. The diagnosis frequently depends on the presence of multiple signs and on the results of several tests accumulated from repeated examinations.

In the treatment of dry eyes we attempt to replace the deficient secretions by topical application of an artificial tear preparation, but results tend to be quite variable. Although tear substitutes can be instilled as frequently as every hour, a major limitation of this approach is the extremely short retention time in the conjunctival sac of all of the commercially available artificial tear formulations. The actual retention time of any of these preparations is, at best, a few minutes only, and often this is simply inadequate to provide a prolonged and satisfactory degree of comfort. Moreover, in many patients with keratoconjunctivitis sicca, there is accumulation of mucus on the ocular surface and in the conjunctival fornices, causing an increase in the viscosity of tears and producing symptoms of irritation, particularly when the mucus adheres to and pulls upon epithelial filaments. Dramatic results in dealing with excess mucus can at times be achieved using the mucolytic agent acetylcysteine in conjunction with tear substitutes. We have obtained equally dramatic therapeutic results in the replacement of insufficient and/or abnormal lacrimal secretions by instillation of an experimental, high viscosity, carboxypolymethylene gel presently under clinical investigation. Details of the treatment of lacrimal insufficiency are presented in Chapter 20.

Trauma: Mechanical, Chemical, Radiational

A wide variety of agents and mechanisms are capable of producing a non-

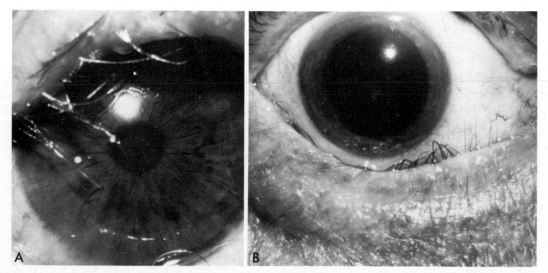

Figure 9–18. Superficial punctate keratopathy resulting from mechanical trauma of the corneal epithelium. A, Trichiasis. B, Entropion of the lower lid.

specific conjunctivitis and an accompanying superficial punctate keratopathy. They include mechanical trauma, chemical toxicity, and radiational injury.[34] Acute episodes are characterized by diffuse hyperemia and at times chemosis of the conjunctiva, a foreign body sensation of varying intensity (described as stinging, burning, etc.), photophobia, excessive lacrimation or watery discharge, and in the more severe cases involuntary closure of the lids. Diffuse punctate epithelial erosions are evident on the corneal surface with the slit-lamp biomicroscope, and often the corneal surface is also speckled with fine, gray dots which presumably are abnormal or dead epithelial cells. These changes stain readily with fluorescein and rose bengal. Chronic cases manifest the same signs and symptoms but generally are less severe and often are accompanied by a papillary conjunctivitis.

Trichiasis is an example of this problem caused by mechanical trauma. The misaligned lashes turn inward and impinge directly upon the cornea. Most often trichiasis is cicatricial in nature; the lash follicles become distorted and are turned inward as a result of scarring due to trauma or inflammation of the lids (Fig. 9–18). However, an identical problem may occur as a result of entropion of the lid, wherein the cause lies

not in the lash or its follicle but in the in-turned lid margin (Fig. 9–18). Contact lens wear is still another apparently traumatic cause of superficial punctate keratopathy. Diffuse, very fine, slightly depressed areas appear in the corneal epithelium of contact lens wearers. Generally they are not visible without the aid of a biomicroscope and the application of fluorescein, which stains the depressions relatively faintly. Presumably the surface epithelial cells are traumatized by the lens and the injured cells desquamate, although it is possible that oxygen deprivation or other interference with cellular metabolism may contribute to epithelial cell injury.

The variety of chemicals known to cause punctate epithelial keratopathy is almost endless.[35] Before adequate ventilation was provided in manufacturing facilities, the problem frequently occurred among workers exposed to toxic chemical fumes and sprays. Reports in the ophthalmic literature indicated that a superficial toxic keratopathy was particularly prevalent among workers in the rayon and sugar beet industries and in those using varnishes and lacquers in confined, inadequately ventilated quarters. Interestingly, a similar, nonspecific toxic keratopathy is associated with the use of household sprays such as hairspray.[36]

Currently, however, ophthalmic medications are a more frequent source of this disorder. Most topically applied ophthalmic drugs can exert toxic effects on the corneal epithelium. Local anesthetics are a typical example.[37] These agents depress respiration and glycolysis of the epithelial cells and interfere with their replication and regeneration. Clinically the corneal surface may appear irregular after application of an anesthetic; it loses its luster and its reflective properties are altered. Biomicroscopic examination demonstrates optic irregularities that are revealed as punctate erosions by fluorescein staining. Similarly, the antiviral antimetabolites interfere with metabolic functions of the corneal epithelium and can cause a nonspecific superficial punctate keratopathy.

Surfactants are compounds characterized by hydrophilic properties at one end of the molecule and lipophilic properties at the other. As a result they are water soluble and also have an affinity for oils and greases. All surfactants lower the surface tension of water. They are frequent components of chemicals used for cleaning and washing, and they are also used in cosmetics and disinfectants. Compounds in this category included benzalkonium chloride (Zephiran), a cationic surfactant, and Ivory soap, an anionic surfactant. Cationic surfactants cause proteins to precipitate, whereas the anionic forms cause cell lysis, so that both types are potentially toxic to the corneal epithelium. A superficial punctate keratopathy often occurs when shampoo or a liquid household detergent accidentally comes in contact with the eye. However, benzalkonium chloride is part of the vehicle formulation of a number of collyria. It is used as a preservative and as a wetting agent to increase the ocular penetration of drugs. A concentration of 1 to 3000 generally is employed; this concentration enhances corneal permeability without producing a clinically detectable injury. However, at a dilution of 1 to 1000 benzalkonium chloride can cause mild discomfort and produce a superficial punctate keratopathy when applied to the human eye. Solutions used for the cleaning and storage of contact lenses contain detergents and surfactants; they can cause a superficial punctate keratopathy if they accidentally come in contact with the eye or if the wearer fails to rinse the lenses properly prior to their insertion.

A large number of chemicals, which collectively can be referred to as tear gases, have an intense lacrimatory action. They are effective at very low concentrations and most are capable of injuring the cornea. They cause an intense stinging and burning sensation in the eyes, a profuse outpouring of tears, and involuntary blepharospasm. In very low concentrations these agents induce a diffuse punctate epithelial keratitis. Higher concentrations can produce severe injury to the corneal stroma with permanent scarring and neovascularization.

Radiation from the invisible portions of the electromagnetic spectrum can cause an acute inflammatory reaction in the conjunctiva and cornea. Infrared rays, such as those produced by the carbon dioxide laser, can injure the cornea,[38] but ultraviolet light gives rise to most cases seen by the ophthalmologist. Photophthalmia can occur under natural conditions or, more commonly, as an accident among those who either work with ultraviolet rays or are otherwise exposed to a source rich in short wavelengths. The wavelength that has the most effect in producing keratitis appears to be 288 mμ, but the action spectrum capable of inciting a photophthalmic reaction is approximately 305 to 250 mμ. Ordinarily sunlight, even when reinforced by the light of a sky free from atmospheric contamination of moisture and dust (which absorb ultraviolet radiation), does not cause photophthalmia. However, these sources may be reinforced by a dazzling reflection from an extensive surface such as the sea, the desert, or particularly a snow or ice field with its high reflection factor. If there is an exposure of several hours to this combined radiational source, the critical threshold of abiotic damage by ultraviolet rays may be exceeded and photophthalmia may result.

Industrial photophthalmia (flash eye) is apt to occur in any occupation in which insufficiently screened sources of light rich in ultraviolet radiation are used. The most acute symptoms generally are encountered among workers with inadequate ocular protection engaged in oxyacetylene or arc welding. Short exposures are additive within a period of up to 24 hours and therefore are cumulatively dangerous. Under conditions of nature the problem is most commonly encountered after exposure to bright sunlight on a snow field (snow-blindness). Regardless of the source of the ultraviolet radiation, the clinical picture is the same. There is always a latent period between exposure and the onset of symptoms. Its length varies directly with the intensity and the duration of the exposure, but most commonly it is about 6 to 10 hours. The first symptom usually is a foreign body sensation ranging in degree from a slight pricking to considerable discomfort likened to an eye full of sand. If the patient has been exposed to moderately intense radiation, as is often the case, frank ocular pain occurs, accompanied by marked photophobia, profuse lacrimation, and striking blepharospasm. In most instances the objective findings are surprisingly mild in view of the patient's particularly miserable and helpless state. The conjunctiva is red and occasionally chemotic, and the pupil tends to be constricted. The corneal surface has lost its luster and appears gray and irregular, but usually the epithelial layer is intact. Application of fluorescein reveals numerous punctate epithelial erosions and gives the epithelium a stippled appearance. The entity usually is self-limited, with most of the discomfort subsiding within 48 hours.[39]

Treatment is dictated by the etiology of the keratopathy. Trichiasis and entropion of the lid require surgical intervention. A hydrophilic contact lens can be used temporarily to protect the corneal epithelium from the trauma of the lashes, but in our experience this has not produced a satisfactory long-term solution to the problem in most cases. The lens tends to become dislodged and/or rapidly coated by meibomian secretions. A punctate epithelial keratopathy secondary to contact lens wear itself requires refitting of the lens and perhaps a lens constructed of an alternative material. If the problem is encountered in a patient with borderline tear production, discontinuation of contact lens wear must be considered.

Prevention is the primary therapeutic approach to a low-grade, chronic chemical keratopathy of industrial or medicinal origin. Ventilation must be improved or other steps taken to eliminate the offending fumes, and ophthalmic medications incriminated as causal must be discontinued. When this is accomplished, the disorder generally subsides spontaneously, but its course often can be hastened by topical instillation of an antibiotic-corticosteroid combination preparation. (The treatment of more severe chemical burns is discussed in Chapter 21.) Photophthalmia is treated by the topical instillation of a mydriatic-cycloplegic agent (to reduce spasm of the ciliary muscle) and an antibiotic (used largely as a prophylactic measure) and the application of a secure pressure dressing over the closed lids. In the more severe cases an orally administered analgesic may be helpful in the initial stages. We re-evaluate the patient 24 hours after the pressure dressing is applied. If discomfort persists or significant epithelial regeneration has not occurred, the topical medications are again instilled and a pressure dressing reapplied.

Exposure Keratopathy

Adequate closure of the eyelids and normal blinking are required for resurfacing and maintenance of the precorneal tear film.[40, 41] Failure of resurfacing to occur with sufficient frequency results in spotwise drying of the precorneal tear film and subsequently in corneal desiccation. Exposure keratopathy describes the cor-

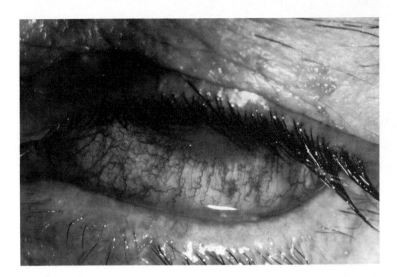

Figure 9–19. Position of lids during attempted forced closure in a case of left seventh nerve palsy, showing exposure of the inferior cornea.

neal changes produced by desiccation. The disorder occurs in a variety of circumstances. It is seen when the globe is proptotic because of an orbital tumor or the exophthalmos of thyroid disease. In the latter instance a paucity of blinking contributes to the resultant corneal desiccation. Paralysis of the orbicularis oculi, resulting from dysfunction of the seventh cranial nerve, causes a deficiency of lid closure (lagophthalmos) (Fig. 9–19). Abnormalities of the lids, such as advanced ectropion or distortion of the lid margin by scarring, similarly can prevent normal closure and can interfere with the normal juxtaposition between lid margin and globe necessary for resurfacing of the tear film. Finally, there are individuals whose facial nerves are intact and whose lids and lid function seem to be completely normal but who fail to close their eyelids fully during sleep (nocturnal lagophthalmos) (Fig. 9–20).[42, 43]

In most cases exposure keratopathy is insidious in onset. The lower third of the cornea is involved, and the epithelium in this area is gray and lusterless (Fig. 9–21). Many fine, punctate, epithelial erosions that stain brightly with fluorescein are observed. Invariably there is a concurrent conjunctivitis, and there

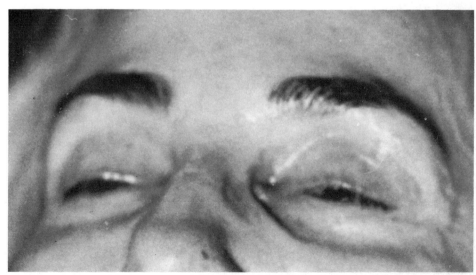

Figure 9–20. Nocturnal lagophthalmos. (Photograph obtained by patient's husband showing position of lids during sleep.)

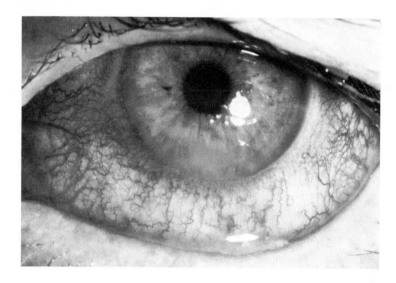

Figure 9–21. Mild exposure keratopathy showing gray, lusterless epithelium (through which iris markings cannot be clearly seen) in lower third of cornea. Fluorescein stain demonstrated many punctate epithelial erosions in this area.

may or may not be a watery discharge. When symptoms are present, an ocular irritation or foreign body sensation, mild photophobia, and blurring of vision are most commonly encountered. In the absence of satisfactory treatment, varying amounts of the involved epithelium are shed (Fig. 9–22), neovascularization occurs, the stroma becomes edematous and infiltrated by inflammatory cells, and, if the epithelial defects persist, bacterial keratitis may occur. Patients with nocturnal lagophthalmos complain of chronic ocular irritation, worse in the morning and improving as the day progresses. The keratopathy is similar to that associated with other forms of this disorder; punctate epithelial changes may involve the lower portion of the cornea or they may occur in a horizontal band across the cornea corresponding to the area exposed during sleep.

The less severe cases of exposure keratopathy often can be successfully treated with topical medications. A bland ophthalmic ointment instilled at bedtime may suffice for nocturnal lagophthalmos, while viscous, artificial tear substitutes and/or a bland ointment instilled more frequently may control mild cases due to proptosis, lid dysfunction, or inadequate apposition of lid to globe. Each instillation of ointment is retained longer in the conjunctival sac and lubricates the cornea for a more

prolonged period than do the liquid tear substitutes, but these advantages are obtained at the expense of a greater interference with vision by the ointment base. The optimal regimen, including frequency of instillation and the preparation to be used, must be determined empirically for each patient. In addition to topical medications, advanced cases of proptosis may require an orbital decompression procedure, and the more severe lid abnormalities often must be treated with a tarsorrhaphy or reconstructive surgery in order to satisfactorily control desiccation of the corneal epithelium induced by exposure.

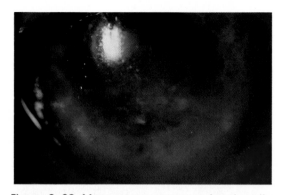

Figure 9–22. More severe exposure keratopathy than illustrated in Figure 9–21. A larger area of epithelium is involved, the epithelium is more ragged, focal areas of epithelium are missing, and there are focal epithelial and subepithelial infiltrates.

Neurotrophic Keratitis

Neurotrophic keratitis is the term used to describe changes in the corneal epithelium resulting from interference with the sensory innervation of the cornea. In 1824 Magendie demonstrated that degenerative changes occur in the cornea when the trigeminal nerve is cut.[44] Numerous studies have subsequently shown that the sensory nerves of the cornea exert a profound influence on the general well-being of the tissue, particularly its epithelial component.[45] The precise nature of this effect and the means by which it is exercised are not known. Loss of corneal sensation, trauma to the insensitive cornea, and diminished blinking and desiccation all appear to be important contributing factors but fail to totally explain the etiology of the entity.

The clinical picture is characteristic. Conjunctival hyperemia generally precedes corneal involvement, and usually there is no significant discharge prior to corneal involvement. Corneal disturbances may occur as early as 24 hours after injury to the trigeminal nerve, and the great majority of cases occur within several months after the injury. Initial corneal changes are a loss of surface luster and microcystic edema of the epithelium (Fig. 9–23). Multiple punctate epithelial erosions then appear in any portion of the cornea and small bullae may occur. The process may persist at this stage for prolonged periods or it may progress.

The more severe forms often are referred to as neuroparalytic keratitis and are characterized by exfoliation of the epithelium (Fig. 9–24); usually all of the central and paracentral epithelium is lost. Epithelial regeneration occurs slowly, if at all, and the stroma then becomes edematous and infiltrated by inflammatory cells. The epithelial defect renders the denervated stroma prone to bacterial invasion. An iritis is often part of the clinical picture. Vision in the involved eye generally is markedly diminished, but there tend to be few other

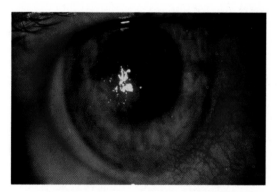

Figure 9–23. Neurotrophic keratitis.

symptoms, largely because of the corneal anesthesia. The disorder is a chronic one and often, despite all therapeutic measures, tends to be slowly progressive.

Treatment of neurotrophic keratitis is nonspecific and has as its primary objective the protection and lubrication of the corneal surface. In its early stages, when the entity is characterized largely by a loss of surface luster and punctate epithelial erosions, topical application of an ophthalmic ointment may successfully accomplish these goals. If the disorder nonetheless shows signs of progression, intermittent application of a pressure dressing (e.g., every second or third day) in addition to the frequent instillation of an ophthalmic ointment often is helpful. A hydrophilic contact lens has been recommended, but our experience with its use in the early stages of neurotrophic keratitis has been variable. At times it appears to be quite useful, affording a gratifying degree of protection to the cornea, but at other times we have observed a loss of large areas of epithelium despite contact lens wear. If necessary, a tarsorrhaphy can be performed, and this tends to be highly successful. We prefer minimal surgical disruption of the lids; often simply abrading the lid margins vigorously and suturing them together is sufficient. As a general rule, the tendency toward epithelial disruption and ulceration decreases with time and the entity becomes increasingly amenable to therapy.

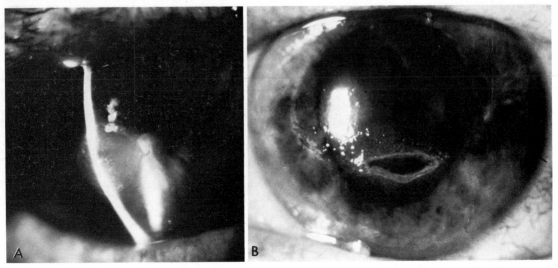

Figure 9–24. Neurotrophic keratitis. *A,* Focal area of gray, lusterless epithelium. *B,* Subsequent exfoliation of most of this area of epithelium.

Thygeson's Superficial Punctate Keratitis

This disorder is characterized by a coarse punctate epithelial keratitis. It involves both eyes, though not necessarily symmetrically or at the same time. All age groups and both sexes may be affected. The cause of the condition is not known; a viral etiology has been proposed but not proven.[46, 47]

A striking feature of Thygeson's superficial punctate keratitis is the absence of an accompanying conjunctivitis. There may be a concurrent mild hyperemia of the bulbar conjunctiva, but the palpebral conjunctiva is not inflamed and there is no discharge or regional adenopathy. Symptoms also are minimal. Typically these include minor discomfort, usually described as burning or irritation, a mild degree of lacrimation and photophobia, and blurring of vision. Rarely does visual acuity decrease below the level of 20/60.

The corneal lesions themselves are coarse, gray epithelial opacities that generally are not visible without magnification (Fig. 9–25). In the authors' experience, they are largely irregular or stellate in shape, but round and oval lesions also occur. The epithelium often is eroded and the lesions stain both with fluorescein and with rose bengal. Individual lesions appear to be formed by numerous tiny dotlike opacities, some of which may be elevated slightly above the corneal surface. A light gray anterior stromal opacity may be seen beneath some of the epithelial lesions; these are transient and do not produce permanent scarring. The total number of epithelial lesions present at a given time is quite variable, but they tend to be numerous; most lie in the central or paracentral cornea. Corneal sensation remains intact.

Thygeson's superficial punctate keratitis tends to have a chronic remittent course. Quiescent, asymptomatic periods, wherein both corneas are clear, are interrupted by episodes of blurred vision and minor ocular irritation. Relapses usually occur insidiously, without an abrupt onset, and multiple spots reappear in the cornea. Individual lesions are transient; each lesion is said to undergo cyclical enlargement and diminution, with concurrent desquamation of its central portion during the latter phase. New spots appear at irregular intervals, so that the distribution of lesions within the cornea changes with time. Typically the entity persists from 1 to several years and then clears spontaneously without any permanent corneal opacification.[48–51] However, a case with an unusually prolonged course (14

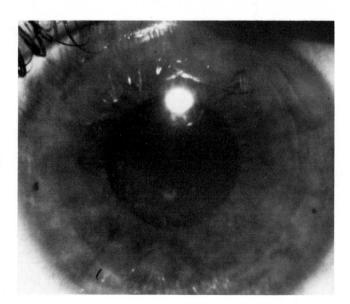

Figure 9–25. Thygeson's superficial punctate keratitis.

years), in which there was permanent subepithelial corneal scarring and elevated lesions resembling Salzmann's nodular degeneration, has been reported.[52]

The lesions of Thygeson's superficial punctate keratitis respond neither to topically administered antibiotics nor to antiviral agents. They are, however, exquisitely sensitive to corticosteroid drops, which rapidly cause both lesions and symptoms to subside. It is our practice to initially treat an acute episode aggressively and then to taper and discontinue the medication, usually over a 3- to 4-week interval. Unfortunately, corticosteroids do not alter the natural course of the disease. Recurrences are encountered, but each acute attack remains responsive to corticosteroid instillation.

Superior Limbic Keratoconjunctivitis

Superior limbic keratoconjunctivitis is a recurrent disorder of unknown etiology, first described by Theodore.[53] It is characterized by inflammation of the tarsal conjunctiva of the upper lid and of the upper bulbar conjunctiva and by an apparent proliferation of the bulbar conjunctiva adjacent to the superior limbus (Fig. 9–26). Fine punctate epithelial erosions are present in the superior cornea,

and these stain readily with fluorescein and rose bengal; the involved superior bulbar conjunctiva also demonstrates fine punctate staining. In some cases epithelial filaments are present in the upper cornea (Fig. 9–26); the filaments may intermittently disappear and reappear.

The condition usually is of several years' duration, its course characterized by remissions and exacerbations, but ultimately it tends to clear spontaneously with few if any permanent residua. Most commonly there is bilateral involvement, although unilateral cases have been reported. Moreover, only one eye may be affected during a given episode, and in bilateral cases findings may be significantly more severe on one side than on the other. Symptoms include varying degrees of discomfort ranging from a burning sensation to frank pain, photophobia, and moderate blepharospasm. The disorder occurs in adults of all ages and seems to be more prevalent among women. An abnormality of thyroid function has been found in a substantial percentage of patients with superior limbic keratoconjunctivitis, but its role in the pathogenesis of the condition has not been established.

Clinically there is often a raised, fleshy zone at the superior limbus (Fig. 9–26). This thickened roll of tissue is tightly adherent to the underlying

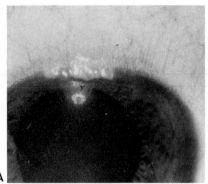 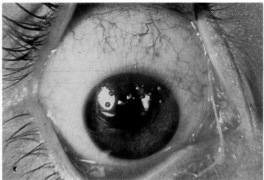

A   B

Figure 9–26. Superior limbic keratoconjunctivitis. *A*, Proliferation of bulbar conjunctiva at upper limbus. *B*, Inflammation of upper bulbar conjunctiva and epithelial filaments in the superior cornea. (*B* courtesy of Frederick H. Theodore, M.D.)

structures. Histopathologic examination shows thickening and cornification of the superficial epithelium. There are large, pale, swollen conjunctival epithelial cells containing few cytoplasmic organelles and at times large empty nuclei. An increase in glycogen granules has also been noted. Electron microscopy does not reveal any viral particles. The subconjunctival tissue is edematous and contains only a scanty infiltrate of neutrophils, lymphocytes, and plasma cells. During a period of remission the clinically evident superior limbic pathology can disappear completely within a short period of time.[53–57]

Not surprisingly, since its etiology is unknown, there is no effective specific therapy for superior limbic keratoconjunctivitis. In most cases tear secretion is normal and tear substitutes afford relief of neither signs nor symptoms. Only infrequently will corticosteroid instillation produce a degree of symptomatic relief. The effect is not generally long lasting, and corticosteroids are not particularly useful in the treatment of this entity. A hydrophilic contact lens may be helpful in providing symptomatic relief in cases with filaments on the corneal surface. Application of 0.5 per cent silver nitrate to the upper bulbar and tarsal conjunctiva (followed by irrigation with normal saline or balanced salt solution) is the most effective form of medical therapy. This can be repeated at intervals to treat acute exacerbations, and published reports indicate a sub-

stantial incidence of therapeutic success, though this approach has not been universally effective. Surgical recession of the bulbar conjunctiva adjacent to the upper limbus also is said to produce relief.[57, 58]

Allergy

In sensitized individuals the conjunctiva may become inflamed shortly after re-exposure to the offending allergen. The pollen of grasses and flowers is a common culprit. Typically the conjunctiva becomes swollen, chemotic, and hyperemic; the severity of these signs depends on the degree of hypersensitivity and the strength and amount of antigenic exposure. Varying degrees of itching and burning, photophobia, and lacrimation accompany the conjunctival inflammation. The conjunctival reaction is basically papillary in type, but in the less severe, more chronic cases, follicles may develop in the lower palpebral conjunctiva. Scrapings of the conjunctiva often show a predominance of eosinophils. The more severe cases of allergic conjunctivitis may be accompanied by corneal involvement, which takes the form of a diffuse, fine, punctate epithelial keratopathy. The epithelial lesions stain lightly with fluorescein. Allergic keratoconjunctivitis shows a varying degree of response to topically applied decongestants and antihistamines as well as to oral antihistamines. However,

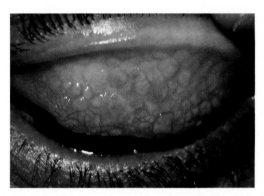

Figure 9–27. Vernal keratoconjunctivitis—tarsal form. Large cobblestone-like papillae on the upper tarsal conjunctiva.

topically administered corticosteroids produce a dramatic suppression of both signs and symptoms, and short-term instillation of a relatively weak preparation (e.g., prednisolone acetate 0.125 per cent) is our treatment of choice for the acute disabling phase of this disorder.

Vernal Keratoconjunctivitis

This entity is a chronic, recurrent, bilateral inflammation of the conjunctiva.[59, 60] Characteristically it produces large papillae resembling cobblestones on the upper tarsal conjunctiva (Fig. 9–27) and/or a gelatinous hypertrophy of the limbal conjunctiva (Fig. 9–28). The thickened limbal conjunctiva contains discrete gray nodules with vascular cores, which are papillae like the pal-

pebral lesions. A pannuslike infiltration of the peripheral cornea may occur, and chalky-white Horner-Trantas spots (Fig. 9–28) may appear within the raised, gelatinous limbal tissue. These signs tend to be associated with conjunctival hyperemia, intense itching, and profuse lacrimation. A relatively scanty, mucinous discharge may be present, and conjunctival scrapings generally contain a preponderance of eosinophils and/or many free eosinophilic granules.

The incidence and activity of vernal conjunctivitis have a striking relationship to a warm environment. The disorder occurs much more commonly in warm, humid areas; in temperate zones it tends to be active during the warm spring and summer months and relatively quiescent during the fall and winter. It is essentially a disease of youth and tends to resolve spontaneously after the age of 40. The preference of vernal conjunctivitis for the young, the seasonal nature of acute attacks, the demonstration of eosinophils in secretions and conjunctival scrapings, and the presence of an allergic history in many of those afflicted with the disorder all strongly suggest an allergic etiology. However, this has not been established with certainty, and vernal conjunctivitis remains a disease of unknown etiology.

A superficial punctate keratopathy is a frequent accompaniment of this disorder, particularly the palpebral form of the disease. Biomicroscopy reveals mul-

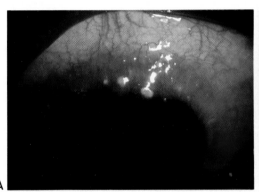
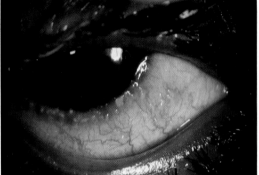

A   B

Figure 9–28. Vernal keratoconjunctivitis—limbal form. *A,* superior limbus, *B,* inferior limbus. The entire limbal circumference may be involved by a gelatinous hypertrophy of the limbal conjunctiva, a pannuslike infiltration of the peripheral cornea, and chalky-white Horner-Trantas spots.

tiple discrete gray spots in the epithelium. These tend to occur more frequently in the upper half of the cornea, but the entire cornea may be involved. Seemingly the spots are formed by degenerate epithelial cells, and punctate epithelial erosions also are encountered.

Topically applied corticosteroids are by far the most effective agent for the treatment of vernal keratoconjunctivitis and provide considerable relief to those affected by this disorder. Unfortunately, the chronic nature of the problem furnishes ideal circumstances in which to encounter the undesirable side effects of local corticosteroids (particularly glaucoma and cataracts). Aggressive corticosteroid instillation (e.g., prednisolone acetate 1.0 per cent every 2 hours while the patient is awake) usually can bring an acute attack under control within 48 hours. The medication then is rapidly tapered (both in terms of the frequency of instillation and the potency of the steroid), and it is discontinued as soon as possible. A therapeutic goal is to use as little corticosteroid as infrequently as possible. In temperate climates it is often possible to eliminate the drug during the fall and winter, and in less severe cases it may be possible to administer the corticosteroid only intermittently during warmer months when the disease becomes active.

We have had some limited success in reducing steroid dosage by the concomitant topical administration of nonsteroidal anti-inflammatory agents, but we have not been impressed by the efficacy of the latter as primary therapeutic agents in vernal keratoconjunctivitis. Unfortunately, ophthalmic nonsteroidal anti-inflammatory agents are not readily available. Contrary to reports in the literature, our experience with disodium cromoglycate has been disappointing. Instillation of astringents, decongestants, and antihistamines has not been useful except, perhaps, in very mild cases. If punctate epithelial erosions persist, topical antibiotics may be instilled prophylactically, although their efficacy in this situation has not been established. When antibiotics are used, we rotate the antibacterial agent every 4 to 6 weeks in the hope of preventing the evolution of a resistant organism.

Rosacea

Rosacea is a disorder of unknown etiology affecting the skin of the face, particularly the cheeks and nose. It is a chronic disease, initially characterized by intermittent vasodilatation, which ultimately persists with the formation of permanent telangiectasis. There is a disturbance in secretion of the sebaceous glands, so that along with the dermal erythema the involved area is characterized by papules and pustules. Persistent vascular stasis and low-grade inflammation stimulate a generalized hypertrophy. The skin becomes thickened and purplish in appearance, and in extreme cases a rhinophyma develops.

Ocular involvement, which occurs only in a small percentage of patients with rosacea, is commonly manifested as a relatively mild blepharoconjunctivitis. Less often a keratitis occurs, and this may have serious visual consequences. An episcleritis also has been reported, but this is rare. Most often the dermal lesions precede the appearance of ocular signs and symptoms, but ocular involvement may be the initial sign of the disorder, or alternatively the eyes and facial skin may be affected simultaneously. Moreover, the ocular lesions may progress or diminish independently of the dermal lesions. Ocular involvement tends to be bilateral, although one eye often is initially involved before the other.

Rosacea frequently is accompanied by hyperemia of the lid margin without a true blepharitis. However, this may progress in severity so that a scaly desquamation of the superficial layers of the skin occurs at the lid margins. Fortunately the blepharitis tends to remain relatively mild; although thickening of the lid margins is not uncommon, scarring, distortion of the lid margins or lashes, and trichiasis do not generally occur. Often the condition spreads and

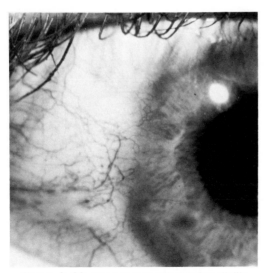

Figure 9–29. Rosacea keratoconjunctivitis.

involves the conjunctiva (Fig. 9–29). Both the bulbar and the palpebral conjunctiva become diffusely hyperemic and edematous. The patient complains of varying degrees of ocular irritation and photophobia, and there is a watery secretion, although typically it is not profuse. Dilated, engorged, conjunctival vessels characterize this disorder; they may appear as telangiectases or as true varicosities, and they are seen most often adjacent to the limbus in the interpalpebral area.

The blepharoconjunctivitis of rosacea predisposes to secondary bacterial infection, particularly by staphylococci, and to the formation of chalazia. The blepharoconjunctivitis may or may not be accompanied by corneal involvement. When it occurs, a rosacea keratitis is characterized initially by vascular invasion of the peripheral cornea. Presumably this is a direct extension of the conjunctivitis, with the dilated perilimbal vessels growing into the superficial lamellae of the adjacent stroma. At first neovascular ingrowth proceeds only about 1 mm. central to the limbus. It may involve the entire circumference but tends to be more prominent inferiorly. There may be an associated superficial punctate keratopathy, again with involvement tending to be more prominent inferiorly. Typically the epithelial lesions are coarse punctate erosions that

stain brightly with fluorescein. Small, gray, well-circumscribed subepithelial infiltrates, round or oval in shape, appear primarily in the lower half of the cornea. Their appearance may precede erosion of the overlying epithelium. The superficial keratopathy usually is bilateral, and, typically, quiescent periods of variable length are interspersed between acute attacks. The latter are characterized by considerable discomfort and visual disability. Continued progression of corneal involvement results in deeper stromal infiltration and ulceration, advancing neovascularization, scarring, and visual loss.[61, 62]

Local ocular therapy is at best only palliative and must be combined with treatment of the facial lesions. Corticosteroid and antibiotic drops are the primary agents used to treat rosacea blepharoconjunctivitis and keratitis, but therapeutic results are extremely variable. At times these drugs seem to ameliorate the disorder; topically applied corticosteroids in particular are apt to yield impressive short-term results. Equally often, however, topical therapy has no apparent effect at all on the course of the disease, especially on a long-term basis. Orally administered tetracycline is of considerable benefit in the control of the dermatitis, and the keratitis also has been observed to improve as a result of this treatment.[63, 64]

Reiter's Disease

Reiter's disease is a syndrome characterized primarily by urethritis, polyarthritis, and conjunctivitis. It is encountered most often in males between the ages of 20 and 40 but occurs in both sexes and in virtually all age groups. Although bacterial cultures and smears are negative, it is suggested that the disorder has an infectious etiology. *Chlamydia* has been incriminated as the causal agent, but this has not been documented with certainty, nor has it been established that the urethritis is of venereal origin, a factor that helps distinguish Reiter's disease from gonorrhea. This differentiation is of importance since gonococcal infection can also produce urethritis, polyarthritis, and conjunctivitis.

Typically there is a mild to moderate febrile response, and most often the urethritis is the presenting sign. It is uncommon for the major triad of signs to present simultaneously, but in most cases they evolve during an acute attack. The disease is characterized by exacerbations and remissions, each acute episode generally persisting for a period of months. Although in some instances the disorder may be self-limiting and not recur after the initial attack, it is a chronic problem in most cases with intermittent flareups for a period of years. Ultimately most cases clear spontaneously. The arthritis generally is polyarticular and tends to be the most persistent and disabling component of the disease. Most frequently the large or weight-bearing joints and the base of the spine are involved. The urethritis is quite variable in the symptomatology it produces. Though it is usually mild and relatively asymptomatic, it can at times be quite painful, particularly in the male. Mucous membranes other than the conjunctiva and those of the genitalia are affected much less often and less severely, but involvement of the mucous membranes of the mouth and intestine have been described. Cutaneous lesions tend to appear late, are characteristically hyperkeratotic, and have a preference for the hands, feet, face, and penis.

The conjunctivitis generally is mild and clears after varying periods without scarring or other permanent sequelae. Characteristically it is a bilateral, nonspecific, smooth, hyperemic infiltration of the mucosa accompanied by a mucopurulent exudate. A superficial keratitis may develop subsequent to the appearance of the conjunctivitis. Most commonly this is characterized by superficial erosions of the epithelium that tend to be most dense in the inferior corneal periphery. In addition, microcystic epithelial edema and punctate infiltrates at or beneath Bowman's membrane have been described. In a considerable number of cases ocular involvement is manifested as an iridocyclitis, which seems to occur independently of the conjunctivitis. Generally it is nongranulomatous, is not associated with a hypopyon, and tends to be transient but recurrent.[65, 66]

Fortunately, from an ophthalmologic standpoint, the disease is relatively benign and tends to be self-limited. In the more severe and persistent cases of anterior uveitis secondary glaucoma may occur, but few other serious ocular sequelae are encountered. The anterior uveitis generally responds to treatment with topical corticosteroids, and mydriatic-cycloplegic agents prevent the formation of posterior synechiae. However, these agents do not appear to alter the course of the keratoconjunctivitis favorably. Treatment with oral tetracyclines has been recommended,[65] but even in patients with a documented chlamydial infection this does not appear to abort the acute attack or reduce the incidence of recurrence.

CLINICAL APPROACH TO THE PATIENT

The existence of superficial punctate keratopathy generally becomes evident during biomicroscopic examination of the cornea. Nonetheless, a comprehensive ocular examination should be completed to uncover any contributory findings and to document the presence or absence of any coexisting (but not necessarily related) abnormalities. A methodical evaluation of the superficial punctate keratopathy, designed to establish its etiology, then is in order. We have found the following approach to be helpful.

Note the distribution of the epithelial lesions. Although several authors have stressed the importance of their location in establishing an etiology, we believe that this point has been overemphasized. Exceptions to the classic patterns will be encountered with great frequency, particularly if the patient has received topical medications prior to evaluation. Nonetheless, the presentation of epithelial lesions in a characteristic pattern represents an important diagnostic finding. Typically the punctate lesions are diffusely and randomly spattered over the entire corneal surface in the early stages of bacterial and viral conjunctivitis and in keratitis medicamentosa. The inferior corneal periphery (approximately the lower third) is characteristically involved in staphylococcal blepharitis, trichiasis, and inclusion conjunctivitis. In contrast, the epithelial lesions of superior limbic keratoconjunctivitis and vernal keratoconjunctivitis involve the superior corneal periphery. Marginal infiltration or ulceration of the cornea accompanied by punctate staining is suggestive of a staphylococcal infection. Distribution of the epithelial lesions in a band across the interpalpebral portion of the cornea classically occurs in keratoconjunctivitis sicca, in exposure keratopathy due to inadequate blinking, and following exposure to ultraviolet radiation. Thygeson's superficial punctate keratitis characteristically involves the central half of the cornea, whereas the lesions caused by adenovirus infection in epidemic keratoconjunctivitis typically occur in the corneal center and midperiphery but not in the extreme periphery adjacent to the limbus. The punctate lesions of herpes zoster, vaccinia, varicella, and Reiter's syndrome classically are said to have an irregular pattern but are characterized by the involvement of the extreme corneal periphery as well as the central and paracentral cornea. The typical patterns of distribution of epithelial lesions in superficial punctate keratopathy are presented in Table 9–2. Again we stress that exceptions seem to occur as commonly as the typical patterns.

Diagnostic importance also has been attributed to the morphologic configuration of punctate epithelial lesions. With few exceptions, however, we have not been able to arrive confidently at a specific diagnosis based solely or even largely on the appearance of the lesion. Again, this is particularly true if topical medications have been administered before we have had an opportunity to assess the patient. At times, though, the appearance of the epithelial abnormalities in conjunction with the history and/or the ancillary findings does permit one to reach a diagnosis with assurance. Examples include a coarse or areolar punctate epithelial keratopathy in the absence of conjunctival hyperemia in Thygeson's superficial punctate keratitis, a persistent punctate subepithelial keratitis in the face of healing of the epithelial component in adenovirus infection, and the punctate epithelial erosions and epithelial filaments accompanied by a scanty marginal tear strip in keratoconjunctivitis sicca. However, we must stress that various types of lesions can occur in combination in a number of these entities, that their morphologic configurations are affected to a great degree by topical application of all medications, that exceptions to these characteristic appearances are quite prevalent, and that the appearance of individual punctate epithelial lesions generally does not aid us in establishing a specific diagnosis.

After careful evaluation of the corneal changes has been completed, it is incumbent upon the examiner to review the history with specific reference to the differential diagnosis of superficial punctate keratopathy. Specific inquiry should be made about a number of points. Does the patient suffer from arthritis, suggestive of lacrimal insufficiency? Is there a history of skin disease—rosacea, erythema multiforme, Stevens-Johnson syndrome—that might suggest a cause? Has the patient experienced a discharge from the genitourinary tract, implicating a chlamydial infection, Reiter's syndrome, or perhaps even a Neisseria organism? Has the patient been exposed to ultraviolet light or noxious chemicals?

Re-examination of the lids is the next logical step. Is there a nodular lesion consistent with molluscum contagiosum or a verruca at the lid margin? Are there vesicles consistent with herpes zoster, herpes simplex, or other acute viral infection? Are there signs suggestive of infection by staphylococci or other bacteria—e.g., inflammatory collarettes at the orifices of the lash follicles, meibo-

Table 9–2. SUGGESTIVE ETIOLOGIC SIGNIFICANCE OF FINDINGS ASSOCIATED WITH SUPERFICIAL PUNCTATE KERATOPATHY

Location of Corneal Lesions

1. Diffuse, random
   bacterial conjunctivitis
   viral conjunctivitis
   keratitis medicamentosa
   contact lens–induced
     punctate keratopathy
   neurotrophic keratitis
   allergic keratoconjunctivitis

2. Central (interpalpebral area)
   keratoconjunctivitis sicca
   exposure keratopathy
   radiation keratopathy (ultraviolet)
   Thygeson's superficial punctate keratitis
   adenoviral keratitis

3. Superior
   superior limbic keratoconjunctivitis
   vernal keratoconjunctivitis
   trachoma
   molluscum contagiosum

4. Inferior
   staphylococcal blepharitis
   inclusion conjunctivitis
   entropion, trichiasis—lower lid
   keratoconjunctivitis sicca
   nocturnal lagophthalmos
   exposure keratopathy
   rosacea keratitis
   Reiter's disease

Lid Disorders

1. Vesicles
   herpes simplex
   herpes zoster
   vaccinia
   pemphigoid

2. Solid tumors
   molluscum contagiosum
   verruca

3. Marginal blepharitis
   bacterial infection
   rosacea

4. Dermatitis
   psoriasis
   rosacea

Conjunctival Inflammatory Response

1. Nonspecific response
   bacterial infection
   viral infection (including recurrent herpes simplex)
   Reiter's disease
   herpes zoster
   allergy

2. Follicular response
   primary herpes simplex infection
   adenovirus infection
   chlamydial infection
   molluscum contagiosum

3. Papillary response
   vernal keratoconjunctivitis
   keratoconjunctivitis sicca

4. Conjunctival scarring
   trachoma
   mucocutaneous syndromes

5. None
   Thygeson's superficial punctate keratitis

Other

1. Regional lymphadenopathy
   adenovirus infection
   primary herpes simplex infection
   herpes zoster
   chlamydial infection
   vaccinia infection

2. Peripheral corneal neovascularization
   chlamydial infection
   rosacea
   molluscum contagiosum
   verruca
   mucocutaneous syndromes
   vernal keratoconjunctivitis
   keratoconjunctivitis sicca

3. Skin disease
   rosacea
   mucocutaneous syndromes (pemphigoid, erythema multiforme, Stevens-Johnson syndrome)
   psoriasis
   follicular hyperkeratosis of palms and soles

4. Arthropathy
   keratoconjunctivitis sicca
   Reiter's disease
   psoriasis

mian hypersecretion, ulcerative blepharitis, or evidence of previous hordeola? Are there scales adherent to the lashes, suggesting seborrhea? Is the lacrimal punctum dilated and congested so that an actinomycetic or a chronic bacterial infection must be considered? Is entropion or trichiasis present, indicating a traumatic origin for the superficial punctate keratopathy? Is the lid ectropic, contributing to an exposure keratopathy?

One then proceeds to re-evaluate the conjunctiva. A follicular conjunctivitis suggests a viral etiology (particularly adenovirus, herpes simplex, or herpes zoster) or a chlamydial infection (either trachoma or inclusion conjunctivitis). A papillary conjunctivitis is more apt to occur as a result of tear insufficiency, whereas giant papillae most commonly indicate vernal keratoconjunctivitis. If a patient with conjunctival papillae wears contact lenses, the lens must be considered among the etiologic possibilities.[67] Conjunctival inflammation characterized primarily by diffuse hyperemia and chemosis is consistent with a bacterial or viral etiology and with Reiter's syndrome. Conjunctival scarring suggests the more severe mucocutaneous disorders (Stevens-Johnson syndrome, benign mucous membrane pemphigoid, etc.) or trachoma.

The type of discharge accompanying the conjunctival inflammation may be an additional helpful point in establishing the diagnosis. A purulent or mucopurulent discharge often is observed in the more severe bacterial infections, in the acute phase of severe chlamydial infections, in vernal conjunctivitis, and in severe cases of Reiter's syndrome. A mucoid discharge is most suggestive of dry eyes, whereas a serous discharge occurs in less severe bacterial and chlamydial infections and in most virus infections of the conjunctiva. Reflux from the punctum upon application of pressure over the nasolacrimal sac indicates a bacterial etiology.

Finally, the ophthalmologist must be aware of and search for associated signs that may contribute to a specific diagnosis. Is there an endocrine dysfunction, which may produce exophthalmos, lid retraction, inadequate blinking, etc., and cause an exposure keratopathy? Are skin lesions evident, suggesting a keratopathy associated with rosacea or psoriasis? Does palpation reveal the presence of preauricular or submandibular lymph nodes, suggesting a viral etiology or the acute stages of a chlamydial infection? Are there changes at the limbus consistent with vernal conjunctivitis, trachoma, or superior limbic keratopathy?

For the sake of completeness, Table 9–2 lists the findings accompanying a superficial punctate keratopathy that classically are indicative of a specific etiology. The table largely reflects the observations of Jones,[1, 2] to whom credit must be given for whatever semblance of order has been brought to this very confusing clinical problem. Nonetheless, it is evident that a wide range of pathologic processes can cause a superficial punctate keratopathy and that a given etiologic agent can manifest itself in a variety of patterns. Conversely, a single type of superficial corneal lesion can be produced by multiple agents. Clearly, the lesions of superficial punctate keratopathy are more often than not nonspecific. Often it is only by analyzing several factors—the location and morphology of the corneal lesions, the state of the lids and conjunctiva, the presence of medical or dermatologic problems, etc.—that the ophthalmologist can arrive at even a provisional clinical diagnosis. A more definitive diagnosis generally depends on confirmatory laboratory findings, the evolution of the disease with time, and/or its response to therapy.

REFERENCES

1. Jones, B. R.: The differential diagnosis of superficial keratitis. Trans Ophthalmol Soc UK 80:665, 1960.
2. Jones, B. R.: Differential diagnosis of punctate keratitis. Int Ophthalmol Clin 2:591, 1962.
3. Leibowitz, H. M., and Cagle, G. D.: Bacterial conjunctivitis: Geographic variations (abstract). Invest. Ophthalmol Vis Sci 18 (ARVO Suppl):133, 1979.
4. Thygeson, P.: Complications of staphylococcal blepharitis. Amer J Ophthalmol 68:446, 1969.
5. Chignell, A. H., Easty, D. L., Chesterton, J. R., and Thomasitt, J.: Marginal ulceration of the cornea. Brit J Ophthalmol 54:433, 1970.
6. Leibowitz, H. M. and Kupferman, A.: The effect of topically administered corticosteroids on antibiotic-treated bacterial keratitis. Arch Ophthalmol 98:1287, 1980.
7. Leibowitz, H. M., Pratt, M. V., Flagstad, I. J., Berrospi, A. R., and Kundsin, R.: Human conjunctivitis. II. Treatment. Arch Ophthalmol 94:1752, 1976.
8. Editorial: Adenovirus keratoconjunctivitis. Brit J Ophthalmol 61:73, 1977.
9. Dawson, C. R., Hanna, L., Wood, T. R., and Despain, R.: Adenovirus type 8 keratoconjunctivitis in the United States. III. Epidemiologic, clinical and microbiologic features. Amer J Ophthalmol 69:473, 1970.

10. O'Day, D. M., Guyer, B., Hierholzer, J. C., Rosing, K. J., and Schaffner, W.: Clinical and laboratory evaluation of epidemic keratoconjunctivitis due to adenovirus types 8 and 19. Amer J Ophthalmol 81:207, 1976.

11. Darougar, S., Quinlan, M. P., Gibson, J. A., and Jones, B. R.: Epidemic keratoconjunctivitis and chronic papillary conjunctivitis in London due to adenovirus type 19. Brit J Ophthalmol 61:76, 1977.

12. Laibson, P. R., Dhiri, S., Oconer, J., and Ortolan, G.: Corneal infiltrates in epidemic keratoconjunctivitis. Response to double-blind corticosteroid therapy. Arch Ophthalmol 84:36, 1970.

13. O'Day, D. M., and Jones, B. M.: Herpes simplex keratitis. In Duane, T. M. (ed.): Clinical Ophthalmology. Vol. 4. Hagerstown, Md., Harper & Row, 1978.

14. Binder, P.: Herpes simplex keratitis. Surv Ophthalmol 21:313, 1977.

15. Garland, J.: Varicella following exposure to herpes zoster. N Engl J Med 228:336, 1943.

16. Hope-Simpson, R. E.; The nature of herpes zoster. A long term study and a new hypothesis. Proc R Soc Med 58:9, 1965.

17. Esiri, M. M., and Tomlinson, A. H.: Demonstration of virus in the trigeminal nerve and ganglion by immunofluorescence and electron microscopy. J Neurol Sci 15:35, 1972.

18. Pavan-Langston, D., and McCulley, J. P.: Herpes zoster dendritic keratitis. Arch Ophthalmol 89:25, 1973.

19. Piebenga, L. W., and Laibson, P. R.: Dendritic lesions in herpes zoster ophthalmicus. Arch Ophthalmol 90:268, 1973.

20. Pavan-Langston, D.: Varicella-zoster ophthalmicus. Int Ophthalmol Clin 15:171, 1975.

21. Thygeson, P.: Observations on conjunctival neoplasms masquerading as chronic conjunctivitis or keratitis. Trans Amer Acad Ophthalmol Otolaryngol 73:969, 1969.

22. Quill, T. H.: Molluscum contagiosum of eyelid and cornea. Report of a case. Proc Staff Meet Mayo Clin 15:139, 1940.

23. Ellis, P. P., and Winograd, L. A.: Ocular vaccinia. Arch Ophthalmol 68:600, 1962.

24. Petit, T. H.: The poxviruses: Vaccinia and variola. Int Ophthalmol Clin 15:203, 1975.

25. Taylor, H. R., and Turner, A. J.: A case report of fowl plague keratoconjunctivitis. Brit J Ophthalmol 61:86, 1977.

26. Jones, B. R.: Epidemic hemorrhagic conjunctivitis in London 1971: A conjunctival picornavirus infection. Trans Ophthalmol Soc UK 92:625, 1972.

27. Sklar, V. E. F., Patriarca, P. A., Onorato, I. M., Langford, M. P., Clark, S. W., Culbertson, W. W., and Forster, R. K.: Clinical findings and results of treatment in an outbreak of acute hemorrhagic conjunctivitis in southern Florida. Am J Ophthalmol 95:45, 1983.

28. Thygeson, P.: Ocular viral diseases. Med Clin N Amer 43:149, 1959.

29. Florman, A. L., and Agatston, H. J.: Keratoconjunctivitis as a diagnostic aid in measles. JAMA 179:568, 1962.

30. Smolin, G.: Report of a case of rubella keratitis. Amer J Ophthalmol 74:436, 1972.

31. Frederique, G., Howard, R. O., and Boniuk, V.: Corneal ulcers in rubeola. Amer J Ophthalmol 68:996, 1969.

32. Jones, B. R.: Trachoma and allied infections. Trans Ophthalmol Soc UK 81:367, 1961.

33. Schachter, J., and Dawson, C. R.: Human chlamydial infections. Littleton, Mass., PSG Publishing Co., Inc., 1978, pp. 63–120.

34. Duke-Elder, S., and MacFaul, P. A.: System of Ophthalmology. Vol. 14, Injuries. St. Louis, C. V. Mosby Co., 1972.

35. Grant, W. M.: Toxicology of the eye. Springfield, Ill., Charles C Thomas, 1974.

36. MacLean, A. L.: Spray keratitis. A common epithelial keratitis from noncorrosive household sprays. Trans Amer Acad Ophthalmol Otolaryngol 71:330, 1967.

37. Henkes, H. E., and Waublee, T. N.: Keratitis from the abuse of corneal anesthetics. Brit J Ophthalmol 62:62, 1978.

38. Leibowitz, H. M., and Peacock, G. R.: Corneal injury produced by carbon dioxide laser radiation. Arch Ophthalmol 81:713, 1969.

39. Duke-Elder, S., and MacFaul, P. A.: System of Ophthalmology. Vol. 14, Injuries. Part 2, Non-Mechanical Injuries. St. Louis, C. V. Mosby Co., 1972, pp. 918–925.

40. Brown, S. I.: Further observation on the pathophysiology of keratitis sicca of Rollet. Arch Ophthalmol 83:542, 1970.

41. Brown, S. I.: Dry spots and corneal erosions. Int Ophthalmol Clin 13:149, 1973.

42. Katz, J., and Kaufman, H. E.: Corneal exposure during sleep (nocturnal lagophthalmos). Arch Ophthalmol 95:449, 1977.

43. Sturrock, G. D.: Nocturnal lagophthalmos and recurrent erosion. Brit J Ophthalmol 60:97, 1976.

44. Magendie, F.: De l'Influence de la cinquieme paire de nerfs sur la nutrition et les fonctions de l'oeil. J Physiol (Paris) 4:176, 1824.

45. Duke-Elder, S., and Leigh, A. G.: System of Ophthalmology. Vol. 8, Diseases of the Outer Eye. Part 2. St. Louis, C. V. Mosby Co., 1965, pp. 803–810.

46. Braley, A. E., and Alexander, R. C.: Superficial punctate keratitis. Isolation of a virus. Arch Ophthalmol 50:147, 1953.

47. Lemp, M. A., Chambers, R. W., and Lundy, J.: Viral isolate in superficial punctate keratitis. Arch Ophthalmol 91:8, 1974.

48. Thygeson, P.: Superficial punctate keratitis. JAMA 144:1544, 1950.

49. Thygeson, P.: Further observations on superficial punctate keratitis. Arch Ophthalmol 65:158, 1961.

50. Thygeson, P.: Clinical and laboratory observations on superficial punctate keratitis. Amer J Ophthalmol 61:1345, 1966.

51. Jones, B. R.: Thygeson's superficial punctate keratitis. Trans Ophthalmol Soc UK 83:245, 1963.

52. Abbott, R. L., and Forster, R. K.: Superficial punctate keratitis of Thygeson associated with scarring and Salzmann's nodular degeneration. Amer J Ophthalmol 87:296, 1979.

53. Theodore, F. H.: Superior limbic keratoconjunctivitis. Eye Ear Nose Throat Monthly 42:25, 1963.

54. Theodore, F. H.: Further observations on superior limbic keratoconjunctivitis. Trans Amer Acad Ophthalmol Otolaryngol 71:341, 1967.

55. Corwin, M. E.: Superior limbic keratoconjunctivitis. Amer J Ophthalmol 66:338, 1968.

56. Cher, I.: Clinical features of superior limbic keratoconjunctivitis in Australia: A probable association with thyrotoxicosis. Arch Ophthalmol 82:580, 1969.

57. Donshik, P. C., Collin, H. B., Foster, C. S., Cavanaugh, H. D., and Boruchoff, S. A.: Conjunctival resection, treatment and ultrastructural histopath-

ology of superior limbic keratoconjunctivitis. Amer J Ophthalmol 85:101, 1978.

58. Tenzel, R. R.: Resistant superior limbic keratoconjunctivitis. Arch Ophthalmol 89:439, 1973.

59. Neumann, E., Gutman, M. J., Blumenkrantz, J., and Michaelson, I. C.: A review of 400 cases of vernal conjunctivitis. Amer J Ophthalmol 47:166, 1959.

60. Duke-Elder, S., and Leigh, A. G.: System of Ophthalmology. Vol. 8, Diseases of the Outer Eye. Part 2. St. Louis, C. V. Mosby Co., 1965, pp. 475–493.

61. Goldsmith, A. J. B.: The ocular manifestations of rosacea. Brit J Dermatol 65:448, 1953.

62. Borrie, P.: Rosacea with special reference to its ocular manifestations. Brit J Dermatol 65:458, 1953.

63. Jenkins, M. S., Brown, S. I., Lempert, S. L., and Weinberg, R. J.: Ocular rosacea. Amer J Ophthalmol 88:618, 1979.

64. Bartholomew, R. S., Reid, B. J., Cheesbrough, M. J., MacDonald, M., and Galloway, N. R.: Oxytetracycline in the treatment of ocular rosacea: A double-blind trial. Brit J Ophthalmol 66:386, 1982.

65. Ostler, H. B., Dawson, C. R., Schachter, J., and Engleman, E. P.: Reiter's syndrome. Amer J Ophthalmol 71:986, 1971.

66. Mills, R. P., and Kalina, R. E.: Reiter's keratitis. Arch Ophthalmol 87:447, 1972.

67. Allansmith, M. R., Korb, D. R., Greiner, J. V., Henriquez, A. S., Simon, M. A., and Finnemore, V. M.: Giant papillary conjunctivitis in contact lens wearers. Amer J Ophthalmol 83:697, 1977.

VI

INFLAMMATION OF THE CORNEA

Inflammation of the Cornea: Basic Principles

10

HOWARD M. LEIBOWITZ, M.D.

Inflammation is a protective response of tissues to injury, designed to destroy, dilute, eliminate, or wall off the injurious agent. It can be induced by a great number of offending agents. Irrespective of the cause, however, inflammation is essentially an expression of tissue damage through a final common pathway. The inflammatory reaction is a dynamic process, involving an interaction between the offending stimulus and the host that ultimately ends with a reparative or healing phase. Classically, inflammation is described in terms of five clinical signs: *redness* and *heat* due to an increase in the rate and volume of blood flow, an *increase in tissue mass* due to exudation of fluid and cell migration into the injured area, *pain*, and *loss of function*.

Any agent that can initiate or perpetuate an inflammatory response qualifies as an inflammatory stimulus. Inflammatory stimuli can be divided into toxic agents, which generally produce an inflammatory response in a host without previous exposure to that host, and immune agents, which generally require a history of prior exposure if they are to incite inflammation. Toxic inflammatory stimuli are classified as necrotizing if they possess inherent properties that can destroy host tissue (usually by destroying the cell membrane or interfering with intracellular metabolism, with resultant cell lysis), or nonnecrotizing if they alter structural integrity indirectly through intermediary pathways that activate inflammatory cells. Regardless of the type of stimulus or the pathway

through which it acts, the severity of the inflammatory reaction is mediated by the potency, quantity, and duration of the stimulus.

The normal host response is composed of a complicated series of physiologic and morphologic defense mechanisms aimed at interrupting, neutralizing, and eliminating the inflammatory stimulus and at repairing the injured structures. The acute phase of inflammation seems to be related to or initiated by histamine release from basophils (mast cells) and maintained by kinins and other chemical mediators. These chemical mediators (histamine, serotonin, kinins, plasmin, complement, prostaglandins, and leukotrienes) cause smooth muscle contraction (arteriolar constriction) and a local increase in vascular permeability. The latter results from an "opening" of the usually "tight" junctions between adjacent endothelial cells of blood vessels, allowing fluid to leak into the surrounding tissue spaces and leukocytes to actively force themselves between the vascular endothelial cells.

Toxic necrotizing agents tend to be neutralized by the intrinsic chemical structure of the surrounding tissue. Nonnecrotizing toxic agents appear to combine with immune globulins, and this results in neutralization of their toxic properties. Immune stimuli are neutralized by antibody. Clinically, both cellular and humoral components probably participate in most situations to neutralize an antigenic stimulus. A number of secondary reactions, designed to eliminate the neutralized toxic or immune stimulus, then occur. The polymorphonuclear leukocyte acts rapidly to eliminate inflammatory stimuli, whereas the macrophage responds more slowly, removing particulate debris that has accumulated during the inflammatory reaction.

The principal mechanism for the initial type of response is the so-called acute inflammatory pathway (or complement-binding pathway), characterized by chemotaxis and degranulation of the polymorphonuclear leukocyte. Virtually all reactants that bind complement can activate this system. The complex resulting from complement binding becomes chemotactic for the polymorphonuclear leukocyte, causing large numbers of these cells to invade the inflammatory site, where they phagocytize the inciting particles. During phagocytosis of these particles degranulation of the lysosomes in the cytoplasms of the polymorphonuclear leukocytes occurs. The relatively high concentrations of the hydrolytic enzymes (collagenase, elastase, cathepsins, etc.) contained in lysosomes degrade the complex into a form that facilitates phagocytosis. These enzymes are released from degenerating polymorphonuclear leukocytes, and their reaction with the surrounding host tissues results in damage to the tissues.

The pathway resulting in the stimulation of macrophages is less clearly defined. In contrast to the polymorphonuclear leukocyte, the macrophage ingests the stimulating particle, producing minimal secondary parenchymal tissue damage. Structural damage is caused by the destructive effects of the primary reaction on tissue. Some degree of macrophage response occurs following acute inflammation. If the acute inflammatory reaction is mild, the macrophage elimination phase is short-lived. If the reaction is severe, the macrophage elimination phase is protracted. Elimination of "foreign particles" must occur before repair can ensue.

Regeneration and/or repair is the final stage in the host response to an inflammatory stimulus. If regeneration occurs, the injured tissue is replaced by identical, functionally equivalent tissue. When inflammation is limited to the conjunctival or corneal epithelium, regeneration takes place. Repair, on the other hand, replaces the injured tissue with fibrous tissue. A collagen scar, frequently interspersed with blood vessels and an occasional fibrocyte, satisfactorily reconstitutes the structure of the eye but often leaves it with a functional deficiency.

Thus, inflammation often produces scarring and scarring results in structural and functional change of normal host tissues. The duration and severity of the inflammatory reaction determine the degree of structural alteration. When normal structural components are destroyed and are replaced by fibrous tissue and newly formed blood vessels, varying degrees of loss in the normal activity of the tissue occurs. This predisposes the site to recurrent inflammatory episodes, often of progressive severity, or to chronically active inflammatory disease, presumably by facilitating an unduly severe host response to almost any inflammatory stimulus. Structural change has been measured as an increased permeability of ocular vasculature. This enables the involved eye to concentrate inflammatory elements and facilitates the inflammatory reaction. Increased quantities of gamma globulin (antibody) accumulate in the ocular extravascular space to combine with a toxic or immune stimulus. The quantity of stimulus required to produce an inflammatory response in this situation is appreciably less than would be required in normal intact ocular structure.

INFLAMMATION OF THE CONJUNCTIVA

Inflammatory processes in the cornea generally also involve the adjacent conjunctiva. Conversely, conjunctival inflammation, particularly when it is caused by a replicating agent, may progress to involve the cornea. Hence, a discussion of inflammation of the conjunctiva seems appropriate here. The

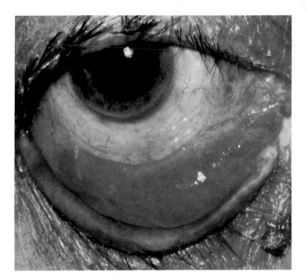

Figure 10–1. Chemosis of the conjunctiva.

essential feature of conjunctival inflammation (conjunctivitis or ophthalmia) is a red eye, visible evidence of dilatation of the conjunctival blood vessels and the resultant hyperemia of the tissue. Edema occurs to varying degrees whenever the conjunctiva is inflamed and hyperemic. There is a transudation of fluid, rich in protein and fibrin, through the walls of the altered conjunctival blood vessels, producing a translucent swelling of the membrane. This causes enlargement of papillae in the tightly adherent tarsal conjunctiva and the formation of redundant folds in the region of the fornices. In the bulbar conjunctiva, where attachment to the underlying globe is lax, large quantities of this serum transudate may accumulate and cause the conjunctiva to balloon away from the globe, a condition referred to as chemosis (Fig. 10–1). In its most pronounced forms the chemotic bulbar conjunctiva bulges over the peripheral cornea and may protrude through the closed lids. There is also an exudation of cellular elements from the blood of the dilated conjunctival vessels. The exudate filters through the conjunctival epithelium, where, along with the tears and secretions of the conjunctival glands, it forms a discharge (Fig. 10–2).

Morphologically the conjunctiva, like all other mucous membranes, consists of two layers, the epithelium and the underlying substantia propria. The epithelium always participates in the in-

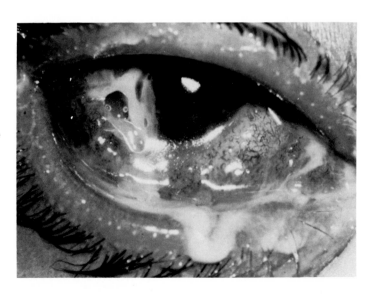

Figure 10–2. Conjunctival discharge.

flammatory process. It becomes edematous, and in many instances hyperplasia occurs. Epithelial cells degenerate, and ultimately desquamation results. In the less severe forms of inflammation, regenerating epithelial cells balance out those that are being shed. Rarely, inflammation may be sufficiently intense to cause conjunctival necrosis with exfoliation of the epithelium.

In the more chronic forms of inflammation there is an increase in the mucus-secreting goblet cells contained within the conjunctival epithelium. There is also a tendency of the epithelium itself to proliferate downward, particularly in the palpebral conjunctiva and adjacent to the limbus. This phenomenon occurs most prominently in those areas where the exudate in the subconjunctival tissue forces the epithelium into papilliform elevations. This active epithelial proliferation is characterized by downward-growing rods of branching cells. These tubular epithelial downgrowths retain a basement membrane and do not invade the adenoid layer of the substantia propria. Canalization frequently results because of necrosis of the central cells, forming gland-like structures whose orifices may become blocked by epithelial debris. Pseudoretention cysts filled with serous, fibrinous, epithelial, and leukocytic debris and mucus are formed largely in the palpebral conjunctiva in this manner (Fig. 10–3). Some may undergo calcareous degeneration and form concretions. If chronic inflammatory changes occur in an exposed area and the conjunctiva is allowed to become dry (as in ectropion of the lid), keratinization of the epithelium occurs. The conjunctival epithelium assumes all the characteristics of skin except for the absence of glands and hair follicles and the occasional presence of mucous cells.

The substantia propria of the conjunctiva consists of two portions, a superficial adenoid layer and a deeper fibrous layer. The adenoid layer consists of a fine connective-tissue reticulum, in the meshes of which lymphocytes lie. Although nodules of lymphocytes are

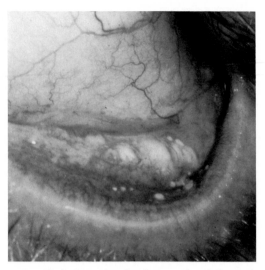

Figure 10–3. Pseudoretention cysts of the conjunctiva.

found in the human conjunctiva, they do not form true follicles. The fibrous layer is generally thicker than the adenoid but is almost nonexistent over the tarsus, with which it is continuous. Actually this layer belongs to the subconjunctival connective tissue rather than to the conjunctiva. The most characteristic feature of inflammation in the substantia propria is the exudation into the tissues. The tarsal and orbital conjunctiva become rough and velvety with exaggerated folds and furrows, which may develop into papilliform structures. In the fornices large folds appear, but the bulbar conjunctiva remains relatively smooth (Fig. 10–4).

The inflammatory cells are derived from two sources. In the acute stage polymorphonuclear leukocytes originate from the blood, and, if the vascular endothelium is sufficiently damaged, erythrocytes escape by diapedesis. Lymphocytes of vascular origin subsequently appear in the subacute stage. In addition, there is a marked increase in lymphocytes in the adenoid layer that originate from the conjunctival tissues themselves. Later, in the more chronic types of conjunctivitis plasma cells are seen, then histiocytes, and finally fibroblasts. As a rule these changes occur diffusely throughout the conjunctival tissue, but occasionally they may be lo-

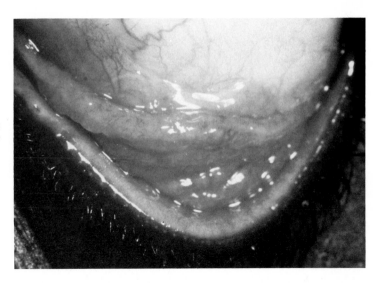

Figure 10–4. Large folds in the inflamed conjunctiva of the lower fornix.

calized. The phlyctenule is an example of the latter (Fig. 10–5). This lesion is characterized by a localized, intense hyperemia and initially an exudation of leukocytes in the center of which necrotic changes take place, to be succeeded by mononuclear cells and plasma cells. Finally, the necrotic infiltrate may break through the epithelium, forming an ulcer, or, alternatively, it may resolve. A true abscess of the conjunctiva is rare, since the delicacy of the epithelium usually leads to the extrusion of a localized inflammatory exudate in its earlier stage. Healing is very effective, and in the absence of extensive ulceration cicatrization rarely occurs.

In addition to edema and hyperemia, the follicle and the papilla are two important signs of inflammation in the palpebral conjunctiva. Follicles represent miniature lymph nodes and are composed of lymphocytes, macrophages, and plasma cells distributed within the adventitial layers of conjunctiva (Fig. 10–6). Conjunctival lymphoid tissue develops during the first few months of life. Its rate of development depends on the degree of irritative stimulus to which the conjunctiva is exposed. True lymphatic follicles are not present in the normal conjunctiva. However, after prolonged irritation of any kind the lymphocytes, which ordinarily crowd the adenoid layer, indiscriminately increase and tend to aggregate into follicles. These resemble lymph nodes or the solitary lymphatic patches found in the

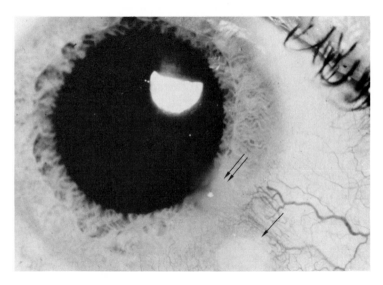

Figure 10–5. Conjunctival (single arrow) and corneal (double arrows) phlyctenules.

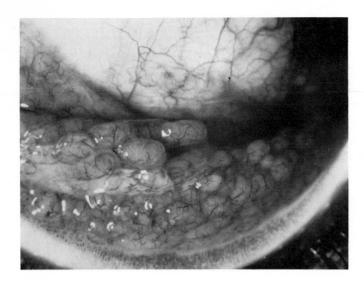

Figure 10–6. Conjunctival follicles.

intestine both in structure and in function. The conjunctival follicle, then, is a tissue reaction to irritation. Histologically, there is no significant difference among the follicles caused by an identifiable irritant (e.g. atropine), those due to an unknown agent (e.g. folliculosis), and those noted in an acute infectious follicular conjunctivitis or early trachoma.

The follicle itself is a dense, localized infiltration of the subepithelial tissues by large lymphocytes with feebly staining nuclei arranged in a central mass. The periphery of the structure is occupied by a dark ring of small, deeply staining lymphocytes, frequently forming secondary nodules. A third characteristic cell type, present in smaller numbers in the interior of the follicle, has been described. It is a very large cell with irregularly shaped, vacuolized cytoplasm capable of phagocytosis. These so-called Leber cells are particularly evident in trachomatous follicles but are not specific for that entity. Plasma cells are rare within follicles but may be common in surrounding tissue. Few polymorphonuclear neutrophils are observed, but mast cells (basophils) may be present in the periphery of the follicle. The whole structure of the follicle is supported by an ill-defined reticulum that becomes more marked at the periphery. Often there is a ring of elongated cells here and the reticulum binds

with the connective tissue fibers of the submucous tissue. There is no true capsule in the early follicle, but in more chronic inflammation (e.g., the later stages of trachoma) dense connective tissue formation precedes cicatricial changes. Enlarged lymphatics are generally found in proximity to the follicle. Even small follicles seem to be nourished by lymph, though true lymphatic spaces with an endothelial lining usually cannot be seen within them.

Follicle size is related to the severity and duration of the inflammatory stimulus. They occur often in the inferior palpebral conjunctiva and in the inferior fornix. Clinically the follicle is discrete and round, varying from approximately 0.5 mm. to 5 mm. in diameter, and is elevated above the smooth conjunctival surface. Its most salient diagnostic feature is its vascular pattern. While blood vessels generally are absent in young follicles, a rich vascular network eventually grows around them from thin-walled endothelium-lined capillaries. These disappear toward the center of the follicle. Therefore, on examination the follicle presents as a discrete mound of cells encircled by a ring of blood vessels. As the number of cellular components increases, the follicle increases in diameter and the blood vessels are displaced peripherally, eventually appearing as a vascular capsule enclosing the base of the follicle.

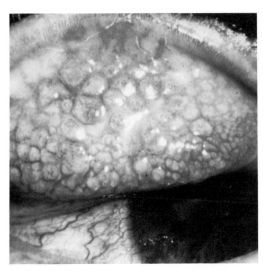

Figure 10-7. Conjunctival papillae.

dermal collagenous tissue, restricting its size and accounting for its polygonal outline. In prolonged inflammation the normal anchoring septa are disrupted mechanically, leading either to papillary confluence, as in bacterial infections, or giant papillae, as in vernal conjunctivitis (Fig. 10–8). The latter phenomenon usually is most highly developed in the richly vascularized area at the proximal border of the tarsal plate.

It is therefore important to differentiate between follicular and papillary reaction. Follicles are new formations of lymphoid tissue with accessory vascularization. Papillae, on the other hand, are essentially vascular formations that have been invaded by inflammatory cells. They characterize the subacute stages of inflammation of varying etiology. Histopathologically, the follicle is a lymphoid response that most likely correlates with cellular antibody production. The papilla is a polymorphonuclear leukocyte (PMN) infiltration that may be superimposed upon the follicle and undoubtedly reflects humoral antibody production and activation of the acute inflammatory pathway.

The progression of severity in active inflammation in the conjunctiva proceeds from follicle to papilla to papillary confluence with exudate formation. As the polymorphonuclear neutrophil reaction progresses, the hydrolytic enzymes released from these cells destroy conjunctival parenchyma, clinically producing an overall confluence of the

Papillae, in contrast, are most frequently encountered on the upper palpebral conjunctiva (Fig. 10–7). They present a fine mosaic pattern of elevated, polygonal hyperemic areas separated by paler channels. A central fibrovascular core is present within each papilla. This gives rise to a central vessel that, upon reaching the surface of the structure, erupts into a spokelike or glomeruluslike vascular pattern that is readily evident on biomicroscopic examination. The papilla additionally is composed of a combination of acute inflammatory cells (polymorphonuclear leukocytes, basophils, etc.), and invariably there is epithelial hypertrophy of the mucous membrane. The connective tissue septa of the papilla are anchored into deeper

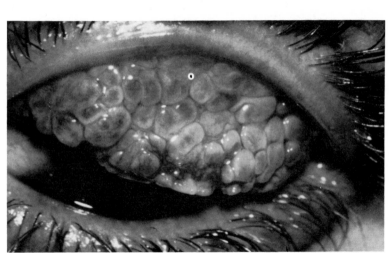

Figure 10-8. Giant papillae.

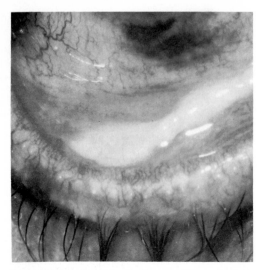

Figure 10–9. Conjunctival pseudomembrane.

papillary reaction (inflammatory swelling) and exudation. The discharge in conjunctivitis is composed of the exudate filtering through the conjunctival epithelium, to which is added epithelial debris, mucus, tears, and the secretion of the other conjunctival glands. At first an increased volume of reflexly secreted tears plus a serous inflammatory exudate produce a watery discharge. With time the secretion of an increased number of goblet cells may give the secretion a mucoid consistency, and eventually the addition of inflammatory cells makes it even thicker and purulent in character (Fig. 10–2). Degenerated epithelial and mucus cells may be added to the exudative elements.

When an exudate rich in fibrin is formed on the surface of the conjunctiva, a pseudomembrane may result (Fig. 10–9). The pseudomembrane consists of little more than a close network of fibrin in the meshes of which are entangled leukocytes and other exudative products. Characteristically, the translucent structure can be easily peeled off, leaving the epithelium intact. If the inflammatory process persists, the pseudomembrane generally is quickly reproduced. In contrast, a true membrane is formed when the inflammatory exudate permeates the superficial layers of the conjunctival epithelium, in addition to being layered out on the surface (Fig. 10–10). As a result the fibrinous network becomes interlaced among the epithelial cells, and attempts to remove it are accompanied by a tearing of the epithelium by the fibrin strands. A raw, bleeding surface results. The involved epithelium ultimately undergoes necrosis, is lifted up by granulation tissue growing beneath it, and is cast off. The granulation tissue usually is ultimately covered by epithelium, but in the most severe cases the subepithelial tissues also may be permeated by the fibrinous network. Extensive scarring may follow, accompanied by symblepharon, lid deformities, trichiasis, and xerophthalmia.

Examination of smears of the conjunctival exudate or epithelial scrapings may provide information of diagnostic value. It is said that in general polymorpho-

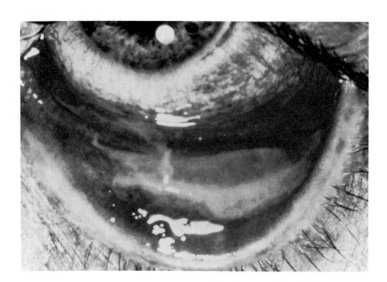

Figure 10–10. A true inflammatory membrane of the conjunctiva.

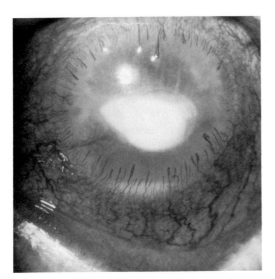

Figure 10–11. Inflammatory infiltrate of the corneal stroma caused by *Staphylococcus aureus* infection.

INFLAMMATION OF THE CORNEA

Active inflammation in the cornea is most readily identified by infiltrates in the stroma (Fig. 10–11). The infiltrates appear as focal granular opacities on biomicroscopic examination and may lie at any level of the stroma, depending on the nature of the inflammatory stimulus. In an avascular cornea a stromal infiltrate is composed predominantly of polymorphonuclear leukocytes. These cellular elements may originate from the limbal vascular arcades and migrate to the site of corneal injury, or, alternatively, they may enter the stroma from the tear film and/or the aqueous humor when defects occur in the limiting cellular layers of the cornea. In vascularized corneas inflammatory cells make their way into the stroma via the new vascular channels, and the infiltrates are composed of mixed cellular components.

Stromal edema almost invariably coexists with the inflammatory infiltrates. This is readily discernible with the slit-lamp biomicroscope by the appearance of vacuoles and optically empty spaces between stromal lamellae and by an increase in corneal thickness measurable by pachymetry. Corneal transparency is decreased as a result. Neovascularization is an additional indicator of active inflammation in the corneal stroma (Fig. 10–12). This is characterized by vascular

nuclear leukocytes predominate in bacterial infections, mononuclear cells in viral infections, and eosinophils in allergic reactions. Additionally, however, a polymorphonuclear response indicates a severe acute inflammatory reaction, whereas a lymphocytic response correlates with more mild disease, so that differences in host response may to a great extent negate the diagnostic usefulness of this technique. While it may be helpful, the cytologic picture is at best often indefinite, and it is by no means invariably sufficient to establish a diagnosis.

Figure 10–12. Neovascularization of the cornea.

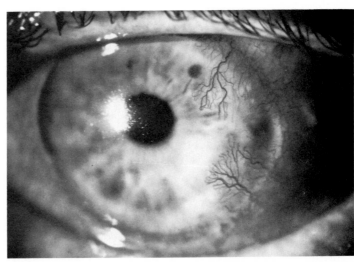

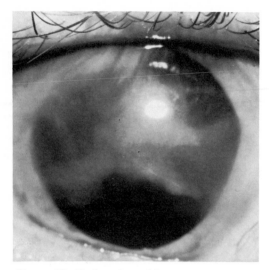

Figure 10–13. Scarring of the corneal stroma.

loops extending from the limbus into the adjacent corneal stroma. The new vessels may lie in the superficial and/or deep corneal stroma, again depending on the nature of the inflammatory stimulus. Cellular elements of the blood often can be visualized flowing through the new vascular network.

Inflammation of the corneal stroma may induce structural alteration characterized by scarring (Fig. 10–13). Whenever the inflammatory process is severe enough to cause tissue destruction, scarring results. This process interrupts the regular lamellar arrangement of the tissue, resulting in loss of transparency. The decrease in corneal clarity may be difficult to distinguish from that produced by chronic stromal edema. However, the loss of optical transparency caused by edema may be reversible, whereas the changes due to corneal scarring generally are irreversible. Translucent stromal scars in young children may clear over extended periods of time, providing one exception to this rule.

Depending on the severity of the inflammatory response and the resulting scarring process, the degree of structural change in the cornea may vary greatly. At one extreme, the damage may be manifested by little more than a decrease in the luster of the light reflex from the corneal surface. At the other extreme,

the normally transparent corneal tissue may be replaced by an opaque, bluish-white lesion. Interspersed between these extremes are multiple gradations of grayish translucency. The scarring process involves the manufacture of new collagen, which contracts as it matures. Thus, corneal thinning results when stromal scarring occurs unless it is offset by concomitant edema of the residual stroma. Pigment, particularly melanin, may be included in the structure of the scar, imparting a coloration other than gray or white to it. As active inflammation subsides and scarring progresses, blood elements decreasingly traverse the new vessels that have invaded the cornea, and so-called ghost vessels are seen; however, true blood vessels remain. If inflammation recurs, they rapidly become engorged and their lumina again fill with blood. Finally, a variety of deposits in the corneal stroma may be observed in cases of long-standing inflammation. Most commonly calcium is deposited in the superficial stromal lamellae following destruction of Bowman's membrane. Although this abnormality may vary widely in appearance, typically it is a fenestrated, gray, sheet-like opacity lying in a horizontal band in the exposed interpalpebral portion of the cornea, separated from the anatomic limbus by a narrow, clear zone (band keratopathy) (Fig. 10–14). Other depos-

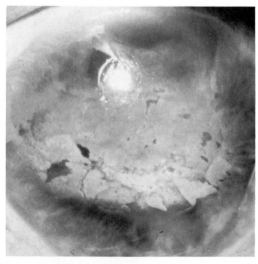

Figure 10–14. Band keratopathy—calcium deposition in the superficial cornea.

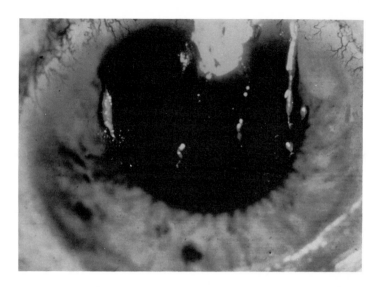

Figure 10–15. Filamentary keratopathy.

its include lipid and proteinaceous material, pigment, and iron.

Because it is capable of rapid regeneration, the corneal epithelium generally does not incur structural change as a result of inflammation. Intraepithelial edema may occur. This is an indirect effect due to involvement of the endothelium by the inflammatory process and a disturbance of its normal dehydrating mechanisms. Clinically it is characterized by optically empty vacuoles within the corneal epithelium and in severe cases by frank vesicle formation. Epithelial filaments also occur in various types of keratitis and are coils of hypertrophied epithelial cells attached to the cornea at their bases (Fig. 10–15).

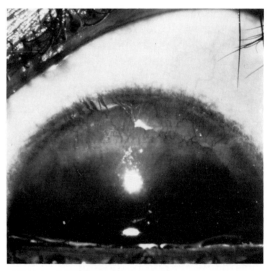

Figure 10–16. Pannus.

On examination with the slit-lamp biomicroscope, they can be seen as comma-shaped opacities with the unattached end hanging downward on the corneal surface and moving with each blink. Although scarring does not involve the epithelium itself, it does occur immediately beneath the epithelium as a pannus (Fig. 10–16). The subepithelial pannus invariably is covered by epithelium.

The corneal endothelium may be involved secondarily by inflammatory processes in the corneal stroma (keratitis) or in the anterior uveal tract (anterior uveitis). In the latter instance inflammatory cells are present in the anterior chamber and can be visualized with the slit-lamp biomicroscope as grayish granular specks circulating in the aqueous humor. Aggregates of these cells may deposit on the endothelial surface of the cornea, where they are referred to as keratic precipitates (KPs) (Fig. 10–17). Several clinical forms of KPs are recognized. In the punctate or granular form the cells are primarily polymorphonuclear leukocytes and lymphocytes. Larger cellular aggregates are known as mutton-fat, greasy, or lardaceous KPs. Macrophages predominate in this type of deposit, and the larger size of the deposit is attributed to the physical properties of the cell membrane of the cytologic components. It is said that monocytes, macrophages, and histiocytes have sticky cell surfaces, allowing

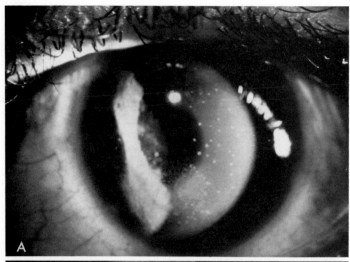

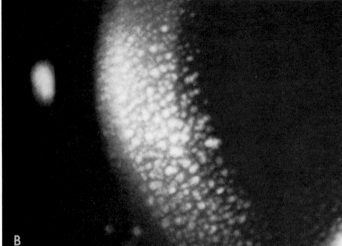

Figure 10–17. Keratic precipitates. *A,* Punctate. *B,* Mutton-fat.

them to adhere readily to one another with the result that larger cell aggregates are formed. Finally, the fibrinous KP, in which the endothelial deposits are composed largely of fibrin with few inflammatory cells, also is recognized. Keratic precipitates usually resolve completely, but residual hyalinized deposits may remain on the posterior cornea.

Retrocorneal membranes, thin, filmy membranes of connective tissue that cover the posterior corneal surface, may be an inflammatory accompaniment (Fig. 10–18) and occur especially following hyphema, penetrating keratoplasty, or corneal perforation due to trauma or infection. These membranes may at times be vascularized or pigmented. It is thought that endothelial cell damage or death precedes proliferation of a re-

trocorneal membrane, and in the great majority of cases its occurrence is accompanied by corneal edema.

Aronson and colleagues applied the term corneal stromal infiltrative disease to inflammation primarily characterized by neutrophilic invasion of the corneal stroma. This in turn was divided into central stromal keratitis and the peripheral infiltrative diseases. Central stromal keratitis referred to all diseases that occurred in the central two thirds of the cornea, so that this group accounts for most cases of corneal visual loss. As stressed earlier in this chapter, all toxic and immune stimuli that produce an infiltrative reaction (i.e., invasion of the corneal stroma by polymorphonuclear leukocytes [PMNs]) are included in this classification. The pathogenesis of these

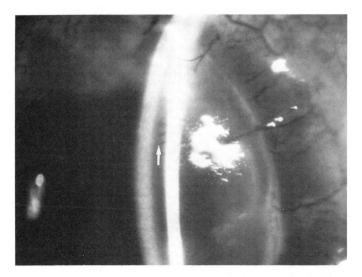

Figure 10–18. Vascularized (arrow) retrocorneal membrane which has separated from the posterior surface of a corneal transplant. (Courtesy of Jay H. Krachmer, M.D. and Peter R. Laibson, M.D.)

disorders involves the acute inflammatory pathway. The inflammatory stimulus (antigen, toxic agent, or cellular degradation products) combines with gamma globulin (antibody), and this complex binds complement. The complement-binding complex is chemotactic for the PMN, attracting large numbers of these cells to the corneal stroma for defense of the injured tissue (Fig. 10–11). The PMNs phagocytize the complement-binding complex, and during this process lysosomal degranulation occurs. That is, the relatively high concentrations of hydrolytic enzymes contained in lysosomes are released and degrade the complement-binding complex into a form that facilitates phagocytosis. In severe reactions, however, excessive quantities of these enzymes may be released, causing autolytic breakdown of the stromal parenchyma. Treatment of these disorders includes both specific therapy (i.e., removal of the stimulating agents) and nonspecific therapy (i.e., removal of the host inflammatory cells that destroy the corneal parenchyma). The latter is accomplished by topical application of corticosteroids (see Chapter 11).

INFLAMMATION OF THE PERIPHERAL CORNEA

Peripheral infiltrative diseases involve the peripheral third of the corneal stroma and the immediately adjacent limbus. In all other respects, including their pathogenesis, they resemble central stromal keratitis and they are treated in a similar manner. The acute inflammatory or complement-binding pathway is operative, and the disorder most frequently presents as subepithelial or stromal opacities of varied sizes and densities (Fig. 10–19). A zone of clear cornea often separates the infiltrate from the limbus, although superficial vascularization (pannus) (Fig. 10–16) may extend from the limbus and encompass it. Punctate staining of the epithelium overlying the infiltrate often can be demonstrated by application of fluorescein.

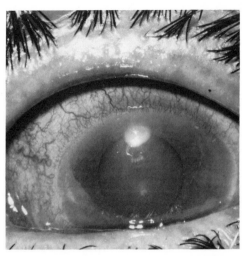

Figure 10–19. Inflammatory infiltrate in the peripheral corneal stroma.

Neovascularization generally signifies chronicity of the inflammatory process, and the peripheral stromal infiltrate often lies at the most central aspect of the fibrovascular membrane. In the most severe types of chronic, progressive inflammation (e.g. atopic keratitis, trachoma) the vascular invasive process may encompass the peripheral infiltrate and extend beyond it to the central cornea, obliterating the normal structure of the entire cornea.

Unfortunately, inflammatory diseases of the peripheral cornea are more complex than central stromal keratitis and include more than just the peripheral infiltrative diseases. Unlike the central stroma, the peripheral cornea and adjacent limbus depend upon the limbal vasculature for normal nutrition and maintenance. This allows a second etiologic mechanism, intravascular clotting, most likely in the paralimbal deep and superficial scleral vascular plexuses, to become operative. The result is a second type of inflammatory disorder, peripheral ulcerative disease, caused by ischemic necrosis of peripheral corneal tissue.

Aronson and coworkers classified the ischemic syndromes as primary and secondary ischemic necrosis of the peripheral cornea (Fig. 10–20). The specific etiology of the primary types, which include a spectrum of disorders ranging in severity from Terrien's senile marginal degeneration to Mooren's ulcer, is not known. However, it is hypothesized that a vasculitis probably originates in the lumen and/or parenchyma of small vessels in the primary form. This is supported by a high incidence of asso-

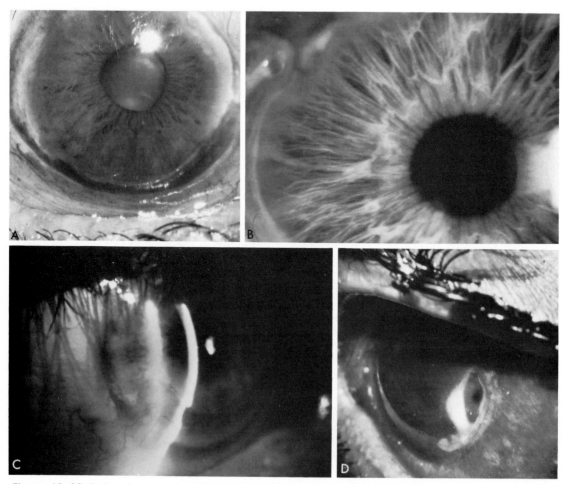

Figure 10–20. Ischemic necrosis of the peripheral cornea. *A* and *B*, Primary type, etiology unknown. *C*, Secondary type, rheumatoid arthritis. *D*, Secondary type, periarteritis nodosa.

ciated collagen disease, which is known to produce vasculitis in many organs and tissues. The prevalent clinical sign is a wasting away of the peripheral corneal stroma in a relatively quiet and often comfortable eye. The initial lesion usually is stromal; breakdown of the epithelium in the involved area is thought to be a secondary manifestation reflecting increased severity of the disease. The most severe forms progress to corneal perforation.

Secondary forms of this entity are differentiated from the primary types only by the presence of an identifiable apparent cause of the ischemia. In contrast to the primary forms, the secondary forms are more likely initiated by an extravascular nidus of inflammation in proximity to the limbal vasculature, which secondarily causes a vasculitis and intravascular clotting. In microbe-induced ischemia, such as that associated with *Pseudomonas* infections, elaboration of endotoxin presumably causes the inflammation that promotes intravascular clotting. In peripheral ischemia associated with chemical trauma the offending chemical either destroys vessels directly or causes sufficient inflammation to produce a vasculitis. Surgical interruption of the vascular supply to the peripheral cornea apparently accounts for ischemia that occurs postoperatively.

Although much of the evidence for the ischemic basis of peripheral ulcerative keratitis lacks firm support, no better etiologic theory is currently available. Moreover, therapy whose rationale is based on an ischemic etiology has produced dramatic instances of success. However, an important caveat must be emphasized here. Ischemia resulting from intravascular clotting is virtually an unequivocal contraindication to the use of local corticosteroids. Corticosteroids promote fibrin accumulation within blood vessels and therefore can intensify an active ischemic process. Once ischemia has been overcome, however, corticosteroids can be carefully used, if necessary, under close observation.

The goals of therapy in primary and secondary ischemic necrosis of the cornea are to arrest inflammation, to restore the integrity of the vascular supply to the limbus, to promote thickening of the eroded corneal stroma, and to restore the integrity of the epithelium. As defined, the primary forms are idiopathic. There is no known stimulus to eliminate or to neutralize, and corticosteroids are contraindicated. These cases are treated with subconjunctivally injected heparin. In secondary forms therapy must be aimed at (1) eliminating or neutralizing the etiologic agent where possible, (2) controlling the inflammatory response, and (3) reversing the intravascular clotting phenomenon. Control of the causal agent is approached in the conventional manner; antibiotics are used for bacterial infections, antiviral antimetabolites for herpes simplex keratitis, initial copious lavage for chemical keratitis, and so forth. Inflammation is controlled with local corticosteroids, just as in infiltrative disease, with the caveat cited above bearing heavily on one's clinical decision. The anti-inflammatory benefit of the corticosteroid must be titrated very carefully against its potential to interfere with reestablishment of the limbal circulation. Clinical decisions regarding the use of corticosteroids and the dose to be employed must be made individually in each case. Whenever possible, we tend to withhold corticosteroids until there is clinical evidence of limbal revascularization. Subconjunctival heparin is used in an attempt to induce the latter.

Heparin is recommended as the treatment of choice with full knowledge that theoretically it is not the optimal drug. A fibrinolytic agent should best promote recanalization of the thrombosed vessels, and there is no evidence that heparin acts in this fashion. Conceptually, a fibrinolytic agent, such as urokinase, would be the drug of choice for initial treatment of intravascular clotting. Unfortunately, it is not available to us, and streptococcal derivatives (e.g., streptokinase), which may function as proenzymes, activating intrinsic fibrinolysins to lyse the clot, are probably too anti-

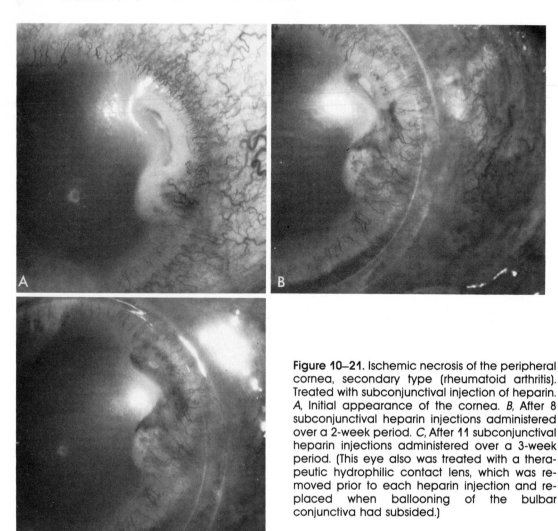

Figure 10–21. Ischemic necrosis of the peripheral cornea, secondary type (rheumatoid arthritis). Treated with subconjunctival injection of heparin. *A,* Initial appearance of the cornea. *B,* After 8 subconjunctival heparin injections administered over a 2-week period. *C,* After 11 subconjunctival heparin injections administered over a 3-week period. (This eye also was treated with a therapeutic hydrophilic contact lens, which was removed prior to each heparin injection and replaced when ballooning of the bulbar conjunctiva had subsided.)

genic to consider for this purpose. Heparin is readily available for clinical use, and experience to date shows it to be quite safe. It probably functions as an indirect fibrinolytic agent. Assuming intravascular clot lysis to be a continuous process, actual clot breakdown is accomplished by intrinsic tissue fibrinolysins. Heparin presumably acts as a fibrin-controlling agent, blocking the fibrinogen-fibrin pathway, thereby preventing reclotting or continuous clotting of the initially thrombosed site.

Heparin is administered subconjunctivally. This places a large quantity of drug in proximity to the lesion. Aqueous heparin, 1000 units per ml., is employed and 0.5 ml. (500 units) is drawn up in a tuberculin syringe to which a 25-gauge needle is attached. Three tenths of a milliliter of lidocaine 2 per cent and 0.2 ml. of physiologic saline are each drawn up in turn and allowed to mix in the 1-ml. tuberculin syringe. Despite the presence of lidocaine in the inoculum, the injection can be painful. Therefore, the ocular surface tissue is first anesthetized with proparacaine hydrochloride 0.5 per cent, one drop instilled at 2-minute intervals for a total of five doses. The injection is performed adjacent to the lesion. Every effort is made to balloon the conjunctiva to the limbus in order to deposit maximal heparin concentration at the affected site.

The frequency with which heparin

injections are performed has been rather arbitrarily determined. During the course of several years we have come to use the following regimen. A subconjunctival injection is administered daily for 5 days. Two days are allowed to elapse, and three additional injections then are performed on alternate days. Two to 3 days are again allowed to pass, and then three more injections are administered on alternate days. If at this point there is no evidence of vascularization of the peripheral ulcer, we generally assume that this mode of therapy will not be effective and the heparin injections are discontinued. If, on the other hand, neovascularization and fi-

broplasia of the ulcer are evident (Fig. 10–21), we continue the heparin injections at a frequency dictated by the clinical response until repair is complete. A successful course of subconjunctival heparin therapy results in the arrest of centripetal and arcuate spread of the ulcerative process as well as cessation of its progress deeper into the corneal stroma, in neovascular or fibrovascular ingrowth into the ulcer bed, in thickening of the corneal stroma in the area of involvement, and in re-epithelialization of the peripheral ischemic ulcer (Fig. 10–22). When heparin is ineffective and peripheral ischemic ulceration continues to progress, surgical intervention

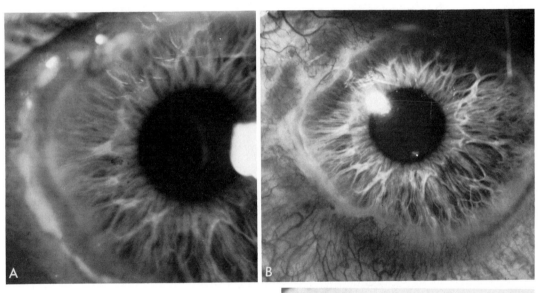

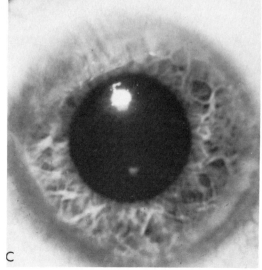

Figure 10–22. Ischemic necrosis of the peripheral cornea, primary type (etiology unknown), treated with subconjunctival injection of heparin. *A,* Initial appearance of the cornea. *B,* After 12 subconjunctival heparin injections administered over a 3-week period. *C,* One year after completion of subconjunctival heparin therapy.

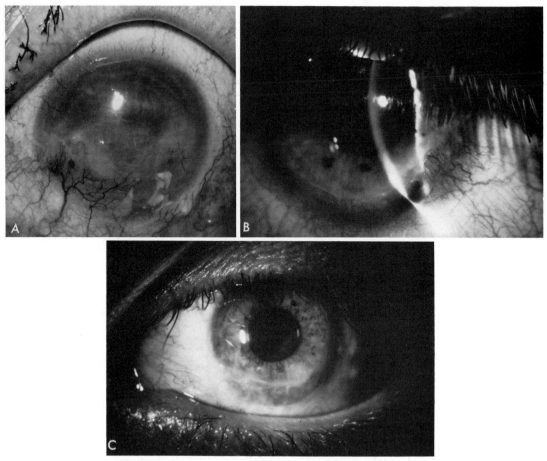

Figure 10–23. Ischemic necrosis of the peripheral cornea. *A,* Secondary type (rheumatoid arthritis) successfully treated with an inlay conjunctival flap in the inferotemporal periphery. *B,* Secondary type (rheumatoid arthritis and systemic lupus erythematosus) with bulging descemetocele. *C,* Same case as *B,* successfully treated with lamellar keratoplasty.

(e.g., segmental inlay conjunctival flap or partial lamellar keratoplasty) is in order (Fig. 10–23).

To the best of our knowledge, only one serious complication of heparin therapy has been reported. This patient inadvertently received 3000 units of aqueous heparin (instead of the intended 300 units) on 3 successive days. Subsequently the ischemic process worsened and the cornea perforated. However, no serious complications have been encountered at the recommended doses. Subconjunctival hemorrhages do occur regularly. Though unsightly, they are of little consequence. However, subconjunctival hemorrhages will invariably frighten the patient and his family, and they must be forewarned that the hemorrhage is expected and that it rep-

resents only a temporary cosmetic problem. Systemic anticoagulation does not occur at the doses we have recommended.

Use of subconjunctival heparin in peripheral infiltrative disease will enhance the infiltrative process. Corticosteroids usually will reverse and control this problem, but correct diagnosis will prevent it altogether. Because of this potential for diagnostic error, only severe cases of peripheral ischemic disease generally are treated with heparin. An additional situation that bears scrutiny is the peripheral ischemic ulcer in which vascularization has been successfully induced by subconjunctival heparin. Infiltrates may appear at the central edge of the invading vessels, a result of the reconstituted vascular supply. Corticosteroid therapy is judiciously initiated here in conjunction with heparin, and the two agents are carefully titrated. Because the corticosteroid can enhance intravascular clotting, the heparin injections must be maintained during this phase of therapy.

EXTERNAL OCULAR RESPONSE

The exposed surface location of the eye ensures its repeated exposure to inflammatory stimuli. However, in the anterior segment the conjunctival and corneal epithelium act as a protective physical barrier to ocular entry of exogenous stimuli. The tears maintain the integrity of these surfaces and further act to neutralize inflammatory stimuli by dilution and by chemical combination of the stimulus with the immune globulins they contain. The enzymatic properties of tears (e.g., lysozyme) probably do not represent a significant additional protective function. The conjunctiva and the limbus also both possess an abundant superficial vascular supply capable of discharging cellular and humoral defense elements.

Nonetheless, the so-called normal eye invariably demonstrates some degree of mild active inflammation. Here, however, the changes wrought by inflammation may be sufficiently mild to predispose the tissue to inflammatory recurrences only minimally or not at all. In such an instance the protective lining regenerates and/or the vascular permeability returns to a normal or nearly normal level. The eye then reacts as if it had never experienced a previous inflammatory episode. If, alternatively, the eye has been exposed to more pronounced inflammatory episodes, vascular permeability may be enhanced to a degree at which previously inadequate stimuli are now capable of initiating an inflammatory response. As a result, although this degree of structural change may be inadequate to perpetuate continuous (chronic) inflammation, the enhancement of vascular permeability may predispose the site to recurrent inflam-

matory episodes. Finally, if structural change is severe enough, it results in chronic inflammation. Here inflammatory inactivity cannot be achieved in the absence of anti-inflammatory therapy. The protective lining (the conjunctival and corneal epithelium) may be so severely altered that exogenous inflammatory stimuli (e.g., bacteria) cannot be adequately excluded from contact with the neutralization phases of the host response.

CLINICAL SEVERITY OF EXTERNAL OCULAR INFLAMMATION

Prevention of structural alteration is a major goal in the treatment of ocular inflammation. To accomplish this goal in dealing with inflammatory disease involving the conjunctiva, the limbus, and the corneal epithelium, it is necessary to recognize and to classify pathogenetically (1) the stages of active inflammation and (2) the degree of structural change evident on clinical examination. Each of these categories can be subdivided into mild, moderate, and severe based on the clinical signs listed in Table 10–1. Not all of the signs described for each stage are necessarily present in a given case.

Active inflammation is classified as mild when any combination of the following is encountered: There is hyperemia of the limbus or the bulbar or palpebral conjunctiva. There also may be low-grade conjunctival chemosis. Small to medium-sized follicles are present in the palpebral conjunctiva overlying the tarsus and the blood vessels at the lid margin are dilated. Only minimal exudate is noted. Changes in the corneal epithelium are limited to stippling or minor erosions and/or intraepithelial infiltrates.

The inflammatory response is said to be moderate when any combination of the following signs is observed: There is confluent hyperemia of the conjunctiva and limbus. There are many medium to large follicles in the palpebral conjunctiva, and the formation of papillae may

Table 10–1. CLINICAL SIGNS OF CONJUNCTIVAL AND CORNEAL INFLAMMATION*

	Active	Chronic
Mild	Hyperemia of limbus or bulbar or palpebral conjunctiva.	Redundancy of conjunctiva in fornix.
	Low-grade chemosis.	Low-grade chemosis.
	Small or medium sized follicles.	Neovascularization and hypertrophy of lid margin.
	Dilatation of vessels at lid margin.	Linear superficial scarring of the palpebral conjunctiva.
	Minimal exudate.	
	Punctate erosions of corneal epithelium or intraepithelial infiltrates.	
Moderate	Confluent hyperemia of conjunctiva and limbus.	Scarring and neovascularization of the lid margin with distortion of the gray line.
	Medium to large follicles.	Stellate conjunctival scarring with distortion of its surface.
	Increased discharge—generally mucinous.	Shrinkage of conjunctival fornices.
	Medium to large erosions of corneal epithelium.	Mild dry eye syndrome.
	Superficial infiltrates in corneal stroma.	Punctate erosions of corneal epithelium.
Severe	Diffuse, marked hyperemia of conjunctival vasculature.	Distortion of lid margins by scarring with madarosis and trichiasis.
	Focal or diffuse subconjunctival hemorrhage.	Distortion of entire lid (entropion or ectropion).
	Coalesced papillae with diffuse hypertrophy of the palpebral conjunctiva.	Shrinkage of conjunctiva with symblepharon formation.
	Copious exudate.	More severe tear insufficiency.
	Pseudomembrane or true conjunctival membrane.	Breakdown of geographic areas of corneal epithelium.
	Extensive ulceration of corneal epithelium.	Infiltrates in corneal stroma.
	Infiltrates involving all layers of the corneal stroma.	Fibroplasia and neovascularization of corneal stroma.
		Limbal pannus formation.

*Modified from Aronson and Elliott, 1972.

be observed. A greater quantity of exudate, generally of a mucinous nature, may be present in the conjunctival sulcus and on the lash margin. At this level of inflammation the changes in the corneal epithelium, if present, consist of medium to large erosions (e.g. dendrite formation) and may be accompanied by subepithelial and superficial stromal infiltrates.

The following clinical signs merit classification of an active inflammatory response as severe: There is diffuse, marked hyperemia of the conjunctival vasculature, frequently accompanied by focal or diffuse subconjunctival hemorrhage. The papillae have coalesced, resulting in diffuse hypertrophy of the palpebral conjunctiva. The exudate is now copious and may combine with extensive fibrin and with ulceration of the epithelial surface of the conjunctiva to form pseudomembranes or true membranes. Corneal changes consist of diffuse ulceration of the epithelium and various-sized inflammatory infiltrates involving all layers of the corneal stroma.

Chronic inflammation reflects permanent structural alteration. It is classified as mild when characterized by any combination of the following changes: There is an apparent redundancy of conjunctival tissue in the fornix. This actually represents a low-grade chemosis of the bulbar conjunctiva. Neovascularization and hypertrophy of the lid margin are present and there is linear superficial scarring of the palpebral conjunctiva.

The changes in structure are said to be moderate when the scarring and neovascularization of the lid margin are accompanied by distortion of the gray line. The linear scarring of the palpebral conjunctiva has progressed to a stellate pattern with resulting distortion of the conjunctival surface. Scarring has produced some shrinkage of the fornices with early symblepharon formation. The conjunctival changes produce the beginnings of a dry eye syndrome, which secondarily may cause punctate changes in the corneal and conjunctival epithelium.

Severe structural alteration is manifested by pronounced scarring. This causes distortion of the lid margin with madarosis and trichiasis and distortion of the entire eyelid (entropion or ectropion). There is shrinkage of the conjunctiva with obliteration of its bulbar component and the fornices. Tear insufficiency becomes increasingly more prominent with breakdown of the corneal epithelium in extensive geographic areas. The corneal stroma is invaded by inflammatory cells and there is frank fibroplasia and neovascularization. The scarring process at the limbus is seen as pannus formation.

BIBLIOGRAPHY

Aronson, S. B., and Moore, T. E., Jr.: Corticosteroid therapy in central stromal keratitis. Amer J Ophthalmol 67:873, 1969.

Aronson, S. B., Elliott, J. H., Moore, T. E., Jr., and O'Day, D. M.: Pathogenetic approach to therapy of peripheral corneal inflammatory disease. Amer J Ophthalmol 70:65, 1970.

Aronson, S. B., Moore, T. E., Jr., and O'Day, D. M.: The effect of structural alteration on anterior ocular inflammation. Amer J Ophthalmol 70:886, 1970.

Aronson, S. B., Fish, M. B., Pollycove, M., and Coon, M. A.: Altered vascular permeability in ocular inflammatory disease. Arch Ophthalmol 85:455, 1971.

Aronson, S. B., and Elliott, J. H.: Ocular Inflammation. St. Louis, C. V. Mosby Co., 1972, pp. 1–73, 99–207.

Duke-Elder, W. S. (ed): System of Ophthalmology. Vol. 8: Diseases of the Outer Eye. Part 1, The conjunctiva. St. Louis, C. V. Mosby Co., 1965, pp. 47–70.

Elliott, J. H., Aronson, S. B., Moore, T. E., Jr., and Williams, F. C.: Heparin therapy of peripheral corneal ischemic syndromes. In Symposium on the Cornea. New Orleans Academy of Ophthalmology. St. Louis, C. V. Mosby Co., 1972, pp. 78–104.

Kimura, S. J., and Thygeson, P.: The cytology of external ocular disease. Amer J Ophthalmol 39:137, 1955.

Leibowitz, H. M., Pratt, M. V., Flagstad, I. J., et al.: Human conjunctivitis. I. Diagnostic evaluation. Arch Ophthalmol 94:1747, 1976.

Meyers, R. L., and Pettit, T. H.: Chemotaxis of polymorphonuclear leukocytes in corneal inflammation. Invest Ophthalmol 13:187, 1974.

Weissman, G.: Mediators of Inflammation. New York. Plenum Press, 1974.

Zweifach, B. W., Grant, L., and McCluskey, R. T. (eds): The Inflammatory Process. 2nd ed. New York, Academic Press, Inc., 1973.

11 Use of Corticosteroids in the Treatment of Corneal Inflammation

HOWARD M. LEIBOWITZ, M.D.
ALLAN KUPFERMAN, Ph.D.

Therapy of inflammatory disease in the cornea is directed at control of the inflammatory response. Ideally it results in the preservation of normal structure and function. Factors able to produce inflammation in the cornea include (1) infections and infestations (by bacteria, viruses, fungi, chlamydia, protozoa, and helminths), (2) immunologic reactions, (3) chemical irritants and noxious agents, (4) toxins, (5) trauma, (6) foreign bodies, (7) tear insufficiency, (8) exposure, (9) compromise of the peripheral nutrient circulation at the limbus, and (10) neoplasms. In addition, there are a substantial number of cases in which the specific etiology cannot be determined.

GENERAL THERAPEUTIC PRINCIPLES FOR CORNEAL INFLAMMATION

Despite the multiplicity of agents capable of causing corneal inflammation, the cornea is limited in its ability to react to an inflammatory stimulus. Therefore, regardless of which of the previously listed factors causes the problem, the basic inflammatory processes within the cornea itself are essentially the same. They include infiltration by inflammatory cells, edema, and neovascularization. Of the three, invasion of the cornea by inflammatory cells is the most important. In most instances the prime culprit producing corneal damage in inflammatory disease is the polymorpho-

nuclear leukocyte (PMN). Large numbers of PMNs invade the inflamed cornea. Many of these cells degenerate and lose the lysosomal granules from their cytoplasm. A number of hydrolytic enzymes are then released from the lysosomal granules and react with the proteins of the cornea. Necrosis of the tissue results, and repair of the tissue damage includes the formation of scar tissue and visual loss.

The similarity of the inflammatory response in the cornea, regardless of its etiology, allows us to apply similar general principles of treatment in each instance. First of all, one employs specific therapy. Whenever possible, treatment is designed to eliminate or to neutralize the causal agent promptly—if it can be identified and if a specific therapeutic agent is available. For example, elimination of bacteria is achieved with antibiotics, elimination of viruses by antiviral antimetabolites, and so forth.

However, since ocular inflammation is an interaction between the inflammatory stimulus and the host response, treatment directed solely at eradication of the stimulus does not immediately alter the clinical course of the inflammatory reaction. Optimal therapy often calls for the concomitant control of the host response. Therefore, in addition to specific therapy, one also uses nonspecific therapy whose primary goal is the elimination of inflammatory cells. This is most frequently accomplished with locally administered corticosteroids. As a general rule, the use of corticosteroids is indicated whenever the structural or functional integrity of the globe is threatened. Thus, these agents are used to treat relatively mild corneal inflammation, whereas they may not be required in moderately severe blepharoconjunctivitis.

Corticosteroids are the most effective of clinically available agents for the nonspecific treatment of corneal inflammation. The polymorphonuclear leukocyte (PMN) is the key to corneal destruction, and corticosteroids control the PMNs. They produce an involution of those inflammatory cells that have invaded the cornea[1, 2] and suppress the migration of additional PMNs to the site of injury.[3, 4] Corticosteroids also inhibit the release of hydrolytic enzymes from inflammatory cells,[5, 6] preventing irreversible structural damage to the cornea and decreasing the chemotactic stimulus that attracts inflammatory cells to the area. Clinically and histologically, the infiltrate in the cornea rapidly disappears in the presence of corticosteroid therapy. It must be emphasized, however, that in all diseases, with the exception of adrenal insufficiency, corticosteroid therapy neither has a specific etiologic effect nor is curative. It is simply nonspecific palliative therapy.

Corticosteroids vary in their inherent anti-inflammatory potency. Table 11–1 summarizes how various *systemically administered* steroids are related with respect to this parameter. Hydrocortisone is the standard against which the list of synthetic corticosteroids is measured, and it is given a relative anti-inflammatory potency value of 1. Cortisone, the other naturally occurring steroid, is slightly less potent with a value of 0.8. Prednisone and prednisolone are essentially four times more potent in their anti-inflammatory effectiveness than is hydrocortisone, and dexamethasone and betamethasone are 25 times more potent than hydrocortisone or approximately six times more potent than prednisolone. Thus, when administering these agents by mouth or parenterally, one can give 20 mg. of hydrocortisone, 5 mg. of prednisone, or 0.75 mg. of dexamethasone and obtain essentially the same anti-inflammatory effect in each case. Unfortunately, topically applied ophthalmic formulations cannot be manipulated in this manner. It is therefore important to stress that the above data on anti-inflammatory potency have been obtained from nonocular experimental models following systemic administration of the drugs and that they are not directly applicable to the topical ophthalmologic use of corticosteroids.

In assessing the consequences of topical instillation of a corticosteroid, one must take into consideration the properties of the conjunctiva and cornea as biologic membranes. One must also consider the influence on conjunctival and corneal absorption of the physical geometry of the eye, blinking of the eyelids, the dynamics of the precorneal tear film and the aqueous humor, and the limitations of the vehicles that can be used in the eye. These factors greatly affect the duration of contact between a topically administered drug and the eye, and consequently they exert great influence on the amount of drug that gains access to ocular tissues and fluids. For practical purposes, the conjunctival sac limits the volume of drug that can be instilled; the ophthalmologist cannot manipulate dosage by altering the volume of drug administered. To a great extent, then, the anti-inflammatory effect that can be obtained in the anterior segment of the eye is determined by the specific corticosteroid compounds com-

Table 11–1. RELATIVE ANTI-INFLAMMATORY POTENCY OF SYSTEMICALLY ADMINISTERED CORTICOSTEROIDS

Compound	Relative Anti-inflammatory Potency	Relative Dose (mg.)
Hydrocortisone	1	20
Cortisone	0.8	25
Prednisone	3.5	5
Prednisolone	4	5
Methylprednisolone	5	4
Triamcinolone	5	4
Dexamethasone	25	0.75
Betamethasone	25	0.75

mercially available as ophthalmic formulations and by the concentration of drug in these formulations.

Ophthalmic corticosteroids vary significantly in their ability to penetrate into the cornea and through the cornea into the anterior chamber. The variability in ocular penetration is attributable to certain properties of the cornea as well as to differences among the corticosteroids. For example, the cellular layers of the cornea, the epithelium and the endothelium, are lipophilic, and therefore they resist penetration by polar or water-soluble molecules. The corneal stroma, on the other hand, is hydrophilic and resists penetration by nonpolar or fat-soluble molecules (Fig. 11–1). Clearly, then, there will be differences in corneal uptake and penetration of various steroid compounds when the epithelium is missing in comparison to those situations in which the epithelium is intact. A fat-soluble corticosteroid will pass readily through the epithelium and endothelium but will encounter substantial resistance to penetration through the stroma. The opposite situa-

tion will occur with a water-soluble steroid. In general, it will not pass through an intact corneal epithelium readily, but if the epithelium is absent, the water-soluble steroid will pass through the hydrophilic corneal stroma with great ease. It therefore follows that if a topically administered corticosteroid preparation is to penetrate through all layers of the cornea, it must be of biphasic polarity. That is, it must have some degree of solubility in both aqueous and lipid media.

TOPICALLY ADMINISTERED CORTICOSTEROIDS

There are at present basically six corticosteroid formulations available in the United States as individual agents for topical ophthalmic use (Table 11–2). Two of these are dexamethasone preparations, both of which are commercially available at a 0.1 per cent concentration. Two others are prednisolone preparations available to the ophthalmologist at a maximum concentration of 1.0 per cent. Ophthalmic dexamethasone can be

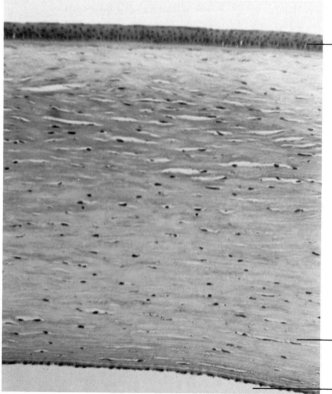

— Epithelium

Figure 11–1. Effect of corneal structure on drug penetration. The epithelium and the endothelium are lipophilic—they allow fat soluble molecules to penetrate and resist penetration by water soluble molecules. The stroma is hydrophilic—it allows water soluble molecules to penetrate and resists penetration by fat soluble molecules. Only molecules with biphasic polarity (some degree of solubility in both lipid and aqueous media) penetrate readily through the intact cornea.

— Stroma

— Endothelium

Table 11–2. WIDELY USED OPHTHALMIC CORTICOSTEROIDS

Corticosteroid Base	Derivative	Formulation	Concentration (Per Cent)	Commercial Product
Prednisolone	Acetate	Suspension	0.125	Econopred Pred Mild AK-Tate 0.125%
			1.0	Econopred Plus Pred Forte AK-Tate 1%
Prednisolone	Sodium phosphate	Solution	0.125	Inflamase AK-Pred 0.125%
			1.0	Inflamase Forte AK-Pred 1%
Dexamethasone	Alcohol	Suspension	0.1	Maxidex
Dexamethasone	Sodium phosphate	Solution	0.1	Decadron Phosphate
		Ointment	0.05	Decadron Phosphate
Fluorometholone	Alcohol	Suspension	0.1	FML
Medrysone	Alcohol	Suspension	1.0	HMS

obtained as an alcohol and as a phosphate, while ophthalmic prednisolone is marketed as an acetate and as a phosphate derivative. The derivative of a steroid base that is used to formulate the commercial ophthalmic product is of considerable importance because this relatively minor chemical alteration substantially affects the ability of the drug to penetrate into and through the cornea.[7, 8] The phosphate preparations are highly soluble in aqueous solution, and therefore dexamethasone sodium phosphate (Decadron) and prednisolone sodium phosphate (Inflamase Forte, AK-Pred 1%) are commercially available as solutions. Alcohol and acetate preparations are sparingly soluble in aqueous solution, and so commercially available dexamethasone alcohol (Maxidex) and prednisolone acetate (Econopred Plus, Pred Forte, AK-Tate 1%) are marketed as suspensions. Of even greater significance is the fact that the acetate and the alcohol preparations are actually biphasic in solubility (particularly the acetate) and therefore are better able to penetrate into and through the intact cornea than are the water-soluble phosphates.

Importance of the Derivative of a Corticosteroid Base

Experimental observations illustrate the importance of these principles. Formulation of three radiolabeled dexamethasone preparations, identical in all respects except for the derivative of the steroid base, permits direct comparison of the drug level produced in the cornea by the phosphate, acetate, and free alcohol forms of dexamethasone[7] (Table 11–3). In the uninflamed cornea with an intact epithelium the biphasic acetate derivative most successfully penetrates into the cornea. The free alcohol form of dexamethasone results in a lower concentration in the cornea, whereas the phosphate form is clearly less able to penetrate through the intact corneal epithelium than are the other two derivatives. On the other hand, removal of the lipophilic epithelium prior to drug administration permits the water-soluble phosphate to penetrate readily into the hydrophilic stroma and to produce the highest corneal drug concentration of the three derivatives. The presence of intraocular inflammation in an eye with an intact epithelium (as determined by

Table 11–3. TOTAL CORTICOSTEROID CONCENTRATION WITH TIME IN THE RABBIT CORNEA FOLLOWING TOPICAL ADMINISTRATION OF 0.1 PER CENT DEXAMETHASONE OINTMENTS*

Corneal Status	Phosphate	Acetate	Alcohol
Epithelium intact, uninflamed eye	0	1,573	348
Epithelium removed, uninflamed eye	3,250	2,588	140
Epithelium intact, inflamed eye	40	1,250	471

*Values expressed in microgram-minutes/gram.

examination with the slit-lamp biomicroscope after instillation of fluorescein) creates still a third situation. Here the acetate derivative again produces the highest concentration. However, the presence of inflammation produced by an experimentally induced anterior and posterior uveitis seemingly results in a partial breakdown of the epithelial barrier to the water-soluble phosphate, allowing it to enter the cornea in a quantity that is intermediate between the amount present when the epithelium has been denuded and the amount detectable when the eye has not been disturbed. The mechanism of this effect is not precisely known.

Suspensions Versus Solutions

Suspensions are said to be superior to solutions. The rationale for this claim is based on the presence of drug particles in the suspension and the assumption that these particles persist in the conjunctival cul-de-sac for prolonged periods. Slow dissolution of the particles is thought to increase the contact time between the drug and the eye, presumably permitting the drug to attain higher levels in ocular tissues and fluid than the comparable drug in solution. Although this thesis seems logical, there is a minimum of experimental data to support it. Undoubtedly of equal or perhaps greater importance is the fact that the corticosteroid derivatives marketed as suspensions, the acetate and the alcohol, are biphasic in solubility, and therefore they are better able to penetrate into and through the intact cornea.

Vehicle

Another factor influencing the corneal drug level attained by topically applied corticosteroids is the vehicle in which the drug is formulated. Contact time of a topically administered drug with the eye plays a major role in the concentration that the drug achieves in the cornea and therefore, within certain limits, in the pharmacologic effect it produces. To

a degree, contact time can be lengthened by increasing the viscosity of the vehicle in which a drug is compounded; the prolongation of contact time produced by ointments forms the basis for the oft-stated teaching that ointments are superior to collyria in terms of the effect they are able to achieve after topical administration to the eye. However, experimental data comparing corneal drug levels attained after instillation of dexamethasone sodium phosphate solution and ointment seemingly contradict this principle. The ointment form of dexamethasone phosphate yielded lower drug levels in the cornea than the solution form.[9–11] Apparently the petrolatum used as a vehicle in the formulation of the ointment fails to release the drug rapidly to the precorneal tear film, so that, despite a prolonged contact time, the drug is not available for penetration into the cornea. Of course, these findings vary for different drugs and vehicles, but these studies serve to emphasize that one cannot routinely assume a greater therapeutic potency for an ointment formulation than for an aqueous preparation of the same drug in equal concentration.

Although commercially available formulations containing water-soluble polymers (e.g., hydroxypropyl methylcellulose) and petrolatum base ointments are more viscous than simple aqueous preparations of ophthalmic drugs, they have not proven to be dramatically more effective. This does not mean that prolongation of contact time between the drug and the eye is not desirable or that the pharmacologic principle stating that it may result in increased bioavailability and enhanced effectiveness is incorrect. However, viscosity of the vehicle is only one factor that influences the ocular contact time of a topically applied drug. Such uncontrollable variables as blink rate, tear secretion, and the rate at which the material exits via the lacrimal drainage system are of considerable importance. Seemingly a major deficiency of all ophthalmic drugs currently in clinical use is their very limited ability to prolong ocular contact time. High-viscosity carboxypolymethylene gels promise to be more effective vehicles in this regard. The material is retained in the conjunctival sac for a period of hours, tending to diminish slowly over time. In the experimental animal, prednisolone acetate formulated in this material yielded markedly higher corticosteroid levels in the cornea and aqueous humor than the comparable commercially available ophthalmic suspension.[12] Administered at 4-hour intervals, the gel form of the corticosteroid demonstrated a level of anti-inflammatory effectiveness that could not be distinguished from hourly administration of the suspension.[13]

At the time this material was written, initial clinical studies of this gel indicated that we can anticipate enhanced bioavailability and therapeutic effect in humans.[14] The material seems well tolerated and productive of few side effects. Pilocarpine formulated in the gel is followed by prolonged miosis and lowering of intraocular pressure. Application only once or twice daily is required to obtain an effect equal to pilocarpine drops administered four times a day. The potential value of this material as the vehicle for an ophthalmic corticosteroid preparation to treat serious inflammatory disease of the anterior segment is apparent. The requirement for less frequent instillation of a corticosteroid will decrease the inconvenience associated with therapy and may therefore increase compliance. The gel vehicle also offers the potential for achieving a given therapeutic effect with much less drug than is needed in suspension form. A concomitant decrease in dose-related steroid ocular toxicity, particularly glaucoma and cataract, represents an exciting therapeutic possibility.

Bioavailability Versus Anti-inflammatory Effectiveness

Examination of in vivo experimental data on the relative ability of four widely used, commercially available, potent ophthalmic corticosteroids to penetrate into the cornea indicates that they are not equivalent (Table 11–4).[8] These differences in the quantity of measurable drug in the cornea suggest corresponding differences in the ability of these ophthalmic corticosteroid preparations to suppress corneal inflammation. However, it must be stressed that this type of *data on corneal bioavailability provides no direct information on the relative ability of these preparations to suppress the inflammatory response once they gain access to the cornea.* Of greater importance to the ophthalmologist is how well these agents work once they reach the cornea. How effectively do they suppress the polymorphonuclear leukocytes that invade the cornea?

Experimentally we can measure anti-inflammatory effectiveness by radiolabeling the polymorphonuclear leukocytes systemically, before they invade the cornea,[15] and then measuring each drug's ability to decrease corneal radioactivity during an inflammatory keratitis. When we do this, we find that *once they gain access to the site of inflammation, topically administered corticosteroids differ in their ability to suppress*

Table 11–4. TOTAL CORTICOSTEROID CONCENTRATION WITH TIME IN THE RABBIT CORNEA FOLLOWING TOPICAL ADMINISTRATION OF COMMERCIALLY AVAILABLE OPHTHALMIC DROPS*

Corneal Status	Dexamethasone Sodium Phosphate 0.1 Per Cent Solution	Dexamethasone Alcohol 0.1 Per Cent Suspension	Prednisolone Acetate 1.0 Per Cent Suspension	Prednisolone Sodium Phosphate 1.0 Per Cent Solution
Epithelium intact, uninflamed eye	0	452	2336	968
Epithelium removed, uninflamed eye	4642	1361	4574	16338
Epithelium intact, inflamed eye	1068	543	2395	1074

*Values expressed in microgram-minutes/gram.

Table 11–5.   MEAN DECREASE IN CORNEAL INFLAMMATORY ACTIVITY FOLLOWING TOPICAL CORTICOSTEROID THERAPY

	Per Cent Decrease
Epithelium Intact	
Prednisolone acetate 1.0% ophthalmic suspension	51
Dexamethasone alcohol 0.1% ophthalmic suspension	40
Fluorometholone alcohol 0.1% ophthalmic suspension	31
Prednisolone phosphate 1.0% ophthalmic solution	28
Dexamethasone phosphate 0.1% ophthalmic solution	19
Dexamethasone phosphate 0.05% ophthalmic ointment	12
Epithelium Absent	
Prednisolone acetate 1.0% ophthalmic suspension	53
Prednisolone phosphate 1.0% ophthalmic solution	47
Dexamethasone alcohol 0.1% ophthalmic suspension	42
Fluorometholone alcohol 0.1% ophthalmic suspension	37
Dexamethasone phosphate 0.1% ophthalmic solution	22

the *inflammatory reaction. Moreover, the level of drug in the cornea does not necessarily equate with its anti-inflammatory effectiveness.* Table 11–5 lists the relative values of the mean decrease in corneal inflammatory activity following topical corticosteroid therapy.

Effectiveness of Specific Ophthalmic Corticosteroids

In an eye with an intact corneal epithelium, the differences between drugs (as shown in Table 11–5) are all statistically significant, and the results indicate that 1.0 per cent prednisolone acetate ophthalmic suspension is the most effective topical anti-inflammatory agent. When the corneal epithelium is absent, the relative values of anti-inflammatory activity are somewhat different. However, the 1.0 per cent prednisolone acetate again produces the greatest mean reduction in polymorphonuclear leuko-

cytic infiltration of the cornea. Overall, therefore, the data indicate that 1.0 per cent prednisolone acetate is the most effective of these agents for the suppression of corneal inflammation.[8, 11, 16, 17] Direct comparison of two commercially available forms of this drug (Econopred Plus and Pred Forte) in the laboratory, relative both to their bioavailability in the cornea and aqueous humor and to their anti-inflammatory effectiveness in the cornea, reveals no significant difference between the two preparations in either of these two parameters.[18] However, evidence has been presented that the two products may differ in their degree of suspension in the usual clinical conditions.[19]

Modification of the derivative of a given corticosteroid base alters its anti-inflammatory effectiveness when the drug is applied topically to the eye. This represents a true change in pharmacologic behavior and is not simply a re-

Table 11–6.   RELATIONSHIP OF THE DERIVATIVE OF AN OPHTHALMIC CORTICOSTEROID BASE TO ITS ANTI-INFLAMMATORY EFFECTIVENESS AND ITS CORNEAL BIOAVAILABILITY FOLLOWING TOPICAL APPLICATION TO THE EYE

Corticosteroid	Anti-inflammatory Effect (Per Cent)	Corneal Bioavailability (μg.-min./gm.)
Epithelium intact		
Dexamethasone acetate 0.1%	55	111
Dexamethasone alcohol 0.1%	40	543
Dexamethasone sodium phosphate 0.1%	19	1068
Epithelium absent		
Dexamethasone acetate 0.1%	60	118
Dexamethasone alcohol 0.1%	42	1316
Dexamethasone sodium phosphate 0.1%	22	4642

flection of the level that the drug reaches at the site of inflammation in the eye (Table 11–6). To date, for reasons that are not totally clear, the acetate derivative of each corticosteroid base studied has been the most effective. The acetate derivative achieves its therapeutic superiority in spite of the fact that the level it reaches in the cornea may be considerably less than that of other derivatives of the same steroid base. Thus, the acetate derivative not only is more effective than other derivatives but also is more potent. For example, a unit amount of dexamethasone acetate in the cornea produces a greater anti-inflammatory effect than a comparable amount of dexamethasone alcohol or dexamethasone sodium phosphate (Table 11–6).[20] Similar data demonstrate the superiority of prednisolone acetate over prednisolone phosphate;[8, 16, 17] it requires almost a four times greater tissue concentration of the phosphate derivative of prednisolone than of the acetate derivative to achieve essentially the same effect (Table 11–7).

Additional evidence that a change in the derivative of a corticosteroid base alters its pharmacologic behavior as an anti-inflammatory agent can be obtained from a comparison of the data derived from the study of varying concentrations of the same corticosteroid base (Table 11–7). An increase in the concentration of prednisolone acetate from 0.125 per cent to 1.0 per cent produced a significant increase both in the corneal concentration of the drug and in its anti-inflammatory effectiveness. This occurred when the corneal epithelium was intact as well as after its removal. However, the same increase in prednisolone sodium phosphate concentration (0.125 per cent to 1.0 per cent) produced a significant increase only in the tissue concentration of the drug, again both in the presence and in the absence of the corneal epithelium. In neither instance was this accompanied by a significant increase in anti-inflammatory effectiveness.[8, 16, 17]

Clearly, then, different derivatives of the same corticosteroid base are not equivalent in their anti-inflammatory properties. The phosphate derivatives of both the corticosteroid bases studied (dexamethasone and prednisolone) appear to be less effective anti-inflammatory agents following topical administration to the eye than other derivatives of the same corticosteroid base. The reason for this is obscure.

Given the fact that 1.0 per cent prednisolone acetate is the drug of choice for topical therapy of corneal inflammation, a question that must be raised is: Does 1.0 per cent represent the optimal concentration of this steroid for ocular use, or would perhaps 2.0 per cent be better? The data in Table 11–8 show that a twofold increase in drug concentration from 1.0 per cent, the maximum commercially available to the ophthalmologist, to 2.0 per cent results in a significant increase in the level of drug in the cornea. Taken alone, these bioavailability data might lead one to conclude that a more effective anti-inflammatory preparation could be obtained simply by in-

Table 11–7. PHARMACOLOGY OF TOPICALLY ADMINISTERED CORTICOSTEROIDS

	Anti-inflammatory Effectiveness (Per Cent)	Corneal Bioavailability (μg.-min./gm.)
Epithelium Intact		
Prednisolone acetate 0.125%	26	464
Prednisolone acetate 1.0%	51	2395
Prednisolone sodium phosphate 0.125%	23	162
Prednisolone sodium phosphate 1.0%	28	1075
Epithelium Absent		
Prednisolone acetate 0.125%	30	461
Prednisolone acetate 1.0%	53	4574
Prednisolone sodium phosphate 0.125%	42	185
Prednisolone sodium phosphate 1.0%	47	16338

Table 11–8. OPTIMAL PREDNISOLONE ACETATE CONCENTRATION FOR TOPICAL THERAPY OF INFLAMMATORY KERATITIS

Drug Concentration (Per Cent)	Corneal Bioavailability* (μg.-min./gm.)	Decrease in Corneal Inflammatory Activity (Per Cent)	
		Epithelium Intact	Epithelium Absent
0.125	629	30	40
1.0	1399	53[†]	57[†]
1.5	—	58[†]	59[†]
2.0	2209	—	—
3.0	—	53[†]	63[†]

*Corneal epithelium intact, uninflamed eye.
[†]No statistically significant difference among these values in the same column.

creasing the concentration of the presently available formulation. However, this conclusion is not borne out by objective measurement of anti-inflammatory effectiveness in the cornea.[21] Even a threefold increase—from 1.0 per cent to 3.0 per cent—is not accompanied by augmentation of anti-inflammatory effect in the cornea. Since there is no significant difference in therapeutic response between the 1.0 per cent and the 3.0 per cent formulations, one must conclude that preparations of prednisolone acetate in a concentration greater than 1.0 per cent carry with them an increased potential for ocular toxicity without a concomitant potential for increased benefit. Thus, their use does not appear to be justified.

Two other corticosteroids are commercially available for topical application to the eye, medrysone and fluorometholone. Medrysone (previously known as hydroxymesterone) is formulated as a 1.0 per cent ophthalmic suspension, but there are very few validated data about this drug available to the ophthalmologist. Clinical experience indicates that it is a very weak anti-inflammatory agent that must be relegated to the treatment of relatively minor conjunctival inflammation. It seemingly has no place in the treatment of serious ocular disease such as inflammatory keratitis. Its major asset appears to be that it is least likely among all ophthalmic corticosteroid formulations to produce a steroid-induced glaucoma.

Fluorometholone is available as a topical ophthalmic formulation only as an alcohol derivative at a 0.1 per cent concentration. There is evidence that it is much less apt to produce an elevation of intraocular pressure following prolonged administration than are the more conventional prednisolone and dexamethasone formulations.[22–24] Although comparatively little fluorometholone penetrates into and through the cornea,[25] the drug is highly potent and therefore produces a moderate suppression of corneal inflammation (Table 11–5).[26] Prednisolone acetate 1.0 per cent is considerably more effective than fluorometholone 0.1 per cent, and the former remains the agent of choice when maximal anti-inflammatory effect is required. However, in view of fluorometholone's apparently lesser potential for elevating the intraocular pressure, it would seem reasonable to substitute this agent for prednisolone acetate 1.0 per cent when the response to treatment of the acute inflammatory reaction is sufficient so that maximum pharmacologic suppression is no longer required. Fluorometholone also appears to be a reasonable choice for treatment of chronic inflammatory conditions requiring extended periods of therapy, a situation in which the incidence of steroid-induced glaucoma increases.

The acetate derivative of fluorometholone has recently become available for investigation. Studies in experimental animals show that this corticosteroid base (i.e., fluorometholone) behaves in the same manner as prednisolone and dexamethasone; the acetate derivative is much more effective as a topical ophthalmic anti-inflammatory agent than is the alcohol derivative.[27] Clinical evaluation of this new fluorometholone derivative is in progress.

Dosage of Topically Administered Corticosteroids

In practice the principal means of regulating the dosage of a topically applied corticosteroid is to vary the frequency with which the medication is instilled. Surprisingly few controlled data are available that relate the frequency of administration to therapeutic effect. With few exceptions, the package insert accompanying ophthalmic corticosteroid products contains a recommendation from the manufacturer that the medication be instilled four times daily. However, we are not told whether this is an average dose regimen, the most effective regimen, or the least toxic regimen, nor do we receive any guidance as to whether this is the recommended treatment for an inflammatory disorder of relatively minor severity or for one with potentially grave visual consequences. For treatment of a keratitis, clinical observation with a slit-lamp biomicroscope is the best means of evaluating therapeutic effectiveness. However, data resulting from our experimental observations provide useful guidelines for treatment[28] (Table 11–9). Hourly instillation of 1.0 per cent prednisolone acetate produces a much greater, more rapid reduction of corneal inflammation than does instillation of the drug every 4 hours. Nonetheless, hourly topical administration does not produce maximal anti-inflammatory effect; instillation of this corticosteroid at 15-minute intervals results in an even greater reduction of the polymorphonuclear leukocytes invading the cornea. (The effect of more frequent instillation was not studied.) However, in our clinical experience administration of topical medications more often than every hour has been impractical. Should this level of anti-inflammatory effect be required on a short-term basis, our experimental data indicate that the delivery of five doses at 1-minute intervals each hour results in a therapeutic effect comparable to that achieved by instillation every 15 minutes. This regimen seems to be more readily implemented in a clinical setting than instillation at 15-minute intervals. A word of caution is in order, however. Though application of prednisolone acetate more frequently than once an hour, or administration of five doses of the medication at 1-minute intervals each hour, is more effective than instillation of a single hourly dose, these regimens may also be more toxic. They should be used in clinical therapy with caution and only for limited periods.

Relevance of Animal Data to Clinical Therapy

The preceding data on bioavailability and therapeutic effectiveness of corticosteroids administered topically to the eye have been obtained in experimental animals under carefully controlled conditions in the laboratory. Unfortunately, in most instances available techniques preclude direct confirmation of this experimental evidence in humans. However, it is possible to safely acquire human data on corneal drug penetration. Topically applied 1.0 per cent prednisolone acetate penetrates rapidly through the human cornea.[29] Substantial amounts can be detected in the aqueous humor 5 minutes after the drug is ad-

Table 11–9. RELATIONSHIP OF FREQUENCY OF TOPICAL ADMINISTRATION OF 1.0 PER CENT PREDNISOLONE ACETATE AND ANTI-INFLAMMATORY EFFECT IN THE CORNEA

Treatment Regimen	Total Doses Delivered	Decrease in Corneal Inflammation (Per Cent)
1 drop every 4 hours	6	11
1 drop every 2 hours	10	30
1 drop every hour	18	51
1 drop every 30 minutes	34	61
1 drop every 15 minutes	66	68
1 drop each minute for 5 minutes every hour	90	72

Table 11–10. PENETRATION OF TOPICALLY ADMINISTERED PREDNISOLONE ACETATE
THROUGH THE CORNEA: COMPARISON OF RABBIT AND HUMAN DATA*

	Rabbit	Human
Peak aqueous humor drug level	1.52 μg./ml.	1.13 μg./ml.
Interval after drug administration peak levels attained	30–45 min.	30–45 min.
Half life of drug in aqueous humor	35 min.	28 min.
Aqueous humor bioavailability	140 μg.-min./ml.	88 μg.-min./ml.

*There is no statistically significant difference (p>0.05) between any of the rabbit and human values.

ministered, the shortest interval measured. Peak concentration in the aqueous humor occurs between 30 and 45 minutes after topical therapy and decreases progressively thereafter. The half life of prednisolone acetate in the human aqueous humor has been calculated to be 28 minutes. Only minimal quantities of the drug are present at intervals greater than 2 hours after instillation. Comparison of the human and rabbit data on corneal penetration of topically applied 1.0 per cent prednisolone acetate ophthalmic suspension demonstrates that there is little difference between the two species. No statistically significant difference could be found in the values for peak aqueous humor drug level, the time at which peak drug level was attained, the half life of the drug in aqueous humor, or the bioavailability value of this corticosteroid in the aqueous humor (Table 11–10).

Perhaps most significant was the finding that the shape of the curve relating aqueous humor concentration to time is the same in the two species[29] (Fig. 11–2). This curve is a graphic representation

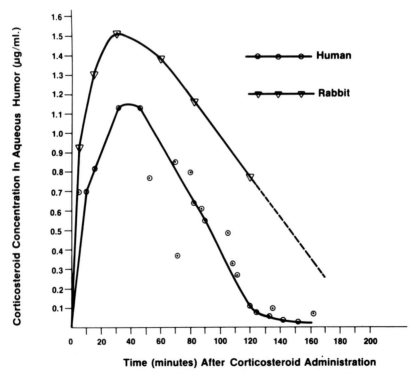

Figure 11–2. Drug concentration in aqueous humor versus time curves for 1.0 per cent prednisolone acetate in rabbit and human eyes. (From Leibowitz, H. M., et al.: Penetration of topically administered prednisolone acetate into human aqueous humor. Published with permission from The American Journal of Ophthalmology 83:402–406, 1977. Copyright by The Ophthalmic Publishing Company.)

of the dynamic interaction among several processes: drug penetration, absorption, distribution, excretion, and metabolism. Although there may well be substantial differences between the two species in one or even in several of these processes individually, the net loss of drug from the anterior chamber is the same in rabbit and man. The remarkable similarity in the shapes of the aqueous humor concentration versus time curves of the two species strongly suggests that the net kinetics of the drug relative to its penetration are the same.

Substantial differences in ocular morphology and physiology exist between the two species (e.g., corneal thickness, blink rate, tear flow dynamics). Nonetheless, we could demonstrate no significant difference in any of the parameters we investigated relating to bioavailability of 1.0 per cent prednisolone acetate in the aqueous humor. This supports the contention that, for this drug at least, the pharmacologic data obtained in quantitative studies in the rabbit can be used to establish meaningful guidelines for use of the drug to treat human disease.

PERIOCULARLY INJECTED CORTICOSTEROIDS

Local therapy of inflammatory keratitis can also be accomplished by administering corticosteroids via the periocular route. There are no commercially available corticosteroid products specifically formulated for periocular injection, but theoretically any compound that is available for administration by either the intramuscular or the intravenous route can be injected subconjunctivally or beneath Tenon's capsule. Our preference is for those compounds that are suitable for intravenous administration, since these represent the most highly purified preparations and are least likely to cause local toxicity. The two most widely used formulations are dexamethasone sodium phosphate (Decadron) and methylprednisolone sodium succinate (Solu-Medrol). Following systemic administration,

dexamethasone is five times more potent in terms of its anti-inflammatory effect than is methylprednisolone (Table 11–1). Therefore, the 4 mg. of dexamethasone contained in 1 ml. of the commercially available Decadron formulation is equivalent to approximately 20 mg. of methylprednisolone. However, 1 ml. of Solu-Medrol contains as much as 62.5 mg., so one would anticipate that the Solu-Medrol would be a more effective anti-inflammatory agent than Decadron when injected periocularly in the same volume. (The volume of material that can be injected periocularly generally is limited to 1 ml.) However, controlled studies of these two drugs and of prednisolone acetate, the preparation most effective after topical instillation, demonstrate quite clearly that the anti-inflammatory effectiveness of steroids in the cornea after periocular injection is not the same as that documented after systemic administration.[30] Neither do the observations on topical corticosteroids relating to changes in anti-inflammatory effect among various derivatives of the corticosteroid base appear to be important in dealing with periocular in-

Table 11–11. MEAN DECREASE IN CORNEAL INFLAMMATORY ACTIVITY FOLLOWING LOCAL STEROID THERAPY

Treatment Protocol	Per Cent Decrease
Topical Application	
Prednisolone acetate 1.0% (Econopred Plus)	52
Subconjunctival Injection	
Prednisolone acetate 25 mg./ml. (Meticortelone)	15
Prednisolone acetate 100 mg./ml. (Durapred)	24
Methylprednisolone sodium succinate 40 mg./ml. (Solu-Medrol)	20
Dexamethasone sodium phosphate 4 mg./ml. (Decadron)	30
Saline 0.9%	1
Combined Topical Application and Subconjunctival Injection	
Prednisolone acetate 1.0% (topical) and methylprednisolone sodium succinate (subconjunctival)	70

jection of the drugs. Moreover, contrary to general opinion, these controlled experiments also demonstrate that topical instillation of a corticosteroid produces a significantly greater reduction in polymorphonuclear leukocytes invading the cornea than does periocular injection of the steroid (Table 11–11). Topical administration over a 30-hour period of 13 drops of 1.0 per cent prednisolone acetate, containing a total of 6.5 mg. of the steroid, reduced corneal inflammatory activity by 52 per cent. Subconjunctival injection of 50 mg. of the same steroid, prednisolone acetate, also given over a 30-hour period yielded only a 15 per cent reduction in corneal inflammation. A fourfold increase in the injected prednisolone acetate to 200 mg. resulted in only a small increment in anti-inflammatory effect, a 24 per cent reduction in PMNs in the cornea. This small increase in therapeutic effect is neither statistically significant nor commensurate with the massive amount of drug injected in proximity to the globe. The maximal therapeutic effect we were able to document following subconjunctival steroid administration, a 30 per cent reduction in corneal inflammation, was achieved by injection of a total of 8 mg. of dexamethasone sodium phosphate during the 30-hour experimental period, still significantly less than that produced after topical steroid instillation.[30] Therefore, the data strongly suggest that *topical administration of corticosteroids should be the primary route of therapy for corneal inflammation.*

The data also appear to indicate that periocular injection of steroid should be reserved for those situations in which an anti-inflammatory effect greater than can be attained by topically administered drugs is necessary. Administration of corticosteroids concurrently by both the topical and the subconjunctival route seemingly produces an additive anti-inflammatory effect. The mean value obtained after concurrent administration via the two routes was essentially equal to the sum of the mean values obtained when the two component drugs were administered individ-

ually (Table 11–11). Clinically, then, *the addition of subconjunctivally injected corticosteroids to a topical regimen may produce a significant increase in therapeutic effect in the cornea.*[30]

ABRUPT CESSATION OF TOPICAL CORTICOSTEROIDS

With regard to the use of local corticosteroids to treat inflammatory keratitis, particularly in high dosage, an additional point merits strong emphasis. It is widely appreciated that abrupt cessation of prolonged high-dose systemic corticosteroid therapy carries with it a significant, potentially life-threatening risk of adrenal insufficiency. However, it does not seem to be widely recognized that abrupt cessation of high-dose topical steroid used to treat corneal inflammation also carries with it a substantial risk. Corticosteroids, like x-rays, remove the more mature leukocytic elements. When white-cell proliferation is allowed to recur, that is, when the steroids are discontinued, the reaction is characterized by proliferation of immature cells (blast or immune recognition cells), which produce great quantities of antibodies to residual antigen in the corneal stroma. Therefore, abrupt discontinuation of corticosteroid therapy can induce a rebound phenomenon and so precipitate an explosive necrotizing inflammatory reaction (Fig. 11–3). This probably represents a massive antigen-antibody reaction between large quantities of residual antigen and unchecked antibody production followed by an overwhelming polymorphonuclear leukocyte reaction. If this sequence of events is not interrupted immediately by the reinstitution of corticosteroid therapy, the cornea may perforate. Therefore, if in the course of treatment of a serious inflammatory reaction of the corneal stroma the need should arise to discontinue topical corticosteroids, this should be done gradually. The frequency with which the corticosteroid is administered should be decreased slowly but progressively and the inflammatory response in

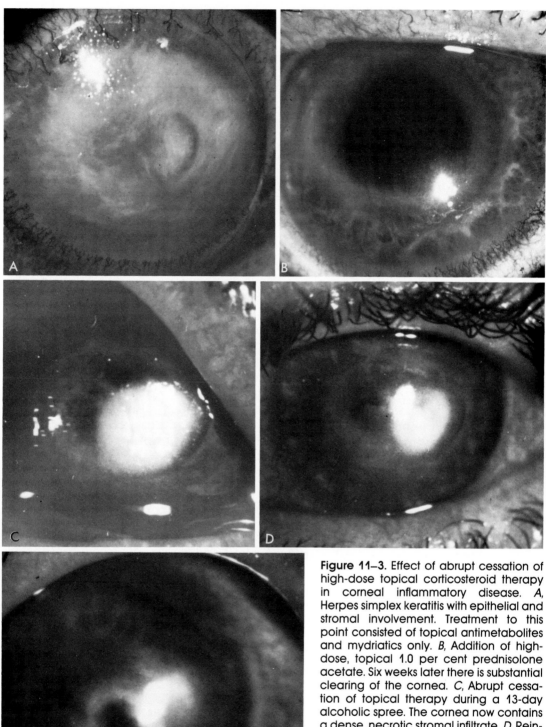

Figure 11–3. Effect of abrupt cessation of high-dose topical corticosteroid therapy in corneal inflammatory disease. *A,* Herpes simplex keratitis with epithelial and stromal involvement. Treatment to this point consisted of topical antimetabolites and mydriatics only. *B,* Addition of high-dose, topical 1.0 per cent prednisolone acetate. Six weeks later there is substantial clearing of the cornea. *C,* Abrupt cessation of topical therapy during a 13-day alcoholic spree. The cornea now contains a dense, necrotic stromal infiltrate. *D,* Reinstitution of topical therapy including high-dose 1.0 per cent prednisolone acetate. Two weeks later the stromal infiltrate shows early signs of resolution. *E,* Abrupt cessation of topical therapy once again, during a second alcoholic spree lasting 6 days. Stromal necrosis with marked tissue loss is evidenced by a bulging descemetocele. Penetrating keratoplasty was required to preserve the integrity of the globe.

the cornea carefully evaluated each time the dose is decreased. Any increase in the severity of a stromal infiltrate must be met with an immediate increase in the corticosteroid dosage. When the corneal inflammatory response is again stable, an attempt is again made to slowly taper the medication.

A hydrophilic contact lens applied to the cornea as a therapeutic device will act as a barrier to topically administered drugs. Corneal bioavailability of a drug will be substantially less than is achieved by the same drug in the absence of the contact lens. Therefore, if a severely inflamed cornea that is being treated with high-dose topically administered corticosteroids is fitted with such a lens, the resultant sudden reduction in corneal steroid levels may be sufficient to allow a rebound of the inflammatory response. We suggest that the stromal inflammatory response first be treated aggressively and brought substantially under control. Tapering of the topical steroid regimen should be well along before a soft contact lens is fitted as a therapeutic adjunct.

COMPLICATIONS

Local administration of corticosteroids significantly decreases the incidence of systemic complications. Indeed, particularly following topical instillation, undesirable systemic side effects of corticosteroids ordinarily do not occur in adults, even when the drug is used for extended periods. Unfortunately, however, local routes of corticosteroid delivery do carry with them a significant potential for local ocular complications. These include (1) enhancement of microbial proliferation, (2) glaucoma, (3) cataract formation, (4) retardation of epithelial regeneration and stromal wound healing, and (5) local intravascular clotting. Since none of these problems constitutes an absolute contraindication to topical corticosteroid administration, a brief discussion of each is in order. Adherence to certain basic principles and

frequent evaluation of the patient permit corticosteroids to be used beneficially in many instances.

Enhancement of Microbial Replication

In the treatment of a keratitis caused by a replicating microorganism, the ophthalmologist must consider the possibility that corticosteroids may enhance microbial replication. Therefore, as a cardinal rule corticosteroids should not be used unless a specific therapeutic agent capable of interfering with replication of the causal organism is available and is administered concurrently. However, a proper discussion of this problem as it relates to the eye requires that different types of microorganisms be considered separately.

In bacterial keratitis we believe that corticosteroids should be used to prevent the structural damage that leads to permanent corneal scarring in cases involving the central and paracentral cornea. Concomitant effective antibiotic therapy is an absolute requirement in all instances. There is experimental evidence in systems other than the eye that a high concentration of corticosteroids impairs phagocytosis and intracellular killing of bacteria,[31-34] so that treatment can interfere with host defense mechanisms and cause clinical worsening of the situation. However, there also is experimental evidence demonstrating that, following concurrent instillation of a bactericidal antibiotic and a corticosteroid, pathogenic bacteria (Staphylococcus aureus, Pseudomonas aeruginosa) are eliminated from the cornea in a manner indistinguishable from that following treatment with the antibiotic alone.[35] Indeed, no apparent difference in bacterial replication in the cornea was observed between eyes that were treated only with corticosteroid drops and eyes that were not treated at all. Enhancement of bacterial replication by corticosteroids was not found. These findings support the conclusion that the addition of a topically applied corticosteroid to an effective topical antibiotic regimen containing a bactericidal agent does not enhance bacterial replication in the cornea if the corticosteroid is not instilled more frequently than the antibiotic.

It appears that when a bactericidal antibiotic and a corticosteroid are instilled concurrently to treat bacterial keratitis, a favorable balance is struck. The antibiotic continues to eliminate the microorganisms from the cornea with no apparent interference from the corticosteroid. In view of this evidence, the use of corticosteroids as part of a therapeutic regimen for central and paracentral bacterial keratitis seems reasonable. Our clinical experience bears this out.

The principles relating to corticosteroid administration in herpes simplex keratitis are more complex, and it is here that the greatest confusion is encountered. Involvement of the corneal epithelium by this organism (e.g., classic dendritic keratitis) is due to infection by live replicating virus, and local corticosteroids will make matters worse. Corticosteroids enhance proliferation of the virus actively replicating within the epithelial cells, causing more severe pathologic alteration of the cornea,[36, 37] a phenomenon well documented both by experimental data and by clinical observation. When corticosteroids are instilled, replicating virus persists and can be cultured for a longer period of time, the epithelial abnormalities run a more prolonged course and tend to be more severe (i.e., geographic defects), and there is a greater incidence of stromal involvement. The undesirable effects of corticosteroids are counteracted to some degree by concomitant administration of one of the antiviral antimetabolites,[38, 39] but the ameliorating effect of the antimetabolite is only partial. Corticosteroids continue to enhance viral proliferation, albeit to a lesser extent. They should not be part of the treatment regimen of an active herpetic dendritic or geographic epithelial keratitis.

On the other hand, there is no solid evidence incriminating replicating virus in chronic stromal herpetic keratitis. It appears obvious that live, replicating viruses must enter the stroma from the epithelium, but seemingly they do not persist within the corneal stroma for any prolonged period in a form capable of replication. Generally virus cannot be successfully cultured from the stromal form of the disease, and although viral material has been demonstrated by electron microscopy,[40] this appears to be made up of incomplete viral particles incapable of replication. Presumably most instances of herpetic disease of the corneal stroma represent a toxic or an immune response to incomplete, nonreplicating viral particles rather than direct damage caused by multiplying live virus. Clinical experience supports this thesis, and we advocate corticosteroids based on the same rationale outlined for bacterial keratitis. Topical corticosteroids eliminate many of the polymorphonuclear leukocytes that invade the stroma, and they substantially lessen the destruction wrought by hydrolytic enzymes released from these inflammatory cells rather than enhance the severity of this form of the disease. Therefore, there seems to be a place for the appropriate use of local corticosteroids in chronic stromal herpetic keratitis. An antiviral agent, usually 0.1 per cent idoxuridine, is administered concurrently on a dose-for-dose basis with the corticosteroid. There is evidence that latent virus persists in the trigeminal ganglion[41] and that periodically reactivation of the latent virus spontaneously occurs.[42] Cultures of the conjunctival sac demonstrate replicating virus at such times; although the antimetabolite penetrates poorly into corneal stroma, it appears to be effective in dealing with these organisms, decreasing the incidence of reinfection of the corneal epithelium.[39]

It seems to be a widely held concept that local corticosteroid therapy may reactivate herpes simplex virus and produce active disease in a cornea previously infected with the organism but quiescent or free of active herpetic disease at the time steroid therapy is initiated. This concept lacks experimental support, and in fact controlled animal experiments demonstrate just the opposite—that is, that local steroids neither reactivate occult or latent virus nor induce herpetic corneal disease in a clinically quiescent eye.[43] Perhaps the best demonstration of this in the human is the almost universal successful use of local steroids following penetrating keratoplasty for herpetic keratitis.

However, this should not be construed as support for the indiscriminate use of corticosteroids in eyes previously infected by herpes simplex virus. As we have stated, occult or latent herpes simplex virus persists in the vicinity of human eyes, apparently in the trigeminal ganglion.[41] Spontaneous shedding of infective viral particles intermittently occurs, and these episodes may be accompanied by recurrent, active epithelial infection. Should such a recurrent epithelial infection occur coincidentally with steroid administration, it seems reasonable to assume that the resultant corneal pathology might be made more severe. Thus, the use of corticosteroids in eyes previously infected by herpes simplex virus undoubtedly entails some degree of risk, and these patients must be followed closely. Nonetheless, the ability of local corticosteroids to control inflammatory processes in stromal herpetic keratitis can be dramatic. In many instances corneal structure can be preserved, transparency restored, and vision saved. The potential for visual preservation offered by corticosteroid therapy justifies its judicious use in this situation.

In the other more common forms of viral keratitis caused by adenovirus (epidemic keratoconjunctivitis) and herpes zoster (herpes zoster ophthalmicus) there is no documented evidence that topically applied corticosteroids enhance viral proliferation. At times they are useful in controlling the resultant inflammatory processes in the cornea. Similarly, local corticosteroids do not cause a worsening of the corneal inflammation resulting from chlamydial infection (e.g., inclusion conjunctivitis). Unfortunately, however, they exert very little positive effect on chlamydial keratoconjunctivitis.

Theoretically those principles applicable to the use of corticosteroids in bacterial keratitis should also apply to fungal keratitis, and evidence that they do has been published.[44] However, in many instances control of the replicating mycotic organisms is difficult or impossible. Either the specific antifungal agent is limited in its effectiveness, or it is not readily available in the United States, or it does not exist. Local corticosteroids should not be used to treat fungal keratitis except, perhaps, by those highly experienced in its management. Even in this instance corticosteroids should be withheld until specific antifungal therapy demonstrates signs of clinical improvement.

Glaucoma

Topically applied corticosteroids can cause glaucoma in susceptible individuals.[45–52] Extensive studies of steroid-induced glaucoma have provided evidence of genetic predisposition for this response.[53–55] However, an additional study at the National Eye Institute of 63 sets of twins indicated that the intraocular pressure response to topical dexamethasone was more consistent between dizygotic twins than between monozygotic twins.[56] This finding, along with evidence presented by Francois and colleagues,[57] seems inconsistent with previous theories of the heredity of steroid-induced glaucoma, and it appears fair to conclude that the mechanism of inheritance of this response is not completely understood. In any event, the best evidence available today indicates that a substantial portion of the total population is susceptible to topically administered corticosteroids and will develop elevated intraocular pressure if the drug is administered long enough.

The response is an insidious one. In normal volunteers the eye remains white and quiet and free of symptoms. In patients with ocular disease symptoms and signs are those of the disease for which they are receiving treatment. The intraocular pressure increases and this is accompanied by a decrease in the facility of outflow of the aqueous humor. Clearly the steroid-induced glaucoma results from interference with the outflow of aqueous humor from the eye.

Generally, susceptible individuals will demonstrate a positive response within 3 or 4 weeks after steroid therapy has been initiated. In our experience it is unusual to obtain a positive response in less than 2 weeks, but we have encountered many patients who do not demonstrate a positive intraocular pressure response until topical corticosteroids have been administered for 6 weeks or considerably longer. (We have also seen a significant steroid-related elevation of intraocular pressure after only 72 hours of topical steroid therapy.) In most instances the intraocular pressure will return to the original levels after topical steroids have been discontinued—usually within a 2- to 4-week period after therapy has been terminated. Unfortunately this is not always the case. There are documented reports of cases in which the glaucoma persisted after the corticosteroid drops had been discontinued.[57, 58] It has been argued that since these patients were steroid responders, they had an inherited predisposition to develop glaucoma and would have developed the disease even if they had not received corticosteroid drops. While perhaps true, this point has not been proved, and it is doubtful that one could convince the patient (or his lawyer) of its validity.

If corticosteroid drops continue to be instilled in those with a positive response, intraocular pressure levels in the 40 to 60 mm. Hg range are not unusual. If only one eye is being treated, the glaucoma response will be confined to that eye. The steroid-induced ocular hypertensive response generally is greater and occurs more rapidly when the drug is applied to an eye with open-angle glaucoma than when it is applied to a normal eye. Steroid-induced glaucoma will cause optic atrophy and permanent visual-field defects similar to those caused by typical open-angle glaucoma.

The intensity of the glaucomatous response depends on the frequency and the duration of corticosteroid administration. It does not seem to be directly related to the anti-inflammatory potency of the corticosteroid compound, either as measured by in vivo suppression of leukocytes in the rabbit cornea[15] or by in vitro inhibition of phytohemagglutinin stimulation of human lymphocyte transformation.[59] Nor does the rise in intraocular pressure appear to be related to the ability of the corticosteroid compound to penetrate into and through the cornea. Cantrill and coworkers found that in ten patients known to have high responses to corticosteroids dexamethasone sodium phosphate 0.1 per cent raised intraocular pressure to significantly higher levels than prednisolone acetate 1.0 per cent.[60] This is somewhat surprising, given the greater in vitro corneal permeability,[61] the greater bioavailability in cornea and aqueous humor of the intact eye,[8] and the greater anti-inflammatory effectiveness in the cornea[8] of prednisolone acetate. However, Mindel and coworkers[62] have presented data that support a totally different conclusion. In their study 54 volunteers with normal intraocular pressure were treated with various commercially available ophthalmic corticosteroids. Compliance was controlled by having nurses administer the drops, an extremely important factor that few, if any, studies have been able to regulate. These investigators found no significant difference between prednisolone acetate and prednisolone phosphate, between dexamethasone phosphate and dexamethasone alcohol, or between prednisolone acetate and dexamethasone phosphate in intraocular pressure elevating response. They concluded that ocular absorption of each of the corticosteroid derivatives exceeded the minimal amounts necessary to maximally elevate intraocular pressure.

Palmberg and coworkers[63] found that the reproducibility of the intraocular pressure response to topically applied dexamethasone phosphate 0.1 per cent was only 73 per cent. They attributed the unexpected results of the identical twin study cited above to the limited precision of the topical corticosteroid response, and it is possible that this also might explain the lack of agreement among reported intraocular pressure responses to different ophthalmic corticosteroids. However, Mindel and associates[62] suggest that lack of compliance with the experimental protocol among subjects is a much more likely explanation for these phenomena, including Palmberg and coworkers' finding of poor reproducibility of the topical steroid intraocular pressure response.

Despite this disparity in the results of clinical studies, it is clear that all available derivatives of prednisolone and dexamethasone are capable of elevating the intraocular pressure when applied topically to the eyes of susceptible individuals. By conventional systemic measurements (see Table 11–1), prednisolone and dexamethasone are potent synthetic anti-inflammatory corticosteroids. Attempts have been made to develop ophthalmic corticosteroids in which there is a separation of the anti-inflammatory and the glaucomatous effects. Fluorometholone in a 0.1 per cent concentration has been most heavily promoted in this regard, and it does appear to have a much lesser propensity to elevate the intraocular pressure than does, for example, prednisolone in a 1.0 per cent concentration.[23, 60] However, the fluorometholone drops have significantly less anti-inflammatory effect in the cornea than do the prednisolone drops, and it is not clear how much the lower incidence of glaucoma induced by fluorometholone administration simply reflects its lower anti-inflammatory effectiveness. For example, if the concentration of dexamethasone phosphate is decreased from 0.1 per cent to 0.005 per cent, the elevation of intraocular pressure produced by the lower concentration is not significantly different from that produced by fluorometholone 0.1 per cent.[60] From a clinical standpoint, perhaps the most important fact to bear

in mind is that, while fewer patients on fluorometholone may develop steroid-induced glaucoma, the problem nonetheless has been caused by this drug; the intraocular pressure of patients using fluorometholone must be monitored as closely as that of patients on other corticosteroids.

As might be expected, the degree of ocular damage is not specifically related to the duration of steroid administration but, rather, to the length of time and to the degree to which the intraocular pressure has been elevated. Steroid-induced glaucoma may be only partly reversed by conventional therapy with epinephrine, miotics, beta blockers, and carbonic anhydrase inhibitors if the topically administered corticosteroid is not discontinued. Conversely, however, should corticosteroid therapy be necessary to control an ocular inflammatory response, conventional glaucoma medications will be helpful in controlling the intraocular pressure, at least in the early stages of a steroid-induced glaucoma, and they will permit the corticosteroid to be administered for a time without irreversible ocular damage occurring. Unfortunately, in most instances the glaucoma medications will become progressively less effective if corticosteroid administration is continued. Discontinuation of the corticosteroid ultimately will be required if intraocular pressure is to be restored to normal levels.

Steroid-induced glaucoma can be caused by subconjunctival injection of corticosteroids.[64, 65] Indeed, following the single inoculation of a depot preparation, the elevated pressure may persist for a considerable period of time.[65] Whether or not steroid-induced glaucoma can be caused by systemically administered corticosteroids is not entirely clear. There are published studies that appear to indicate that systemically administered steroids can produce a statistically significant increase in intraocular pressure and a decrease in outflow facility. It is difficult to evaluate these data with certainty because a truly comparable control group is not available. Perhaps a fair commentary on this aspect of the problem is that, if systemically administered steroids do produce elevation of intraocular pressure in susceptible individuals then long-term administration (probably in excess of a year) is required and the severity of the response is not as dramatic as that observed after local steroid administration.

Cataract

There is evidence that topical steroids may cause posterior subcapsular cataracts.[66-68] Apparently a relatively long period of corticosteroid administration is required. The true prevalence of this problem is difficult to ascertain, since prolonged topical steroid administration frequently is used to treat chronic inflammatory conditions that are themselves cataractogenic.

Posterior subcapsular cataract also may occur as a complication of long-term, high-dose systemic corticosteroid therapy.[69-75] Other than its location beneath the posterior lens capsule, there is nothing specific about the morphologic appearance of a steroid-induced cataract. Clinically it cannot be differentiated from senile posterior subcapsular cataract, from radiation cataracts, or from cataracts associated with intraocular inflammation. The dosage and the duration of systemic steroid administration appear to be the determining factors in the production of posterior subcapsular cataract; the prevalence of the cataract seems to be directly related to the total steroid dose. Apparently these lens opacities do not appear until the patient has received steroids for more than 1 year, and thereafter their prevalence increases directly with the length of time that steroids are administered. The cataracts may increase in density after steroid dosage has been reduced or after the drug has been discontinued.

The weight of evidence indicates that long-term systemic corticosteroid therapy may have a cataractogenic effect.[76] However, much of the data has been obtained from patients with rheumatoid arthritis, and there is an unusually high incidence of posterior subcapsular cataracts among rheumatoid arthritis patients not receiving steroids. Thus, it is important to note that additional evidence supporting a cause-and-effect relationship between systemically administered corticosteroids and posterior subcapsular cataracts is obtained from studies of asthmatic children and adolescents. Among patients in this age group treated with corticosteroids for a year or longer, there is a significant incidence of posterior subcapsular lens opacities.[77, 78]

Wound Healing

Corticosteroids interfere with protein synthesis, decrease collagen deposition, and retard fibroplasia. These effects combine to delay wound healing, but it is difficult to transpose this information accurately to a practical level for the ophthalmologist. A review of the ophthalmic literature produced many controlled studies that support the conclusion that local steroids delay corneal wound healing,[79-83] yet other studies fail to demonstrate that steroids significantly retard wound healing.[84-86] Great variation is encountered in the strength of individual corticosteroid-treated wounds, and much depends on the manner in which the experiment is conducted and in which wound healing is measured. Impairment of corneal wound healing appears to be dose-related; weak or infrequently applied corticosteroids cause little or no alteration of wound strength. Undoubtedly of equal importance is the rapidity with which corticosteroid therapy is instituted. If the initial phases of fibroplasia are allowed to occur prior to the onset of therapy, then it becomes increasingly difficult to demonstrate any retardation of wound healing. Thus, although local corticosteroids undoubtedly retard or slow down the rate of healing of wounds involving the corneal stroma, modern techniques of ophthalmic microsurgery, properly executed, permit substantial quantities of corticosteroids to be instilled, when necessary, with few subsequent wound complications. If the initiation of steroid therapy can be delayed 24 to 48 hours, this should provide the surgeon with an extra margin of safety.

Delayed corneal re-epithelialization may be associated with microbial infections, alkali burns, penetrating keratoplasty, radiation keratoconjunctivitis, toxic keratopathies, dry eyes, and superficial injuries that produce the recurrent erosion syndrome. It is commonly stated that topically administered corticosteroids retard the regeneration of the corneal epithelium, but controlled data to support this statement generally are not cited. Experimental studies in rabbits by Elliott and coworkers[87] have shown that topical instillation of 0.1 per cent dexamethasone sodium phosphate at hourly intervals 16 times daily does indeed significantly retard the rate of epithelial regeneration in comparison to that which occurs when normal saline drops are instilled four times a day. However, dexamethasone sodium phosphate 0.1 per cent given hourly 16 times a day was no more detrimental to the corneal epithelial healing rate than the vehicle alone when it was similarly applied. These workers concluded that their data showed no specific adverse effect of the corticosteroid on the corneal epithelial healing rate. However, the insult of frequent (in this case hourly) topical drops causes a significant slowdown in the rate of regeneration of the corneal epithelium. Presumably most ophthalmic formulations, if administered frequently enough, will retard epithelial regeneration in a similar fashion.

Local Intravascular Clotting

An inflammatory reaction in a vascularized tissue often includes a perivasculitis. This damages the endothelium of the involved blood vessel, causing fibrinogen to accumulate and to polymerize to fibrin. The fibrin deposition causes platelets to aggregate, which in turn leads to thrombus formation and to vascular occlusion. Vascular occlusion can, of course, produce ischemic necrosis. In the cornea this sequence of events is important primarily when it involves the limbal arcade of blood vessels. The patency of these vessels is a requirement for the nutrition and maintenance of the peripheral cornea. If they become occluded as the result of an inflammatory reaction or a collagen vascular disease, ischemic necrosis of the peripheral cornea can occur; this is manifested as a peripheral ringlike ulcer, which can progress to perforation. Vascular ischemia is an unequivocal contraindication to local steroid therapy, since corticosteroids promote fibrin accumulation within blood vessels and thereby can intensify the active ischemic process. However, once such ischemia has been overcome (the use of subconjunctivally injected heparin has been recommended for this purpose), corticosteroids then may be used to treat the inflammation.[88, 89]

Other Complications

Despite their pre-eminent role in the treatment of ocular inflammation, topically administered corticosteroids also have been associated, presumably on a cause-and-effect basis, with the occurrence of an acute anterior uveitis.[62, 90, 91] Invariably the anterior uveitis appeared in a previously uninflamed eye receiving the medication during a provocative test for glaucoma. Most cases had their onset within a few days after discontinuation of the drug, although the uveitis has been reported in subjects still using corticosteroid drops. The great majority of cases have occurred in blacks, while the incidence in men and women has been approximately equal. There is no apparent relationship between the uveitis and intraocular pressure response to topical corticosteroids. Presenting symptoms include ocular pain, photophobia, and blurred vision; presenting signs include conjunctival injection, perilimbal hyperemia, and anterior chamber reaction characterized by cells, flare, and keratic precipitates. There seems to be no relationship between the uveitis and any specific ophthalmic corticosteroid formulation. The anterior chamber inflammatory reaction has occurred after topical instillation of dexamethasone sodium phosphate, dexamethasone alcohol, prednisolone acetate, and triamcinolone acetonide.

Topically administered corticosteroids also may cause a mild blepharoptosis and mild mydriasis.[92] The mechanisms producing these effects are not known.

SUMMARY

Corticosteroids are by far the most frequently used agents to treat ocular inflammation. When administered topically to the eye, different derivatives of the same corticosteroid base are not equivalent in their anti-inflammatory properties. A change in the derivative of a corticosteroid base alters its behavior as an anti-inflammatory agent. To date the acetate derivative of each corticosteroid base studied has been the most effective, and among commercially available ophthalmic formulations 1.0 per cent prednisolone acetate is the drug of choice for maximal anti-inflammatory effect. Hourly instillation produces a greater, more rapid reduction of corneal inflammation than does instillation of the drug every 4 hours, whereas instillation at 15-minute intervals results in an even greater therapeutic effect. Topical delivery of five doses of 1.0 per cent prednisolone acetate at 1-minute intervals each hour results in an anti-inflammatory effect comparable to that achieved by instillation every 15 minutes.

Topical instillation of a corticosteroid produces a greater reduction in inflammatory cells invading the cornea than does periocular injection of a steroid. Administration of corticosteroids concurrently by topical and subconjunctival routes produces an additive anti-inflammatory effect.

Addition of a topically applied corticosteroid to an effective topical antibiotic regimen containing a bactericidal agent does not enhance bacterial replication in the cornea if the corticosteroid is not instilled more frequently than the antibiotic. Corticosteroids enhance viral proliferation and are contraindicated in active epithelial herpetic keratitis. In many instances stromal herpetic keratitis appears to be a toxic or immune response to incomplete, nonreplicating viral particles rather than an alteration of tissue by multiplying live virus, and the judicious use of corticosteroids is advocated along with an antiviral antimetabolite. Because control of replicating fungal organisms by specific antifungal agents is often difficult to achieve, corticosteroids should not be used in the treatment of mycotic keratitis.

Complications associated with local administration of corticosteroids include glaucoma, cataract, enhancement of microbial replication, retardation of epithelial regeneration and stromal wound healing, and intravascular clotting of the limbal circulation with ischemic necrosis of the peripheral cornea. None constitutes an absolute contraindication to use of the drug. Adherence to certain basic principles and frequent evaluation of the patient permits corticosteroids to be used beneficially in many instances.

REFERENCES

1. Cope, C. L.: *Adrenal Steroids and Disease.* Philadelphia, J. B. Lippincott Co., 1964.
2. Dougherty, T. F., and White, A.: Evaluation of alterations produced in lymphoid tissue by pituitary–adrenal cortical secretion. J Lab Clin Med 32:584, 1947.
3. Spain, D. M.: Steroid alterations in the histopathology of chemically induced inflammation. In Mills, L. C., and Moyer, J. W. (eds.): *Inflammation and Diseases of Connective Tissue.* Philadelphia, W. B. Saunders Co., 1961, pp. 514–517.
4. Spector, W. G., and Willoughby, D. A.: *The Pharmacology of Inflammation.* New York, Grune & Stratton, 1968, p. 108.
5. Weissman, G.: Effect on lysosomes of drugs useful in connective tissue disease. In Campbell, E. G. (ed.): *Biological Council Symposium on the Interaction of Drugs and Subcellular Components in Animal Cells.* Vol. 2. Boston, Little, Brown, 1968, p. 203.
6. Weissman, G.: The many-faceted lysosome. In Good, R. A., and Fisher, D. W. (eds.): *Immunobiology.* Stamford, Conn., Sinauer Associates, 1971, pp. 37–43.
7. Kupferman, A., Pratt, M. V., Suckewer, K., and Leibowitz, H. M.: Topically applied steroids in corneal disease. III. The role of drug derivative in stromal absorption of dexamethasone. Arch Ophthalmol 91:373, 1974.
8. Leibowitz, H. M., and Kupferman, A.: Bioavailability and therapeutic effectiveness of topically administered corticosteroids. Trans Amer Acad Ophthalmol Otolaryngol 79:78, 1975.
9. Cox, W. V., Kupferman, A., and Leibowitz, H. M.: Topically applied steroids in corneal disease. I. The role of inflammation in stromal absorption of dexamethasone. Arch Ophthalmol 88:308, 1972.
10. Cox, W. V., Kupferman, A., and Leibowitz, H. M.: Topically applied steroids in corneal disease. II. The role of drug vehicle in stromal absorption of dexamethasone. Arch Ophthalmal 88:549, 1972.
11. Leibowitz, H. M., and Kupferman, A.: Pharmacology of topically applied dexamethasone. Trans Amer Acad Ophthalmol Otolaryngol 78:856, 1974.
12. Schoenwald, R. D., and Boltralik, J. J.: A bioavailability comparison in rabbits of two steroids formulated as high viscosity gels and reference aqueous preparations. Invest Ophthalmol Vis Sci 18:61, 1979.
13. Kupferman, A., Ryan, W. J., and Leibowitz, H. M.: Prolongation of the anti-inflammatory effect of prednisolone acetate: Influence of formulation in a high viscosity gel. Arch Ophthalmol 99:2028, 1981.
14. Goldberg, I., Ashburn, F. S., Jr., Kass, M. A., and Becker, B.: Efficacy and patient acceptance of pilocarpine gel. Amer J Ophthalmol 88:843, 1979.
15. Leibowitz, H. M., Lass, J. H., and Kupferman, A.: Quantitation of inflammation in the cornea. Arch Ophthalmol 92:427, 1974.
16. Leibowitz, H. M., and Kupferman, A.: Anti-inflammatory effectiveness in cornea of topically administered prednisolone. Invest Ophthalmol 13:757, 1974.
17. Kupferman, A., and Leibowitz, H. M.: Anti-inflammatory effectiveness of topically administered corticosteroids in the cornea without epithelium. Invest Ophthalmol 14:252, 1975.
18. Kupferman, A., and Leibowitz, H. M.: Biological

19. equivalence of ophthalmic prednisolone acetate suspensions. Amer J Ophthalmol 82:109, 1976.
19. Apt, L., Henrick, A., and Silverman, L. M.: Patient compliance with use of topical ophthalmic corticosteroid suspensions. Amer J Ophthalmol 87:210, 1979.
20. Leibowitz, H. M., Stewart, R. H., Kupferman, A., and Kimbrough, R. L.: Evaluation of dexamethasone acetate as a topical ophthalmic formulation. Amer J Ophthalmol 86:418, 1978.
21. Leibowitz, H. M. and Kupferman, A.: Kinetics of topically administered prednisolone acetate. Optimal concentration for treatment of inflammatory keratitis. Arch Ophthalmol 94:1387, 1976.
22. Becker, B., and Kolker, A. E.: Intraocular pressure response to topical corticosteroids. In Leopold, I. H. (ed.): *Ocular Therapy: Complications and Management.* St. Louis, C. V. Mosby Co., 1967, pp. 79–83.
23. Fairbairn, W. D., and Thorson, J. C.: Fluorometholone: Anti-inflammation and intraocular pressure effects. Arch Ophthalmol 86:138, 1971.
24. Stewart, R. H., and Kimbrough, R. L.: Intraocular pressure response to topical fluorometholone. Arch Ophthalmol 97:2139, 1979.
25. Leibowitz, H. M., and Kupferman, A.: Penetration of fluorometholone into the cornea and aqueous humor. Arch Ophthalmol 93:425, 1975.
26. Kupferman, A., and Leibowitz, H. M.: Therapeutic effectiveness of fluorometholone in inflammatory keratitis. Arch Ophthalmol 93:1011, 1975.
27. Kupferman, A., Berrospi, A. R., and Leibowitz, H. M.: Fluorometholone acetate: A new ophthalmic derivative of fluorometholone. Arch Ophthalmol 100:640, 1982.
28. Leibowitz, H. M., and Kupferman, A.: Optimal frequency of topical prednisolone administration. Arch Ophthalmol 97:2154, 1979.
29. Leibowitz, H. M., Berrospi, A. R., Kupferman, A., Velez-Restropo, G., Galvis, V., and Arango-Alvarez, J.: Penetration of topically administered prednisolone acetate into human aqueous humor. Amer J Ophthalmol 83:402, 1977.
30. Leibowitz, H. M., and Kupferman, A.: Periocular injection of corticosteroids. Arch Ophthalmol 95:311, 1977.
31. Allison, F., and Adcock, M. H.: The influence of hydrocortisone and certain electrolyte solutions upon phagocytic and bactericidal capacities of leukocytes obtained from peritoneal exudate of rats. J Immunol 92:435, 1964.
32. Crepa, S. B., Magnin, G. E., and Seastone, C. V.: Effect of ACTH and cortisone on phagocytosis. Proc Soc Exp Biol Med 77:704, 1951.
33. Mandell, G. L., Rubin, W., and Hook, E. W.: The effect of an NADH oxidase inhibitor (hydrocortisone) on polymorphonuclear leukocyte bacterial activity. J Clin Invest 409:1381, 1970.
34. Stossel, T. P., Mason, R. J., Hartwig, J., and Vaughan, M.: Quantitative studies of phagocytosis by polymorphonuclear leukocytes: Use of emulsions to measure the initial rate of phagocytosis. J Clin Invest 51:615, 1972.
35. Leibowitz, H. M., and Kupferman, A.: The effect of topically administered corticosteroids on antibiotic-treated bacterial keratitis. Arch Ophthalmol 98:1287, 1980.
36. Kaufman, H. E., and Maloney, E.D.: Experimental

herpes simplex keratitis: The effect of corticosteroids and epithelial curettage. Arch Ophthalmol 66:99, 1961.

37. Takahashi, G. H., Leibowitz, H. M., and Kibrick, S.: Topically applied steroids in active herpes simplex keratitis. Arch Ophthalmol 85:350, 1971.

38. Kaufman, H. E., and Maloney, E. D.: IDU-hydrocortisone in experimental herpes simplex keratitis. Arch Ophthalmol 68:396, 1962.

39. Patterson, A., and Jones, B. R.: The management of ocular herpes. Trans Ophthalmol Soc UK 87:59, 1967.

40. Dawson, C., Togni, B., and Moore, T. E., Jr.: Structural changes in chronic herpetic keratitis. Arch Ophthalmol 79:740, 1968.

41. Nesburn, A. B., Cook, M. L., and Stevens, J. G.: Latent herpes simplex virus: Isolation from rabbit trigeminal ganglia between episodes of recurrent ocular infection. Arch Ophthalmol 88:412, 1972.

42. Nesburn, A. B., Elliott, J. H., and Leibowitz, H. M.: Spontaneous reactivation of experimental herpes simplex keratitis in rabbits. Arch Ophthalmol 78:523, 1967.

43. Kibrick, S., Takahashi, G. H., Leibowitz, H. M., and Laibson, P. R.: Local corticosteroid therapy and reactivation of herpetic keratitis. Arch Ophthalmol 86:694, 1971.

44. Aronson, S. B., and Elliott, J. H.: *Ocular Inflammation.* St Louis, C. V. Mosby Co., 1972, p. 161.

45. Francois, J.: Cortisone et tension oculaire. Ann Oculist 187:805, 1954.

46. Goldman, H.: Cortisone glaucoma. Arch Ophthalmol 68:621, 1962.

47. Briggs, H. H.: Glaucoma associated with the use of topical corticosteroid. Arch Ophthalmol 70:312, 1963.

48. Bernstein, H. N., Mills, D. W., and Becker, B.: Steroid induced elevation of intraocular pressure. Arch Ophthalmol 70:15, 1963.

49. Armaly, M. F.: Effect of corticosteroids on intraocular pressure and fluid dynamics. I. The effect of dexamethasone on the normal eye. Arch Ophthalmol 70:482, 1963.

50. Becker, B., and Mills, D. W.: Corticosteroids and intraocular pressure. Arch Ophthalmol 70:500, 1963.

51. Armaly, M. F.: Effect of corticosteroids on intraocular pressure and fluid dynamics. III. Changes in visual function and pupil size during topical dexamethasone application. Arch Ophthalmol 71:636, 1964.

52. Lerman, S.: Steroid therapy and secondary glaucoma. Amer J Ophthalmol 56:31, 1963.

53. Becker, B., and Hahn, K. A.: Topical corticosteroids and heredity in primary open angle glaucoma. Amer J Ophthalmol 57:543, 1964.

54. Armaly, M. F.: Statistical attributes of the steroid hypertensive response in the clinically normal eye. Invest Ophthalmol 4:187, 1965.

55. Armaly, M. F.: The heritable nature of dexamethasone-induced ocular hypertension. Arch Ophthalmol 75:32, 1966.

56. Schwartz, J. T., Reuling, F. H., Jr., Feinlieb, M., Garrison, R. J., and Collie, D. J.: Twin heritability study of the corticosteroid response. Trans Amer Acad Ophthalmol Otolaryngol 77:126, 1973.

57. Francois, J., Heintz-DeBree, C., and Tripathi, R. C.: The cortisone test and the heredity of primary open-angle glaucoma. Amer J Ophthalmol 62:844, 1966.

58. Spiers, F.: A case of irreversible steroid-induced rise in intraocular pressure. Acta Ophthalmol 43:419, 1965.

59. Bigger, J. F., Palmberg, P. F., and Becker, B.: Increased cellular sensitivity to corticosteroids in primary open angle glaucoma. Invest Ophthalmol 11:832, 1972.

60. Cantrill, H. L., Palmberg, P. F., Zink, H. A., Waltman, S. R., Podos, S. M., and Becker, B.: Comparison of in vitro potency of corticosteroids with ability to raise intraocular pressure. Amer J Ophthalmol 79:1012, 1975.

61. Hull, D. S., Hine, J. E., Edelhauser, H. F., and Hyndiuk, R. A.: Permeability of isolated rabbit cornea to corticosteroids. Invest Ophthalmol 13:457, 1974.

62. Mindel, J. S., Goldberg, J., and Tavitian, H. O.: Similarity of the intraocular pressure response to different corticosteroid esters when compliance is controlled. Ophthalmology 86:99, 1979.

63. Palmberg, P. F., Mandell, A., Wilensky, J. T., Podos, S. M., and Becker, B.: The reproducibility of the intraocular pressure response to dexamethasone. Amer J Ophthalmol 80:844, 1975.

64. Kalina, R. E.: Increased intraocular pressure following subconjunctival corticosteroid administration. Arch Ophthalmol 81:788, 1969.

65. Herschler, J.: Intractable intraocular hypertension induced by repository triamcinolone acetonide. Amer J Ophthalmol 74:501, 1972.

66. Burde, R. M., and Becker, B.: Corticosteroid induced glaucoma and cataracts in contact lens wearers. JAMA 213:2075, 1970.

67. Wood, D. C., Contaxis, I., Sweet, D., Smith, J. C., and Van Dolah, J.: Response of rabbits to corticosteroids. Amer J Ophthalmol 63:841, 1967.

68. Tarkkanen, A., Esilia, R., and Liesmaa, M.: Experimental cataracts following long term administration of corticosteroids. Acta Ophthalmol 44:665, 1966.

69. Oglesby, R. B., Black, R., von Sallman, L., and Bunim, J. J.: Cataracts in patients with rheumatoid diseases treated with corticosteroids. Arch Ophthalmol 66:625, 1961.

70. Giles, C. L., Mason, G. L., Duff, I. F., and McLean, J. A.: The association of cataract formation and systemic corticosteroid therapy. JAMA 182:719, 1962.

71. Wiesinger, H., and Irby, R.: Posterior subcapsular cataract (PSC) in patients with rheumatoid arthritis treated with corticosteroids. Invest Ophthalmol 2:295, 1963.

72. Oglesby, R. B., Black, R. L., von Sallman, L., and Bunim, J. J.: Cataracts in rheumatoid arthritis patients treated with corticosteroids. Further observations. Arch Ophthalmol 66:97, 1961.

73. Crews, S. J.: Posterior subcapsular lens opacities in patients on long term corticosteroid therapy. Brit Med J 1:644, 1963.

74. Havre, D. C.: Cataracts in children on long term corticosteroid therapy. Arch Ophthalmol 73:818, 1965.

75. Braver, D. A., Richards, R. D., and Good, T. A.: Posterior subcapsular cataracts in steroid treated children. Arch Ophthalmol 77:161, 1967.

76. Pfahl, S. B., Makley, T. A., Rothermich, N., and McCoy, F. W.: The relationship of steroid therapy and cataracts in patients with rheumatoid arthritis. Amer J Ophthalmol 52:831, 1961.

77. Bihari, N., and Grossman, B. J.: Posterior subcapsular cataracts related to long term corticosteroid treatment in children. Am J Dis Child 116:604, 1968.

78. Rooklin, A. R., Lampert, S. I., Jaeger, E. A., McGrady, S. J., and Mansmann, H. C.: Posterior sub-

capsular cataracts in steroid-requiring asthmatic children. J Allergy Clin Immunol 63:383, 1979.

79. Ashton, N., and Cook, C.: Effect of cortisone on healing of corneal wounds. Brit J Ophthalmol 35:708, 1951.

80. Palmerton, E. S.: The effect of local cortisone on wound healing in rabbit corneas. Amer J Ophthalmol 40:344, 1955.

81. Gasset, A. R., Lorenzetti, D. W. C., Ellison, E. M., and Kaufman, H. E.: Quantitative corticosteroid effect on corneal wound healing. Arch Ophthalmol 81:589, 1969.

82. McDonald, T. O., Borgmann, A. R., Roberts, M. D., and Fox, L. G.: Corneal wound healing. Invest Ophthalmol 9:703, 1970.

83. Polack, F. M., and Rosen, P. N.: Topical steroids and tritiated thymidine uptake. Arch Ophthalmol 77:400, 1967.

84. Beams, R., Linaberg, L., and Grayson, M.: Effect of topical corticosteroids on corneal wound strength. Amer J Ophthalmol 66:1131, 1968.

85. Basu, P. K.: Effect of different steroids on the healing of nonperforating corneal wounds in rabbits. Arch Ophthalmol 59:657, 1958.

86. Fink, A., and Baras, I.: Effect of steroids on tensile strength of corneal wounds. Amer J Ophthalmol 42:759, 1956.

87. Ho, P. C., and Elliott, J. H.: Kinetics of corneal epithelial regeneration. II. Epidermal growth factor and topical corticosteroids. Invest Ophthalmol 14:630, 1975.

88. Aronson, S. B., Elliott, J. H., Moore, T. E., Jr., and O'Day, D. M.: Pathogenetic approach to therapy of peripheral corneal inflammatory disease. Amer J Ophthalmol 70:65, 1970.

89. Elliott, J. H., Aronson, S. B., Moore, T. E., and Williams, F. C.: Heparin therapy of peripheral corneal schemic syndromes. In *Symposium on the Cornea*. New Orleans Academy of Ophthalmology. St. Louis, C. V. Mosby Co., 1972, pp. 78–104.

90. Krupin, T. LeBlanc, R. P., Becker, B., Kolker, A. E., and Podos, S. M.: Uveitis in association with topically administered corticosteroid. Amer J Ophthalmol 70:883, 1970.

91. Martins, J. C., Wilensky, J. T., Asseff, C. F., Obstbaum, S. A., and Buerk, K. M.: Corticosteroid induced uveitis. Amer J Ophthalmol 77:433, 1974.

92. Becker, B.: The side effects of corticosteroids. Invest Ophthalmol 3:492, 1964.

VII

INFECTION OF THE CORNEA

A. Therapeutic Agents

Antibiotics	**12**

HOWARD M. LEIBOWITZ, M.D.
ALLAN KUPFERMAN, Ph.D.

The purpose of this chapter is to review the pharmacology of antibiotics used in the treatment of bacterial infections of the cornea. The discussion generally will be limited to those agents available for local administration to the eye—that is, to those agents delivered by topical application or by periocular injection.

Antibiotics are substances produced by microorganisms, or they are a chemical modification of such substances. When present in high dilution, they are antagonistic to the growth or life of other microorganisms.[1] The sulfonamides are not true antibiotics because they are not normally produced by microorganisms but rather are synthetic chemical substances. Therefore, they are classified as chemotherapeutic agents. Since several antibiotics now are produced partially or completely by synthetic means,[2–5] the classic separation of antimicrobial agents into these two categories, antibiotics and chemotherapeutic agents, is largely an academic distinction and has no clinical importance. Indeed, the terms antibiotics, antibacterials, antimicrobials, and chemotherapeutic agents often are used interchangeably to describe any substance that is clinically useful in the treatment of infectious diseases. In this sense the sulfonamides will be included in this presentation because of their historical interest and because at times they may be useful inhibitors of bacterial growth in the eye.

Some antibiotics are bactericidal; that is, they interfere with the viability of sensitive organisms. Other antibiotics are bacteriostatic, indicating that they interfere with the ability of the organism to replicate but do not directly terminate its viability. However, bacteriostatic antibiotics at times will act as bactericidal agents if administered in sufficient quantity.[6–9] Moreover, some antibiotics usually described as bacteriostatic may actually exert a bactericidal effect against some species of pathogenic bacteria.[9–10] Which mechanism of action prevails for these presumed bacteriostatic agents at the levels attained in the human cornea after local administration of the drug is not generally known.

MECHANISM OF ACTION

Antibiotics may interfere with bacterial growth by several mechanisms.[11–15] These include (1) inhibition of bacterial cell wall synthesis, (2) alteration of bacterial cell membrane permeability, (3) inhibition of protein synthesis through action on bacterial ribosomes, (4) alteration of bacterial nucleic acid metabolism, and (5) interference with bacterial metabolism. Irrespective of its specific mechanism of action, however, the principle underlying the chemotherapeutic action of all antibiotics is one of selective toxicity.[16] That is, the drug must be quite toxic for pathogenic bacteria but relatively nontoxic to cells of the host. Ideally, the two effects would be independent, but in practice these agents exert varying degrees of toxicity on mammalian cells. Interestingly, the antibiotic that most frequently comes close to achieving this chemotherapeutic ideal is penicillin, a drug that is rarely used topically by the ophthalmologist because of the risk of systemic sensitization. Nonetheless, the ability of the ophthalmologist to administer antibiotics locally, thereby achieving relatively high levels of the drug at the site of infection with relatively low total dose, enables him to avoid much of the inherent toxicity of antibiotic to mammalian cells.

Inhibition of Cell Wall Synthesis

To implement the principle of selective toxicity, bacterial and mammalian cells must differ in some fundamental respect. This is perhaps best illustrated by those antibiotics that exert their effect by inhibition of bacterial cell wall synthesis (Table 12–1). Bacteria contain an outer cell wall and, internal to this, a lipoprotein membrane, which limits the interior of the cell. In contrast, the mammalian cells of the host lack a cell wall; only the cell membrane delimits the cell. Because it is completely absent in human cells, the cell wall is the target that permits certain antibiotics to approximate the theoretical ideal of selective toxicity. The outer bacterial cell wall is a thick, rigid structure that maintains

Table 12–1. ANTIBIOTICS THAT EXERT THEIR EFFECT BY INHIBITION OF BACTERIAL CELL WALL SYNTHESIS

1. The penicillins
2. The cephalosporins
3. Cycloserine
4. Vancomycin
5. Ristocetin
6. Bacitracin
7. Novobiocin

the shape of the organism. It contains a mucopeptide ground substance, and it is this material that provides rigid mechanical stability to the cell because of its many cross-linkages.[17]

Certain antibiotics, the best documented of which is penicillin, exert their effect by interfering with mucopeptide synthesis,[18] an action that results in the production of a deficient cell wall. Normally the cell wall protects the organism from osmotic damage in body fluids. The internal pressures of pathogenic bacteria tend to be higher than serum and other extracellular fluids, and the organism imbibes water, swells, and bursts if the cell wall is defective. In sensitive organisms penicillin therapy gives rise to imperfect cell walls that are not capable of protecting the bacterial cell from osmotic action. As a consequence the cell swells, ruptures, and dies, a bactericidal action that occurs only when the cell is actively dividing.[19]

The ability to kill multiplying bacterial cells but not organisms that are not actively dividing is an important feature of penicillin action. During growth, gaps occur in the mucopeptide of the bacterial cell wall and the gaps are filled in with new structural units. These units are incorporated into the mucopeptide by a transpeptidation (cross-linking) reaction that can be blocked by penicillin. As a result, gaps remain in the mucopeptide of the cell wall, and the cell membrane protrudes through these gaps. The membrane ruptures under osmotic stress, and the cell dies. Cells that are not undergoing multiplication can survive in the presence of penicillin because their mucopeptide is unbroken and there is no reparative cross-linking activity for the penicillin to block.[20]

The other antibiotics listed in Table 12–1 also act by inhibiting bacterial cell wall synthesis. However, in this group of antibiotics there are differences in specific modes of action.[12, 21–23] Moreover, the composition of the cell wall varies among bacteria. For example, the mucopeptide ground substance makes up about 65 per cent of the cell wall of *Staphylococcus aureus* but only 1 to 10 per cent of the cell wall of *Escherichia coli*. The mucopeptide is at least four times thicker in Gram-positive cells than in Gram-negative cells.[24] It is possible that differences in mucopeptide composition and content and their relation to the lipoprotein cell membrane are major factors in determining the differences in response of Gram-positive and Gram-negative bacteria to this group of antibiotics. In any event, cell wall synthesis of Gram-positive bacteria is more easily disrupted by these agents than that of Gram-negative bacteria, accounting for the greater effectiveness of these agents against Gram-positive organisms.[23, 25]

Alteration of Cell Membrane Permeability

Beneath the cell wall lies a membrane, composed of lipid (primarily phospholipids in bacteria) and protein structural elements, that completely encloses the cytoplasm of the bacterial cell. The cytoplasmic membrane functions as a barrier, and it is the phospholipids in the membrane that account for its selective permeability to water, ions, and nutrients. Antibiotics that alter or interfere with the permeability of the bacterial cell membrane (Table 12–2) do so primarily because of their ability to act as cationic detergents that react with the phosphate groups of the cell membrane phospholipids.[26, 27] The structure of antibiotics in this group is complex; they contain both lipophilic and lipophobic groups. The antibiotic orients itself between the lipid and protein films of the microbial membrane by inserting the lipophilic portion of its molecule into

the membrane lipid.[28] This disrupts the membrane, and the cell is unable to maintain its integrity; it dies as a result of osmotic shock, loss of cellular constituents, and an inability to transport necessary cellular metabolites.[29]

There is a stoichiochemical relationship between the number of molecules of antibiotic and the number of cells that the antibiotic will kill.[26, 27] Bacteria that are sensitive to these antibiotics are those which permit the antibiotic to be absorbed within the layers of the cell membrane. Nonsensitive organisms have the ability to prevent the antibiotic from penetrating the cell membrane. In general, disruption of the cell membrane produces a greater adverse effect on Gram-negative than on Gram-positive organisms.

Of the antibiotics that disrupt bacterial cell membrane function, polymyxin B is the best known and most widely used in ophthalmology. Bacteria sensitive to polymyxin B are those with a high percentage of phosphorus in the lipid of their cell walls, while those that are resistant have a higher concentration of nitrolipids in their cell walls.[26, 27] The cell membranes of fungi contain sterols that are not present in bacterial cell membranes. Amphotericin B and other polyene antibiotics alter the permeability of organisms whose membranes contain sterols. Hence, they do not affect bacteria; they are limited in their action to certain yeasts, fungi, and amebas.[24, 30]

Inhibition of Protein Synthesis Through Action on Bacterial Ribosomes

Bacterial ribosomes are spherical cytoplasmic particles that differ from those in mammalian cells both in number and in physical characteristics. They act as an assembly line where amino acids are linked to form peptide chains and proteins.[31] Genetic instruction for protein synthesis is coded in the structure of the DNA of the cell nucleus. DNA directs the production of template or messenger RNA containing the same information. The messenger RNA becomes bound to

Table 12–2. ANTIBIOTICS THAT EXERT THEIR EFFECT BY ALTERATION OF BACTERIAL CELL MEMBRANE PERMEABILITY

1. The polymyxins
2. Colistin
3. Novobiocin
4. The polyene antifungal agents (amphotericin, nystatin)
5. Gramicidin

Table 12–3. ANTIBIOTICS THAT EXERT THEIR EFFECT BY INHIBITION OF PROTEIN SYNTHESIS BY BACTERIAL RIBOSOMES

1. Chloramphenicol
2. The tetracyclines
3. The aminoglycosides (streptomycin, kanamycin, neomycin, gentamicin, tobramycin)
4. The macrolides (erythromycin, oleandomycin, spiromycin)
5. Lincomycin, clindamycin

ribosomes in the cytoplasm and forms a template for the assembly of amino acids in a specified sequence.[32, 33] Ribosomal binding of messenger RNA, as well as the biochemical processes used by bacteria to produce long chains of amino acids in their ribosomes, differ from those of mammalian cells, providing another mechanism for selective toxicity to function. Antibiotics that inhibit the growth of microorganisms by disrupting protein synthesis at the ribosomal level (Table 12–3) make selective use of these differences by interfering with the sequence of events primarily in bacterial cells. The result is a failure of the organism to grow, not a termination of its viability, though exceptions occur (e.g., the aminoglycosides). Thus, inhibition of protein synthesis may produce a bacteriostatic effect; the elimination of the pathogenic organism and the resolution of the infection then depend upon the host's defense system. Agents included in this group are chloramphenicol, the tetracyclines, the aminoglycosides (e.g., neomycin, gentamicin, tobramycin, streptomycin), and the macrolide antibiotics (e.g., erythromycin). They tend to have a wide spectrum of action, adversely affecting the growth of many Gram-positive and Gram-negative organisms.

Alteration of Bacterial Nucleic Acid Metabolism

The information that determines the amino acid sequence in a given protein is coded in DNA and transcribed into messenger RNA. Messenger RNA be-comes bound to ribosomes, where the code is translated into protein synthesis. Antibiotics interfering with the translation process act on the ribosomes and have been discussed in the previous section. Antibiotics that alter bacterial nucleic acid metabolism act on the transcription process. During transcription the two polynucleotide chains of DNA, which normally are twisted about each other in the form of a double helix, unwind and separate. One strand serves as a specific template upon which a complementary strand of RNA is synthesized. Antibiotics that obstruct the transcription process can do so by interfering with either the separation of DNA strands or the synthesis of RNA.

There are no antibiotics commonly available for local ophthalmic use that act by inhibiting bacterial nucleic acid metabolism. The agents in this category available for systemic use are listed in Table 12–4. In general the enzymes involved in nucleic acid metabolism in bacterial and mammalian cells differ, rendering the action of the antibiotics relatively specific for microbial organisms.[14] Other drugs active against protozoa and viruses act by interfering with transcription. Chloroquine, an antiprotozoal agent, inhibits nucleic acid synthesis by interfering with the ability of DNA to act as a template.[34] The antiviral agent idoxuridine is incorporated into viral DNA instead of thymidine.[35] Normally deoxyuridilic acid is converted into thymidilic acid by the enzyme thymidilic acid synthetase. Idoxuridine inhibits this enzyme so that insufficient thymidine phosphate is available for DNA synthesis. Strands of DNA containing idoxuridine instead of thymidine are more easily broken and may result in the production of nonfunctional protein that cannot be assembled into viral particles.[36]

Interference with Bacterial Metabolism

There is a group of drugs that alter the biochemical environment of bacteria and exert their therapeutic effect by in-

Table 12–4. ANTIBIOTICS THAT EXERT THEIR EFFECT BY ALTERING BACTERIAL NUCLEIC ACID METABOLISM

1. Rifampin
2. Nalidixic acid

terfering with bacterial metabolism (Table 12–5). The sulfonamides are the principal ophthalmic agent in this group and historically are of great interest in bacterial chemotherapy. Folic acid derivatives are essential for purine and ultimately for DNA synthesis in both humans and bacteria. Whereas humans are able to absorb and utilize preformed folic acid from their diet, certain bacterial cells are impermeable to folic acid and must synthesize it de novo from para-aminobenzoic acid. Sulfonamides are chemically very similar to para-aminobenzoic acid and compete with it for the microbial enzyme dihydropteroate synthetase. This competition between the sulfonamides and the para-aminobenzoic acid results in a deficiency in folic acid production within bacterial cells (Fig. 12–1).[37] Folic acid metabolism in patients is not affected by sulfonamides, nor do sulfonamides produce a folic acid deficiency within mammalian cells, since these cells cannot synthesize folic acid. Conversely, the preformed dietary folic acid necessary for mammalian cell metabolism does not interfere with the action of sulfonamide drugs, since bacteria cannot transport exogenous folate into their cells. As a general rule, organisms that must synthesize folic acid are susceptible to sulfonamide action; organisms that use existing folic acid are not. However, breakdown of cells in pus may produce a considerable accumulation of thymidine, purines, methionine, and serine, substances that reverse the inhibitory

Table 12–5. ANTIBIOTICS THAT EXERT THEIR EFFECT BY INTERFERING WITH BACTERIAL METABOLISM

1. The sulfonamides
2. Trimethoprim
3. Aminosalicylic acid
4. The sulfones

effect of sulfonamides on bacteria by replenishing the end products of folic acid metabolism. Therefore, sulfonamides may lose their therapeutic effectiveness in the presence of a copious purulent exudate.[38]

TOPICAL OPHTHALMIC ANTIBIOTICS

Among the large number of chemical compounds documented to be therapeutically effective against bacterial infections, only ten individual antibiotics currently are commercially available in the United States for topical administration to the eye. Alphabetically they are bacitracin, chloramphenicol, chlortetracycline, colistin, erythromycin, gentamicin, neomycin, polymyxin B, tetracycline, and tobramycin. Chloramphenicol, chlortetracycline, erythromycin, and tetracycline are generally classified as bacteriostatic drugs, and the others are bactericidal.

Bacitracin

Bacitracin is a mixture of polypeptides (the most important of which is bacitracin A) produced by a strain of *Bacillus subtilis*. Like the penicillins, bacitracin contains a thiazolidine ring, but it does not have their beta-lactam ring (Fig. 12–2). It is a bactericidal antibiotic that achieves its antibacterial effect through inhibition of cell wall synthesis. Since its action is enhanced by metal ions, particularly zinc, it is formulated as zinc bacitracin. Bacitracin is not absorbed by the oral route and is extremely nephrotoxic when given parenterally. With the availability of less toxic bactericidal antibiotics, it virtually has no place in systemic therapy; its clinical usefulness is limited to topical applications.

Bacitracin is supplied commercially as an ophthalmic ointment at a concentration of 500 units per gm. It is highly active against many species of Gram-positive bacteria as well as against pathogenic *Neisseria* species. Its principal usefulness in treating corneal infections

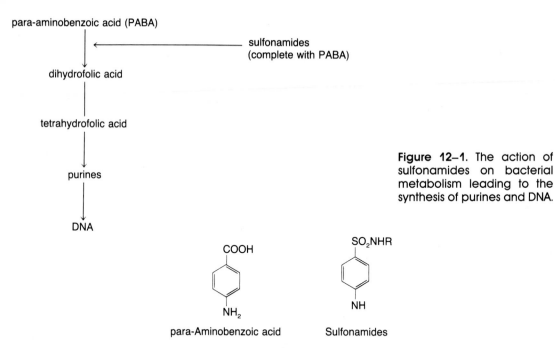

Figure 12–1. The action of sulfonamides on bacterial metabolism leading to the synthesis of purines and DNA.

para-Aminobenzoic acid

Sulfonamides

results from its effectiveness against *Staphylococcus aureus*, including most penicillinase-producing strains, and against streptococci, including *Streptococcus pneumoniae*. Although strains of *Staphylococcus aureus* usually are sensitive to this drug, they are less sensitive than most other Gram-positive bacteria. Group A hemolytic streptococci are so much more sensitive than other groups of streptococci that bacitracin sensitivity can be used as a screening test for identification of group A streptococci.

Chloramphenicol

Chloramphenicol is a broad-spectrum antibiotic that originally was isolated from the fungus *Streptomyces venezuelae* but is now prepared synthetically. Several forms of chloramphenicol have

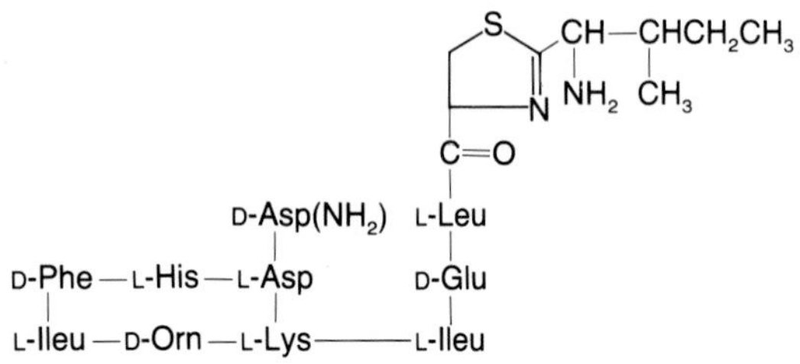

Figure 12–2. Bacitracin.

been available for parenteral administration; presently the sodium succinate ester is regarded as most satisfactory. It is highly soluble and is suitable for administration by either the intramuscular or the intravenous route. Consequently, it can be administered by periocular injection. This ester of chloramphenicol has no antibacterial activity, but after administration most of it undergoes rapid hydrolysis in tissues with the liberation of active chloramphenicol.[39] The topical ophthalmic formulations are available as a 0.5 per cent solution and as a 1.0 per cent ointment; both contain active chloramphenicol, not the ester.

Chloramphenicol is a potent inhibitor of bacterial protein synthesis.[40] It is classified as a bacteriostatic agent because in vitro this drug usually arrests the multiplication of bacteria but does not reduce the number of organisms. However, in high concentration chloramphenicol may be bactericidal to some organisms; indeed, it is bactericidal to *Hemophilus influenzae*, a highly sensitive organism, in relatively low concentration.[6] Experimental data following topical ophthalmic application suggest that it functions as a bacteriostatic agent against susceptible *Staphylococcus aureus* infecting the cornea.[41]

Unlike most other antibiotics, chloramphenicol crosses the blood-ocular and blood-brain barriers with relative facility.[42] It penetrates both the aqueous humor and the vitreous humor after systemic administration and penetrates the cerebrospinal fluid even in the absence of meningitis. Chloramphenicol is the only naturally occurring antibiotic with nitrobenzene in its structure (Fig. 12–3), and this chemical group probably accounts for its toxicity to both bacteria and patients. Its well-known tendency to produce blood dyscrasias, including irreversible aplastic anemia, presumably is explained by its benzene ring, a component of many organic substances known to have similar hematologic toxicity.[24]

Hematologic side effects seemingly can result from the topical application of chloramphenicol to the eye. Though it is an apparently rare complication, at least four cases strongly suggesting this association have been reported;[43–46] two were cases of fatal aplastic anemia.[45,46] Additional instances supporting a probable relationship between topically instilled ophthalmic chloramphenicol preparations and adverse hematologic effects have been reported to the National Registry of Drug-Induced Side Effects.[47] In no instance has the association between topical ophthalmic chloramphenicol and aplastic anemia definitely been proved; to the best of our knowledge, all cases have had other possible explanations for the hematologic abnormality. Nonetheless, even the possibility of inducing a potentially fatal side effect is of sufficient gravity to merit its thoughtful consideration among the factors that determine the risk-benefit ratio of this drug.

Optic neuritis also has been described as a complication in a small number of patients receiving chloramphenicol systemically, at times progressing to optic atrophy and blindness.[48,49] Many of these patients were children with cystic fibrosis receiving prolonged treatment for pulmonary infection. In some instances blindness occurred without recognizable fundus changes. Partial return of vision may occur after cessation of the antibiotic, but this is not invariable. We are unaware of this complication occurring after topical administration or periocular injection of chloramphenicol.

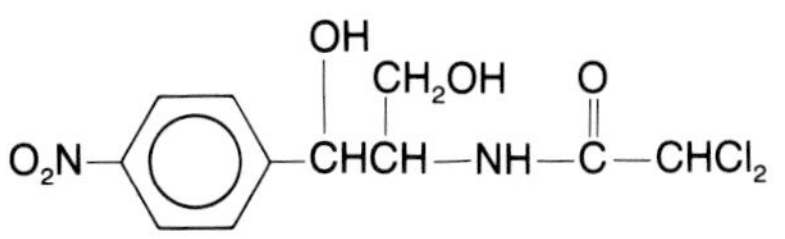

Chloramphenicol is an active agent against a wide variety of both Gram-positive and Gram-negative bacteria. Among the Gram-negative organisms many of the enterobacteriaceae are susceptible, including *Escherichia coli*, *Klebsiella pneumoniae*, *Proteus* species, and *Serratia marcescens*; all are known corneal pathogens. Other Gram-negative bacteria also are sensitive to chloramphenicol, including *Neisseria gonorrhoeae*, *Neisseria meningitidis*, and *Hemophilus influenzae*. *Pseudomonas aeruginosa* is always resistant. The Gram-positive cocci and Gram-positive bacilli usually are susceptible. Among the cocci that are sensitive to chloramphenicol are *Staphylococcus aureus* (including penicillinase-producing strains), *Staphylococcus epidermidis*, *Streptococcus pyogenes*, *Streptococcus pneumoniae*, *Streptococcus viridans*, and *Streptococcus faecalis*. Chloramphenicol also is effective against rickettsiae and chlamydiae.

Chlortetracycline and Tetracycline

Chlortetracycline, a compound derived from the fungus *Streptomyces aureofaciens*, is an antibiotic whose spectrum of bacterial inhibition is similar to that of chloramphenicol. Tetracycline is produced semisynthetically by catalytic reduction of chlortetracycline. Both drugs belong to a group of antibiotics collectively called the tetracyclines because their common hydronaphthacene nucleus contains four fused rings (Fig. 12–4). There usually is cross-resistance among the various tetracyclines, and in practice only one member of the group,

$$O_2N-\bigcirc-\underset{\underset{OH}{|}}{C}H\underset{\underset{CH_2OH}{|}}{C}H-NH-\overset{\overset{O}{||}}{C}-CHCl_2$$

Figure 12–3. Chloramphenicol.

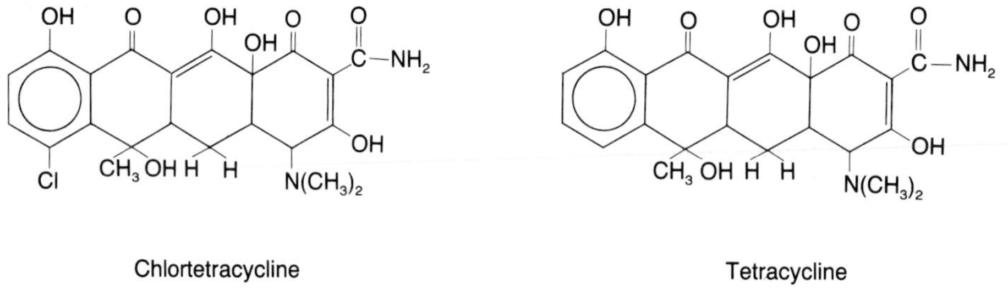

Chlortetracycline   Tetracycline

Figure 12–4. Chlortetracycline and tetracycline.

often tetracycline, is used for sensitivity testing. (Minocycline, which is not available as an ophthalmic formulation, differs somewhat in regard to cross-resistance.) Similarly, the difference in antibacterial activity among individual tetracyclines is relatively minor, and usually their activity does not differ by more than twofold. With the exception of Gram-positive cocci, chlortetracycline is slightly less active against most bacteria than is tetracycline. On the other hand, the tetracyclines are more active in vitro against Gram-positive cocci than is chloramphenicol. Experimental observations suggest that this is also the case in the cornea when either of the two drugs is administered topically.[41]

Chlortetracycline is available as a 1.0 per cent ophthalmic ointment, and tetracycline is supplied both as a 1.0 per cent ophthalmic suspension in oil and as a 1.0 per cent ophthalmic ointment. Both drugs are generally effective against Gram-positive cocci such as Staphylococcus aureus (including penicillinase-producing strains), Staphylococcus epidermidis, Streptococcus pyogenes, Streptococcus pneumoniae, Streptococcus viridans, Streptococcus faecalis, and anaerobic streptococci. Gram-positive bacilli also are generally susceptible. However, many of these organisms may acquire resistance to the tetracyclines. Staphylococci readily become resistant, especially hospital-acquired strains, and strains of Streptococcus pyogenes and Streptococcus pneumoniae resistant to tetracycline have been encountered.[50–53] Among Gram-negative organisms, the tetracyclines are active against pathogenic

Neisseria species, Hemophilus influenzae, and many of the Enterobacteriaceae, including Escherichia coli and Klebsiella pneumoniae. Proteus species and Serratia marcescens usually are resistant, whereas Pseudomonas aeruginosa invariably is resistant. Rickettsiae and chlamydiae both are susceptible to tetracycline therapy. Lower concentrations of both drugs generally are required to inhibit Gram-positive organisms than are required to inhibit Gram-negative organisms.[54]

Tetracyclines inhibit bacterial protein synthesis[55] and usually are described as bacteriostatic. However, they are bactericidal in low concentrations against some bacterial species in vitro.[10] Included in this category are two known corneal pathogens, Streptococcus pyogenes and Streptococcus pneumoniae. There is also experimental evidence suggesting that topically applied chlortetracycline and tetracycline are bactericidal against Staphylococcus aureus in the cornea.[41]

Tetracyclines may be deposited in the deciduous teeth of children if they receive the drug systemically early in life or if the mother is treated with it during pregnancy (since the drug crosses the placenta).[56, 57] They can also produce a lifelong discoloration of the permanent teeth in children up to about the age of 6. The type of discoloration varies somewhat depending upon the tetracycline compound used; chlortetracycline tends to produce gray-brown teeth, whereas tetracycline causes yellowish discoloration. This side effect has not been reported following topical ophthalmic administration or periocular injection.

Colistin and Polymyxin B

The polymyxins are a group of cyclic polypeptide antibiotics produced by a spore-forming, aerobic soil bacterium, *Bacillus polymyxa*. Different polymyxins, named A, B, C, D, and E, are obtained from different strains of the bacillus. Initially only polymyxin B in the form of its sulfate (Fig. 12–5) was commercially available, and for treatment of infections of the external eye and adnexa this compound remains the most widely used member of the group. Polymyxin B is not available in a pure form, and therefore its activity and dosage often are measured in units. One milligram of pure polymyxin B is equivalent to 10,000 units; commercial preparations usually contain approximately 6,000 units per mg. It is supplied as a sterile powder and is generally reconstituted as an ophthalmic solution containing 25,000 units per ml.

Colistin initially was believed to be a new antibiotic but subsequently was shown to be identical to polymyxin E (Fig. 12–5).[58] This drug is supplied primarily as a methane sulfonate. A new unit of activity was adopted for this compound which was one third of the value of that used for polymyxin B. One milligram of pure polymyxin E is equivalent to 30,000 units, but commercial preparations of colistin contain 12,500 units per mg. At present polymyxin B and E are both available for nonophthalmic use either as sulfates or as methane sulfonates. While the methane sulfonate form of each of these drugs is less toxic than the comparable sulfate, it also has inferior antibacterial activity. Each sulfate has about eight times more activity than the methane sulfonate against *Pseudomonas aeruginosa*. The activity of these four compounds against *Pseudomonas aeruginosa* is directly related to their toxicity; an equally toxic dose of each achieves about the same antibacterial effect.[59, 60]

For ophthalmic use colistin formerly was available only as the sulfate (Coly-Mycin S ophthalmic). It was not a marketed ophthalmic product but could be obtained directly from the manufacturer for topical ophthalmic use when required for treatment of a specific case that was unresponsive to other antibiotics. It was provided as a sterile powder along with the appropriate diluent for reconstitution as a 0.12 per cent ophthalmic preparation. Following the introduction of ophthalmic gentamicin its usefulness declined, and at the present time it is no longer available as an ophthalmic formulation.

The antibacterial spectra of polymyxin B sulfate and colistin sulfate are very similar. The two drugs are active against nearly all species of Gram-negative bacteria, including many strains of *Pseudomonas aeruginosa*. Important exceptions include all *Proteus* species, the pathogenic *Neisseria* species (gonococci and meningococci), and *Serratia marcescens*. Gram-positive bacteria are all resistant to polymyxins. Both of these agents are bactericidal. They bind to the bacterial cell membrane, where they act as a cationic detergent whose surface active properties damage and alter the osmotic permeability of the cell membrane. This allows intracellular constituents to escape, killing the organism. Although their importance has been largely superseded by gentamicin and

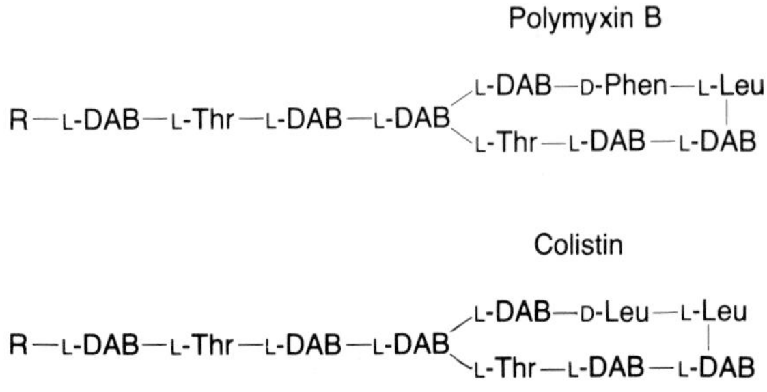

Figure 12–5. Polymyxin B (polymyxin B₁ and polymyxin B₂) and colistin (polymyxin E₁ and polymyxin E₂). In polymyxin B₁ and polymyxin E₁, R = (+)-6-methyloctanoyl; in polymyxin B₂ and polymyxin E₂, R = 6-methylheptanoyl. DAB = α, γ-diaminobutyric acid.

Polymyxin B

R—L-DAB—L-Thr—L-DAB—L-DAB
  ⟨L-DAB—D-Phen—L-Leu
  ⟨L-Thr—L-DAB—L-DAB

Colistin

R—L-DAB—L-Thr—L-DAB—L-DAB
  ⟨L-DAB—D-Leu—L-Leu
  ⟨L-Thr—L-DAB—L-DAB

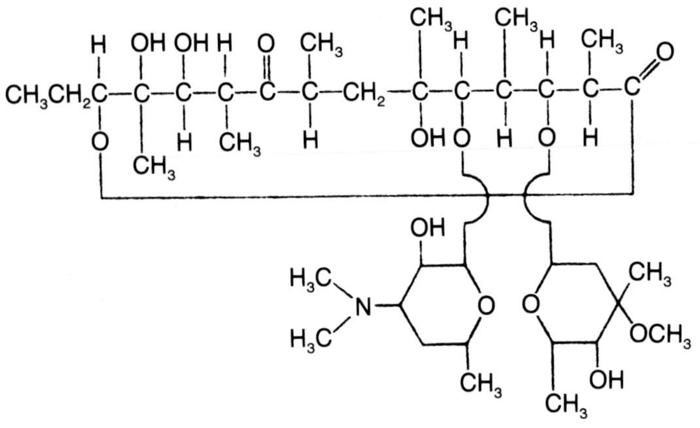

Figure 12–6. Erythromycin.

tobramycin, the polymyxins are alternatives for the treatment of *Pseudomonas aeruginosa* keratitis. Bacteria usually sensitive to the polymyxins do not readily acquire resistance, although when a resistant strain of *Pseudomonas aeruginosa* is encountered, it invariably shows complete cross-resistance between polymyxin B and colistin. However, the polymyxins are particularly suitable for topical therapy because development of bacterial resistance to this drug is uncommon. Although they are toxic compounds when administered systemically, toxicity is not a problem with topical ophthalmic instillation. Therefore, the polymyxin derivative with the greatest therapeutic activity (i.e., the sulfate) should always be used for this purpose.

Erythromycin

Erythromycin, isolated from the fungus *Streptomyces erythreus*, belongs to a group of antibiotics known as the macrolides, which have in common a large lactone ring (Fig. 12–6). It is marketed for ophthalmic use in the form of its base as a 0.5 per cent ointment. Erythromycin is highly active against Gram-positive cocci such as *Staphylococcus aureus* (including penicillinase-producing strains), *Staphylococcus epidermidis*, *Streptococcus pyogenes*, *Streptococcus pneumoniae*, *Streptococcus viridans*, and *Streptococcus faecalis*. Resistant strains of *Staphylococcus aureus*, *Streptococcus pyogenes*, and *Streptococcus pneumoniae* have been encountered, particularly staphylococci in hospital environments, so sensitivity testing is advisable. The drug is also active against Gram-positive bacilli, but among Gram-negative organisms the only important susceptible pathogens are *Neisseria gonorrhoeae*, *Neisseria meningitidis*, and *Hemophilus influenzae*. The Enterobacteriaceae, including *Pseudomonas aeruginosa*, are erythromycin-resistant. Chlamydiae, the etiologic agent of trachoma and inclusion conjunctivitis, and rickettsiae are sensitive to erythromycin.

Erythromycin achieves its effect by interfering with bacterial protein synthesis at the ribosomes.[40] It is generally classed as a bacteriostatic drug, but in vitro it is bacteriostatic at low concentrations and bactericidal at high concentrations.[6] Available experimental evidence suggests that at the concentration reached by topical administration erythromycin may act as a bactericidal agent against *Staphylococcus aureus* in the cornea.[41]

Gentamicin

Gentamicin is an aminoglycoside antibiotic structurally related to the other members of the group, streptomycin, neomycin, and kanamycin. The commercial antibiotic consists of three closely related components, gentamicins C_1, C_2, and C_{1A} (Fig. 12–7). Unlike the

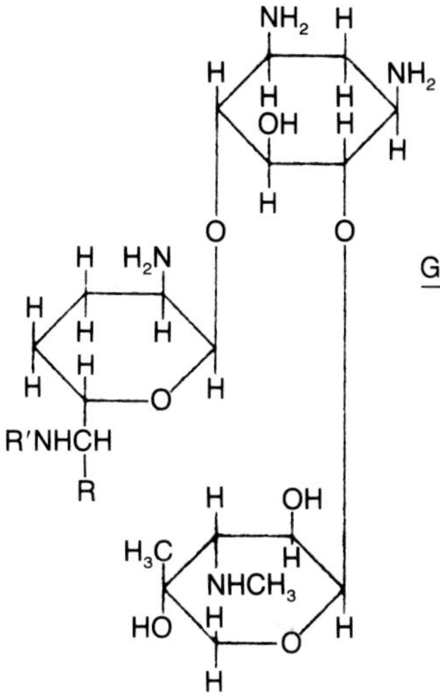

Gentamicin	R	R'
C$_1$	CH$_3$	CH$_3$
C$_2$	CH$_3$	H
C$_{1A}$	H	H

Figure 12–7. Gentamicin.

other aminoglycosides, which are derived from different species of *Streptomyces*, gentamicin is produced by a species of *Micromonospora purpurea*. It is a broad-spectrum antibiotic whose primary usefulness in bacterial keratitis is against Gram-negative organisms. *Pseudomonas aeruginosa* is quite sensitive, and activity against this organism is one of the most important features of gentamicin. Based on its bactericidal spectrum, its stability, its intraocular penetration, its efficacy, and its low degree of toxicity following local ocular use, gentamicin is one of the preferred antibiotics for use against unidentified Gram-negative organisms in the cornea. The other is tobramycin, which will be discussed later in this chapter. Gentamicin is active against nearly all of the Gram-negative bacilli that normally inhabit the human bowel. However, the *Neisseria* species are only moderately sensitive (the degree of sensitivity varying with individual strains), and *Hemophilus influenzae* similarly is only moderately sensitive. Although not classified as a primary antistaphylococcal agent, gentamicin is active in vitro against penicillinase- and nonpenicillinase-producing staphylococci and has been clinically effective in the treatment of staphylococcal infections.[61] Unfortunately, other Gram-positive cocci, such as *Streptococcus pyogenes* and *Streptococcus pneumoniae*, have only a low

degree of sensitivity to gentamicin or are completely resistant to it. As a result, gentamicin is not a suitable antibiotic for the treatment of streptococcal and pneumococcal keratitis; the minimal inhibitory concentration of gentamicin for these two bacterial species often is more than 100 times higher than drugs recommended primarily for Gram-positive organisms (e.g., bacitracin or erythromycin).

Gentamicin is commercially available to the ophthalmologist as a solution and as an ointment. Both are formulated at a 0.3 per cent concentration. Available data fail to demonstrate any superiority of one form over the other following topical administration for treatment of bacterial keratitis.[41] Gentamicin achieves its effect by interference with bacterial protein synthesis[62] and generally is bactericidal at the concentrations achieved in the cornea. An important property is that, along with tobramycin, it is one of only two topical ophthalmic antibiotics that are active both against the *Proteus* species and against *Pseudomonas aeruginosa*. Its activity usually is equal to or greater than the polymyxins against the latter organism. Gentamicin and colistin appear to have an additive effect against *Pseudomonas aeruginosa*, and gentamicin and ampicillin similarly seem to have an additive effect on *Proteus* organisms. Strains of *Staphylococcus aureus* resistant to both methicillin and to cephalosporins have been shown to be sensitive to gentamicin, further supporting its use for the treatment of staphylococcal keratitis. Moreover, strains of *Staphylococcus aureus* resistant to neomycin usually are sensitive to gentamicin.[63] Naturally acquired neomycin resistance does not seem to be accompanied by resistance to gentamicin, and allergic reactions from topical gentamicin are encountered far less often than with neomycin.

Neomycin

Neomycin (Fig. 12–8) is an aminoglycoside antibiotic available as a 0.5 per

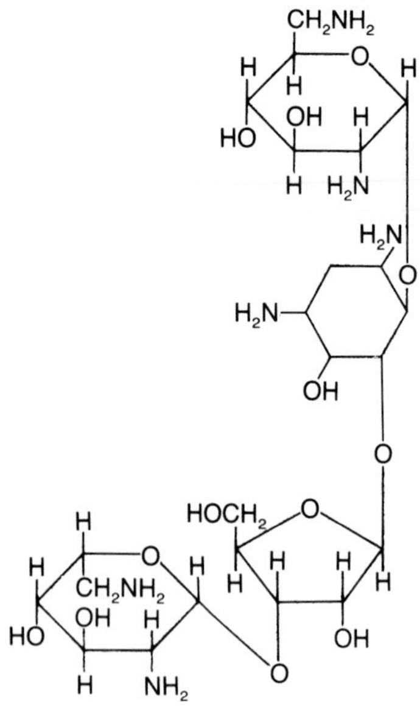

Figure 12–8. Neomycin.

cent ophthalmic solution. It is quite toxic following systemic administration, and as a result it is not used systemically. Its clinical use is limited to topical administration, for which purpose it is formulated as a sulfate since in this form it is stable in water. Like the other aminoglycosides, neomycin achieves its effect by inhibiting bacterial protein synthesis. It is a highly effective bactericidal agent against staphylococci (including penicillinase-producing strains), and this is its area of greatest usefulness in treating bacterial keratitis. All streptococci (including *Streptococcus pneumoniae*) and the Gram-positive bacilli are relatively resistant.[64] Neomycin-resistant staphylococcal strains occur, and the majority also show resistance to penicillin, erythromycin, and tetracyclines. Some reports indicate that these staphylococcal strains also become resistant to bacitracin, an antibiotic sometimes used in combination with neomycin in topical formulations.[65, 66] Most of the medically important Gram-negative bacilli are relatively sensitive to neomycin in the corneal concentrations achieved by topical administration; the major exception is *Pseudomonas aeruginosa*. For practical purposes, however, gentamicin demonstrates greater activity against this group of ocular pathogens in most instances.

Tobramycin

Tobramycin (Fig. 12–9), the most recent ophthalmic antibiotic, is commercially available as a 0.3 per cent ophthalmic solution and ointment of tobramycin sulfate. It is an aminoglycoside antibiotic derived from *Streptomyces tenebrarius*, whose spectrum of activity is similar to that of gentamicin. Like gentamicin, the Gram-positive spectrum of tobramycin is, for practical purposes, limited to the staphylococci. Both *Staphylococcus aureus* (including penicillinase-producing strains) and *Staphylococcus epidermidis* are susceptible. The majority of isolates of *Staphylococcus aureus* are inhibited in vitro by a concentration of less than 1 µg./ml. of tobramycin. In contrast, the minimum inhibitory concentration of tobramycin in vitro against *Streptococcus pyogenes* and *Streptococcus pneumoniae* is usually greater than 20 µg./ml. Gram-negative bacilli are inhibited by low concentrations of tobramycin. The majority of strains of *Proteus mirabilis*, indole-positive *Proteus*, *Escherichia coli*, *Klebsiella pneumoniae*, and *Acinetobacter* are inhibited by a concentration of 1.5 µg./ml. or less. Tobramycin is more active than the other aminoglycosides, including gentamicin, against *Pseudomonas aeruginosa* by at least two- to fourfold; for the treatment of bacterial

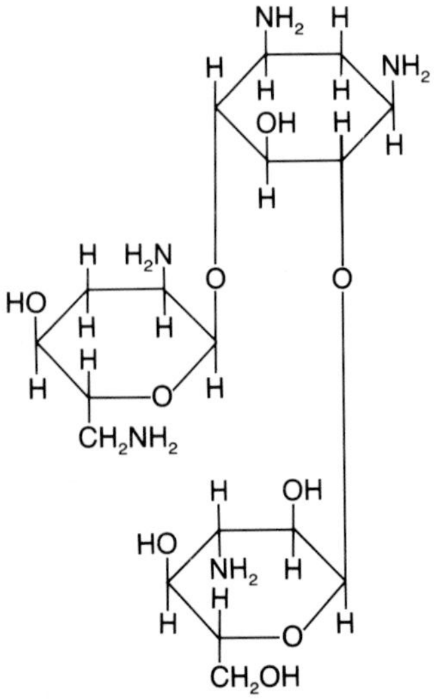

Figure 12–9. Tobramycin.

keratitis this represents its greatest potential advantage. The in vitro activities of tobramycin and gentamicin are similar against the more fastidious Gram-negative coccal and bacillary organisms such as *Neisseria* and *Hemophilus*. Neither agent can be considered a first-line drug for treatment of a keratitis caused by these bacteria. Like the other aminoglycosides, tobramycin produces its antibacterial activity by inhibiting bacterial protein synthesis. It binds irreversibly to a ribosomal subunit, causing that subunit to be removed from the ribosomal pool. As a result, protein synthesis is inhibited in a bactericidal manner.[67]

TOPICAL OPHTHALMIC ANTIBIOTIC COMBINATION FORMULATIONS

Many combination antibiotic formulations are available to the ophthalmologist. Most of these combination preparations contain, at the very least, neomycin sulfate and polymyxin B sulfate. Both are bactericidal drugs in the corneal concentrations achieved after topical administration. General pharmacologic principles state that a bactericidal antibiotic in combination with another bactericidal antibiotic may be synergistic.[68] Whether such an effect occurs in the cornea is not known. In any event, these combination drugs are applied to the eye not so much to intensify antibiotic action but to broaden the antibacterial coverage to include most of the likely pathogenic organisms. These preparations combine the antistaphylococcal and Gram-negative properties of neomycin with the Gram-negative spectrum of polymyxin B (which includes *Pseudomonas aeruginosa*). Their major weakness is the lack of satisfactory coverage for the relatively common Gram-positive corneal pathogens *Streptococcus pyogenes* and *Streptococcus pneumoniae*. To avoid this pitfall, other combination preparations add a third antibiotic, most commonly bacitracin or gramicidin. Bacitracin has been discussed above. Gramicidin is a bacteri-

cidal peptide antibiotic active against most strains of aerobic and anaerobic Gram-positive bacteria. Pneumococci and hemolytic streptococci are most sensitive, whereas staphylococci tend to be relatively resistant. Gram-negative bacilli are completely resistant to gramicidin, whereas *Neisseria* are sensitive to high concentrations only. Thus, the addition of gramicidin or bacitracin has theoretical merit; it extends the Gram-positive coverage of the formulation. Whether the combination of the two drugs with substantial antistaphylococcal properties (i.e., neomycin and bacitracin) is superior in its effect against susceptible strains of staphylococci in the cornea to that of either drug alone has not been determined. Moreover, if one carefully examines the labels of the many available brands of the combination preparations, one finds differences in the concentrations of the antibiotics contained therein. The practical significance of these differences in drug concentration on relative antibacterial effect in vivo in the cornea is not known.

TOPICAL OPHTHALMIC SULFONAMIDES

Several ophthalmic sulfonamide preparations are commercially available, but these contain only two specific sulfonamide agents. Sodium sulfacetamide (Fig. 12–10), a short-acting, highly soluble sulfonamide of low antibacterial activity, is available as a 10 per cent solution and ointment, as a 15 per cent solution, and as a 30 per cent solution and ointment marketed under a number of proprietary names. Sulfisoxazole diolamine (Gantrisin, Fig. 12–10) is available as a 4 per cent solution and ointment. The sulfonamides have a broad spectrum of antibacterial activity and classically are effective against many of the Gram-positive and some of the Gram-negative organisms known to cause corneal infections. However, although the sulfonamides originally had a wide range of activity, their antibacterial spectrum has been seriously restricted by acquired bacterial resistance.

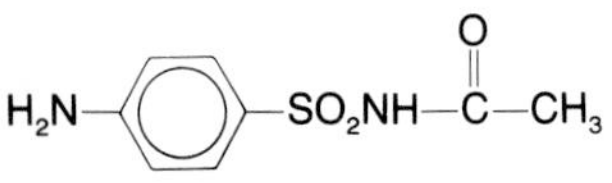

Figure 12–10. Ophthalmic sulfonamides.

Sulfacetamide

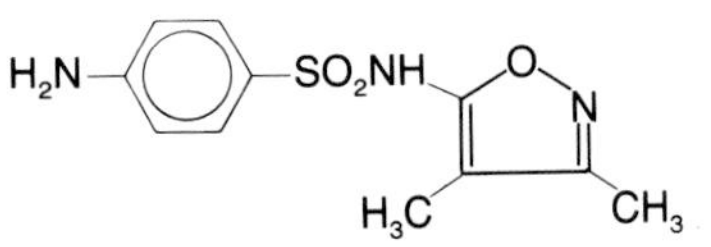

Sulfisoxazole

They are not effective against *Pseudomonas aeruginosa*. Although they can be bactericidal in high concentrations,[69, 70] the mode of action of the sulfonamides is largely bacteriostatic (Fig. 12–1). In pus, secretions, and organic debris that collect on the surface of a bacterial corneal ulcer and in the adjacent fornices there may be considerable accumulation of thymidine, purines, methionine, and serine. These substances impede the inhibitory effect of sulfonamides on bacteria by replenishing the end products of folic acid metabolism, causing these agents to lose their therapeutic effectiveness.[38] As a result, sulfonamides rarely are used to treat serious corneal infections. Interestingly, however, there are very few hard data to document the appropriate role of topical sulfonamides in bacterial infection of the outer eye and adnexa.

ANTIBIOTICS FOR PERIOCULAR INJECTION

Treatment of the more severe forms of bacterial keratitis may include the inoculation of large quantities of antibiotics adjacent to the globe in an effort to increase the levels that these drugs attain in the cornea. Specific preparations are not formulated for this purpose. In each instance a parenteral form of the antibiotic is used, and the material intended for intramuscular or intravenous use is injected subconjunctivally or beneath Tenon's capsule. A number of antibiotics have been recommended for this purpose. Several of these drugs are the same as those delivered by the topical route, including the most commonly used ones, gentamicin and tobramycin. In addition, several antibiotics not commercially available for topical ophthalmic instillation are a part of the

periocular antibiotic armamentarium still advocated by some authorities to treat severe bacterial keratitis. For the most part these agents are penicillins or cephalosporins.

Penicillin G (Benzylpenicillin)

All of the penicillins share a common 6-aminopenicillanic acid nucleus. This is a cyclic dipeptide of L-cysteine and D-valine arranged in a basic structure consisting of a thiazolidine ring joined to the beta-lactam ring. Individual penicillins differ only with respect to the side chains attached to the common nucleus (Fig. 12–11). The early penicillin was a mixture of several penicillin compounds designated as F, G, X, and K; of these, penicillin G (benzylpenicillin) was found to be the most satisfactory. Several relatively stable salts of this drug are used clinically; sodium penicillin G (sodium benzylpenicillin), a highly soluble salt, is used for periocular injection. Its dosage is still commonly expressed in units. One unit of activity is equal to 0.6 µg. of pure sodium penicillin G.

Penicillin G is highly active against many Gram-positive cocci, particularly *Streptococcus pyogenes* and *Streptococcus pneumoniae*. However, many strains of staphylococci are resistant to penicillin G. This phenomenon usually is attributable to the production of penicillinase by the resistant organism. The enzyme hydrolyzes and destroys penicillin G. Gram-positive bacilli are consistently sensitive to penicillin G. *Neisseria gonorrhoeae* and *Neisseria meningitidis* also are sensitive to penicillin G, although resistant gonococcal strains are encountered with increasing frequency. Gram-negative bacilli are invariably resistant. Among sensitive organisms penicillin is a selective inhib-

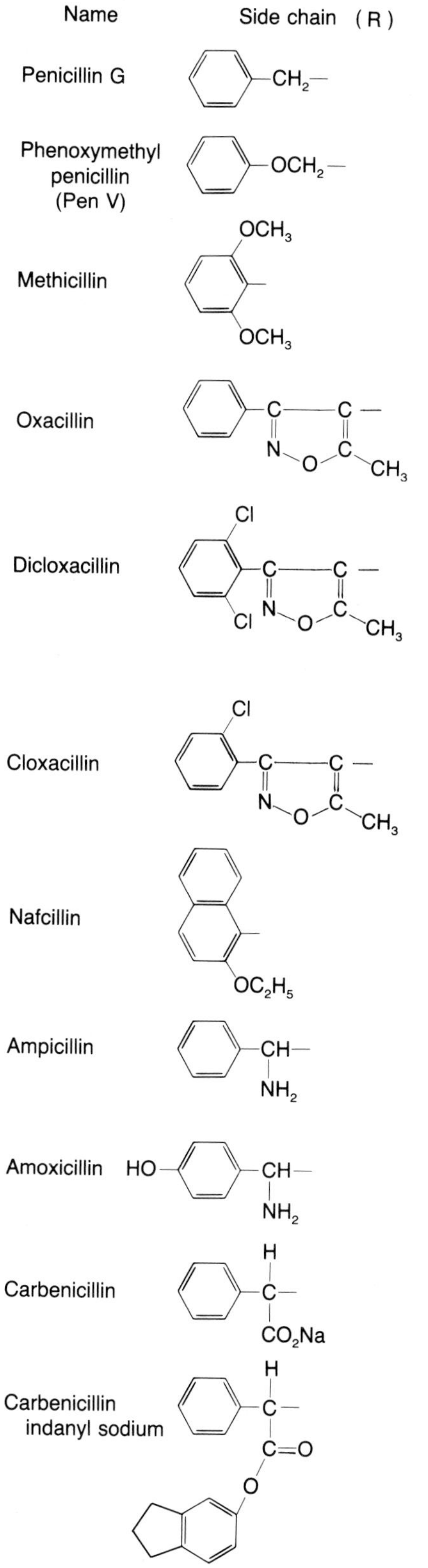

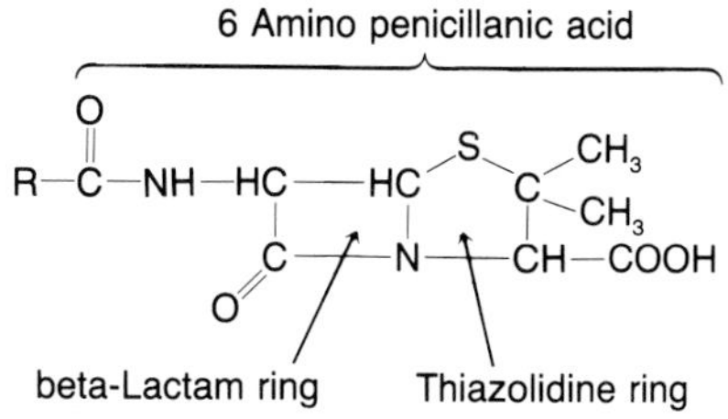

Name	Side chain (R)

Figure 12–11. Structure of the penicillins.

itor of bacterial cell wall synthesis in multiplying bacteria through its capacity to inhibit formation of cross-linkages in the mucopeptide lattice. This inhibition of cell wall synthesis is not in itself lethal, but body fluids normally are hypotonic in comparison to the interior of bacteria, an osmotic relationship that facilitates lysis of affected organisms. Penicillin G is therefore classified as a bactericidal agent.

Methicillin

Methicillin is a semisynthetic penicillin derived from the nucleus shared by all penicillins, 6-aminopenicillanic acid. Its antibacterial spectrum is similar to that of penicillin G. That is, it is active against Gram-positive bacteria and also against the Gram-negative cocci *Neisseria gonorrhoeae* and *Neisseria meningitidis*. The major advantage of methicillin is that it is not hydrolyzed by penicillinase. It remains active in the presence of this enzyme and so is effective against penicillinase-producing strains of staphylococci that are resistant to penicillin G. However, bacterial strains resistant to methicillin have been encountered with increasing use of the drug.[71, 72] Methicillin resistance is due not to destruction of the antibiotic by a bacterial enzyme but to tolerance of the bacterial cell.[73] There is some evidence suggesting that the cell walls of resistant strains differ from those of susceptible strains.[74] In any case, methicillin-resistant staphylococci also are frequently resistant to penicillin G, erythromycin, the cephalosporins, tetracycline, and chloramphenicol, and thus their treatment may be difficult.[73]

Like all penicillins, methicillin inhibits formation of the mucopeptides in bacterial cell walls. It inhibits the growth of both penicillin G–sensitive and penicillinase-producing staphylococci. However, it must be emphasized that penicillin G is approximately 50 times more active than methicillin against penicillin-sensitive staphylo-

cocci and streptococci.[75] Therefore, methicillin has an advantage and is indicated only for the treatment of staphylococcal infections (proven or suspected) when the staphylococcus is a penicillinase producer and so is resistant to penicillin G. Methicillin should not be used for infection by organisms susceptible to penicillin G, because the latter is both more effective and cheaper. Methicillin seems to be one of the penicillins bound least by serum proteins, a factor that may be of importance when it is administered via the periocular route in the treatment of bacterial keratitis.

Oxacillin

Oxacillin is one of several isoxazolyl penicillins which, like methicillin, resist inactivation by penicillinase. Its antibacterial spectrum is similar to that of methicillin. It is active against Gram-positive cocci such as staphylococci and streptococci (including *Streptococcus pneumoniae*) and against Gram-positive bacilli. The *Neisseria* species are the only Gram-negative organisms sensitive to this drug. Oxacillin is primarily of use for the treatment of penicillinase-producing staphylococci resistant to penicillin G. Methicillin-resistant staphylococci are also resistant to oxacillin.

In vitro oxacillin is at least four times more active than methicillin against staphylococci. However, additional in vitro studies have shown that oxacillin, like other isoxazolyl penicillins, is highly bound to serum proteins. About 93 per cent of the drug appears to be protein-bound, and only 7 per cent remains free.[76, 77] There is evidence that the protein-bound part of the drug has little or no antibacterial activity. If the effectiveness of oxacillin is tested in 95 per cent human serum instead of in nutrient broth, its minimum inhibitory concentration increases about tenfold.[78] Therefore, the greater intrinsic activity of oxacillin, compared with methicillin, may be compromised by serum protein binding. It is not clear to what degree the protein binding of any penicillin affects its therapeutic effectiveness, because often the bond is loose and readily reversible in vivo. Oxacillin and methicillin demonstrate about equal activity when tested in the presence of serum, and clinically neither has been shown to be clearly more effective. There is no information on how this reversible protein binding and inactivation affects the in vivo efficacy of these drugs when they are injected periocularly to treat a bacterial keratitis. Somewhat arbitrarily, we tend to look upon these two penicillin compounds as equally efficacious. At present, in part through habit, we use oxacillin when this family of antibiotics is indicated. Like methicillin, oxacillin is less active than penicillin G against bacteria sensitive to penicillin G. Cloxacillin, another isoxazolyl penicillin whose chemical structure differs from oxacillin only by the addition of a chlorine atom, can cause corneal opacities in rabbits when the drug is injected subconjunctivally.[79] To our knowledge, this complication has not been reported with oxacillin.

Ampicillin

Ampicillin is a semisynthetic penicillin derived from the penicillin nucleus, 6-aminopenicillanic acid. It is active against most of the Gram-positive bacteria sensitive to penicillin G. Penicillin G is more effective against these organisms, but its superiority over ampicillin is not great. Ampicillin is destroyed by staphylococcal penicillinase; thus, many staphylococcal strains are ampicillin-resistant just as they are penicillin G–resistant.

Ampicillin also is active against Gram-negative bacteria, many of which are penicillin G–resistant. *Neisseria gonorrhoeae, Neisseria meningitidis,* and *H. influenzae* are ampicillin-sensitive. *Proteus mirabilis* is usually sensitive, but the other *Proteus* species are resistant. Although some strains of *Escherichia coli* are sensitive, the other enterobacteriaceae generally are resistant. *Pseudomonas aeruginosa* is always resistant.

Carbenicillin

Carbenicillin is a semisynthetic penicillin with activity against *Pseudomonas aeruginosa.* Although its effectiveness against this organism is of a relatively low order, it is the most important feature of carbenicillin. For systemic infections this antibiotic can be administered in sufficient dosage to obtain serum concentrations exceeding 50 to 60 µg./ml., a level that will inhibit many *Pseudomonas aeruginosa* strains. Unfortunately, a substantial proportion of *Pseudomonas aeruginosa* strains are not inhibited by carbenicillin concentrations as high as 200 µg./ml. Moreover, carbenicillin-resistant variants readily emerge in the face of therapy with this antibiotic.[80–82] Carbenicillin resistance may arise not only by genetic mutation but also by transfer of resistance factors from *Escherichia coli* to *Pseudomonas aeruginosa* and vice versa.[83] Therefore, it is likely that the prevalence of highly resistant *Pseudomonas aeruginosa* strains will increase with the continuing use of the antibiotic.

Compared with ampicillin, carbenicillin has a relatively high activity against indole-positive *Proteus* species (*Proteus vulgaris, Proteus rettgeri,* and *Proteus morganii*). Its action against other Gram-negative bacteria is comparable to that of ampicillin; it is effective against *Neisseria gonorrhoeae, Neisseria meningitidis, Hemophilus influenzae, Proteus mirabilis,* and to a degree against *Escherichia coli.* Ampicillin is used in preference to carbenicillin for treatment of infections due to these bacteria because it is the more active of the two. Penicillinase-producing staphylococci are resistant to carbenicillin. Nonpenicillinase-producing staphylococci, *Streptococcus pyogenes,* and *Streptococcus pneumoniae* are sensitive, but ampicillin and penicillin G are much more effective for the treatment of infection caused by these microorganisms.

Carbenicillin should not be used alone to treat *Pseudomonas aeruginosa* infections, because bacterial resistance tends to develop rapidly.[81] The combination of gentamicin sulfate and carbenicillin disodium has been recommended on the basis of in vitro and in vivo evidence of synergism in their antibacterial effect against *Pseudomonas aeruginosa*.[84-87] However, mixing of these two drugs in vitro results in the inactivation of gentamicin.[88] The ratio of carbenicillin to gentamicin in vitro influences the rate of inactivation. At a relative concentration of 20 to 1 the half-life of gentamicin is 4 hours; at a relative concentration of 100 to 1 its half-life is only 45 minutes. Prior treatment of carbenicillin with penicillinase eliminates this effect even at the 100 to 1 ratio, indicating that the inactivation of gentamicin by carbenicillin is dependent upon the integrity of the beta-lactam ring in the penicillin molecule. Carbenicillin and gentamicin interact to form a conjugate linked between the amino groups in the sugars of gentamicin and the beta-lactam ring of the penicillin. This type of conjugate inactivates the antimicrobial action of both molecules. A similar reaction occurs with other analogues of penicillin. The rate of inactivation also is influenced by the fluid into which the two drugs are placed. In solutions for intravenous administration, gentamicin inactivation occurs rapidly, but in serum the half-life of gentamicin with carbenicillin is 24 hours. In treated patients (except those with renal insufficiency) the rate of inactivation of gentamicin was the same as in serum.[88] In vivo the effect of gentamicin on *Pseudomonas* organisms appears to take place before any significant loss of activity through interaction with carbenicillin can occur. No specific data are available on the effect of this drug combination following periocular injection, but based on the evidence at hand the use of the regimen seems reasonable if physical mixing of the drugs in vitro is avoided.

Other Penicillins

Penicillins remain among the most reliable and nontoxic of all medicines. Through structural modifications new drugs with increased antibacterial activity and a broader antibacterial spectrum of action continue to be produced. A molecular side chain modification produced ticarcillin, a drug with greater activity against *Pseudomonas aeruginosa* than carbenicillin. Azlocillin is an acylureido penicillin with activity similar to that of ticarcillin except that it is about four times more active against *Pseudomonas aeruginosa*. Mezlocillin is also an acylureido penicillin similar to ticarcillin except that it has greater activity against *Streptococcus faecalis*, *Klebsiella* species, and *Bacteroides fragilis*.

Piperacillin is a unique piperazine penicillin with activity against *Pseudomonas aeruginosa* of about the same order of magnitude as that of azlocillin. Unlike the acylureido penicillins, however, piperacillin has a level of activity against Gram-positive organisms comparable with that of ampicillin. It also is the most effective of all penicillins against *Bacteroides* species. Because of its extremely wide spectrum of activity and its apparent low toxicity, piperacillin may well become a first-line agent.

Mecillinam is an amidinopenicillin with a fairly narrow spectrum of activity against *Escherichia coli* and *Klebsiella*, *Enterobacter*, and *Citrobacter* species. It is active against many ampicillin-resistant *Shigella* and *Salmonella* species but is much less active than ampicillin against the Gram-positive organisms *Hemophilus influenzae* and *Neisseria* species. To date none of these newer penicillins has had extensive ocular use. Their specific role, if any, in the treatment of bacterial infections of the eye and especially of bacterial keratitis remains to be established.

Cephalosporins

The cephalosporins are all semisynthetic antibiotics derived from cephalosporin C, a natural antibiotic produced by a strain of the mold *Cephalosporium acremonium*. The nucleus of cephalosporin C is closely related to the penicillin nucleus, 6-aminopenicillanic acid, but differs by having a six-membered dihydrothiazine ring instead of a five-membered thiazolidine ring attached to the beta-lactam ring (Fig. 12–12). The active nucleus is known as 7-amino-cephalosporanic acid. The basic advantages of the cephalosporin nucleus are its innate resistance to staphylococcal penicillinase and its relative safety in patients allergic to penicillin. The cephalosporin antibiotics, like the penicil-

lins, are bactericidal and, like them, achieve their effect by inhibition of cell wall synthesis.

In the past cephalothin, the parent cephalosporin compound, and cephaloridine have been administered by periocular injection to treat ocular infections. However, cephalothin is irritating and capable of local tissue destruction, and cephaloridine is associated with severe renal toxicity. Cefazolin, a somewhat newer cephalosporin derivative,

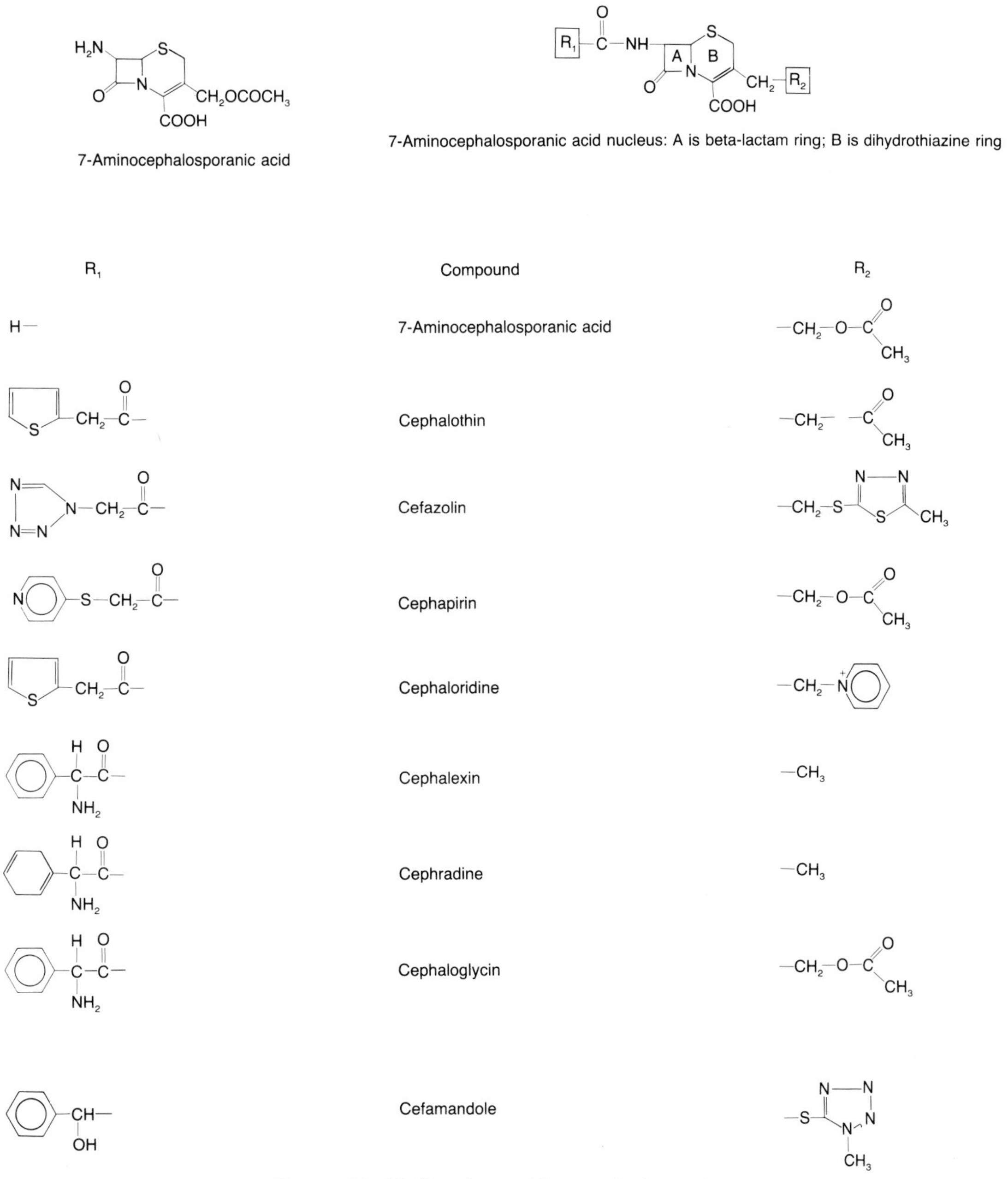

7-Aminocephalosporanic acid

7-Aminocephalosporanic acid nucleus: A is beta-lactam ring; B is dihydrothiazine ring

Figure 12–12. Structure of the cephalosporins.

presently is the cephalosporin of choice for periocular injection. Overall, it offers essentially the same spectrum of bacterial coverage as the older derivatives. Most Gram-positive cocci, including penicillinase- and nonpenicillinase-producing staphylococci, Streptococcus pyogenes, and Streptococcus pneumoniae, are sensitive to cefazolin. So, too, are Gram-positive bacilli. Streptococcus faecalis and methicillin-resistant staphylococci usually are resistant. Among Gram-negative bacteria, the Neisseria species (gonococci and meningococci) and Escherichia coli usually are sensitive, but resistant strains do occur. Proteus mirabilis is the only Proteus species commonly sensitive to cefazolin. The susceptibility of the Klebsiella species varies; Klebsiella pneumoniae is usually sensitive, Klebsiella aerogenes less often so. Pseudomonas aeruginosa is always resistant. This is due to the production of beta-lactamases, which destroy cephalosporin compounds.

Although cefazolin exhibits some degree of effectiveness against these Gram-negative organisms, it shows high intrinsic activity only against the Gram-positive cocci. This is where its usefulness lies in the treatment of corneal infections. Cefazolin is an effective alternative to the penicillins for the treatment of staphylococcal, streptococcal, and pneumococcal infections. On the assumption that they are poorly cross-allergenic with the penicillins, cephalosporins frequently are recommended for treatment of severe infections in penicillin-allergic patients.[89, 90] However, approximately 8 per cent of penicillin-sensitive patients react to cephalosporin C derivatives,[91] and all cephalosporins should be avoided in patients with a history of anaphylaxis to a penicillin derivative.

A major advantage of cefazolin in systemic use is that it produces a higher serum level than cephalothin and cephaloridine following intramuscular injection. The significance of this observation relative to periocular injection and the resulting corneal and intraocular drug levels is not known. Cefazolin also is said to be less painful than other cephalosporin derivatives following intramuscular injection. Based on limited experience, periocularly injected cefazolin seems less irritating than cephaloridine.

The first generation cephalosporins (e.g., cefazolin) are effective primarily against aerobic, Gram-positive bacteria. Second generation cephalosporins (e.g., cefamandole, cefoxitin, cefaclor) tend to be somewhat less active against Gram-positive cocci but have a broader spectrum of action. They tend to be relatively resistant to the beta-lactamases produced by Gram-negative organisms and are therefore more effective than the first generation cephalosporin derivatives against such organisms as Hemophilus influenzae and Enterobacteriaceae strains. The most recent, third generation, cephalosporin derivatives (e.g., cefotaxime, moxalactam, cefoperazone, cefsulodin) show even greater resistance to beta-lactamases and, therefore, greater activity against Gram-negative organisms, including Pseudomonas aeruginosa.[92] However, in comparison with the earlier cephalosporins they are weakly potent against Gram-positive pathogens,[92] and none seems to be the ultimate antipseudomonal drug. The role of the third generation cephalosporins, if any, in the treatment of bacterial keratitis remains to be defined.

Vancomycin

Vancomycin is a relatively toxic antibiotic that for systemic use can only be administered intravenously. Consequently, it is generally regarded as a "reserve drug" for the treatment of severe staphylococcal infections. Its role in the treatment of bacterial keratitis is essentially the same. Vancomycin is highly effective against Gram-positive cocci, including Staphylococcus aureus, Staphylococcus epidermidis, Streptococcus pyogenes, Streptococcus pneumoniae, Streptococcus viridans, and Streptococcus faecalis. Gram-positive bacilli also are sensitive. For practical purposes all Gram-negative bacteria are resistant.

Vancomycin is a bactericidal drug that interferes with the synthesis of bacterial cell walls by a mechanism different from that of the penicillins and cephalosporins.[93] It also differs from these drugs in that it inhibits the growth of spheroplasts, possibly by an additional action on the bacterial cell membrane.[94] These differing mechanisms of action seem to explain the effectiveness of vancomycin not only against penicillinase-producing strains of staphylococci but also against methicillin-resistant strains whose cell wall synthesis is unaffected by the penicillins and cephalosporins. The emergence of resistant staphylococci has not been observed during the treatment of patients with this drug. There is no cross-resistance between vancomycin and other antibiotics.

THERAPEUTIC APPLICATIONS

Table 12–6 lists a number of bacterial pathogens and a number of antibiotics useful in ophthalmology. With specific reference to bacterial keratitis and its treatment with topically applied antibiotics, it presents a semiquantitative evaluation of the probable effectiveness of each drug against each organism. This table is offered only as a guide; treatment

Table 12–6. GUIDE TO ANTIBIOTIC EFFECTIVENESS IN LOCAL THERAPY OF BACTERIAL KERATITIS*

	Amikacin	Bacitracin	Cefazolin	Chloramphenicol	Erythromycin	Gentamicin	Neomycin	Polymyxin B	Tobramycin	Vancomycin
Gram-Positive Cocci										
Staphylococcus aureus	G	G	G	G	G	G	G	P	G	G
Streptococcus pneumoniae	P	G	G	G	G	P	P	P	P	G
Streptococcus pyogenes	P	G	G	G	G	P	P	P	P	G
Streptococcus faecalis	P	F	P	G	G	P	P	P	P	G
Gram-Negative Cocci										
Neisseria gonorrhoeae	P	G	F	G	G	P	F	P	P	P
Neisseria meningitidis	P	G	F	G	G	P	F	P	P	P
Gram-Negative Rods										
Acinetobacter	G	P	P	G	P	G	G	G	G	P
Enterobacter	G	P	P	G	P	G	G	G	G	P
Escherichia coli	G	P	F	G	P	G	G	G	G	P
Hemophilus species	P	P	F	G	G	P	F	G	P	P
Klebsiella species	G	P	F	G	P	G	G	G	G	P
Moraxella species	G	P	F	F	P	G	G	G	G	P
Proteus mirabilis	G	P	F	G	P	G	F	P	G	P
Indole-positive Proteus	G	P	P	G	P	G	F	P	G	P
Pseudomonas aeruginosa	G	P	P	P	P	G	P	G	G	P
Serratia species	G	P	P	G	P	G	G	P	G	P

*G = good; F = fair; P = poor.

of bacterial keratitis is discussed in detail in Chapter 15. In using Table 12–6 it is important to bear in mind that it does not replace careful culturing and sensitivity testing. Particularly in Gram-negative infections, the antibiotic sensitivity of the organism must be determined. Antibiotic sensitivity of an organism often differs among various strains of that organism and often varies considerably from one geographic location to another. These factors, along with the location of the infection within the cornea and with its severity, will affect the choice of the antibiotic. Nonetheless, it is our hope that Table 12–6 will provide some clarification of a complex clinical problem, even if some of the specifics offered therein are controversial.

REFERENCES

1. Bowman, W. C., Rand, M. J., and West, G. B.: *Textbook of Pharmacology.* Oxford, Blackwell Scientific Publications, 1968, p. 924.
2. Chain, E. B.: Penicillinase resistant penicillins and the problem of the penicillin resistant staphylococci. In DeReuck, A. V. S., and Cameron, M. P. (eds.): *Resistance of Bacteria to the Penicillins.* (Ciba Foundation Study Group No. 13.) Boston, Little, Brown, 1962, pp. 3–19.
3. Klein, J. O., and Finland, M.: The new penicillins. N Engl J Med 269:1019, 1963.
4. Weinstein, L.: Antibiotics. V. Miscellaneous antimicrobial agents. In Goodman, L. S., and Gilman, A. (eds.): *The Pharmacological Basis of Therapeutics.* 3rd ed. New York, Macmillan Co., 1965, p. 1260.
5. Bartz, Q. R.: Isolation and characterization of chloromycetin. J Biol Chem 172:445, 1948.
6. Garrod, L. P., and Waterworth, P. M.: Methods of testing combined antibiotic bactericidal action and the significance of the results. J Clin Pathol 15:328, 1962.
7. Barker, B. M., and Prescott, F.: *Antimicrobial Agents in Medicine.* Oxford, Blackwell Scientific Publications, 1973, p. 36.
8. Weinstein, L.: Antimicrobial agents: Streptomycin, gentamicin and other aminoglycosides. In Goodman, L. S., and Gilman, A. (eds.): *The Pharmacological Basis of Therapeutics.* 5th ed. New York, Macmillan Co., 1975, p. 1167.
9. Weinstein, L.: Antimicrobial agents: Miscellaneous antibacterial agents; Antifungal and antiviral agents. In Goodman, L. S., and Gilman, A. (eds.): *The Pharmacological Basis of Therapeutics.* 5th ed. New York, Macmillan Co., 1975, p. 1224.
10. Steigbigel, N. H., Read, C. W., and Finland, M.: Susceptibility of common pathogenic bacteria to seven tetracycline antibiotics in vitro. Amer J Med Sci 255:179, 1968.
11. Feingold, D. S., Hsu Chen, C. C., and Sud, I. J.: Basis for the selectivity of the polymyxin antibiotics on cell membranes. Ann NY Acad Sci 235:480, 1974.
12. Strominger, J. L.: The action of penicillin and other antibiotics on bacterial wall synthesis. Johns Hopk Med J 133:63, 1973.
13. Pestka, S.: Inhibitors of ribosome functions. Ann Rev Microbiol 25:487, 1971.
14. Goldberg, I. H., and Freedman, P. A.: Antibiotics and nucleic acids. Ann Rev Biochem 40:775, 1971.
15. Hash, J. H.: Antibiotic mechanisms. Ann Rev Pharm 12:35, 1972.
16. Albert, A.: *Selective Toxicity.* 4th ed. London, Methuen and Co., Ltd., 1968.
17. Bayer, M. E.: Ultrastructure and organization of the bacterial envelope. Ann NY Acad Sci 235:6, 1974.
18. Blumberg, P. M., and Strominger, J. L.: Interaction of penicillin with the bacterial cell: Penicillin-binding proteins and penicillin sensitive enzymes. Bact Rev 38:291, 1974.
19. Park, J. T., Edwards, J. R., and Wise, E. M., Jr.: In vivo studies on the uptake and binding of β-lactam antibiotics in relation to inhibition of wall synthesis and cell death. Ann NY Acad Sci 235:300, 1974.
20. Greenwood, D.: Mucopeptide hydrolases and bacterial "persisters." Lancet 2:465, 1972.
21. Perkins, H. R., and Nicto, M.: The chemical basis for the action of the vancomycin group of antibiotics. Ann NY Acad Sci 235:348, 1974.
22. Storm, D. R.: Mechanisms of bacitracin action: A specific lipid-peptide interaction. Ann NY Acad Sci 235:387, 1974.
23. Blumberg, P. M.: Penicillin binding components of bacterial cells and their relationship to the mechanisms of penicillin action. Ann NY Acad Sci 235:310, 1974.
24. Braude, A. I.: *Antimicrobial Drug Therapy.* Philadelphia, W. B. Saunders Co., 1976, pp. 1–37.
25. Davis, B. D., Dulbecco, R., Eisen, H. N., Ginsberg, H. S., and Wood, W. B., Jr.: *Microbiology.* New York, Hoeber Medical Division, 1968, pp. 147–166.
26. Newton, B. A.: *Surface Active Bactericides in Strategy of Chemotherapy.* Vol. 8. London, J. and A. Churchill, Ltd., 1958, pp. 62–93.
27. Newton, B. A.: The properties and mode of action of the polymyxins. Bact Rev 20:14, 1956.
28. Sebek, O. K.: Polymyxin and circulin. In Gottlieb, D., and Shaw, P. D. (eds.): *Antibiotics.* Vol. 1. *Mechanism of Action.* Berlin, Springer Verlag, 1967, pp. 142–152.
29. Few, A. V.: Interaction of polymyxin E with bacterial and other lipids. Biochim Biophys Acta 16:137, 1955.
30. Kinsky, S. C.: Nystatin binding by protoplasts and a particulate fraction of *Neurospora crassa*, and a basis for the selective toxicity of polyene antifungal antibiotics. Proc Nat Acad Sci USA 48:1049, 1962.
31. Nomura, M: Ribosomes. Sci Amer 221:28, 1969.
32. McGilvery, R. W.: *Biochemistry: A Functional Approach.* Philadelphia, W. B. Saunders, 1970, pp. 17–49.
33. Watson, J. D.: The synthesis of proteins upon ribosomes. Bull Soc Chem Biol 46:1399, 1964.
34. Hahn, F. E., O'Brien, R. L., Ciak, J., Allison, J. L.,

and Olenick, J. G.: Studies on modes of action of chloroquine, quinacrine and quinine and on chloroquine resistance. Milit Med 131(Suppl):1071, 1966.

35. Kaplan, A. S., and Ben-Porat, T.: Differential incorporation of iododeoxyuridine in the DNA of pseudorabies virus–infected and noninfected cells. Virology 31:734, 1967.

36. Appleyard, G.: Chemotherapy of viral infections. Brit Med Bull 23:114, 1967.

37. Bass, A. D.: Chemotherapy of bacterial infections. II. Sulfonamides. In DiPalma, J. R. (ed.): Drill's Pharmacology in Medicine. New York, McGraw-Hill, 1965, pp. 1300–1311.

38. Feingold, D. S.: Antimicrobial chemotherapeutic agents: The nature of their action and selective toxicity. N Engl J Med 269:957, 1963.

39. McCrumb, F. R., Snyder, M. J., and Hicken, W. J.: The use of chloramphenicol acid succinate in the treatment of acute infections. Antibiot Ann 1957-58, p. 837.

40. Goldberg, I. H.: Mode of action of antibiotics. II. Drugs affecting nucleic acid and protein synthesis. Amer J Med 39:722, 1965.

41. Kupferman, A., and Leibowitz, H. M.: Topical antibiotic therapy of staphylococcal keratitis. Arch Ophthalmol 95:1634, 1977.

42. Woodward, T. E., and Wisseman, C. L., Jr.: Chloromycetin (chloramphenicol). New York, Medical Encyclopedia, Inc., 1958.

43. Rosenthal, R., and Blackman, A.: Bone marrow hypoplasia following use of chloramphenicol eye drops. JAMA 191:136, 1965.

44. Carpenter, G.: Chloramphenicol eye drops and marrow aplasia. Lancet 2:326, 1975.

45. Abrams, S. M., Degnan, T. J., and Vinciguerra, V.: Marrow aplasia following topical application of chloramphenicol eye ointment. Arch Intern Med 140:576, 1980.

46. Fraunfelder, F. T., Bagby, G. C., Jr., and Kelly, D. J.: Fatal aplastic anemia following topical administration of ophthalmic chloramphenicol. Amer J Ophthalmol 93:356, 1982.

47. Fraunfelder, F. T., and Bagby, G. C., Jr.: Ocular chloramphenicol—Aplastic anemia. JAMA 247:18, 1983.

48. Leading Article: Chloramphenicol blindness. Brit Med J 1:1511, 1965.

49. Cocke, J. G., Jr., Brown, R. E., and Geppert, L. J.: Optic neuritis with prolonged use of chloramphenicol. J Pediatrics 68:27, 1966.

50. Sabath, L. D.: Drug resistance of bacteria. N Engl J Med 280:91, 1969.

51. Mitchell, R. G., and Baber, K. G.: Infections by tetracycline resistant hemolytic streptococci. Lancet 1:25, 1965.

52. Hansman, D., and Andrews, G.: Hospital infection with pneumococci resistant to tetracycline. Med J Aust 1:498, 1967.

53. Schaedler, R. W., Choppin, P. W., and Zabriskie, J. B.: Pneumonia caused by tetracycline-resistant pneumococci. N Engl J Med 270:127, 1964.

54. Weinstein, L.: Antibiotics. IV. The tetracyclines: Chlortetracycline, oxytetracycline, tetracycline, and demethylchlortetracycline. In Goodman, L. S., and Gilman, A. (eds.): The Pharmacological Basis of Therapeutics. 3rd ed. New York, Macmillan Co., 1965, pp. 1242–1243.

55. Suarez, G., and Nathans, D.: Inhibition of aminoacyl-s RNA binding to ribosomes by tetracycline. Biochem Biophys Res Comm 18:743, 1965.

56. Kline, A. H., Blattner, R. J., and Lunin, M: Transplacental effect of tetracyclines on teeth. JAMA 188:178, 1964.

57. Weyman, J.: The clinical appearances of tetracycline staining of the teeth. Brit Dent J 118:289, 1965.

58. Wilkinson, S.: Identity of colistin and polymyxin E. Lancet 1:922, 1963.

59. Eickhoff, T. C., and Finland, M.: Polymyxin B and colistin: In vitro activity against Pseudomonas aeruginosa. Amer J Med Sci 249:172, 1965.

60. Nord, N. M., and Hoeprich, P. D.: Polymyxin B and colistin: A critical comparison. N Engl J Med 270:1030, 1964.

61. Richards, F., McCall, C., and Cox, C.: Gentamicin treatment of staphylococcal infections. JAMA 215:1297, 1971.

62. Hahn, F. E., and Sarre, S. G.: Mechanism of action of gentamicin. J Infect Dis 119:364, 1969.

63. Barber, M., and Waterworth, P. M.: Activity of gentamicin against Pseudomonas and hospital staphylococci. Brit Med J 1:203, 1966.

64. Barker, B. M., and Prescott, F.: Antimicrobial Agents in Medicine. Oxford, Blackwell Scientific Publications, 1973, pp. 54, 241–245.

65. Leading Article: Staphylococci resistant to neomycin and bacitracin. Lancet 2:421, 1965.

66. Rountree, P. M., and Beard, M. A.: The spread of neomycin resistant staphylococci in a hospital. Med J Aust 1:498, 1965.

67. Neu, H. C.: Tobramycin: An overview. J Infect Dis 134(Suppl):53, 1976.

68. Jawetz, E., and Gunnison, J. B.: Studies on antibiotic synergism and antagonism: A scheme of combined antibiotic action. Antibiot Chemother 2:243, 1952.

69. Weinstein, L.: Chemotherapy of microbial diseases: Sulfonamides. In Goodman, L. S., and Gilman, A. (eds.): The Pharmacological Basis of Therapeutics. 3rd ed. New York, Macmillan Co., 1965, p. 1147.

70. Barker, B. M., and Prescott, F.: Antimicrobial Agents in Medicine. Oxford, Blackwell Scientific Publications, 1973, p. 76.

71. Barrett, F. F., McGehee, R. F., and Finland, M.: Methicillin-resistant Staphylococcus aureus at Boston City Hospital. N Engl J Med 279:441, 1968.

72. Benner, E. J., and Kayser, F. H.: Growing clinical significance of methicillin-resistant Staphylococcus aureus. Lancet 2:741, 1968.

73. Leading Article: The staphylococcus and methicillin resistance. Med J Aust 2:1189, 1968.

74. Sabath, L. D., Leaf, C. D., Gerstein, D. A., and Finland, M.: Cell walls of methicillin resistant Staphylococcus aureus. Antimicrob Agents Chemother 1969, p. 73.

75. Knox, R.: A new penicillin (BRL 1241) active against penicillin resistant staphylococci. Brit Med J 2:690, 1960.

76. Sutherland, R., Croydon, E. A. P., and Rolinson, G. N.: Flucloxacillin, a new isoxazolyl penicillin compared with oxacillin, cloxacillin, and dicloxacillin. Brit Med J 4:455, 1970.

77. Marcy, S. M., and Klein, J. O.: The isoxazolyl penicillins: Oxacillin, cloxacillin, and dicloxacillin. Med Clin N Amer 54:1127, 1970.

78. Barber, M., and Waterworth, P. M.: Pencillinase resistant penicillins and cephalosporins. Brit Med J 2:344, 1964.

79. Knudsen, E. T., Brown, D. M., and Rolinson, G. N.: A new orally effective penicillinase—Stable penicillin BRL 1621. Lancet 2:632, 1962.

80. Holmes, K. K., Clark, H., Silverblatt, E., and Turck,

M.: Emergence of resistance in *Pseudomonas* during carbenicillin therapy. Antimicrob Agents Chemother 1969, p. 391.

81. Lowbury, E. J. L., Kidson, A., Lilly, H. A., Ayliffe, G. A. J., and Jones, R. J.: Sensitivity of *Pseudomonas aeruginosa* to antibiotics: Emergence of strains highly resistant to carbenicillin. Lancet 2:448, 1969.

82. Darrell, J. H., and Waterworth, P. M.: Carbenicillin resistance in *Pseudomonas aeruginosa* from clinical material. Brit Med J 3:141, 1969.

83. Roe, E., Jones, R. J., and Lowbury, E. J. L.: Transfer of antibiotic resistance between *Pseudomonas aeruginosa*, *Escherichia coli*, and other gram negative bacilli in burns. Lancet 1:149, 1971.

84. Brumfitt, W., Percival, A., and Leigh, D. A.: Clinical and laboratory studies with carbenicillin. A new penicillin active against *Pseudomonas pyocyaneae*. Lancet 1:1289, 1967.

85. Smith, C. B., Dans, P. F., Wilfert, J. N., and Finland, M.: Use of gentamicin in combination with other antibiotics. J Infect Dis 119:370, 1969.

86. Sonne, M., and Jawetz, E.: Combined action of carbenicillin and gentamicin on *Pseudomonas aeruginosa* in vitro. Appl Microbiol 17:893, 1969.

87. Andriole, V. T.: Synergy of carbenicillin and gentamicin in experimental infection with pseudomonas. J Infect Dis 124:46, 1971.

88. Riff, L. J., and Jackson, G. G.: Laboratory and clinical conditions for gentamicin inactivation by carbenicillin. Arch Intern Med 130:887, 1972.

89. Apicella, M. A., Perkins, R. L., and Saslaw, S.: Treatment of bacterial endocarditis with cephalosporin derivatives in penicillin-allergic patients. N Engl J Med 274:1002, 1966.

90. Steigbigel, N. H., Kislak, J. W., Tilles, J. G., and Finland, M.: Clinical evaluation of cephaloridine. Arch Intern Med 121:24, 1968.

91. Editorial: Cross-allergenicity of penicillins and cephalosporins. JAMA 199:495, 1967.

92. Murray, B. E., and Moellering, R. C., Jr.: Cephalosporins. Ann Rev Med 32:559, 1981.

93. Strominger, J. L., and Tipper, D. J.: Bacterial cell wall synthesis and structure in relation to the mechanism of action of penicillins and other antibacterial agents. Amer J Med 39:708, 1965.

94. Riley, H. D., Jr.: Vancomycin and novobiocin. Med Clin N Amer 54:1277, 1970.

Antiviral Agents | 13

DENIS M. O'DAY, M.D.

In 1976, 3 per cent vidarabine eye ointment was officially approved and released by the Food and Drug Administration. Thus, after a lapse of 15 years, including 6 years for clinical testing, an alternative to idoxuridine (IDU) was finally available. The development of antiviral drugs has been agonizingly slow, as evidenced by the fact that a third ophthalmic antiviral antimetabolite, trifluridine, was not officially released by the FDA for clinical use until 1981. These agents have the potential to selectively interfere with and alter biosynthetic mechanisms in mammalian cells. On this account oncogenicity and teratogenicity must be carefully excluded before the agent can be considered safe. Then, too, there is a lesser but still serious problem of local toxicity that may become apparent only on prolonged testing. The future of a number of compounds with good antiviral activity is uncertain in the light of such considerations. Indeed, it is likely, as concern mounts over the problems of iatrogenic genetic alterations, that even more stringent criteria will be applied in assessing these newer drugs.

ROLE OF ANTIVIRAL AGENTS IN OCULAR VIRAL INFECTIONS

Against this background it is highly pertinent to re-examine the role of specific antiviral therapy in diseases of the external eye. Herpes simplex, adenovirus, and herpes zoster are the viruses of major interest as far as the conjunctiva and cornea are concerned. If we rank these viruses in terms of blindness and morbidity, herpes simplex is clearly the most important, followed by herpes zoster. However, it should be remembered that adenoviral keratoconjunctivitis, though rarely responsible for visual loss, may be accompanied by severe and prolonged morbidity.

Herpes simplex causes disease in the corneal epithelium. The familiar dendritic or ameboid ulcer is a direct result of viral replication in epithelial cells; the lesion is formed as the diseased cells desquamate. It can be argued that the dendritic ulcer is one of the best examples of a disease process due entirely to viral replication. It is not surprising that antiviral measures are highly effective and that therapy intended to modulate the host response may be deleterious.[1] In the corneal stroma the process is more complicated. Despite the lack of an effective antiviral agent, we know that corticosteroids can be highly effective.[2] Virus particles are present in the stroma in stromal keratitis due to herpes simplex but appear to be defective and have rarely been cultured despite numerous attempts by many workers.[3] All this would suggest that the disease process in the stroma is an immunopathologic inflammation, and laboratory evidence in support of this hypothesis is slowly accumulating. It seems likely that viral replication is no longer a major consideration by the time stromal inflammation develops. Rather, it is thought that the virus replicates at some undetermined time earlier, depositing a variety of antigens in the stroma, including large and insoluble viral fragments, that then initiate the later inflammatory response.[4] In zoster keratitis the process appears to be similar; replicating virus cannot be cultured except perhaps at the very outset of the disease. Keratoconjunctivitis, due to adenoviral infections, can probably be divided into two stages. Viral replication occurs in the conjunctiva and possibly in the corneal epithelium for a relatively brief period, and virus can rarely be recovered after the twelfth day of the disease.[5] The disease persists, however, for a considerably longer time—in some cases for a year or more. Again an immunologic basis is postulated and supported by an excellent response to local corticosteroid therapy. Thus, of the three viruses, herpes simplex continues to be the major concern in the search for effective antiviral agents. Indeed, antiviral therapy so far has no place in the treatment of zoster or adenoviral infections.

For disease in the corneal epithelium due to herpes simplex infection, local antiviral therapy clearly is indicated, but for the corneal stromal infection the issue is less clear. Although current antiviral agents do not penetrate the stroma significantly, we do have effective therapy in the form of corticosteroids to treat the inflammation when it occurs. The search that is now in progress for more potent and more soluble antivirals to treat stromal disease would appear to be inappropriate unless they can be demonstrated to be virtually nontoxic both locally and systemically. In order to treat any infrequent or intermittent episodes of viral replication in the corneal stroma, these drugs would have to be administered for prolonged periods of time. A better approach might be a therapeutic attack on the trigeminal ganglion, where the virus is latent between episodes of spread to peripheral target tissues. At this time such a development appears remote.

ANTIVIRAL ANTIMETABOLITES FOR HERPES SIMPLEX INFECTIONS

Idoxuridine (IDU)

The first agent demonstrated to have antiviral activity and released for general use was idoxuridine (IDU). IDU is a substituted pyrimidine nucleoside. Because it is similar to the thymine molecule, one of the bases of the DNA molecule, it is readily incorporated into the viral DNA. This renders the newly formed viral particles noninfective.[6] IDU is poorly soluble in water, achieving a maximum concentration of 0.1 per cent. It is active in the corneal epithelium but is rapidly degraded to an inactive metabolite (2'-deoxyuridine) and does not penetrate into the corneal stroma in significant amounts. IDU is available as a 0.1 per cent drop or as a 0.5 per cent ointment. Standard treatment regimens include hourly drops during the day with ointment at night, and ointment five times daily.

IDU is toxic in tissue culture systems and might be expected to exert a similar effect on normal human cells. Fortunately, IDU is preferentially incorporated into virus-infected cells due to the elaboration of an enzyme, thymidine kinase. This effect delays the onset of toxicity; nonetheless, in a majority of patients signs of toxicity (Table 13–1)

Table 13–1.   CLINICAL FEATURES OF IDU TOXICITY

Cornea
  Fine punctate keratopathy
  Filamentary keratitis
  Retardation of epithelial healing
  Perilimbal filaments
  Perilimbal edema
Conjunctiva
  Punctate staining with rose bengal
  Congestion
  Lower tarsal follicles
  Perilimbal filaments
  Perilimbal edema
Lid Margins
  Punctal edema—occlusion
  Edema of orifices of meibomian glands
Lids
  Ptosis

can be recognized after 2 weeks of relatively intense therapy, when a sensation of stinging and burning on administration of the drug can develop. Rarely, local hypersensitivity may appear. Although punctal edema and stenosis are commonly quoted as evidence of toxicity, these are late signs. More important are the corneal changes. These include a diffuse punctate keratopathy and the development of an indolent, nonhealing epithelial ulceration with hypertrophic margins. Actual hypertrophy of the corneal epithelium, mimicking a true dendritic ulcer in shape, can occur, and with prolonged administration subepithelial and stromal opacification and neovascularization may be seen. The changes are slow to progress and can cause considerable confusion in the management of the underlying keratitis. The lids also show destructive changes. The margins become edematous with pouting of the meibomian gland orifices; these changes may be of considerable long-term significance, contributing to future chronic lid disease.

In addition to the problem of toxicity, viral strains resistant to idoxuridine have emerged, causing management of herpetic keratitis to be more difficult. This has prompted the search for alternative, and it is hoped more effective, antimetabolic agents. IDU resistance and toxicity are major factors that defeat the aims of antimetabolic therapy of stromal keratitis when the drug is used to cover possible concurrent viral replication in the corneal epithelium during treatment with corticosteroids. Thus, alternative antiviral agents are a necessity.[7]

Idoxuridine initially was shown to be an effective agent for treatment of epithelial forms of herpetic keratitis in open uncontrolled trials,[8–10] and its effectiveness was later confirmed in uncoded and coded randomized clinical trials. IDU is more effective than placebo therapy[11–13] and as effective as carbolization[1] and proflavine photoinactivation.[14] It is as effective as vidarabine[15] but seemingly less effective than trifluridine.[16] Herpes simplex virus is not completely eradicated from the corneal epithelium after a short course of IDU,[17] so that, if treatment is stopped when the herpetic lesion heals, some lesions may recur within a short time (recrudescent ulcer).[9, 18] Topical IDU therapy should be continued for several days after the herpetic lesion has healed to avoid recrudescent ulceration.

Vidarabine

Vidarabine, formerly known as adenine arabinoside (Ara-A) is a substituted purine nucleoside first synthesized in the early 1960s. The mechanism of action has not been fully elucidated, but, like IDU, it attacks the virus during its most vulnerable phase, the replicative cycle. The agent does not appear to inactivate virus through direct contact, nor does it prevent viral attachment or entry into the cell. Several possible modes of action have been postulated.[19] Vidarabine is metabolized to hypoxanthine arabinoside, causing the preferential inhibition of viral DNA polymerase, of virus-induced ribonucleotide reductase, or of some other virus-specific enzyme in the pathway of viral DNA synthesis. The viral enzymes are more sensitive to the inhibitor (vidarabine) than the corresponding host cell enzymes. Vidarabine is rapidly deaminated in the cornea to the hypoxanthine compound, Ara-Hx, by an adenine deaminase. Hypoxanthine arabinoside has antiviral activity, although it is inferior to that of the parent compound. The in vitro antiviral activity of vidarabine itself can be enhanced fivefold by the simultaneous use of a deaminase inhibitor that prevents the formation of Ara-Hx.[19] Ara-A is poorly soluble, but the hypoxanthine component is more soluble and readily penetrates the cornea. Ara-A monophosphate is still another derivative of adenine arabinoside, with up to 30 times more antiviral activity than the parent compound. Unfortunately, it is too toxic for human use, causing neovascularization and even corneal perforation.[20] The ready penetration of these compounds into the eye raises questions of toxicity that have not hitherto been encountered, since the early compounds were purely surface active.

Vidarabine has been approved as a 3 per cent ointment for ophthalmic use. It is usually applied five times daily. Collaborative studies in the United States and overseas have indicated that vidarabine and IDU are about equally effective in the therapy of epithelial herpetic disease.[15, 21] Similarly, the data from clinical trials show no significant difference in effectiveness between vidarabine and trifluridine in the treatment of dendritic ulcers,[22, 23] but trifluridine is apparently more effective in healing geographic ulcers.[22]

As with IDU, resistant strains are seen but cross-resistance has not been observed. Vidarabine is well tolerated but is not free from side effects, principally in the form of punctate keratopathy.[24, 25] Hypersensitivity reactions also have been seen occasionally, and hypertrophic epithelial changes similar to those seen with IDU occur. With expanded use of the drug, further toxicity undoubtedly will be encountered.

Trifluridine

Trifluridine (Viroptic), formerly known as trifluorothymidine, is a halogenated pyrimidine synthesized in an effort to provide a pyrimidine nucleoside that would theoretically interfere with or replace thymidine in the synthesis of DNA. The agent is a potent inhibitor of thymidylate synthetase, and as a consequence it inhibits DNA synthesis. In addition, however, it is incorporated into viral DNA directly, rendering the viral particle noninfective.[26] Trifluridine is also incorporated into mammalian cells, and the question of teratogenicity remains unresolved; conflicting results appear in the literature.[27, 28] The compound is ten times more soluble in water than IDU, and, in view of the possibility

of greater ocular penetration, the issue of teratogenicity is being investigated further.

Clinically trifluridine is an effective drug for epithelial herpetic keratitis.[16, 22, 23] As stated above, it apparently is more effective than IDU in the treatment of dendritic and geographic ulcers, equally effective as vidarabine in the treatment of dendritic ulcers, and superior to vidarabine as treatment for geographic ulcers. Evidence has been presented that trifluridine is more effective than other available antimetabolites in healing recalcitrant steroid-treated ulcers.[29, 30] It is available as a 1.0 per cent solution whose ocular instillation is recommended every 2 hours while the patient is awake (for a maximum daily dosage of nine drops) until the corneal ulcer has re-epithelialized. The drug is then tapered and discontinued. Interestingly, in many of the early clinical studies of trifluridine the drug was administered in less than the currently recommended dose, so that it may be even more effective than these studies indicate. However, as the drug is used in higher doses for more prolonged periods, toxicity becomes evident, primarily in the form of a punctate keratopathy.[31, 32] Other adverse responses to trifluridine include contact dermatitis, filamentary keratopathy,[31] edema of the corneal stroma, and ocular irritation.

Herpetic epithelial corneal ulcers may fail to resolve despite treatment with IDU[28, 30] or vidarabine.[22, 29, 30, 32, 33] The lesions may remain unaltered, fail to epithelialize, progress, or recur after initial healing while the patient is still on antiviral therapy. Some such therapeutic failures may be due not to continued viral replication but to toxicity of the antiviral drug or to concurrent stromal disease that prevents epithelial regeneration. Nonetheless, at least some of these cases represent true drug resistance wherein the antimetabolite fails to control viral replication. Cases resistant to IDU have responded satisfactorily to vidarabine and trifluridine, and, similarly, cases unresponsive to vidarabine have been successfully treated with trifluridine.[16, 30, 32, 34] There seems to be little, if any, cross-intolerance or cross-resistance among IDU, vidarabine, and trifluridine. As a result, trifluridine represents an attractive alternative for use in patients who are either hypersensitive to or intolerant of other antiviral antimetabolites, and it is often effective in cases resistant to the other agents.

Acycloguanosine

One other agent currently being evaluated has intriguing possibilities. 9-(2 hydroxy ethoxy methyl) guanine (acyclovir) has potent in vitro and in vivo antiviral capabilities. It appears nontoxic in animal studies, since it requires the presence of a virus-elaborated thymidine kinase for incorporation into DNA. Normal mammalian cells are thus unaffected by this compound, but infected cells become the target of a specific antiviral therapy. Studies are continuing with this agent for both systemic and topical use.[35, 36] Although there has been considerable interest in this compound because of its potential for eradicating latent infection, data so far have been inconclusive. In addition, although the agent is attractive for topical use because of its efficacy and lack of toxicity, a significant drawback appears to be the rapid emergence of resistant strains. It seems unlikely that this agent will be released as a topical ophthalmic preparation in the near future.

These, then, are the major specific antiviral drugs that may be effective in the treatment of herpes simplex infection of the corneal epithelium. There are other promising agents under investigation, including Ac$_2$IDU, BVDU, and thymidine arabinoside, but the data on their effectiveness is still preliminary[37] and they are unavailable for routine clinical use.

PHOTODYNAMIC INACTIVATION

The technique of photodynamic inactivation received attention several years ago as a possibly effective method of treating certain viral lesions.[38] Photodynamic inactivation is a light-sensitized auto-oxidation reaction; it may be defined as the photosensitization of a biologic system by a substance that serves as a light absorber for a photochemical reaction in which molecular oxygen takes part. These substances, known as photoactive dyes, include a number of well-known compounds that have been used in medicine for many years (e.g., methylene blue, toluidine blue, acriflavine, proflavine, and rose bengal). A wide variety of biologic substances can be destroyed by this technique, including amino acids, protein, nucleic acids, plant and animal viruses, bacteria, red cells, and fungi. In the case of herpesvirus the photoactive dye binds actively replicating viral DNA at its guanine base. Subsequent exposure to light disrupts the DNA molecule and renders the virus noninfective.[39] Animal and clinical studies have shown the technique to have some promise, with a cure rate comparable to IDU.[14, 40] However, major toxicity problems, such as a photosensitized punctate epithelial keratopathy and anterior uveitis, have halted clinical trials of this technique, and it is not currently in use for the treatment of human disease.

INTERFERONS

Interferons are small soluble glycoproteins elaborated by cells infected by almost any of the RNA and DNA viruses. Their presence can be detected both in animals and in tissue culture. When a virus infects a cell, it gives rise to complete virus particles, incomplete forms, and interferon. The interferon is then taken up by adjacent healthy cells, and this inhibits subsequent viral replication if the interferon level is sufficiently high. Interferon induced by one virus may inhibit multiplication of a broad range of interrelated viruses, and production can be stimulated by a wide variety of related synthetic and naturally occurring substances, including double and multiple stranded RNA.

There has been enormous interest in interferon in the past few years. Initially it was hoped that active lesions would be treatable. This hope has not been fulfilled to date despite numerous attempts both with powerful interferon inducers and with animal and human interferons. Attention then was directed to investigating the role of interferon as a prophylactic agent for the prevention of recurrent epithelial herpes. Initial studies in rabbits with poly-IC, a double-stranded RNA, raised hopes that recurrence rates could be reduced. However, when the technique was applied to humans, using the interferon inducers or either human or monkey interferon, the results were disappointing. Part of the problem has been the lack of availability of interferon in sufficiently high concentrations to produce a clinical effect. A study by Jones and colleagues with human leukocyte interferon at a concentration of 11×10^6 units per ml. has shown that one dose per day significantly reduces the incidence of recurrent herpes in individuals with recent active disease.[41] The ability to control the recurrence of herpetic epithelial disease would be a crucial breakthrough in the management of this blinding disorder. Interferon is still under intensive study but is not available for general use. Recent advances in the methods used to manufacture interferon lead us to be hopeful that this approach may yet become clinically useful.

CRYOTHERAPY

This technique experienced a brief period of popularity several years ago. In one study it was shown that freezing dendritic corneal ulcers with a cryoprobe at $-80°$ C led to a cure rate superior to that of IDU.[42] The procedure is painful, and significant stromal inflammation may develop subsequently. In fact, cryotherapy seems to be little more than a rather elaborate way of performing debridement. Its practical value is questionable.

DEBRIDEMENT

Debridement is the oldest method of treatment of acute herpetic epithelial lesions and still perhaps the most effective. It takes advantage of the fact that there is a disruption of intercellular bridges among infected cells, so that the involved cells adhere poorly to one another and to the underlying basement membrane.[43] Controlled removal of the lesion is best achieved by gently debriding the margins of the epithelial ulcer with a tightly rolled cotton-tipped applicator. The virus-infected cells brush off easily, whereas the surrounding normal cells separate only with great difficulty and are left intact.[44] The removal of epithelium containing replicating virus markedly reduces the source of infection for adjacent healthy cells and the stimulus for stromal inflammation.

Debridement is best performed under magnification at the slit-lamp biomicroscope or under the operating microscope. Topical anesthesia (proparacaine hydrochloride 0.5 per cent or tetracaine hydrochloride 0.5 per cent) usually is adequate. A knife blade or other sharp instrument should not be used because of the risk of damage to Bowman's membrane, which could provide a portal of access to the stroma for viral particles[45] or result in a subsequent recurrent erosion problem.

Recrudescence of active epithelial lesions may occur after debridement.[41, 44] Small focal lesions are seen from which virus can be isolated. If left untreated, some of these lesions progress to form dendritic ulcers. These events make it necessary for the ophthalmologist to follow mechanical treatment with topical antiviral therapy. The number of viral particles present in the focal recurrences is probably small, so that the dose of the antimetabolite need not approach the toxic range. Chemical virucidal agents, such as phenol 10 per cent, have been advocated to sterilize the freshly debrided ulcer margins but are probably unnecessary. "Scrubbing" the bare surface is injurious, and iodine is damaging, especially to a diseased corneal stroma.[46]

Debridement is effective; the technique produces an excellent response and healing is rapid. Clinical study has demonstrated that herpetic epithelial ulcers debrided with a cotton-tipped applicator heal faster than a control group treated with IDU.[46] Debridement has one major advantage: It is free from the toxicity of antimetabolic drugs. Unfortunately, it is inconvenient, both to the ophthalmologist and to the patient, and is also somewhat traumatic to the latter. Debridement cannot be carried out in children and is potentially hazardous in the presence of large geographic ulcers or significant stromal keratitis.

CONCLUSION

The ophthalmologist has at his command several antiviral agents and a number of peripheral techniques and modalities that have therapeutic potential. In addition, there is again optimism about the role of interferon as a prophylactic agent. These are significant advances from the point of view of local therapy, but the problem of herpetic infection needs to be placed in perspective. Although the cornea is the target tissue for herpesvirus during episodic attacks, it is the trigeminal and other spinal ganglia that harbor life-long latent reservoirs of virus. An effective solution to the problems of recurrent herpetic corneal disease must, therefore, await an understanding of trigeminal involvement, the phenomenon of latency, and the interactions that occur between the virus and its host.

REFERENCES

1. Patterson, A., and Jones, B. R.: The management of ocular herpes. Trans Ophthalmol Soc UK 87:59, 1967.
2. Aronson, S. B., and Moore, T. E., Jr.: Corticosteroid therapy in central stromal keratitis. Amer J Ophthalmol 67:873, 1969.
3. Dawson, C., Togni, B., and Moore, T. E., Jr.: Structural changes in chronic herpetic keratitis. Arch Ophthalmol 79:740, 1968.
4. O'Day, D. M., and Jones, B. R.: Herpes Simplex Keratitis. In Duane, T. (ed.): Clinical Ophthalmology. Vol. 4. Harper & Row, 1976.
5. Dawson, C., Hanna, L., Wood, T. K., and Despain, R.: Adenovirus type 8 infection in the United States. III. Epidemiologic, clinical and immunological features. Amer J Ophthalmol 69:473, 1970.
6. Jones, B. R.: Prospects in treating viral diseases of the eye. Trans Ophthalmol Soc UK 87:537, 1967.
7. O'Day, D. M., Poirier, R. H., Jones, D. B., and Elliott, J. H.: Vidarabine therapy of complicated herpes simplex keratitis. Amer J Ophthalmol 81:642, 1976.
8. Kaufman, H. E., Martola, E. L., and Dohlman, C. H.: Use of 5-iodo-2'-deoxyuridine (IDU) in treating herpes simplex keratitis. Arch Ophthalmol 68:235, 1962.
9. Gordon, D. M., and Karnofsky, D. A.: Chemotherapy of herpes simplex keratitis. Amer J Ophthalmol 55:229, 1963.
10. Luntz, M. H., and MacCallum, F. O.: Treatment of herpes simplex keratitis with 5-iodo-2'-deoxyuridine. Brit J Ophthalmol 47:449, 1963.
11. Burns, R. P.: A double-blind study of IDU in human herpes simplex keratitis. Arch Ophthalmol 70:381, 1963.
12. Laibson, P. R., and Leopold, I. H.: An evaluation of double-blind IDU therapy in 100 cases of herpetic keratitis. Trans Amer Acad Ophthalmol Otolaryngol 68:21, 1964.
13. Patterson, A., Fox, A. D., Davies, G., Jones, B. R., Cobb, B., Maguire, C., Holmes-Sellers, P. J., and Wright, P.: Controlled studies of IDU in the treatment of herpetic keratitis. Trans Ophthalmol Soc UK 83:583, 1963.
14. O'Day, D. M., Jones, B. R., Poirier, R., Pilley, S., Chisholm, I., Steele, A., and Rice, N. S. C.: Proflavine photodynamic viral inactivation in herpes simplex keratitis. Amer J Ophthalmol 79:941, 1975.
15. Pavan-Langston, D., and Dohlman, C. H.: A double-blind clinical study of adenine arabinoside therapy of viral keratoconjunctivitis. Amer J Ophthalmol 74:81, 1972.
16. Laibson, P. R., Arentsen, J. J., Mazzanti, W. D., and Eiferman, R. A.: Double controlled comparison of IDU and trifluorothymidine in 33 patients with superficial herpetic keratitis. J Amer Ophthalmol Soc 75:316, 1977.
17. Underwood, G. E., Elliott, G. A., and Buthala, D. A.: Herpes keratitis in rabbits: Pathogenesis and effect of antiviral nucleosides. Ann NY Acad Sci 130:151, 1965.
18. McKinnon, J. R., McGill, J., and Jones, B. R.: A summary code for ocular herpes simplex. Brit J Ophthalmol 59:539, 1975.
19. Shannon, W. M.: Adenine arabinoside: Antiviral activity in vitro. In Pavan-Langston, D., Buchanan, R. A., and Alford, C. S. (eds.): Adenine Arabinoside: An Antiviral Agent. New York, Raven Press, 1975, pp. 1–42.

20. Foster, C. S., and Pavan-Langston, D.: Corneal wound healing and antiviral medication. Arch Ophthalmol 95:2062, 1977.
21. Pavan-Langston, D.: Clinical evaluation of adenine arabinoside and idoxuridine in treatment of routine and idoxuridine-complicated herpes simplex keratitis. In Pavan-Langston, D., Buchanan, R. A., and Alford, C. A. (eds.): *Adenine Arabinoside: An Antiviral Agent.* New York, Raven Press, 1975, pp. 345–356.
22. Coster, D. J., Jones, B. R., and McGill, J. I.: Treatment of amoeboid herpetic ulcers with adenine arabinoside or trifluorothymidine. Brit J Ophthalmol 63:418, 1979.
23. Van Bijsterveld, O. P., and Post, H.: Trifluorothymidine versus adenine arabinoside in the treatment of herpes simplex keratitis. Brit J Ophthalmol 64:33, 1980.
24. Jones, B. R.: Rational regimens of administration of antivirals. Trans Amer Acad Ophthalmol Otolaryngol 79:104, 1975.
25. Pavan-Langston, D., and Buchanan, R. A.: Vidarabine therapy of herpetic keratitis. Trans Amer Acad Ophthalmol Otolaryngol 81:OP813, 1976.
26. Prusoff, W. H., and Goz, B.: Potential mechanisms of action of antiviral agents. Fed Proc 32:1679, 1973.
27. Kury, G., and Crosby, R. J.: The teratogenic effect of 5-trifluoromethy-2'-deoxyuridine in chicken embryos. Toxicol Appl Pharmacol 11:72, 1967.
28. Itoi, M., Gefter, J. W., Kaneko, N., Ishii, Y., Ramer, R. M., and Gasset, A. R.: Teratogenicities of ophthalmic drugs. I. Antiviral ophthalmic drugs. Arch Ophthalmol 93:46, 1975.
29. McKinnon, J. R., McGill, J. I., and Jones, B. R.: A coded clinical evaluation of adenine arabinoside and trifluorothymidine in the treatment of ulcerative herpetic keratitis. In Pavan-Langston, D., Buchanan, R. A., and Alford, C. A. (eds.): *Adenine Arabinoside: An Antiviral Agent.* New York, Raven Press, 1975, pp. 401–410.
30. McGill, J. I., Holt-Wilson, A. D., McKinnon, J. R., Williams, H. P., and Jones, B. R.: Some aspects of the clinical use of trifluorothymidine in the treatment of herpetic ulceration of the cornea. Trans Ophthalmol Soc UK 94:342, 1974.
31. Coster, D. J., McKinnon, J. R., McGill, J. I., Jones, B. R., and Fraunfelder, F. T.: Clinical evaluation of adenine arabinoside and trifluorothymidine in the treatment of corneal ulcers caused by herpes simplex virus. J Infect Dis 133:A17, 1966.
32. Hyndiuk, R. A., Charlin, R. E., Alpren, T. V. P., and Schultz, R. O.: Trifluridine in resistant human herpetic keratitis. Arch Ophthalmol 96:1839, 1978.
33. McGill, J. I., Coster, D. J., Fraunfelder, F. T., Holt-Wilson, A. D., Williams, H., and Jones, B. R.: Adenine arabinoside in the management of herpetic keratitis. Trans Ophthalmol Soc UK 95:246, 1975.
34. Pavan-Langston, D., and Foster, C. S.: Trifluorothymidine and idoxuridine therapy of ocular herpes. Amer J Ophthalmol 84:818, 1977.
35. McCulley, J. P., Binder, P. S., Kaufman, H., O'Day, D. M., and Poirier, R. H.: A double-masked multicenter clinical trial of acyclovir versus idoxuridine in treating herpes simplex keratitis. Ophthalmology 89:1195, 1982.
36. Pavan-Langston, D., Lass, J., Hettinger, M., and Udell, I.: Acyclovir and vidarabine in the treatment of ulcerative herpes simplex keratitis. Amer J Ophthalmol 92:829, 1981.
37. Hettinger, M. E., Pavan-Langston, D., Park, N.-H., Albert, D. M., De Clercq, E., and Lin, T.-S.: Ac₂IDU, BVDU, and thymidine arabinoside therapy in experimental herpes keratitis. Arch Ophthalmol 99:1618, 1981.
38. Wallis, C., and Melnick, J. L.: Photodynamic inactivation of animal viruses: A review. Photochem Photobiol 4:159, 1966.
39. Freifelder, D., and Uretz, R. B.: Mechanism of photoinactivation of coliphage T-7 sensitized by acridine orange. Virology 30:97, 1966.
40. Tara, C. S., Stanley, J. A., Kucera, L. S. and Hollis, S.: Photodynamic inactivation of herpes simplex keratitis. Arch Ophthalmol 92:51, 1974.
41. Jones, B. R., Coster, D. J., Falcon, M. G., and Cantell, K.: Topical therapy of ulcerative herpetic keratitis with human interferon. Lancet 2:128, 1976.
42. Fulhorst, H. W., Richards, A. B., Bowbyes, J., and Jones, B. R.: Cryotherapy of epithelial herpes simplex keratitis. Amer J Ophthalmol 73:46, 1972.
43. Hollenberg, M. J., Wilkie, J. S., Hudson, J. B., and Lewis, B. J.: Lesions produced by human herpesviruses 1 and 2. Morphologic features in rabbit corneal epithelium. Arch Ophthalmol 94:127, 1976.
44. Coster, D. J., Jones, B. R., and Falcon, M. G.: Role of debridement in the treatment of herpetic keratitis. Trans Ophthalmol Soc UK 97:314, 1977.
45. Kimura, S. J.: *Herpes Simplex Keratitis in Infectious Diseases of the Conjunctiva and Cornea.* St. Louis, C. V. Mosby Co., 1963, p. 124.
46. Whitcher, J. P., Dawson, C. R., Hoshiwara, I., Daghfoud, T., Messadi, M., Triki, F., and Oh, J.: Herpes simplex keratitis in a developing country. Natural history and treatment of epithelial ulcers in Tunisia. Arch Ophthalmol 94:587, 1976.

Antifungal Agents | 14

DENIS M. O'DAY, M.D.

Fungal infection of the cornea has been considered until recently to be a rare and unusual event. The last decade, however, has seen a seemingly dramatic increase in the frequency of these infections. Indiscriminate use of antibiotics and corticosteroids has been blamed by some for this phenomenon, but this has not been substantiated by one large series of reported cases.[1] It is perhaps more likely that increased awareness by the clinician along with improved diagnostic methodology in the laboratory have combined to increase recognition of this type of infection.

Fungi are complex organisms. A typical fungus is composed of a mass of branched, tubular filaments (hyphae) known as mycelium. The hyphal wall is not a passive envelope but serves to regulate the interchange of substances between the fungus and its environment as well as to elaborate enzymes that break down large insoluble molecules into simpler molecules that can then be absorbed directly. Antifungal agents effect their action either by altering the hyphal cell membrane in some way or by interfering with internal biosynthetic mechanisms. It is important to recognize that all antifungals developed to date are inhibitory at levels that can usually be obtained in man.

THE POLYENES

The first major group of antifungal agents to be discovered was the polyene antibiotics. Since the initial discovery of nystatin by Hazen and Brown in 1950,[2] more than 60 members of this class have been described. Only amphotericin B, amphotericin methyl ester, and natamycin (pimaricin) are of practical interest as far as ocular fungal infections are concerned.

The basic structure of polyene antibiotics is a large, conjugated, double-bond system linked to an amino acid sugar, mycosamine. Various members of the group are classified on the basis of the number of double bonds. The polyene antibiotics selectively bind to a sterol (ergosterol) present in the plasma membrane of susceptible fungi. This interferes with its permeability so that leakage of potassium and essential metabolites occurs.[3] As a group the polyenes are unstable in oxygen, light, heat, water, and extremes of pH. The plasma membranes of mammalian cells also contain sterols; therefore, to some degree all polyenes also are toxic to mammalian cells when administered systemically. However, the sterol in mammalian cells is mainly in the form of cholesterol. Polyenes appear to have a higher affinity for ergosterol than cholesterol, and this may limit mammalian cell toxicity to some extent.[4]

Amphotericin B

Amphotericin B was discovered in 1955 and was the first polyene to be effective when given systemically in experimental and deep human mycoses. The molecule contains seven double bonds (hep-

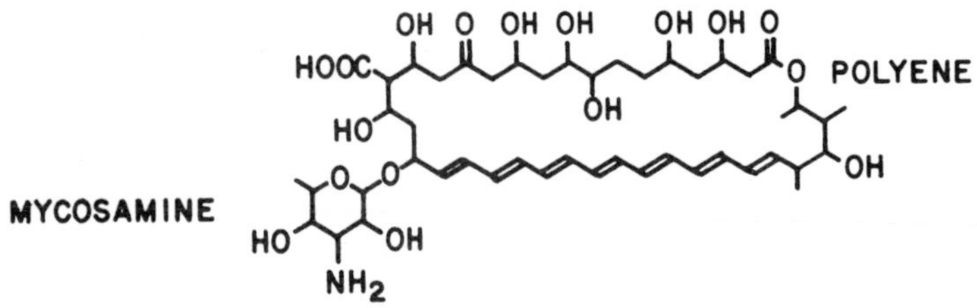

Figure 14–1. Structure of amphotericin B.

taene) (Fig. 14–1). It is insoluble in water, is unstable at 37° C, and is poorly absorbed from the gastrointestinal tract. When amphotericin B is given intravenously, satisfactory plasma levels can be achieved, although there is a significant binding to plasma lipoprotein with a subsequent slow release after the drug is discontinued.[5] The plasma half life is approximately 24 hours.

The only preparation of this agent approved for general use in the United States is amphotericin B (Fungizone) for IV injection. This consists of a sterile lyophilized powder containing 50 mg. of amphotericin B, 41 mg. of sodium desoxycholate, and 25 mg. of sodium phosphate buffer. Sodium desoxycholate acts as a solubilizer. The powder contained in the vial is dissolved by shaking in 10 ml. of sterile water before use. Sodium chloride or preservatives should not be used because they cause precipitation.

When administered intravenously, amphotericin B can be quite toxic, and this has severely limited its therapeutic effectiveness. Hypersensitivity reactions, including anaphylaxis, thrombocytopenia, flushing, generalized pain, and convulsions have been reported. Additional toxic effects that may be encountered with this drug include chills, fever, phlebitis, headache, anemia, and decreased visual function. Almost half the patients receiving amphotericin B intravenously will develop chills and fever; the fever may range as high as 40° C. Decreased renal function also is associated with amphotericin B and seems to be caused by renal vasoconstriction as well as by a direct toxic effect on the renal tubules.[6, 7] Fortunately, these changes usually are reversible upon cessation of the drug; provided renal function returns to normal, they do not con-

stitute a contraindication to the further use of amphotericin B. Occasionally, however, there is permanent impairment, and irreversible renal failure may occur after administration of large doses of the drug.

The data on ocular penetration of amphotericin B are sketchy, but penetration of the drug into the eye generally is considered to be poor.[8] In an effort to reduce toxic side effects, a variety of treatment regimens have been recommended. Should amphotericin B be necessary for treatment of an ocular fungal infection, my preference is for the regimen devised by Drutz and associates,[9] which aims at a dose of 0.5 mg./kg./day. The agent is administered daily by slow intravenous infusion over 4 to 6 hours, using a small pediatric scalp vein needle placed in a new vein each day. The contents of one ampule of amphotericin B (Fungizone) are dissolved in 10 ml. of sterile water and diluted in 500 ml. of 5 per cent dextrose in water to which 10 mg. of heparin have been added. The initial dose is 1 mg., rising in increments over the following days, to 3 mg., 5 mg., and so forth until a daily dose of 20 to 40 mg. is slowly reached. Daily estimations of pre- and postinfusion levels in the blood, optimally maintaining amphotericin B in the 0.75 to 1.5 mg./ml. range, aid in the decision concerning the optimal dosage. Patient intolerance and signs of toxicity may necessitate a slower infusion and a more gradual rise to optimal blood levels.[9]

In an attempt to augment ocular drug levels, topical, subconjunctival, and intraocular injections have been advocated. Drops can be formulated from the intravenous preparation at a concentration of 0.5 to 1.0 mg./ml., but toxicity is a problem. The topical preparation incites ocular inflammation, probably due largely to the presence of desoxycholate, and the treated eye may actually become icteric.[10] Similarly, subconjunctival injection of more than 300 mg. of the preparation can produce long-lasting periocular inflammation, and repeated injections can lead to epithelial ulceration.[11] Injection directly into the anterior chamber or into the vitreous cavity has been attempted, with conflicting results as far as toxicity is concerned. In doses of 25 µg., repeated injections into the anterior chamber have been well tolerated in one patient, although other authors have found that doses as low as 1 µg. into the vitreous humor have produced histopathologic lesions in the retina.[12]

Amphotericin B is effective against yeast infections, particularly the *Candida* species, *Cryptococcus*, and some filamentous fungi, notably *Aspergillus*. Its efficacy against other fungi has been limited (Table 14–1).

The treatment of corneal fungal infections with amphotericin B is, therefore, complicated by toxicity irrespective of the route of administration. The drug must be used with great caution, especially since prolonged therapy is indicated in such cases.

Amphotericin Methyl Ester

The problems of toxicity and lack of water solubility with amphotericin B, in the face of promising in vitro activity, have led to the synthesis of a new compound, amphotericin methyl ester. This agent is considerably less toxic and more water soluble. Experimental data and some limited human experience indicate that a higher therapeutic ratio can probably be obtained with this drug. In preliminary animal studies fungicidal levels of the drug have been achieved by topical and subconjunctival injection without the significant toxicity accompanying amphotericin B. Further studies will be needed to determine the precise role of this drug in ocular mycotic infections.[13]

Natamycin (Pimaricin)

Natamycin is a polyene antibiotic with four double bonds (Fig. 14–2) that was

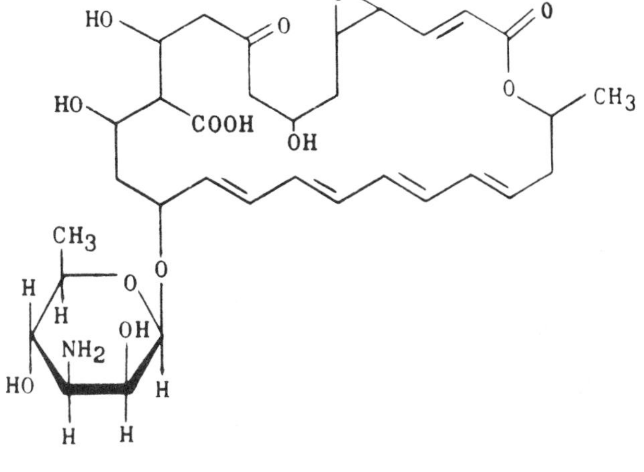

Table 14–1. RANGE OF SUSCEPTIBILITY OF OCULAR ISOLATES TO AMPHOTERICIN B AND NATAMYCIN

| Organism | Minimal Inhibitory Concentration (µg./ml.) | |
	Amphotericin B	Natamycin
Candida albicans	0.10–0.20	3.12–12.5
Torulopsis glabrata	0.39	0.39–3.12
Paecilomyces species	25–50	12.5–25
Penicillium species	0.10–3.12	0.78–1.56
Fusarium solani	0.78–3.12	1.56–6.25
Fusarium oxysporum	0.78–3.12	3.12–25
Aspergillus species	0.10–1.56	3.12–25
Cladosporium species	0.10–0.20	0.78–1.56

Figure 14–2. Structure of natamycin.

first isolated in 1958. Like the other polyenes, it is characterized by instability and a lack of solubility. It is believed to cause irreversible lytic changes in the cell membrane. Natamycin has a broad range of antifungal activity against filamentous fungi, particularly *Fusarium* species, although resistant strains are seen. *Candida* species tend to be less sensitive (Table 14–1). The compound is unsuitable for parenteral administration, and very little is absorbed from the gastrointestinal tract. A 5 per cent ophthalmic suspension currently is available (Alcon Laboratories, Inc., Fort Worth, Texas) for the treatment of corneal infections, and considerable experience has accumulated regarding its effectiveness in these infections.[14] However, deeper tissue penetration is probably limited and subconjunctival injection is valueless. In view of the in vitro and clinical experience, natamycin appears to be the prime drug for therapy of *Fusarium* infections of the cornea as well as the initial drug of choice for filamentous fungal infections of unidentified species. Although the agent is considered to be nontoxic, low-grade inflammation may develop with prolonged use.

Nystatin

Nystatin, the first polyene to be discovered, has very little applicability in the treatment of ocular mycoses. The agent is too toxic for parenteral administration. Experience with topical application has been disappointing because of toxicity and poor tissue penetration.

FLUCYTOSINE (5-FLUOROCYTOSINE)

Flucytosine (5-fluorocytosine, 5-FC) was synthesized in 1957 as an antimetabolite for the treatment of leukemia. As such it was totally ineffective. However, its antifungal activity was rapidly recognized, and today it has a proven place in the therapy of selected mycotic infections. Flucytosine, a fluorinated pyrim-

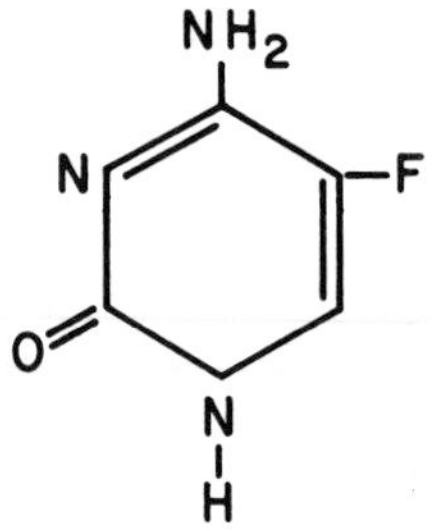

Figure 14–3. Structure of 5-fluorocytosine (5-FC).

idine (Fig. 14–3), is a white powder moderately soluble in water and readily absorbed from the gastrointestinal tract.

In contrast to the polyenes, flucytosine appears to act as an antimetabolite. In sensitive organisms the agent is transported across the cell membrane by a specific permease. Fungi lacking this enzyme are resistant to the drug.[15] Once inside the cell, flucytosine is converted to a 5-fluorouracil, which interferes with pyrimidine and nucleic acid synthesis. Flucytosine is not metabolized by mammalian cells; up to 95 per cent of the drug is excreted. However, recent studies have shown that gastrointestinal microorganisms can convert flucytosine to fluorouracil, which is then absorbed.

Following oral administration the serum half life is usually 6 hours. However, this is prolonged in patients with poor renal function and can be calculated by multiplying the serum creatinine level (in mg./100 ml.) by six.[16] Flucytosine is a drug of low toxicity, but side effects do occur. Nausea and diarrhea are seen uncommonly and skin rashes have been reported on occasion. Hematopoietic and hepatic toxicity may follow administration of this agent. These complications appear to be dose-related and reversible on cessation of therapy.[16] Regular hematologic evaluations and liver function tests are advisable during therapy.

Flucytosine is available as Ancoban in 250 mg. and 500 mg. capsules. The adult dose is 50 to 150 mg./kg. body weight.[17] Following oral administration the drug is well distributed in tissues, including the eye. The few reported studies of intraocular penetration indicate high levels in the anterior chamber and in vitreous humor following standard oral dosage.[11] Flucytosine also may be administered in drop form as a 1 per cent solution that is well tolerated. This preparation is not available in the United States. The sparse data available suggest that the topically applied drug does not penetrate into the anterior chamber in appreciable amounts, and the value of subconjunctival injection is not known.

Unfortunately, flucytosine has a relatively narrow range of antifungal activity. Among the pathogenic yeasts, *Candida*, *Cryptococcus*, and *Torulopsis* are generally sensitive, although resistant strains do occur. Resistance also may be induced during treatment. As far as the filamentous fungi are concerned, the *Cladosporium* species and some strains of *Aspergillus* have been found to be sensitive (Table 14–2).

True synergism appears to exist between flucytosine and amphotericin B, so that the combined use of these agents is being increasingly advocated. It is postulated that amphotericin facilitates the passage of flucytosine through the cell wall.[18] The use of both agents may prevent the emergence of resistant strains during therapy.

IMIDAZOLES

The discovery in 1965 that the antihelminthic compound thiabendazole, a substituted benzamidazole, had antifungal activity has led to the development of this new class of therapeutic agents with great potential for the treatment of keratomycoses.

Table 14–2. RANGE OF SUSCEPTIBILITY OF OCULAR ISOLATES TO FLUCYTOSINE

Organism	Minimal Inhibitory Concentration (μg./ml.)
Candida species	<0.50->50
Torulopsis glabrata	<0.50-0.20
Paecilomyces species	>50
Penicillium species	0.20-12.5
Fusarium solani	>50
Fusarium oxysporum	>50
Cladosporium species	<0.50->50
Aspergillus species	1.56-50

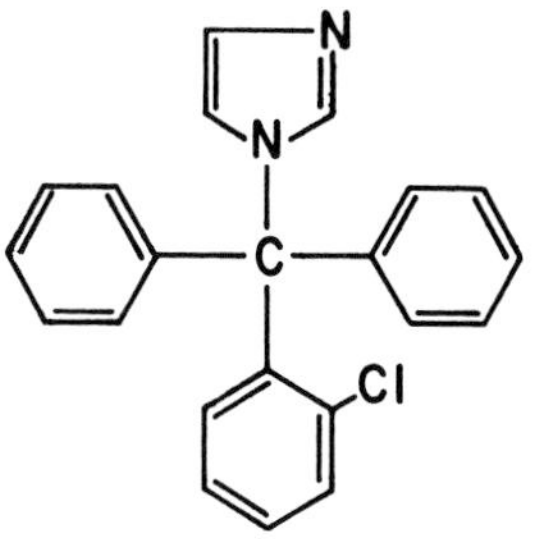

Figure 14–4. Structure of clotrimazole.

Clotrimazole

Clotrimazole is a chlorinated trityl imidazole (Fig. 14–4) first synthesized by Bayer Research Laboratories in Germany in 1967. Its precise mode of action is unknown, but it appears to bind selectively to the fungal cell membrane. This causes changes in permeability that result in leakage of small molecules and electrolytes. Except at high concentrations not usually obtainable in man, the changes are reversible, so that clotrimazole's main action is fungistatic.[19] Although this mechanism of action is broadly similar to that of the polyenes, there is nonetheless an important difference. The sterol content of the fungal cell membrane does not appear to be as critical, so that clotrimazole is considerably less toxic to mammalian cells.

Clotrimazole is poorly soluble in water and parenteral administration is not feasible. By mouth the drug is rapidly absorbed and produces satisfactory blood levels during the first week or two of therapy. Unfortunately, clotrimazole is a potent inducer of microsomal drug-metabolizing enzymes, so that blood levels fall rapidly thereafter despite continued administration. At times nausea and vomiting also are significant side effects, and reversible abnormalities in liver function tests (SGOT and alkaline phosphatase) may develop. There is no indication of renal or hematopoietic toxicity.[20]

Clotrimazole has broad antifungal activity (Table 14–3) but appears to be of greatest value in the treatment of *Aspergillus* infections (Table 14–4). It may be the drug of choice for these infections.

Table 14–3. RANGE OF SUSCEPTIBILITY OF OCULAR ISOLATES TO CLOTRIMAZOLE

Organism	Minimal Inhibitory Concentration μg./ml.
Candida albicans	0.50–6.25
Torulopsis glabrata	0.39–3.12
Paecilomyces species	3.25–25
Fusarium solani	3.12–25
Fusarium oxysporum	6.25–12.5
Aspergillus species	0.10–0.78
Cladosporium species	3.12–12.5

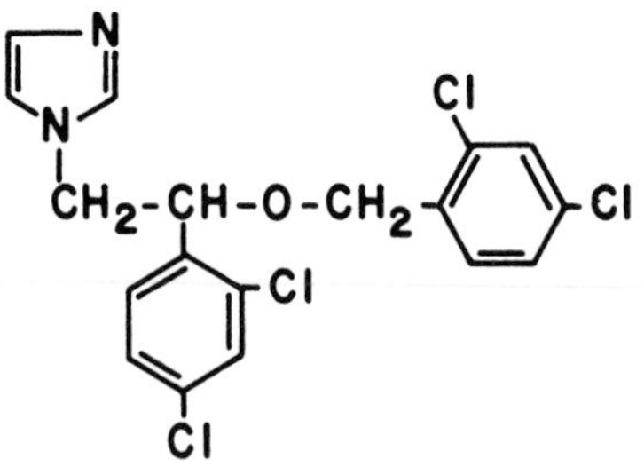

Figure 14–5. Structure of miconazole.

In superficial corneal infections the topical preparation in 1 per cent arachis oil or the Bayer preparation (Canesten) has been shown to be useful.[21] In the United States the topical preparation is under study; oral preparations are not available. The degree of intraocular penetration is unknown.

Miconazole

Miconazole is a phenethyl imidazole synthesized in Belgium in 1969 (Fig. 14–5). The antifungal activity results primarily from alterations in the plasmalemma and cell wall that induce permeability changes. It has a broad spectrum of activity against yeasts and filamentous fungi, though individual strains may be resistant (Table 14–5). Interestingly, it is as active as benzyl penicillin against Gram-positive bacteria. Miconazole is soluble in organic solvents and is moderately well absorbed from the gastrointestinal tract. It may be administered intravenously in normal saline after dissolving in cremophor EL. There has been considerable interest in this agent for the treatment of deep systemic mycoses because of the lack of serious side effects and the absence of enzyme induction.

Miconazole administered intravenously and topically has been used with success in the treatment of corneal fungal infections.[11] The miconazole base, either as a 1 per cent drop in arachis oil or as a 2 per cent cream, has been well tolerated in the limited number of cases treated. The nitrate salt shows identical antifungal activity but appears too toxic for prolonged use. Neither of the topical ocular preparations is available in the United States, though a 2 per cent cream has been released for dermatologic and vaginal use (MicaTin, Johnson & Johnson). Monistat, the intravenous prepa-

Table 14–4. ORGANISMS AND MINIMAL INHIBITORY CONCENTRATIONS (MIC) OF CLOTRIMAZOLE IN 15 CASES OF OCULOMYCOSIS*

Case Number	Genus	Species	MIC (μg./ml.)
2	Aspergillus	fumigatus	0.75
3	"	"	0.75
4	"	"	1.5
5	"	"	0.75
6	"	"	1.5
7	"	"	3.7
8	"	flavus	0.75
9	"	wentii	N.D.†
10	"	flaviceps	N.D.†
11	Candida	albicans	0.75
12	"	"	1.5
13	"	tropicalis	0.75
14	Fusarium	moniliforme	6.0
15	Paecilomyces	variotii	0.75
16	Dreschlera	rostrata	0.35

*Each patient was successfully treated with clotrimazole. Data from Jones, B. R., et al.: The place of Canesten in the management of oculomycosis. Münch Med Wochenschr *118*(Suppl 1):97, 1976.
†N.D. = not determined.

Table 14–5. RANGE OF SUSCEPTIBILITY OF OCULAR ISOLATES TO MICONAZOLE AND ECONAZOLE

Organism	Minimal Inhibitory Concentration µg./ml.	
	Miconazole	*Econazole*
Candida albicans	0.10–6.25	0.20–6.25
Torulopsis glabrata	0.50–1.56	0.10–0.39
Paecilomyces species	0.78–12.5	1.56–25
Fusarium solani	3.12–25	0.78–25
Fusarium oxysporum	12.5–50	12.5–25
Aspergillus species	0.10–0.78	0.05–1.56
Cladosporium species	0.20–0.78	0.10–0.78

ration, is available and can be administered topically (10 mg./ml.) or by subconjunctival injection (5 to 10 mg.). Both routes of administration are well tolerated, and both have been reported to produce therapeutic levels in the cornea.[22]

Econazole

Econazole is a dichlorimidazole similar to miconazole with a similar mode of action. This agent has a wide spectrum of activity against filamentous organisms in vitro but appears to be less effective than miconazole against *Candida* species (Table 14–5). Econazole is well tolerated in the eye as a 1 per cent watery suspension and has been effective in the therapy of a variety of keratomycoses.[11] Unfortunately there are no plans to market the drug in the United States.

CONCLUSION

From this brief review of the available and experimental antifungal agents, it is apparent that developments in this field of antimicrobial therapy are occurring rapidly. In the past we have been accustomed to antifungal agents with great toxicity and limited potential. However, the newer agents afford reasonable hope of an improved ratio of therapeutic to toxic effects. It is sobering to realize that, despite their demonstrated efficacy, most of these agents remain beyond the reach of the practicing ophthalmologist. Although natamycin has been released for ophthalmic use, prospects for availability of the other agents are not good. Meanwhile, newer ways of exploiting established drugs need to be investigated further. The phenomenon of synergism would seem to offer significant potential in this regard.

REFERENCES

1. Forster, R. K., and Rebell, G.: The diagnosis and management of keratomycoses. I. Cause and Diagnosis. Arch Ophthalmol 93:975, 1975.
2. Hazen, E., and Brown, R.: Two antifungal agents produced by a soil actinomycete. Science 112:423, 1950.
3. Kinsky, S. C.: Antibiotic interactions with model membranes. Ann Rev Pharmacol 10:119, 1970.
4. Kotler-Brastburg, J., Price, H. D., Medoff, G., Schlessinger, D., and Kobayashi, G. S.: Molecular basis for the selective toxicity of amphotericin B for yeast and filipin for animal cells. Antimicrob Agents Chemother 5:377, 1974.
5. Bindschadler, D. D., and Bennett, J. E.: A pharmacologic guide to the clinical use of amphotericin B. J Infect Dis 170:427, 1969.
6. Douglas, J. B., and Healy, J. K.: Nephrotoxic effects of amphotericin B including renal tubular acidosis. Amer J Med 46:154, 1969.
7. Bergess, L., and Binhall, R.: Nephrotoxicity of amphotericin B with emphasis on changes in renal tubular function. Amer J Med 53:77, 1972.
8. Green, W. R., Bennett, J. E., and Goos, R. D.: Ocular penetration of amphotericin B. Arch Ophthalmol 73:769, 1965.
9. Drutz, D. J., Spickard, A., Rogers, D. E., and Koenig, M. G.: Treatment of disseminated mycotic infections—A new approach to amphotericin B therapy. Amer J Med 45:405, 1968.
10. O'Day, D. M., Moore, T. E., and Aronson, S. B.: Deep fungal corneal abscess. Arch Ophthalmol 86:414, 1971.

11. Jones, B. R.: Principles in the management of oculomycosis. Amer J Ophthalmol 79:719, 1975.
12. Mosher, M. A., Lusk, B., Pettit, T. H., Howard, D. H., and Rhodes, J.: Fungal endophthalmitis following intraocular lens implantation. Amer J Ophthalmol 83:1, 1977.
13. Jones, D. B., Bonner, D. P., Mechlinski, W., Schaffner, C. P., Gentry, L. O., and Wallis, C. H.: Pharmacokinetics and chemotherapeutic activity of amphotericin B methyl ester. Presented at the Association for Research in Vision and Ophthalmology meeting, Sarasota, Florida, May, 1975.
14. Jones, D. B., Forster, R. K., and Rebell, G.: *Fusarium solani* keratitis treated with natamycin (pimaricin): 18 consecutive cases. Arch Ophthalmol 88:147, 1972.
15. Bennett, J. E.: Chemotherapy of systemic mycosis. N Engl J Med 290:320, 1974.
16. Dawborn, J. K., Page, M. D., and Schavone, D. J.: Use of 5-fluorocytosine in patients with impaired renal function. Brit Med J 4:382, 1973.
17. Kucers, A., and Bennett, N.: *The Use of Antibiotics.* 2nd ed. Philadelphia, J. B. Lippincott Co., 1975. p. 581.
18. Smith, J. W.: Synergism of amphotericin B with other antimicrobial agents. Ann Intern Med 78:450, 1973.
19. Iwata, K., Yamaguchi, H., and Hiratoni, T.: Mode of action of clotrimazole. Sabouraudia 11:158, 1973.
20. Tettenborn, D.: Toxicity of clotrimazole. Postgrad Med J 50(Suppl 1):17, 1974.
21. Jones, B. R., Clayton, Y. M., Jones, D. B., O'Day, D. M., and Poirier, R. H.: The place of Canesten in the management of oculomycosis. Münch Med Wochenschr 118(Suppl 1):97, 1976.
22. Foster, C. S., and Stefanszyn, M.: Intraocular penetration of miconazole in rabbits. Arch Ophthalmol 97:1763, 1979.

B. Clinical Entities

Bacterial Keratitis | 15

HOWARD M. LEIBOWITZ, M.D.

The external eye and the surrounding tissue harbor bacteria throughout life. The organisms cultured from the conjunctival sac usually are similar to those found on the periocular skin, the lid margins, and the upper respiratory tract. Less frequently organisms (primarily Gram-negative bacilli) that commonly inhabit the gastrointestinal tract are isolated from the conjunctiva of the normal eye.[1] *Staphylococcus aureus, Staphylococcus epidermidis,* and *Corynebacterium* species (diphtheroids) are the bacterial organisms found most often in the conjunctival sac.[2-5] Streptococci, including *Streptococcus pneumoniae,* and a variety of Gram-negative bacilli are present infrequently in the normal conjunctival flora, and a number of anaerobic organisms also inhabit the area.[6] Generally the normal flora of both eyes of an individual are identical.[1]

The presence of these microorganisms in the normal, uninfected conjunctival sac provides a constant reservoir of potentially pathogenic bacteria capable of causing serious ocular infections. Bacterial organisms in the meibomian glands, on the lid margins, and in the canaliculi and lacrimal sac similarly may be a primary source of infection. For reasons that are largely obscure, these organisms develop the capability of colonizing the adjacent tissues and causing conjunctivitis and keratitis.

Although many bacterial species are capable of invading and proliferating in the cornea, few are able to penetrate through an intact corneal epithelium. Thus, the epithelial layer represents a formidable barrier to the entrance of bacteria into the cornea. It follows, then, that most cases of bacterial keratitis are traumatic in origin and involve a break in the epithelium. Often the traumatic episode is minor and goes unnoticed; it may be nothing more than a minute abrasion caused by airborne debris or a small foreign body (Fig. 15–1A). On the other hand, the initiating traumatic episode may be of more major proportions. Misdirected lashes, conjunctival concretions or scarring, or a contact lens (Fig. 15–1B) can erode the epithelium and provide an entry for infectious bacteria. Alternatively, conditions such as bullous keratopathy, tear insufficiency, exposure or neuroparalytic keratopathy, and keratomalacia can result in an interruption of the intact epithelium and are therefore associated with an increased incidence of bacterial keratitis. So, too, are debilitating chronic illness, malnutrition, alcoholism, and advanced age. In these latter instances a deficiency or weakening of normal host defenses presumably renders the corneal stroma more susceptible to infection and permits normally saprophytic bacteria to become pathogenic invaders.

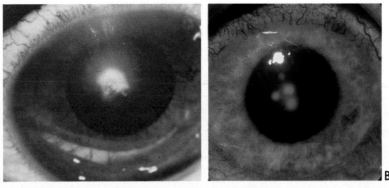

Figure 15–1. Localized staphylococcal anterior stromal infiltrates in areas of epithelial abrasion caused by a small, steel foreign body *(A)* and a contact lens *(B)*.

CLINICAL CHARACTERISTICS

In general, an acute bacterial infection of the cornea is characterized by the following sequence of events. A break occurs in the epithelium, through which varying numbers of organisms enter the stroma and proliferate. This initiates an inflammatory response in which large numbers of inflammatory cells, primarily polymorphonuclear leukocytes, are chemotactically attracted to the area. An abscess is formed, visible biomicroscopically (and often grossly) as a grayish-white infiltrate in the stroma (Fig. 15–2). If effective therapy is not instituted, lytic enzymes are released by the leukocytes and by certain strains of bacteria, causing necrosis of the involved

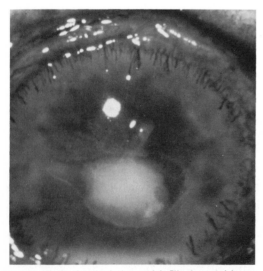

Figure 15–2. Central stromal infiltrate and hypopyon due to infection by *Staphylococcus aureus.*

stroma. Bowman's membrane and the anterior stromal lamellae are destroyed and subsequently are sloughed, leaving an ulcer of varying depth. The ulcer commonly is round or oval in shape, and its sides and floor usually are gray and ragged. It may be difficult to assess the degree of tissue loss accurately at this stage, for both the involved and the contiguous stroma are thickened by the imbibition of fluid and the massive infiltration of leukocytes. In most instances these inflammatory cells have already invaded the stroma underlying the ulcer and are visible for a considerable distance around the ulcer. If the infection is not halted effectively, the ulcerative process will progress. It may spread radially to involve a larger area of the cornea or posteriorly to involve the deeper stromal lamellae. In the latter case the inflammatory infiltrate can involve the entire thickness of the corneal stroma, and all of the stromal lamellae may desquamate in the subsequent ulcerative process.

Thus, in severe bacterial corneal ulcers Descemet's membrane may be the only corneal structure that remains intact (Fig. 15–3). That it does so is testimony to its inherent structural strength, which is greater than that of the stroma. Neither leukocytes[7, 8] nor blood vessels[9, 10] are able to penetrate Descemet's membrane, and it is resistant to digestion by proteolytic enzymes.[11] However, in spite of its remarkably resistant structure, Descemet's membrane is not indestructible. Leukocytic en-

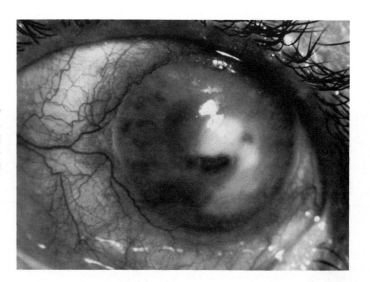

Figure 15–3. Secondary infection by *S. aureus* of a stromal herpes simplex keratitis. Much of the involved necrotic stroma has sloughed, leaving only an intact, slightly bulging Descemet's membrane.

zymes can destroy it,[12] and fungi can penetrate an intact Descemet's membrane.[13] The intraocular pressure ultimately causes distention of Descemet's membrane, and the outward, blisterlike bulging of the structure is referred to as a descemetocele. Destruction of Descemet's membrane, either by leukocytic enzymes or by progressive distention, results in perforation of the globe.

The active stage of bacterial keratitis is characterized by ocular pain, photophobia, excessive lacrimation, and blepharospasm. Vision is lost to a varying degree, depending on the location and the severity of the infectious process. If the ulcer involves the central or paracentral cornea, the visual disturbance is caused by the infiltrate and the irregularity of the corneal surface. More peripheral ulcers may be accompanied by edema, and the resulting loss in corneal transparency causes a visual deficit. The involved eye is invariably red, a reflection of a reactive dilatation of the conjunctival vessels. The hyperemia also involves the circumcorneal network of vessels (ciliary injection) and the iris vasculature. In most instances iris involvement can be readily established by comparison with the opposite eye. The involved iris is swollen (as reflected by a blurring of its surface markings) and presents a purplish discoloration, and the pupil is constricted. The hyperemia

is accompanied by an increased permeability of the involved vessels. Substantial quantities of serum components and cells exude from these vessels, producing the purulent exudate found in the conjunctival sac (Fig. 15–4) and on the surface of the ulcer itself as well as the anterior chamber cells, proteinaceous flare, fibrinous exudates, and hypopyon that commonly accompany a bacterial corneal ulcer. Few bacterial organisms are able to pass through Descemet's membrane; therefore, if this structure is intact, the inflammatory reaction in the anterior chamber almost invariably is sterile. Inflammation in the anterior

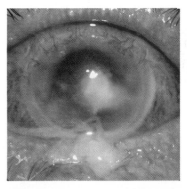

Figure 15–4. *S. aureus* keratitis showing a typical stromal infiltrate, conjunctival hyperemia, and purulent exudate.

chamber subsides when the corneal inflammatory response resolves.

The most severe ulcers are accompanied by corneal neovascularization. Limbal blood vessels invade the corneal stroma, most often in the superficial lamellae, to widely varying degrees. The extent and location of neovascularization are largely dependent upon the longevity of the untreated or inadequately treated infectious process, the position of the ulcer, and the virulence of the causal organism. In general, the longer the active infection is present, the more peripheral the location of the corneal ulcer, and the more virulent the infecting bacteria, the greater the degree of neovascularization that is induced.

With appropriate therapy one obtains regression of the necrotizing processes. At the cellular level there is an involution of the leukocytes that have invaded the cornea, and additional inflammatory cells cease to be attracted there. Clinically the corneal infiltrate begins to disappear. Necrotic material is shed and the ulcer may become larger. The walls and floor of the ulcer become smoother and more transparent. This, coupled with a decrease in (and often resolution of) corneal edema and with re-epithelialization of the ulcerated area, results in a less sharply demarcated border between involved and uninvolved corneal tissue. There is a more gradual transition between the ulcer site and the surrounding normal cornea. Unfortunately, cicatrization occurs as part of the healing process. New connective tissue is laid down in an irregular manner, with the result that the scar is not optically transparent (Fig. 15–5). If central in location, this optical density will cause a visual defect that persists unless the scar is replaced surgically with transparent cornea. Any residual irregularities or facets left on the corneal surface by the ulcerative process will accentuate the degree of visual loss. Residual complications may also include anterior and posterior synechiae, adherent leukoma, glaucoma, cataract, and anterior ectasia of the cornea.

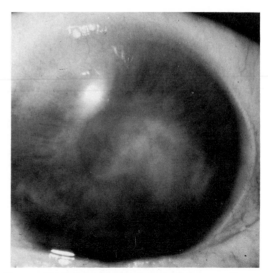

Figure 15–5. Translucent irreversible scar, the residuum of an *S. aureus* keratitis.

ETIOLOGIC ORGANISMS

A majority of the organisms cultured from infections of the corneal stroma (Table 15–1) are of the same species that normally are present in the conjunctival sac, on the lids or periocular skin, or in

Table 15–1. CHARACTERISTICS OF BACTERIAL CORNEAL PATHOGENS IN A GRAM-STAINED SMEAR

Gram-Positive Cocci
　　Staphylococcus aureus
　　Staphylococcus epidermidis
　　Streptococcus pneumoniae
　　Streptococcus pyogenes
　　Streptococcus viridans
　　Streptococcus faecalis

Gram-Positive Rods
　　Bacillus species
　　Corynebacterium species (diphtheroids)

Gram-Negative Cocci
　　Neisseria gonorrhoeae
　　Neisseria meningitidis

Gram-Negative Diplobacilli
　　Moraxella species

Gram-Negative Rods
　　Pseudomonas aeruginosa
　　Proteus species
　　Klebsiella pneumoniae
　　Escherichia coli
　　Serratia marcescens
　　Acinetobacter

the adjacent nasal passages. Although selected series indicate that their incidence may vary geographically, *Staphylococcus, Pseudomonas, Streptococcus pneumoniae* (pneumococcus), and *Moraxella* appear to be the predominant causes of bacterial ulcers in the United States at the present time.[14-17] A *Pseudomonas* keratitis often can be recognized clinically by the rapidly progressive and extensive corneal involvement, the liquefactive type of stromal necrosis, and the yellowish-green, adherent, mucopurulent discharge. However, the morphologic characteristics of keratitis due to *Staphylococcus, Streptococcus pneumoniae,* or *Moraxella* generally are not sufficiently distinct from one another to permit identification of the causal organism with any degree of accuracy on the basis of clinical examination alone. Nonetheless, an understanding of the attributes and biologic properties of the more common corneal pathogens is helpful.

Staphylococci

Staphylococci are among the hardiest of all non–spore-forming bacteria, and in this writer's experience they have been the most common cause of bacterial keratitis. During the present era of antibacterial chemotherapy the prevalence of this organism as an ocular pathogen seems to have increased dramatically, presumably because of the frequency with which it becomes resistant to antibiotics. Most of the virulent and more pathogenic strains of *Staphylococcus* form golden colonies and are named *Staphylococcus aureus*. These strains are surrounded by a wide zone of clear hemolysis on blood agar and they are able to ferment mannitol. However, some highly pathogenic strains do not produce golden pigment, so it has become customary to classify as *Staphylococcus aureus* all strains that elaborate coagulase. Coagulases are enzymes that cause citrated (or oxalated) plasma to coagulate. Apparently staphylococci are the only bacteria able to produce these

enzymes. The ability to produce coagulase has generally been considered to be the best laboratory evidence that a given strain of *Staphylococcus* is potentially pathogenic for man. However, there is no evidence that coagulase is directly involved in pathogenicity; its correlation with virulence appears to be coincidental.[18-20] Moreover, the pathogenicity of coagulase-negative strains is well documented both clinically and experimentally. *Staphylococcus epidermidis,* though less virulent and less pathogenic to man, has been implicated as a causal agent of bacterial keratitis, seemingly with increasing frequency in recent years.[15, 21] This species does not produce coagulase, is nonhemolytic on blood agar, and does not ferment mannitol.

Staphylococcus aureus and *Staphylococcus epidermidis* cannot be distinguished morphologically by their microscopic appearance on a Gram-stained smear. Both are Gram-positive cocci that characteristically grow in clusters on solid media but also commonly are seen singly or in pairs on microscopic examination. *Staphylococcus aureus* can be characterized by bacteriophage typing; coagulase-negative *Staphylococcus epidermidis* strains rarely are sensitive to the typing phages. Evidence has been presented that it is unusual to find more than one phage type of *Staphylococcus aureus* among the organisms isolated from an individual. Although a large variety of staphylococci are obtained from human isolates, a given individual usually carries only a single strain of *Staphylococcus aureus* (as determined by phage typing), and this strain often is present in the nose, in the throat, and on the skin.[22] The phage types of *Staphylococcus* recovered from both infected and uninfected eyes are the same as those present in contiguous areas of the face and upper respiratory tract of the individual. Moreover, the phage types recovered from infected eyes are similar to those in uninfected eyes. In instances in which preoperative cultures have been available, postoperative infection has been shown to be caused by the same phage type present in the eye before operation. Other cases have been documented in which the infection was due to a staphylococcus of the same phage type as was isolated from the opposite uninfected eye. It can be concluded that in the great majority of instances, *Staphylococcus aureus* ocular infections are caused by an organism normally carried by the patient.

Staphylococci release a number of extracellular proteins that are associated with a variety of toxic effects. Among these exotoxins are several immunologically distinct hemolysins, a nonhemolytic leukocidin, and various enterotoxins. The alpha toxin (alpha-hemolysin) is injurious to human leukocytes and apparently accounts, at least in part, for the ability of staphylococci, particularly *Staphylococcus aureus*, to resist phagocytosis. This factor is also dermonecrotic. The delta toxin is a nonantigenic protein with detergentlike activity. Erythrocytes, macrophages, lymphocytes, neutrophils, and platelets all are damaged by delta toxin. The Panton-Valentine leukocidin produced by most pathogenic staphylococci attacks polymorphonuclear leukocytes and macrophages. In the presence of calcium large amounts of protein derived from the cytoplasmic granules of these leukocytes are secreted; this degranulation can be observed microscopically. Certain strains of staphylococci also elaborate an exfoliative toxin (epidermolytic toxin) that causes exfoliation of the epidermis. Its role in eye disease is not known.[18-20]

In addition, coagulase-positive staphylococci produce a number of extracellular enzymes, including lipases, hyaluronidase, staphylokinase, and a nuclease. The lipases are lipid-hydrolyzing enzymes active on a variety of substrates, including fats and oils that accumulate on the surface of the skin. Their production seems essential to the organism's ability to effect the invasion of healthy skin. Lipases permit staphylococci to utilize skin fats and oils, an action that has survival value for the organism. Presumably this explains the propensity of staphylococci to colonize areas of substantial sebaceous activity, including the meibomian glands.[18-20]

Hyaluronidase hydrolyzes the hyaluronic acid present in the intercellular ground substance of connective tissue. More than 90 per cent of the *Staphylococcus aureus* strains produce this enzyme, which presumably facilitates the spread of infection. However, since inflammation antagonizes this effect, its importance probably is limited to the very early stages of infection. Staphylokinase is a proteolytic enzyme with fibrinolytic activity, whereas the nuclease can cleave both DNA and RNA. The latter enzyme is elaborated by 90 per cent or more of coagulase-positive strains but is absent in coagulase-negative strains.[18-20]

In the eye staphylococcal exotoxins, undoubtedly acting in concert with several of the extracellular enzymes, can cause necrosis of the corneal epithelium and produce a sterile infiltrate in the underlying stroma. As a result there are two types of staphylococcal keratitis. The first generally accompanies a staphylococcal marginal blepharitis or conjunctivitis and is an inflammatory response to the toxins (and/or enzymes) released by replicating organisms infecting these contiguous tissues. It has a rather typical morphologic appearance characterized by one or several small, well-circumscribed, peripheral, anterior stromal infiltrates that initially are free of replicating bacteria (Fig. 15–6). The second is an inflammatory response to replicating staphylococci within the cornea. Here the infiltrate generally is more central, larger, and more severe (see Figs. 15–2, 15–4).

The hallmark of staphylococcal disease is suppuration. Once staphylococci gain a foothold in the corneal stroma, they cause necrosis, abscess formation, and ulceration. The presence of a silk suture or other foreign body enhances the potential for staphylococci to infect the cornea and produce necrosis. So, too, does prior corneal disease. *Staphylococcus epidermidis*, an opportunistic pathogen, rarely seems to infect a previously healthy cornea. However, it has

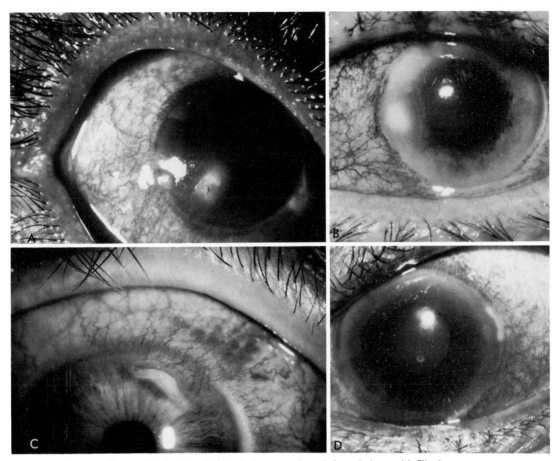

Figure 15–6. *A* to *D*, Staphylococcal peripheral stromal infiltrates.

been isolated and identified as a cause of bacterial keratitis in eyes with previous corneal disease. Examples include bullous keratopathy and stromal keratitis produced by herpes simplex keratitis.[15, 22] In all cases much of this tissue damage is irreversible and leads to permanent scarring.

Pseudomonas

Pseudomonas aeruginosa is the most common and most severe Gram-negative pathogen. Like the staphylococcus, this microorganism has risen to greater pathogenic importance during the antibiotic era. Because of its widespread distribution and its resistance to many antibiotics, it often becomes dominant when more susceptible bacteria are suppressed. Hence, following the introduction of broad-spectrum antibiotics *Pseu-*

domonas aeruginosa has come to be recognized as a major agent of hospital-acquired infections, especially in persons debilitated by chronic illness and those treated with wide-spectrum antibiotics. The organism is a slender, Gram-negative rod commonly found in soil and water. It is a resident of the intestinal tract in only about 10 per cent of healthy individuals and is also found sporadically in moist areas of the human skin (e.g., axilla, groin) and in the saliva. Many strains synthesize a bluish-green phenazine pigment (pyocyanin) as well as a greenish-yellow fluorescein pigment. As a result, the exudate accompanying a *Pseudomonas* keratitis fluoresces in the ultraviolet light of a Wood's lamp (but not in the cobalt-blue light of the slit-lamp biomicroscope).[23] Serologic typing, standardized bacteriophage typing, and a system of typing by pyocyanin production all have been used to identify specific strains. However, there are few available data correlating specific strains with virulence in the cornea.

Pseudomonas has remarkably simple nutritional requirements. It can use ammonia as a source of nitrogen and it can metabolize a large variety of carbon sources. This allows it to replicate in almost any moist environment containing even trace amounts of organic compounds. It grows in a variety of eye drops, weak antiseptic solutions, irrigating solutions, and cosmetics as well as on sinks, humidifiers, and anesthesia and resuscitation equipment. It has even been known to multiply in stored distilled water. The mechanism by which *Pseudomonas* causes disease in man is not entirely clear, but the organism produces endotoxin, a number of extracellular enzymes (including at least two types of proteases and a lipase), and at least three exotoxins that may be of pathogenic significance. In addition, the pyocyanin pigment may contribute to the overall disease process through its effect on oxygen uptake of tissue cells, including leukocytes. However, the virulence of *Pseudomonas aeruginosa* in the cornea seems largely related to the intracellular production of a calcium-activated protease that is capable of producing extensive destruction of the corneal stroma.[24] Earlier studies suggested that this enzyme was a collagenase,[25-27] but more recent data indicate that the cornea-destroying protease of *Pseudomonas aeruginosa* is a proteoglycanolytic enzyme.[28] Proteoglycan is a major

noncollagenous solid component of the cornea presumably responsible for maintaining the order and interfibrillar attachments of the corneal collagen fibrils. Degradation of the proteoglycan seemingly frees and disperses the fibrils and results in corneal liquefaction without destroying the collagen.[28] Irrespective of its mechanism of action, however, it is clear that *Pseudomonas aeruginosa* elaborates an enzyme that is able to rapidly liquefy the corneal stroma (Fig. 15–7).

Streptococcus pneumoniae (Pneumococcus)

In older reported series *Streptococcus pneumoniae* (pneumococcus) was the most common cause of bacterial keratitis. Its prevalence as an etiologic agent seems to have been superseded both by *Staphylococcus* and by *Pseudomonas* in more recent times. Nonetheless, *Pneumococcus* continues to be isolated frequently from bacterial corneal ulcers, a finding that undoubtedly reflects its normal habitation of the upper respiratory tract, lacrimal drainage apparatus, and at times the conjunctiva.

Typically *Streptococcus pneumoniae* are encapsulated Gram-positive, lancet-shaped diplococci. In sputum, pus, and ocular secretions they may be observed in short chains and occasionally as individual cocci. Pneumococcal capsules are composed of large polysaccharide polymers that form hydrophilic gels on

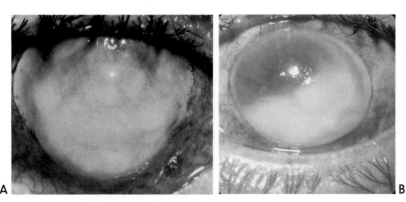

Figure 15–7. *A* and *B,* Liquefactive stromal necrosis of *Pseudomonas aeruginosa* keratitis.

the surface of the organisms. More than 80 serologic types of pneumococci have been differentiated by their immunologically distinct capsular polysaccharides, but ocular infections do not seem to be caused by any particular pneumococcal types. No type or types are typical of ocular isolates. On the contrary, a diverse number of pneumococcal serotypes have been isolated from the eye.[29]

However, the capsular antigens of *Streptococcus pneumoniae* are related to the pathogenicity of the organism. For any given type of pneumococcus, virulence appears to be roughly correlated with capsular size. Intermediate variants that produce small capsules are less virulent than fully encapsulated strains of the same type but more virulent than rough variants that produce no capsule at all. However, pneumococci of different types with capsules of the same size may vary widely in virulence.[18-20] Rough, avirulent strains have been recovered from the external eye.[29]

Streptococcus pneumoniae, like *Staphylococcus,* is an invasive pathogen (Fig. 15–8) that tends to produce an acute purulent infection. However, the organism is an extracellular parasite capable of damaging the tissues of the host only as long as it remains outside the phagocyte itself. Once ingested, it is promptly destroyed. Protection against phagocytosis is provided by the capsule, which exerts an antiphagocytic effect.

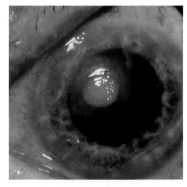

Figure 15–8. *Streptococcus pneumoniae* keratitis. Forty-eight hours earlier, before topical therapy had been instituted, a hypopyon had been present along with purulent secretions on the surface of the infiltrate and in the conjunctival sac.

The physicochemical factors that operate at the interface between the leukocyte and the capsule to impede the process of ingestion have not been defined.

Moraxella

Moraxellas are Gram-negative unencapsulated diplobacilli. Although they are rods, they tend to be short and plump and on microscopic examination are easily confused with *Neisseria gonorrhoeae* and *Neisseria meningitidis*. Moreover, some strains tend to retain crystal violet stain and appear to be Gram-positive in scrapings obtained from a corneal ulcer;[15] in this instance they may initially be mistaken for *Streptococcus pneumoniae*. The older ophthalmic literature stressed that there were two major species of *Moraxella* that produced ocular infections.[30] *Moraxella liquefaciens* (the diplobacillus of Petit) was said to cause central hypopyon keratitis and was said to be different from *Moraxella lacunata* (the diplobacillus of Morax-Axenfeld), which caused angular conjunctivitis and at times mild marginal corneal ulcers. The important features that presumably differentiated *Moraxella liquefaciens* from *Moraxella lacunata* was the ready growth of the former on ordinary laboratory media and its ability to liquefy gelatin at room temperature. However, this separation was not well founded on either clinical or bacteriologic grounds and is of historical interest only; modern taxonomy no longer recognizes *Moraxella liquefaciens* as a separate species. Cases of central corneal ulcer with hypopyon due to *Moraxella lacunata* have been documented.[15, 31, 32] In addition, less common species of this genus, *Moraxella non-liquefaciens* and *Moraxella osloensis*, have been isolated from corneal ulcers.[14, 15] These strains are part of the normal flora of the mucous membranes of the upper respiratory and genitourinary tracts of man. The *Moraxella* species are opportunistic pathogens and are thought to produce ulcerative keratitis more commonly in alcoholic and debilitated persons (Fig. 15–9).

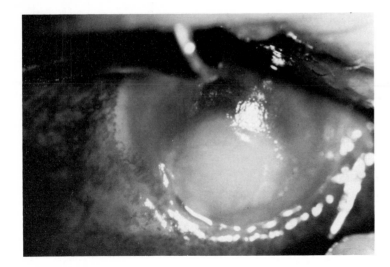

Figure 15–9. Initially neglected *Moraxella* keratitis in a debilitated, chronic alcoholic.

Other Bacteria

Although most bacterial ulcers are caused by *Staphylococcus, Pseudomonas, Streptococcus pneumoniae,* and *Moraxella* organisms, a great number of other bacterial species can invade and proliferate in the cornea.[14-17] In a majority of instances this occurs in a susceptible cornea (i.e., a cornea with pre-existent disease or belonging to a debilitated individual) with a break in its epithelium. Mention has been made that *Staphylococcus epidermidis,* though less pathogenic than *Staphylococcus aureus,* can cause corneal ulceration. Among Gram-positive cocci, *Streptococcus* species also are encountered (Fig. 15–10). Alpha hemolytic streptococci (*Streptococcus viridans*) seem to be more common corneal pathogens than the more virulent beta hemolytic strains (*Streptococcus pyogenes*) presumably because the former are normal inhabitants of the upper respiratory tract. The nonhemolytic enterococcus (*Streptococcus faecalis*), a common inhabitant of the human gastrointestinal tract, occasionally causes a corneal ulcer if transmitted to the periocular area following epithelial injury or in the presence of impaired host resistance.

Gram-positive, spore-forming, aerobic bacilli have been isolated from the conjunctival sac of persons engaged in the processing and handling of hay and related materials or involved in the care of stables and horses. In one study a total of seven positive cultures were obtained from 40 eyes. *Bacillus cereus* was isolated from four eyes, and *Bacillus megaterium, Bacillus pumilus,* and *Bacillus coagulans* were isolated from one eye each.[33] The same investigators reported two cases of corneal ulcers caused by *Bacillus coagulans* and *Bacillus brevis,* respectively. Among Gram-positive rods, *Corynebacterium* species have been implicated infrequently in keratitis.[21]

Although less destructive than *Pseudomonas aeruginosa,* presumably because of the absence of a protease, *Pseudomonas fluorescens* has also infrequently produced ulcerative keratitis.[14] Similarly, many of the Enterobacteriaceae, a large group of Gram-negative rods that are normal constituents of the intestinal flora, if afforded the opportunity, will invade the corneal stroma. Though relatively uncommon, cases caused by *Escherichia coli, Aerobacter aerogenes, Proteus morganii, Klebsiella pneumoniae, Serratia marcescens,* and *Acinetobacter lwoffi (Mima polymorpha)* have been documented. The keratitis is of varying severity, depending on the specific organism that is involved. *Proteus morganii* can produce a rapidly evolving, highly destructive corneal ulcer reminiscent of *Pseudomonas aeruginosa* (Fig. 15–11). The keratitis caused

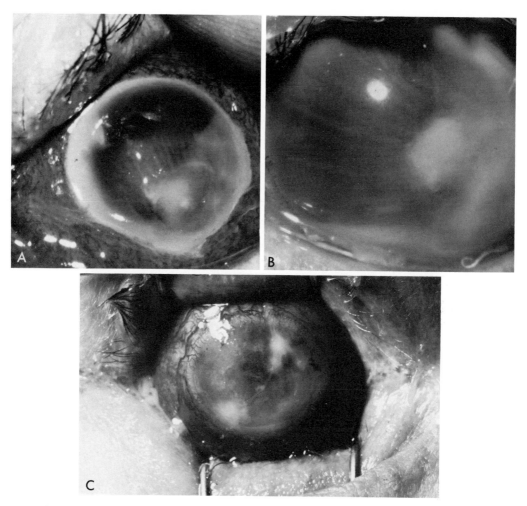

Figure 15–10. Streptococcal keratitis: *A, S. viridans. B, S. pyogenes. C, S. faecalis.*

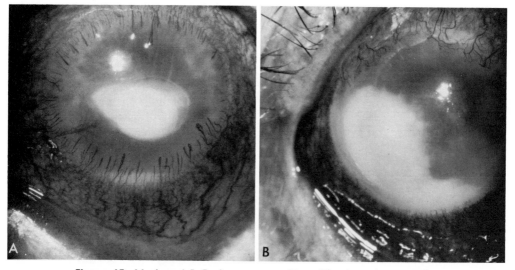

Figure 15–11. *A* and *B, Proteus morganii* keratitis of varying severity.

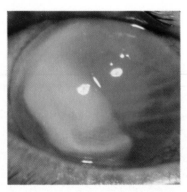

Figure 15–12. *Klebsiella pneumoniae* keratitis.

by *Klebsiella pneumoniae* also tends to be severe (Fig. 15–12). *Serratia marcescens*, which until recently was looked upon as a harmless saprophyte, is now known to be an opportunistic pathogen capable of producing a keratitis of variable severity. There is evidence that this organism *(Serratia)* produces extracellular proteases capable of causing rapid and extensive liquescent necrosis of the cornea.[34]

The Gram-negative diplococci, *Neisseria gonorrhoeae* and *Neisseria meningitidis*, also are infrequent causes of ulcerative keratitis. Either may invade the cornea following an untreated or inadequately treated conjunctivitis. Particular care must be rendered in the treatment of cases of conjunctivitis caused by these organisms because of their ability to penetrate an intact corneal epithelium. (The diphtheria bacillus also can penetrate an intact corneal epithelium.)

Mycobacterium fortuitum, an atypical mycobacterium, is a rare corneal pathogen. Almost all cases in which this organism has been isolated from an ulcerative keratitis have involved corneal injury by a foreign body. The ulcers caused by *Mycobacterium fortuitum* tend to have a slowly progressive, chronic course accompanied by mild anterior chamber reaction. The ulcers remain superficial for a considerable period of time and tend to heal slowly after invasion of superficial blood vessels. Atypical mycobacteria resemble *Corynebacterium* species (diphtheroids) on Gram stain; an acid-fast stain is required for diagnosis. Isolates are generally resistant to all antibiotics, but the prognosis is nonetheless said to be good.[35]

Anaerobic bacteria normally inhabit human skin and mucous membranes. They have been isolated from the conjunctivae of both normal eyes and eyes with active conjunctivitis.[6] It is therefore not surprising that on rare occasions they have been incriminated as the causal agent of a bacterial keratitis. *Peptococcus morbillorum* and *Peptococcus variabilis*, both Gram-positive cocci, as well as *Propionibacterium acnes*, a Gram-negative rod, have been reported.[15, 21]

CLINICAL DIAGNOSIS

There are certain distinctive clinical features that should prompt the examiner to suspect strongly that the keratitis he is inspecting with the slit-lamp biomicroscope is due to bacterial infection. Invariably there is a dense, necrotic-appearing stromal infiltrate, most often grayish-white in color (Fig. 15–2). The overlying epithelium usually is absent, the epithelial border of the ulcer is sharply demarcated, and the stromal infiltrate generally extends beyond the borders of the epithelial defect. The eye is red because of conjunctival injection. Purulent material often is present in the conjunctival sac (Fig. 15–4), and additional mucopurulent material may be adherent to the surface of the corneal ulcer. The cornea surrounding the ulcer generally is edematous, and there is a variable degree of anterior chamber reaction. If a reliable history of trauma or other incident consistent with bacterial inoculation of the cornea can be obtained, the interval between this incident and the onset of the above findings is usually 24 to 72 hours.

However, it must be stressed that although there may be typical features associated with certain bacteria, it is impossible to make an absolute etiologic diagnosis with the slit-lamp biomicroscope. The Gram-positive cocci, particularly *Staphylococcus aureus* (Figs. 15–2 and 15–4) and *Streptococcus pneumoniae* (Fig. 15–8), tend to form localized, round or oval, grayish-white, suppurative ulcers. The surrounding uninvolved cornea tends to remain relatively clear and free of infiltration. There is a varying degree of reaction in the anterior chamber, and a hypopyon may or may not be present. *Pseudomonas aeruginosa* produces the most pathognomonic corneal ulcer (Fig. 15–7). It generally evolves more rapidly and involves more of the cornea than an ulcer caused by the Gram-positive cocci. Yellow-green purulent material may be adherent to the ulcer surface, and the necrotic stroma often appears more "mushy" or "soupy" than that of Gram-positive ulcers. A hypopyon generally accompanies the more severe cases. A *Moraxella* corneal ulcer (Fig. 15–9) is most often paracentral or perilimbal. This organism tends to be less virulent than the Gram-positive cocci. Consequently, the corneal ulcers they produce tend to be smaller, less destructive to the corneal stroma (and therefore somewhat more gray than white in appearance), and slower to spread than those caused by the Gram-positive cocci. The occurrence of a hypopyon is quite variable.

Unfortunately, in all cases these findings can vary substantially. The clinical appearance of a corneal ulcer is determined not only by the species of responsible bacteria and the virulence of the particular causative strain but also by the size of the original inoculum, the duration of the infection, pre-existing corneal disease, concomitant systemic disease or debility, and antibiotic and corticosteroid therapy. Each of these factors can modify the clinical picture considerably. Similar features also may be present in viral and fungal infections, and neurotrophic keratitis, exposure keratitis, and keratitis sicca all are able to mimic morphologic characteristics of bacterial infection. Indeed, these corneal disorders may be complicated by a secondary bacterial infection; their potential for this complication is augmented by persistent epithelial defects, by a decrease in corneal sensation, by abnormal tear flow, and by exposure.

Thus, the corneal changes produced by infecting bacteria are too varied to provide a reliable and accurate basis for an etiologic diagnosis. They tend to be an even less helpful guide to appropriate therapy. This frequent inability to make a specific diagnosis and to institute rational treatment on the basis of clinical morphology alone makes it imperative that a meticulous laboratory investigation be undertaken in each case of ulcerative keratitis. A single protocol designed to identify a causal agent should be followed in the evaluation of every case of corneal ulcer.

LABORATORY DIAGNOSIS

Our initial procedure is to obtain material for culture from the conjunctiva and lid margin. Whenever the patient is cooperative enough, this maneuver is carried out without the use of a topical anesthetic; the preservatives in the anesthetic formulation may decrease the recovery of bacterial pathogens. The lower lid of the involved eye is everted and a sterile swab is wiped along the entire lower cul-de-sac. We prefer swabs of calcium alginate, a fiber made from alginic acid. The material is inert, has soft characteristics, and is soluble, making quantitation possible.[36] The more common cotton swabs may contain some fatty acids that inhibit bacterial growth,[37, 38] but their use is acceptable. Swabs constructed of Dacron polyester also are satisfactory. The applicator is first moistened in trypticase soy broth; then the lower tarsal conjunctiva is swabbed (Fig. 15–13), and the swab is directly plated onto one half of a blood agar, a chocolate agar, and a Sabouraud's dextrose agar plate and used to inoculate supplemental thioglycolate broth. The lower and then the upper lid margins are everted in turn, and the lid margins are wiped with another sterile, moistened swab (Fig. 15–13). This is used to inoculate the second half of the same

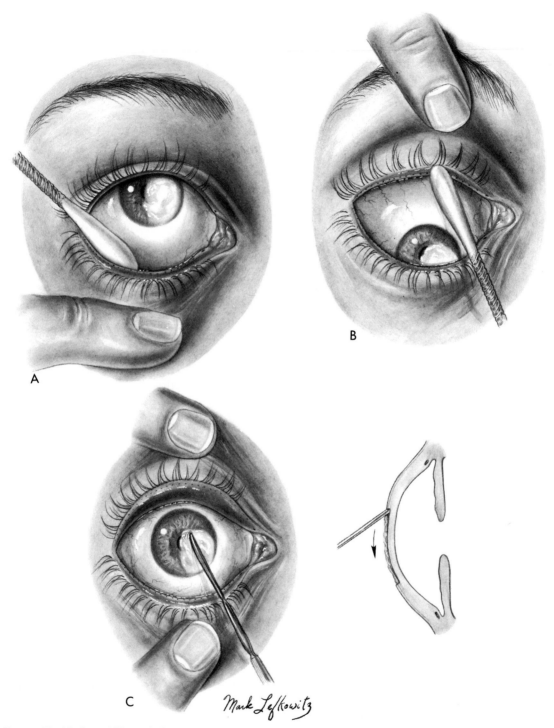

Figure 15–13. Acquisition of diagnostic specimens in bacterial keratitis. *A,* Conjunctival specimen. A sterile calcium alginate swab, premoistened in trypticase soy broth, is wiped along the lower cul-de-sac. *B,* Lid margin specimen. A second identical sterile moistened swab is wiped along the everted margins of the upper and lower lids. *C,* Corneal specimen. The base and edges of the corneal ulcer are scraped with a sterile platinum spatula.

agar plates and an additional tube of supplemental thioglycolate broth. It is not our routine practice to take cultures from the lid margins and conjunctiva of the opposite eye, although on occasion they are obtained for comparative purposes. Next the cornea and conjunctiva are anesthetized with topically administered 0.5 per cent proparacaine hydrochloride. Under direct visualization through either the slip-lamp biomicroscope or the operating microscope the ulcer is scraped with a sterile Kimura platinum spatula (Fig. 15–13). We do not use a sterile applicator to obtain diagnostic corneal material; this has not proved to be of value.

It has been pointed out that viable replicating members of some bacterial species, such as *Streptococcus pneumoniae*, are more apt to be found at the active edge of a corneal ulcer, whereas other species, such as *Moraxella*, are more likely to be isolated from the depths of the ulcer crater. Therefore, it is imperative that scrapings be obtained from and that each culture medium be inoculated with material from both the central area and the advancing edges of the ulcer. Multiple scrapings are required, and the platinum spatula is sterilized in an alcohol lamp flame prior to each corneal curettage. Extreme care must be exercised to ensure that the edge of the spatula makes contact only with the corneal ulcer; it should not be allowed to touch the lid margins or conjunctiva. Use of a sterile wire lid speculum is helpful in obtaining corneal scrapings, especially in poorly cooperative patients. The speculum is positioned after cultures of the lid margins and conjunctiva have been obtained.

Often, particularly in the case of small, fresh infiltrates, sufficient material cannot be obtained from a corneal ulcer to prepare all of the slides and cultures that are desirable. Similarly, in occasional patients with very deep ulcers (or an impending descemetocele), particularly those who are unable or unwilling to cooperate fully, it is prudent to limit the number of applications of the spatula to the ulcer for fear of inducing corneal perforation. It is therefore our practice to prepare the specimens in the sequence listed in Table 15–2. The initial material is inoculated directly onto a blood agar plate. Additional material from corneal scraping is spread onto a precleaned glass slide for staining with Gram stain. The material is spread over a small area of the glass slide to ensure its concentration and to facilitate its detection during microscopic examination. Repeated scrapings of the corneal ulcer are carried out whenever possible, and the material obtained is in turn inoculated directly onto chocolate agar and Sabouraud's dextrose agar plates and spread onto a second slide for staining with Giemsa stain. Material from the platinum spatula then is transferred to a calcium alginate swab, which is then inserted into the bottom of a tube containing supplemental thioglycolate broth. If additional material can be obtained from the corneal ulcer, it is spread onto glass slides so that a duplicate slide for Gram stain can be prepared and special stains can be employed as indicated.

Fungi are encountered infrequently as a causal agent of ulcerative keratitis in our locale (Boston). However, in warmer, more humid climates where mycotic keratitis is more common, a slide stained with periodic acid–Schiff stain and a culture in brain-heart infu-

Table 15–2. USUAL SEQUENCE IN THE PREPARATION OF DIAGNOSTIC SPECIMENS IN CASES OF BACTERIAL KERATITIS*

Blood agar culture
Gram-stained smear
Chocolate agar culture
Sabouraud agar culture
Giemsa-stained smear
Thioglycolate broth culture

Additional smears for special stains

PAS-stained smear
Brain-heart infusion broth culture

Acid-fast–stained smear
Löwenstein-Jensen agar culture

*Procedures listed below the double line are not routinely carried out; they are done only if there is a strong clinical suspicion that the keratitis is of fungal or mycobacterial etiology.

sion broth are helpful in identifying a fungal agent and would assume increasing importance. Atypical mycobacteria, particularly *Mycobacterium fortuitum*, are identified in an acid-fast stained slide and by culture in Löwenstein-Jensen medium. We do not carry out these procedures routinely. Because of the infrequency with which these entities appear in our patient population, they are done only if there is a strong clinical suspicion that the keratitis is of fungal or mycobacterial etiology.

A brief commentary on the media used to isolate bacteria from the external eye and its adnexa is in order (Table 15–3). Blood agar is used extensively since it readily supports the growth of the great majority of corneal pathogens. In essence it is composed of trypticase soy agar to which 5 to 10 per cent defibrinated sheep blood has been added aseptically. It is inexpensive and may be

Table 15–3. CULTURE MEDIA USED IN THE DIAGNOSTIC EVALUATION OF BACTERIAL KERATITIS*

Medium	Purpose
Routine	
Blood agar plate	Aerobic and facultatively anaerobic bacteria, fungi
Chocolate agar plate	Aerobic and facultatively anaerobic bacteria; enhances the isolation of *Moraxella, Neisseria, Hemophilus*
Sabouraud dextrose agar plate with chloramphenicol or gentamicin (50 µg./ml. of medium)	Fungi
Supplemented Thioglycolate broth	Aerobic and anaerobic bacteria
Supplemental	
Brain-heart infusion broth with gentamicin (50 µg./ml. of medium)	Fungi
Löwenstein-Jensen agar slant	Mycobacteria, *Nocardia*
Thayer-Martin agar plate	*Neisseria*

*Sabouraud dextrose agar and brain-heart infusion broth are incubated at 25° C. All other media are incubated at 37° C in an atmosphere of 3 to 10 per cent CO_2.

stored for a week at refrigeration temperature without deteriorating.

Chocolate agar is used to enhance the isolation of *Moraxella, Neisseria,* and *Hemophilus* species. This medium is basically a polypeptone agar to which 5 to 10 per cent sterile defibrinated or citrated blood has been added; the mixture is heated until the blood becomes brown or chocolate in color. Chocolate agar is also enriched with a chemically defined supplement. As a general rule, all bacteria that grow readily on blood agar will also grow on chocolate agar, though the reverse is not true. It has been our practice to use both media in our evaluation of corneal ulcers. The hemolysis pattern around colonies of blood agar often permits certain bacterial differentiations to be made at an early stage. Similar information is not afforded by chocolate agar.

Sabouraud's agar, a combination of glucose, peptone, and agar, is used to isolate fungi. Since the B complex vitamins are an important nutritional requirement for most fungi, 0.1 per cent yeast extract often is added. So, too, is a broad-spectrum antibiotic (e.g., chloramphenicol or gentamicin) to avoid bacterial contamination. Cyclohexamide, an inhibitor of saprophytic fungal growth and a component of some commercially available fungal media, is to be avoided, since most cases of fungal keratitis are caused by so-called saprophytes.

Brain-heart infusion broth is an alternative medium for cultivation of fungi. Thioglycolate broth permits the growth of anaerobic and microaerophilic bacteria under the usual technique of incubation used for aerobes and is perhaps the most practical method of recovering these organisms. Sodium thioglycolate, a reducing substance, produces an environment of low oxidation-reduction potential. However, a blood agar plate placed immediately in an anaerobic jar (which provides a high CO_2 atmosphere) is preferable; the necessary apparatus is commercially available as a disposable product. Finally, if a mycobacterial infection is suspected, Löwenstein-Jensen medium can be used to isolate these organisms. The infrequency with which we encounter mycobacterial keratitis makes it impractical for us to run this culture routinely, and we tend to rely on the fact that these organisms also grow on routine blood agar cultures.

All of the media used for the evaluation of bacterial corneal ulcers are generally stored under refrigeration. They should be brought to room temperature prior to inoculation with corneal samples. Bacterial cultures are incubated at 37° C, whereas fungal cultures are grown at 25° to 27° C. Each of the solid media that are used should be streaked in a routine manner; this permits identification of the location from which the organisms are cultured.

We use the methods described by Jones[14] and Wilson.[15] As described previously, the upper part of a plate is used to inoculate the sample from the conjunctival sac and is streaked in the pattern of an undulating line. The lower portion of the same plate is used to inoculate the specimen from the lid margin. It is streaked in the form of a capital letter R if the sample has been obtained from the right lids, L if it originates from the left lids (Fig. 15–14). The corneal scrapings are inoculated directly onto a separate plate by lightly streaking both sides of the spatula over the agar surface in a series of parallel rows of C-shaped streaks. Each row of C-streaks represents inoculation of the media with a separate corneal scraping. The spatula should not penetrate the agar; recognition and isolation of microorganisms in cut streaks of agar are difficult.

Bacterial growth on two or more of these C-streaks generally is interpreted to signify that the isolate is the cause of the corneal ulcer. Growth of the same organism on the inoculation marks from the conjunctival or lid margin specimens or in the thioglycolate broth confirms its etiologic role. Growth of the C-streaks only (on the corneal plate) or growth of aerobic bacteria in the thioglycolate broth (but not on the solid media) usually represents contaminants. Growth from the conjunctiva and lid margin cultures only (corneal cultures are negative) must be interpreted with great caution because such isolates are not necessarily the cause of the corneal ulcer. In this instance, if the culture results are consistent with the findings of the Gram-stained smear of the corneal scrapings, we assume as a working diagnosis that this is the etiologic organism. Nonetheless, because of our lack of certainty, we often will continue wider-spectrum antibiotic therapy than required to treat this organism alone.

The cultures do not provide the clinician with any information for a minimum of 12 to 18 hours. Often 24 to 48 hours elapse before definitive data are forthcoming. Therefore, the corneal scrapings and the smears obtained from the conjunctival sac and the lid margins are stained to allow visualization of various structures by microscopic examination (which is performed promptly). Of these preparations the Gram stain is the most useful in the evaluation of a bacterial corneal ulcer, in which one's primary interest is the causal organism

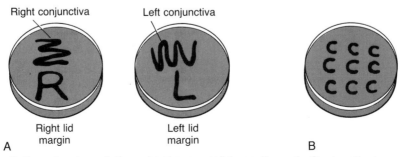

Figure 15–14. Pattern for inoculating streaks on solid medium: *A,* Conjunctival and lid margin specimens. *B,* Corneal specimens. Each row of C-shaped inoculations represents a separate sample.

Table 15–4. STAINING TECHNIQUE FOR SMEARS

Gram Stain
1. Fix slide by gently flaming (or in 95 per cent methanol for 5 minutes)
2. Flood with gentian violet for 30–60 seconds
3. Rinse with tap water
4. Flood with Gram's iodine for 30–60 seconds
5. Rinse with tap water
6. Tilting the slide, allow 95 per cent ethanol (decolorizing solution) to run over the slide until the purple color ceases to be washed off
7. Rinse with tap water
8. Flood with safranin for 30 seconds
9. Rinse with tap water
10. Gently blot dry

Giemsa Stain
1. Fix slide in absolute methyl alcohol for 5 minutes
2. Add 1 ml. of Giemsa stain and 2 ml. of Paragon buffer to 47 ml. of distilled water in a Coplin staining jar
3. Immerse slide in stain solution for 1 hour
4. Rinse by rapidly dipping the slide twice in 95 per cent ethyl alcohol
5. Air dry

(Table 15–4). Although frequently there is a poor correlation between the organisms seen in the Gram-stained smear and those identified by culture,[21, 39] the smear generally provides the only objective diagnostic information available when the initial therapeutic decisions must be made.

Preparation of the Gram-stained smear begins with the application of crystal violet, a basic dye that penetrates the bacterial cell, where it reacts with acidic components of the protoplasm. An iodine solution subsequently is applied, and this forms a complex with the crystal violet. All bacteria are stained blue or purple at this stage; the crystal violet–iodine complex is attached to the protoplast (a bacterial organism from which the cell wall has been removed) either inside the organism or at the surface. A decolorizer, alcohol or acetone, then is added. The Gram-positive organisms retain the crystal violet–iodine complex and remain blue. The cell wall in this class of organisms seems to act as a barrier that prevents the extraction of the crystal violet–iodine complex by the decolorizer. Gram-negative organisms, on the other hand, are rapidly decolored by the alcohol or acetone, presumably because their higher cell wall lipid content is soluble in the decolorizer. Finally, a counterstain, such as safranin, is applied; the decolorized Gram-negative organisms take on the contrasting red color of this dye.

The Gram stain provides a prompt and valuable technique for differentiating bacteria (Table 15–1). However, mycobacteria are difficult to differentiate from diphtheroids in the Gram-stained smear and are best identified with the Ziehl-Nielsen acid-fast stain. In contrast, the Giemsa stain classically is used to characterize the predominant cell types in inflamed tissues and in the accompanying discharge. It also permits detection of cytoplasmic inclusions associated with chlamydial infections. When used for these purposes, the Giemsa stain generally is more helpful in the diagnostic evaluation of conjunctivitis. However, it does stain fungi, including the cross-walls of hyphae, a morphologic characteristic that is important in fungal differentiation, and this perhaps is the major value of the Giemsa stain in the assessment of an active keratitis. A potassium hydroxide (KOH) preparation also is used to identify hyphal fragments, and the periodic acid–Schiff (PAS) stain may be helpful in fungal identification.

Mention must be made of the limulus lysate assay for bacterial endotoxin. The cell walls of Gram-negative bacteria contain a soluble lipopolysaccharide endotoxin that is elaborated into the tissues and fluids surrounding a site of infection. In the horseshoe crab, *Limulus polyphemus*, the natural response to Gram-negative bacterial infection is disseminated intravascular coagulation.[40] Only one formed element, the amebocyte, is present in the circulatory system of the horseshoe crab, and the creature's entire coagulation pathway appears to be contained within this cell. Minute quantities of endotoxin can activate this coagulation pathway in vitro, causing the isolated granular portion of these blood cells to form a firm clot in a test tube.[41] This reaction has been adapted as an in vitro assay for the presence of bacterial endotoxin and is the most sensitive method clinically available for its detection.

The test is highly reliable and is capable of detecting subnanogram quantities of bacterial endotoxin after an incubation period of 1 hour or less. Evidence of its diagnostic value in bacterial keratitis and endophthalmitis has been published.[42-44] The results of the limulus lysate assay have a high correlation with the results of bacterial culture and seem to be more reliable than Gram-stained smears for prompt recognition of Gram-negative organisms in corneal ulcers. There appears to be a gratifying absence of false-positive reactions in corneal infections due to Gram-positive bacteria, fungi, and herpes simplex virus and a low incidence of false-negative reactions in cases of Gram-negative bacterial keratitis. Moreover, the assay is unaffected by the presence of antibiotics and permits accurate diagnosis of partially treated patients. The test promises to be a useful adjunct to the traditional methods of smear examination and culture for rapidly establishing a diagnosis of Gram-negative corneal infection.

TREATMENT

Therapy of bacterial keratitis has two major goals: (1) the elimination of viable bacteria from the cornea, and (2) the suppression of the inflammatory response elicited by the invading organisms. For a given organism the extent of corneal damage and the resultant visual impairment generally are inversely proportional to the speed with which these therapeutic goals are accomplished.

Bacterial elimination is accomplished by the administration of antibiotics. A satisfactory objective experimental model for quantifying the therapeutic effect of specific antibiotics in the cornea is now available.[45, 46] Prior to the availability of this model most attempts to assess therapeutic effectiveness approached the problem indirectly by measuring the quantity of antibiotic reaching the affected tissue after a given regimen had been administered. Indeed, many investigators studied anterior chamber drug concentrations, assuming they accurately reflected the concentration of drug simultaneously present in the cornea. However, experimental evidence indicates that this is not the case, and at best aqueous humor drug concentration furnishes only a very rough guide to the concentration of drug in the cornea.

Other important factors that influence therapeutic effectiveness in the eye appear to have been studied very little or not at all. One such factor is protein binding of antibiotics. This phenomenon results in reversible inactivation of antibiotics,[47, 48] and it has been suggested that the protein-bound part of the drug has little or no antibacterial activity.[49-52] Albumin, the constituent responsible for protein binding, is present in the cornea, in the inflammatory debris present in corneal ulcers and in the adjacent fornices, and in the aqueous humor of inflamed eyes.[53] The degree to which different antibiotics are bound by protein varies greatly,[54] but how and to what degree the phenomenon affects the antibacterial properties of antibiotics administered locally to the eye is not known.

An additional point that deserves emphasis is that it may not be necessary to maintain bactericidal drug levels in blood or tissue fluids continuously to effect a therapeutic success. Investigation of several treatment schedules of penicillin G in scarlet fever led to the conclusion that as long as the drug is detectable in the blood for 6 hours a day, clinical as well as bacteriologic cures result.[55, 56] Numerous clinical experiences suggest that this is undoubtedly true in other types of infection, including bacterial keratitis. How long and at what intervals measurable antibiotic levels must be maintained in the cornea to obtain optimal antibacterial effects are not known. Obviously this information will not be gleaned from studies that measure drug levels only. In the past most published recommendations of the frequency and route of drug administration for optimal effectiveness were based solely on such measurements.[57] However, with our present ability to directly quantify therapeutic effect in the cornea,[45, 46] more definitive data are available and the older recommendations are subject to revision.

ROUTE OF ANTIBIOTIC ADMINISTRATION

To achieve an optimal therapeutic effect, one attempts to deliver large concentrations of the appropriate antibiotics to the site of infection in the cornea without toxic side effects. The ophthalmologist is fortunate that most antibiotics are intrinsically active; they do not first have to undergo metabolic changes in some organ distant from the eye in order to exert an antibacterial effect. Consequently, high corneal concentrations of an antibiotic can be attained and its efficacy in that tissue can be assured without great risk of systemic side effects by simply administering the medication directly or adjacent to the infected cornea.

Therefore, for treatment of bacterial keratitis most authorities recommend that antibiotics be delivered principally by topical instillation and by subconjunctival or sub-Tenon's injection. Topical application of the drug, especially to the avascular cornea, produces a high concentration locally, where its pharmacologic effect is desirable, with substantially lower concentrations in other tissues, particularly those at a distance from the site of administration. Delivered by this route, an antibiotic is virtually free of systemic toxicity. On the other hand, animal studies indicate that periocular injection of antibiotics may produce higher corneal drug levels than frequent topical application of the same medication, and this provides the rationale for use of this route of drug administration in the treatment of bacterial corneal ulcers. Fundamentally, however, periocular injection is an atypical form of systemic administration; both

measurable circulating drug levels[58-61] and systemic pharmacologic effects[62] have been detected following its use. Nonetheless, since substantially lower doses are required, there is considerably less risk of generalized toxicity with periocular injection than is incurred with systemic administration. It must be stressed, however, that although periocular injection may produce higher antibiotic levels in the cornea than topical application, it does so at the expense of higher systemic levels, greater patient apprehension, more subsequent inflammation and pain, greater inconvenience and expense, and risk of inadvertent intraocular administration.[63-65]

A direct, comparative evaluation of topical application versus subconjunctival injection is difficult because of the different total quantities of drug administered, the inability to assess the degree of injury to ocular barriers during injection, the arbitrary selection of frequency of topical administration, the variable status of the corneal epithelium in bacterial keratitis, and a variety of additional factors. No quantitative human data are available, and, indeed, the ophthalmic literature is not clear on what constitutes optimal antibiotic therapy for bacterial keratitis. However, several points are well documented experimentally. The topical route is highly effective; controlled animal studies demonstrate that viable bacteria are rapidly eliminated from the cornea.[66-69] Moreover, topical administration is the most efficient mode of treatment. The total quantity of drug required to eradicate bacteria from the cornea is considerably less than that administered by other routes. In contrast, some experimental studies cast doubt on the usefulness of periocularly injected antibiotics in the treatment of bacterial keratitis.[70, 71] Other investigators have found that periocularly injected antibiotics eradicate bacteria from the cornea but that they are not more effective than topical antibiotics.[72, 73] These differences perhaps reflect variations in experimental technique (e.g., differences in leakage from the subconjunctival depot, disparate methods of inducing the bacterial keratitis), as discussed by Hyndiuk.[73]

What is perhaps most important to the clinician is that all of the authorities who have studied the question appear to be in agreement that topically applied antibiotics, especially concentrated formulations, are highly effective in eradicating bacteria from the cornea. None of these investigators has produced evidence suggesting that periocularly injected antibiotics achieve this goal more effectively than the same drugs applied topically, nor are we able to find any evidence documenting that periocularly injected antibiotics enhance the effectiveness of topical therapy if concentrated formulations are used. Thus, available evidence leads us to conclude without doubt that topical instillation must be considered the primary route of antibiotic therapy for bacterial keratitis. Viable bacteria are rapidly eliminated from the cornea and minimal amounts of drug are required. Since quantities of antibiotic far in excess of what is delivered topically fail to produce a superior therapeutic effect when injected periocularly in an experimental situation, we rely on aggressive topical antibiotic therapy as our principal mode of treatment.

Initially a concentrated formulation of the medication is instilled hourly 24 hours a day. At times, when confronted with a severe ulcer, particularly one caused by a Gram-negative organism, we order the antibiotics instilled more frequently, every 15 to 30 minutes, for the first 6 hours of treatment. Unfortunately, compliance with this order tends to be erratic, and our experience indicates that this regimen is not practical for routine use in a general hospital. Experimental studies of topically applied prednisolone acetate have shown that instillation of five doses at 1-minute intervals each hour produces a therapeutic effect equal to that achieved by administration of the drug every 15 minutes.[74] We have administered topical antibiotics according to this regimen during the first 6 to 8 hours of therapy in a small group of patients with bacterial keratitis.

Although no definitive comparative data are available, we have the distinct impression that the technique is highly effective and that it is more readily implemented than instillation of antibiotic drops at 15-minute intervals.

When there is clinical evidence of improvement, treatment is limited to the waking hours, and the concentrated antibiotic formulation is instilled hourly from 7 a.m. to 11 p.m. inclusive. As additional signs of recovery become evident, the frequency of antibiotic instillation gradually is decreased, first to 2-hour intervals, then to 3-hour intervals, and so forth. The rapidity with which topical antibiotics are tapered is governed by the clinical course of the corneal ulcer. Subsequently the ophthalmologist can obtain a progressive decrease in dosage by continuing to decrease the frequency of instillation of the concentrated antibiotic formulation or by substituting the lower concentration commercial preparation.

The decision about whether or not to also inject antibiotics periocularly is based upon the severity of the corneal ulcer, upon the presumptive nature of the causal organism, and upon its response to topical therapy. In view of the experimental evidence indicating a lack of effectiveness of periocularly injected antibiotics in bacterial keratitis,[70, 71] we rarely use this mode of drug delivery. However, if we are confronted with an extensive corneal infiltrate or ulcer that is not responding satisfactorily to topical therapy and initial evaluation indicates that its probable cause is a Gram-negative rod, then in desperation additional antibiotics may be injected periocularly. It is important to note, however, that our view of the role of periocularly injected antibiotics in the treatment of bacterial keratitis is not universally shared by others, and some authorities continue to recommend their routine use. Therefore, we shall comment on this mode of drug delivery.

There are no antibiotic preparations specifically compounded for periocular injection, but any formulation suitable for administration by either the intramuscular or the intravenous route theoretically can be injected subconjunctivally or beneath Tenon's capsule. When they are available, we prefer the intravenous preparations since they are the most highly purified and are least likely to cause local toxicity. Periocular injection of these antibiotic formulations into the inflamed tissues surrounding a bacterial keratitis can be painful. Multiple instillations of 0.5 per cent proparacaine hydrochloride often will provide satisfactory anesthesia; five topical doses of this anesthetic at 2-minute intervals are recommended. If substantial pain is encountered nonetheless, 0.2 ml. of 2 per cent lidocaine should be injected subconjunctivally in the same quadrant in which the antibiotic is to be administered. The anesthetic can be added to the antibiotic solution and injected simultaneously or it can be inoculated prior to the antibiotic. In the latter instance gentle pressure can be applied to the globe through the closed lids to disseminate the anesthetic. This will help to insure both its pharmacologic effect and that there is sufficient subconjunctival space to accommodate a full 1 ml. volume of antibiotic. At times pain may occur following the injection despite these attempts to obtain local anesthesia. Moreover, for many individuals a periocular injection represents a traumatic event of considerable magnitude. In these instances administration of 75 mg. of meperidine or a comparable analgesic 45 minutes prior to the injection is beneficial.

Whenever a periocular injection of antibiotic is performed, we attempt to inject up to 1 ml. of the medication anteriorly, ballooning up the bulbar conjunctiva adjacent to the limbus in the meridian closest to the ulcer. A 25-gauge or smaller needle attached to a tuberculin syringe is employed. If the lesion is central, the initial injection is performed arbitrarily in the quadrant in which the least technical difficulty is encountered; subsequent injections are rotated in successive quadrants. Additional injections are performed at 24-hour intervals, depending upon the severity of the clinical problem. As indicated, we rarely employ subconjunctivally injected antibiotics, and then only as a supplement to a topical regimen, never as the sole source of treatment. Since periocular injection is not without risk, is often a source of considerable apprehension and pain, and is of questionable effectiveness in bacterial keratitis, it is discontinued as soon as the keratitis shows a definite response. Control of the infection then is maintained with topical medications alone. The degree of conjunctival edema and hyperemia accompanying a severe bacterial keratitis can be expected to increase with each subconjunctival antibiotic injection. Bleeding from the injection site and pain are more apt to be encountered following each additional inoculation, factors that often limit the use of this route to about 3 days. Fortunately, there frequently is evidence of clinical improvement within this interval, and effective therapy can be maintained solely by topical agents.

We consider the use of intravenously administered antibiotics for the treatment of bacterial keratitis an ineffective desperation measure, and we therefore limit the use of this route to cases in which there is a concurrent suspected or documented intraocular infection. Ocular inflammation accompanying the more severe cases of bacterial keratitis results in increased intraocular penetration of systemically administered antibiotics through the blood-ocular barriers.[75-78] However, the degree of enhancement varies considerably among antibiotics,[79-81] and it is not known how the alteration in the blood-ocular barriers by inflammation affects antibiotic levels in the cornea. Most available data concern the penetration of systemically administered antibiotics into the aqueous humor. This information indicates that for the penicillins, at least, the degree of penetration of the eye following systemic administration appears to be a function of serum concentration. Over the dose ranges studied there are no consistent differences in the proportion of the drug that enters the anterior chamber.[75, 78, 82, 83] The penetration ratio (i.e., the percentage of peak serum level) appears to remain relatively constant despite variations in peak serum level, dose, and mode of delivery. Thus, following systemic administration the highest absolute concentration in the aqueous humor occurs when a quantity of drug is given in a manner that produces the highest serum level. Based on these observations, rapid intravenous injection seems to be the optimal systemic route. Greater antibiotic penetration into the aqueous humor is demonstrable after "pulse" injection than after continuous intravenous infusion,[84] and we employ this approach whenever systemic antibiotics are used.

However, the principle underlying the chemotherapeutic action of antibiotics is one of selective toxicity. That is, the drugs are quite toxic for pathogenic bacteria but are relatively nontoxic to the cells of the host. Ideally these two effects would be independent, but in practice antibiotics exert a varying degree of toxicity on mammalian cells. Systemic administration of antimicrobial compounds results in more severe and more varied toxic reactions than does local administration of the same compounds. Limited primarily only by its physicochemical properties, a systemically administered drug gains access to many body compartments; noninfected tissues are exposed to the drug and can be adversely affected. Despite this risk of generalized toxicity, systemic administration yields comparatively low levels of drug in the affected ocular tissue. Reliable data on drug levels in the cornea following intravenous administration are not available. However, there is evidence indicating that aqueous humor drug concentrations represent only a small percentage of the systemic dose and that the quantity of antibiotic reaching the aqueous humor after systemic administration is considerably less than the levels produced by local administration of the same drug.[85] There is no reason to assume that drug levels in the cornea are higher than those in the aqueous humor. An increase in ocular levels can be gained only with a substantially larger increase in the quantity of drug administered systemically and, therefore, only at the expense of a considerably increased risk of generalized toxicity. However, even this maneuver appears to be futile and therefore unwarranted. There is no evidence that intravenously administered antibiotics augment the corneal drug levels that result from local administration, while experimental studies show that antibiotics administered intravenously at doses in excess of that recommended for the most severe human infections fail to eliminate bacteria from the cornea.[70]

Continuous antibiotic lavage either via a catheter passed through the upper lid or by means of an infusion contact lens type of device has been recommended for treatment of severe ulcers caused by *Pseudomonas aeruginosa* or Gram-negative organisms of comparable virulence. The continuous flow of antibiotic solution over the corneal surface presumably results in higher antibiotic levels in the cornea than intermittent topical applications. It keeps the corneal surface and the conjunctival sac free of mucopurulent discharge that might contain lytic enzymes and in which bacterial organisms might thrive. This method is said to put less of a demand on nursing personnel, but the difficulties frequently encountered in containment and collection of fluid after ocular irrigation call this claim into question. Moreover, the technique is not without disadvantage. When antibiotics are maintained in solution for many hours, there is always the risk of significant deterioration of the drug before it reaches the infected tissue. Similarly, if one mixes two or more antibiotics for continuous infusion, there is substantial risk of drug incompatibility. If a catheter is used, it requires that a surgical incision be made in the lid adjacent to an infected area. If a constant infusion type of contact lens is used, it is a large, scleral type of device that may become dislodged or may be uncomfortable. In either case the patient is immobilized, the continuous flow of drug may interfere with epithelial regeneration, and there may be sufficient systemic absorption to be worrisome. To avoid the latter complication, low dilutions of the antibiotic, 0.05 per cent to 0.1 per cent in Ringer's solution, are recommended, and continuous irrigation of the ulcer surface is obtained at a flow rate of six to eight drops a minute. We have not found this technique to be practical and have no clinical experience with it.

To summarize, our approach to the treatment of bacterial keratitis calls for the use of only concentrated, topically applied antibiotics in the great majority of cases. We have now used this approach clinically for more than 5 years with great success. In a small number of cases, those characterized by extensive infiltration and ulceration of the cornea caused by a highly virulent bacterial pathogen that is unresponsive to topical antibiotic therapy, additional antibiotic is injected periocularly in a desperate attempt to augment the bactericidal effect. When used, periocularly injected antibiotics are always administered as a supplement to the topical regimen, never as the sole mode of therapy.

SPECIFIC ANTIBIOTICS

At present the antibacterial activity of an antibiotic is determined in vitro for clinical purposes. Inhibition of bacterial growth can be measured by serial dilution or by diffusion of antibiotics.[86] In the dilution tests the antibiotic is diluted serially in broth or agar and the results are expressed as the lowest concentration that inhibits growth of a standard bacterial inoculum at $37°$ C. This method provides a more quantitative evaluation of antibiotic effect than the diffusion tests. Nonetheless, the method most widely used clinically is a diffusion test, the disk test. A known concentration of the antibiotic is incorporated into filter paper disks or tablets, and these are placed on the surface of a solid culture medium inoculated with the organism under examination. Results are interpreted on the basis of inhibition of growth of the organism around the disk. Theoretically, the minimum inhibitory concentration (MIC) can be calculated indirectly from the diameter of the inhibitory zone around the disk, but such an approach is subject to substantial inaccuracy. Commonly only a qualitative interpretation is made of whether the organism is susceptible or resistant to a given antibiotic, and this seems adequate for most clinical purposes. The ease with which the method can be executed, its comparatively low cost, and the speed with which the results are obtained combine on a practical level to offset its relative lack of accuracy.

At best, then, the usual sensitivity tests provide only a qualitative guide to the choice of an antibiotic; agreement between in vitro tests and clinical results is only approximate. A concentration of antibiotics insufficient to prevent growth in a test tube may, because of the interplay of host factors, prove to be effective in the body. Moreover, in the eye a sufficient quantity of antibiotic often can be administered topically, and thus the drug concentration achieved in the cornea is greater than that produced in agar by the commonly used, commercially available sensitivity disks. Since drugs used for topical ophthalmic therapy may be highly toxic when given systemically (e.g., neomycin, bacitracin), sensitivity disks for these drugs are not included in the routine battery of sensitivity tests run by the diagnostic laboratory. Clearly, definitive data reflecting antibacterial effect in the cornea can be obtained only by in vivo measurements within the cornea itself. The routine in vitro procedures used in diagnostic laboratories for testing of bacterial sensitivity to antibiotics seem far removed from those encountered in the infected cornea. Nonetheless, recent studies have documented that in general there appears to be surprisingly good correlation between in vivo clinical effectiveness in the cornea and in vitro inhibitory concentrations.[66, 68]

Whenever it is commercially available, we use an aqueous antibiotic preparation (i.e., a solution or a suspension) rather than an ointment formulation. It is commonly taught that an ophthalmic ointment is superior to the same drug in an aqueous preparation for topical therapy of an anterior segment disorder. The rationale for this thesis is based upon the observation that the ointment vehicle prolongs contact time of the drug with the eye. Higher drug levels are thought to occur in ocular tissues following the application of an ointment, and greater pharmacologic effects presumably result. However, we know of no evidence that demonstrates the superiority of an antibiotic ointment over a comparable aqueous formulation. Gentamicin is commercially available in the same concentration (0.3 per cent) as an ophthalmic solution and as an ophthalmic ointment in petrolatum vehicle. Experimental studies have shown that both forms yield comparable in vivo antibacterial suppression in the cornea.[66] The same experiments produced data that indicated that commercially available chloramphenicol ointment was significantly more effective than the commercial ophthalmic solution, but it must be emphasized that the ointment (1.0 per cent) contains twice as much active drug as the solution (0.5 per cent). When a 1.0 per cent solution was formulated, its antibacterial capabilities were indistinguishable from those of the ointment. In addition to lacking any apparent therapeutic advantages, ointments have several distinct disadvantages: they are messy, they do not lend themselves to frequent administration (i.e., there is an accumulation of ointment base in the conjunctival cul-de-sac and on the lid margins), and their concentration of antibiotic cannot be increased readily in the absence of major manufacturing facilities.

The concentration of active ingredient in most commercially available ophthalmic antibiotic preparations is based upon questionable experimental data or, in some instances, on no experimental data at all. Jones[14] and Wilson[15] have suggested that the commercially available preparations of ophthalmic antibiotics contain an insufficient concentration of drug to produce maximal inhibition of bacterial growth in the cornea following topical administration. They have suggested that the ophthalmologist himself formulate higher concentrations of these antibiotics using standard parenteral preparations and commercially available hydroxypropyl methylcellulose as a vehicle. Use of these concentrated or fortified antibiotic preparations is based on the observation that up to a point the amount of drug that penetrates into and through the cornea increases as the concentration of the formulation increases, and presumably this results in greater antibacterial effect. These fortified antibiotic preparations have been said to produce superior therapeutic results in bacterial keratitis, and laboratory studies support these claims.[67, 87] In rabbits concentrated antibiotic formulations containing approximately four times the quantity of drug found in commercial preparations eliminated pathogenic bacteria from the cornea more rapidly and more effectively than did the commercial preparations. The concentrated preparations tend to be more irritating than the commercial formulations, but to date we are not aware of any serious toxicity resulting from their use, and we administer them as initial treatment for all but the most minor peripheral bacterial corneal ulcers. Instructions for their preparation appear in Table 15–5.

As of this writing, we have not had extensive clinical experience with the limulus lysate test. Therefore, selection of specific antibiotics for initiation of treatment prior to the availability of culture and sensitivity data is based on the Gram stain of the corneal scraping and on a knowledge of the general etiologic prevalence of various bacterial species in our area. If no bacteria are seen in the Gram-stained smear, then our decision is guided by the fact that the two most commonly encountered pathogens are *Staphylococcus* and *Pseudomonas*. Since less than 50 per cent of ocular *Staphylococcus* isolates are said to be sensitive to penicillin G,[14] we empiri-

Table 15–5. PREPARATION OF CONCENTRATED TOPICAL OPHTHALMIC ANTIBIOTICS

Bacitracin 10,000 units/ml.
Remove 9 ml. from a 15-ml. bottle of Tears Naturale and add 3 ml. of the tear substitute to each of 3 vials of sterile bacitracin powder for intramuscular use (50,000 units/vial). Return the 9 ml. of solubilized bacitracin to the plastic squeeze bottle. Final concentration 150,000 units/15 ml. or 10,000 units/ml. of tear substitute.

Cefazolin 33 mg./ml.
Remove 2 ml. from a 15 ml. bottle of Tears Naturale and discard. Solubilize the contents of one vial of cefazolin for parenteral use (500 mg.) with 2 ml. of sterile physiologic saline and add the 2 ml. of reconstituted drug to the plastic squeeze bottle. Final concentration 500 mg./15 ml. or 33 mg./ml.

Erythromycin Lactobionate 10 mg./ml.
Remove 1.5 ml. from a 15-ml. bottle of Tears Naturale and discard. Solubilize the contents of one vial of erythromycin lactobionate (500 mg.) with 5 ml. of sterile water for injection. Add 1.5 ml. of the reconstituted drug to the plastic squeeze bottle. Final concentration 150 mg./15 ml. or 10 mg./ml.

Gentamicin 14 mg./ml.
The parenteral form of gentamicin is packaged in a 2-ml. vial containing 40 mg./ml. Add 2 ml. of parenteral gentamicin (containing 80 mg.) to the 5-ml. dropper bottle of commercial ophthalmic gentamicin 0.3 per cent (containing 15 mg.). Final concentration of gentamicin = 95 mg./7 ml. or 13.6 mg./ml.

Polymyxin B 33,000 units/ml.
Remove 2 ml. from a 15-ml. bottle of Tears Naturale and discard. Solubilize the contents of one vial of polymyxin B sulfate for parenteral administration (500,000 units) in 2 ml. of sterile physiologic saline and add the 2 ml. of reconstituted drug to the plastic squeeze bottle. Final concentration 500,000 units/15 ml. or 33,000 units/ml.

Tobramycin 14 mg./ml.
The parenteral form of tobramycin is packaged in a 2-ml. vial containing 40 mg./ml. Add 2 ml. of parenteral tobramycin (containing 80 ml) to the 5-ml. dropper bottle of commercial ophthalmic tobramycin 0.3 per cent (containing 15 mg.). Final concentration of tobramycin = 95 mg./7 ml. or 13.6 mg./ml.

Vancomycin 50 mg./ml.
Remove 3 ml. from a 15-ml. bottle of Tears Naturale and discard. Solubilize the contents of two vials of vancomycin hydrochloride intravenous (500 mg./vial) with 2 ml. of sterile water for injection per vial. Add 3 ml. (1.5 vials) of reconstituted drug to the plastic squeeze bottle. Final concentration 750 mg./15 ml. or 50 mg./ml.

cally use a drug that is effective against penicillinase-producing staphylococci. Other Gram-positive cocci also are likely etiologic candidates, so the initial regimen must provide for this contingency. Routine coverage against *Pseudomonas* is mandatory, not only because of its current prevalence but also because the rapidity with which it can devastate the cornea makes it likely that an erroneous failure to do so will be met with disaster. It is the ophthalmologist's good fortune that the antibiotics effective against *Pseudomonas* also provide excellent coverage for most of the other Gram-negative corneal pathogens.

When confronted with a negative Gram stain from what we believe clinically to be a bacterial corneal ulcer, it has been our practice to begin topical antibiotic therapy with tobramycin solution 1.4 per cent (or gentamicin solution 1.4 per cent) and bacitracin solution 10,000 units per ml. Tobramycin is used principally because of its wide range of activity against Gram-negative rods, including *Pseudomonas aeruginosa*, but it also provides excellent coverage against staphylococci, including penicillinase-producing strains. However, neither tobramycin nor the other available ophthalmic aminoglycosides, gentamicin or neomycin, provide adequate coverage against streptococcal species, including *Streptococcus pneumoniae*. Bacitracin generally is relied upon to combat these organisms; it possesses marked bactericidal activity against a variety of Gram-positive organisms and also against *Neisseria* species but has little effect against Gram-negative bacteria.

Most authorities recommend that a concentrated preparation of a cephalosporin derivative be formulated and administered in this situation to provide optimal coverage for Gram-positive pathogens. Cefazolin, at a concentration of 33 mg./ml., is the most commonly used agent at present. We agree that this represents an excellent therapeutic choice. However, we have had years of successful experience with bacitracin and it continues to produce gratifying therapeutic results in our hands. This experience, the small potential for side effects with cephalosporins among penicillin-sensitive individuals, and the lesser potential for bacterial resistance of an antibiotic not used systemically have caused us to continue the use of bacitracin as our primary agent to combat Gram-positive organisms. Perhaps the advent of third-generation cephalosporins with their extremely broad spectrum of action will cause us to reassess this area.

Alternatively, a concentrated solution of erythromycin lactobionate 10 mg./ml. can be used instead of bacitracin as part of the initial regimen when the nature of the causal organism is unknown. This recommendation is based on our therapeutic success with concentrated tobramycin in cases of staphylococcal ulcers, the demonstration of substantially greater in vitro sensitivity of a large number of ocular pneumococcal isolates to erythromycin than to bacitracin,[29] the limited demonstration of significant in vivo effectiveness in the cornea of erythromycin against penicillinase-producing Staphylococcus aureus,[66] and an incidence of in vitro sensitivity of erythromycin equal to bacitracin among ocular staphylococcal isolates from our patient population. Erythromycin generally is classified as a bacteriostatic antibiotic, whereas bacitracin is bactericidal, a factor that unquestionably explains why use of the latter is much more frequently recommended. However, evidence is available indicating that erythromycin, although bacteriostatic at low concentrations, is bactericidal at high concentrations.[88, 89] Which mechanism of action prevails at the levels attained in the human cornea after topical application of the drug is not definitely known. Nevertheless, there are experimental data showing that topically administered erythromycin can rapidly eliminate at least one strain of penicillinase-producing Staphylococcus aureus from the cornea, suggesting that at least in some instances it functions as a bactericidal agent.[66]

If the initial Gram stain of the corneal scrapings shows Gram-positive cocci or rods, we use a solution of bacitracin 10,000 units per ml. topically. In most cases we also instill tobramycin 1.4 per cent or gentamicin 1.4 per cent, not only because of its effectiveness against many strains of staphylococci but also because

of our unwillingness to completely trust the Gram stain and ignore the possibility of a Gram-negative etiology prior to the availability of culture results. When Gram-negative cocci are seen on the Gram-stained slide, suggesting Neisseria as the etiologic agent, bacitracin, cefazolin, or erythromycin solution is instilled topically. In this instance, because of the ability of the gonococcus to invade and penetrate the intact corneal epithelium, penicillin G 2,000,000 units per ml. (or erythromycin lactobionate 100 mg./ml. in penicillin-sensitive individuals) is injected subconjunctivally, and the patient is treated for gonorrhea with the full recommended dose of antibiotics administered by mouth or intramuscularly. Gram-negative rods are treated initially with tobramycin solution 1.4 per cent; a concentrated solution of polymyxin B (33,000 units per ml.) is added if necessary. We have not had occasion to use carbenicillin (6.0 mg./ml.) or ticarcillin (6.0 mg./ml.) in conjunction with the aminoglycoside, as many authorities have recommended.

Antibiotic therapy may be modified as the results of culture and sensitivity testing become known. In some instances, within 24 to 48 hours after therapy has been initiated we have been confronted with data from the laboratory indicating that the treatment in progress should not be effective, yet clinically the ulcer is responding well. In such an instance we are loathe to alter therapy and tend to disregard the laboratory findings; the antibiotic regimen in use is maintained and the patient is kept under close observation. Often, however, identification of the organism and its in vitro antibiotic sensitivities are accorded major importance in the ultimate selection of antibiotic therapy. If clinically the ulcer is not responding satisfactorily, additional antibiotics are applied or the therapeutic regimen is altered as dictated by the laboratory findings. Table 12–6 provides a guide to the general effectiveness of various antibiotics. Table 15–6 lists recommended topical antibiotics. For those instances in which they may be useful, Table 15–7 provides a guide to the for-

Table 15–6. TOPICAL ANTIBIOTIC THERAPY BASED ON FINDINGS OF GRAM-STAINED SMEAR

	Recommended Drugs	Alternatives
No organism	Bacitracin 10,000 units/ml. Tobramycin 14 mg./ml.	Erythromycin lactobionate 10 mg./ml. Cefazolin 33 mg./ml. Gentamicin 14 mg./ml.
Gram-positive cocci	Bacitracin 10,000 units/ml. Cefazolin 33 mg./ml.	Erythromycin lactobionate 10 mg./ml. Vancomycin 50 mg./ml.
Gram-negative cocci	Bacitracin 10,000 units/ml. Erythromycin lactobionate 10 mg./ml.	Cefazolin 33 mg./ml.
Gram-negative diplobacilli	Polymyxin B 33,000 units/ml. Neomycin 33 mg./ml.	Gentamicin or tobramycin 14 mg./ml. Cefazolin 33 mg./ml.

Gram-negative rods	Tobramycin 14 mg./ml.	Gentamicin 14 mg./ml.
		Polymyxin B 33,000 units/ml.
		  (not generally active against *Proteus*
		  species; substitute neomycin 33 mg./ml.)
		Carbenicillin 6 mg./ml. ⎱ To be used with
		Ticarcillin 6 mg./ml. ⎰ aminoglycoside

mulation and dosage of periocularly injected antibiotics.

The duration of antibiotic therapy is determined by the clinical response of

Table 15–7. PREPARATION OF ANTIBIOTICS FOR SUBCONJUNCTIVAL INJECTION*

Cefazolin 100 mg. (0.5 ml.)
 Solubilize one vial of lyophilized cefazolin sodium (500 mg.) with 2.5 ml. of sterile normal saline. Draw up 0.5 ml. for subconjunctival injection.

Carbenicillin 100 mg. (0.5 ml.)
 Solubilize one vial of carbenicillin disodium (1000 mg.) with 5 ml. of sterile water for injection. Draw up 0.5 ml. for subconjunctival injection.

Erythromycin Lactobionate 50 mg. (0.5 ml.)
 Solubilize one vial of erythromycin lactobionate (500 mg.) with 5 ml. of sterile water for injection. Draw up 0.5 ml. for subconjunctival injection.

Gentamicin 40 mg. (1.0 ml.)
 Each vial of gentamicin injectable contains 80 mg. in 2 ml. of diluent. Draw up 1 ml. (40 mg.) for subconjunctival injection.

Oxacillin 100 mg. (0.5 ml.)
 Solubilize one vial of oxacillin sodium for injection (1000 mg.) with 5 ml. of sterile saline for injection. Draw up 0.5 ml. for subconjunctival injection.

Tobramycin 40 mg. (1.0 ml.)
 Each vial of tobramycin injectable contains 80 mg. in 2 ml. of diluent. Draw up 1 ml. (40 mg.) for subconjunctival injection.

Vancomycin 25 mg. (0.5 ml.) (may cause sloughing of the conjunctiva)
 Solubilize one vial of vancomycin hydrochloride intravenous (500 mg.) with 10 ml. of sterile saline for injection. Draw up 0.5 ml. for subconjunctival injection.

*A subconjunctival injection is generally limited to 1 ml. total volume.

the corneal ulcer and the virulence of the pathogen. Ulcers caused by Gram-negative organisms generally require treatment for longer periods than those caused by Gram-positive organisms. As a conservative guideline, antibiotics can be discontinued safely 7 to 10 days after the corneal infiltrate has cleared and epithelial continuity has been restored. Particular caution is advised in cases of *Pseudomonas* ulcers. Instances of reactivation and recurrence have been described despite effective antibiotic therapy for what seemed to be an appropriate length of time. In the management of *Pseudomonas aeruginosa* keratitis we discontinue topical corticosteroids when the corneal infiltrate has cleared or there is no further observable anti-inflammatory effect, and we continue topical antibiotics for approximately 3 weeks thereafter. A total antibiotic course of 6 to 8 weeks is not unusual in our experience, and, indeed, it is recommended.

CORTICOSTEROIDS

While the elimination of replicating bacteria with antibiotics is in progress, the normal host response is in motion, reflected by the leukocytic infiltration of the cornea. We have stressed that the damage caused by lysosomal enzymes released by inflammatory cells, predominantly polymorphonuclear leukocytes, is paramount among the events that lead to irreversible corneal opacification in bacterial keratitis. Termination of bacterial replication in the cornea does not result in the prompt cessation of the corneal inflammatory response. Leukocytes capable of contributing to stromal destruction continue to be chemotactically attracted to the cornea for varying periods of time to participate in the elimination of bacterial particles and tissue debris. Suppression of the inflammatory response, therefore, represents the second major goal in the treatment of bacterial keratitis. This is best accomplished with topical corticosteroids.

It is this writer's recommendation that topical corticosteroids be used in the treatment of bacterial infections whenever the inflammatory process involves the central or paracentral cornea. Corticosteroids control the damage produced by invading polymorphonuclear leukocytes and thereby preserve normal corneal structure and transparency. However, in systems outside the cornea there is experimental evidence that high concentrations of corticosteroids impair phagocytosis and intracellular killing of bacteria.[90-93] Thus, although corticosteroids preserve the normal structure and transparency of the cornea, they also have the potential to interfere with host defense mechanisms which represent the natural response to infection.

It is imperative, then, that a balance be struck between the desirable and undesirable effects of corticosteroids, and experimental studies show that concurrent topical administration of an antibiotic and a corticosteroid produces a favorable outcome.[69, 87] The antibiotic continues to eliminate the microorganism from the cornea with no apparent interference from the corticosteroid. It is important to note that these experimental data indicate that corticosteroids do not enhance bacterial replication when administered concurrently with an effective bactericidal antibiotic. One cannot be certain that similar findings would be obtained following concurrent administration of a corticosteroid and a bacteriostatic antibiotic. Although the bacteriostatic antibiotic suppresses bacterial replication, the actual elimination of the organism is largely dependent on the host response. Since the corticosteroid nonspecifically suppresses the host response, it is possible that the administration of a corticosteroid along with a bacteriostatic antibiotic might produce a different outcome, though—rather surprisingly—in the rabbit hourly instillation of the corticosteroid alone for as long as 48 consecutive hours did not enhance microbial replication in comparison with simultaneously run untreated controls.[87] Thus, conservative interpretation of available data supports the conclusion that the addition of a topically applied corticosteroid to an effective topical antibiotic regimen containing a bactericidal agent does not enhance bacterial replication if the corticosteroid is not instilled more frequently than the antibiotic.

Clinically we prefer to follow a conservative course, and we treat bacterial keratitis solely with concentrated, topically applied antibiotics for approximately a 24-hour period in an attempt to ensure control of bacterial replication. If there is no clinical evidence of progression, we generally interpret this as a sign of a positive therapeutic response, and we then institute treatment with corticosteroids. If the corneal ulcer is especially severe, or if the scrapings demonstrate Gram-negative rods, we occasionally continue therapy with antibiotics alone for an additional 24 hours despite the absence of progression of the ulcerative process and then initiate topical steroid therapy. Our results with this regimen have been gratifying. Others begin concurrent antibiotic and corticosteroid therapy from the outset with equal success,[94] and experimental data support the validity and efficacy of this latter approach. Most frequently steroid therapy consists of 1.0 per cent prednisolone acetate ophthalmic suspension administered topically with the same frequency as the topical antibiotics are being instilled; in no instance is the corticosteroid instilled more frequently than the antibiotic in the treatment of an active bacterial keratitis. As a general rule, topical corticosteroids are tapered on a dose-for-dose basis with the antibiotics.

GENERAL THERAPEUTIC PRINCIPLES

In addition to antibiotics and corticosteroids, bacterial corneal ulcers are routinely treated with a long-acting parasympatholytic mydriatic-cycloplegic solution (e.g., atropine 1 per cent, scopolamine 0.25 per cent) administered topically two to four times daily. This agent deters the formation of posterior synechiae and reduces the discomfort of ciliary muscle spasm induced by the anterior uveitis that accompanies most cases of bacterial keratitis. We have not found collagenase inhibitors to be of practical value in the treatment of bacterial corneal ulcers. Most of the collagenolytic enzymes that play a role in the ulcerative processes accompanying bacterial infection presumably are of leukocytic origin. Neutralization of these many diverse enzymatic substances with clinically available collagenase inhibitors (e.g., acetylcysteine, disodium ethylenediaminetetraacetate [EDTA]) has proven therapeutically ineffective in our hands. We believe it more appropriate to attack these enzymes at their source and to prevent their elaboration. This requires the elimination of invading leukocytes, a function that is effectively accomplished with corticosteroids. Collagenase inhibitors have also been recommended for the management of *Pseudomonas aeruginosa* keratitis to inhibit the enzymes released by many strains of this organism. Our own experience with using collagenase inhibitors for this purpose has been disappointing, and there is no well-documented evidence that these agents exert a beneficial effect on the clinical course of severe *Pseudomonas* keratitis.

Hydrophilic contact lenses have a limited but useful role in the treatment of bacterial keratitis. When stromal necrosis has resulted in substantial tissue loss with marked, localized thinning, the diseased cornea is subject to mechanical trauma by the lid margins during blinking and to desiccation resulting from abnormal tear distribution over the irregular corneal surface. Both factors can contribute to the inflammatory process, causing additional stromal necrosis and tissue loss and initiating a sequence of events leading to perforation. A soft contact lens can be fitted and worn on the damaged cornea continuously 24 hours a day for varying lengths of time, effectively interrupting this disastrous cycle. The hydrogel device acts as an optical bandage, protecting the cornea from the trauma of the blinking lids and helping to maintain a moist film over its irregular surface. It facilitates re-epithelialization and at times promotes fibroblastic proliferation so that stromal repair and thickening occur.[95, 96]

In the management of the most severe of bacterial ulcers, in which the entire thickness of the corneal stroma has become necrotic and has sloughed and only Descemet's membrane remains intact, a hydrophilic contact lens can be extremely useful. It provides sufficient structural reinforcement of Descemet's membrane to prevent its distention by the intraocular pressure while maintaining it in a moist state and shielding it from trauma. A hydrogel lens can be worn continuously on a diseased cornea containing a descemetocele for extended periods of time and will prevent perforation in a high proportion of cases.[97] We prefer to use the device only on culture-negative cases, but there is no evidence that its use is contraindicated in the presence of active infection. Anti-infective and anti-inflammatory therapy are administered while the lens is in place. The hydrophilic contact lens acts as a barrier to penetration of topically administered drugs; this must be considered in the determination of the appropriate dosage of all medications that are being used.

In every case of bacterial keratitis the

lacrimal passages must be evaluated to ascertain whether or not a chronic dacryocystitis is present and contributing to the pathogenesis of the corneal infection. When a dacryocystitis is present, the patency of the lacrimal passages must be re-established, generally through surgical intervention (i.e., dacryocystorhinostomy), to ensure the eradication of infection in the lacrimal sac. Commonly antibiotic therapy is first instituted in an attempt to stabilize the infectious processes in the cornea. However, the futility of attempting to resolve a bacterial corneal ulcer or avoid a recurrence in the presence of an infected lacrimal sac that is continuously discharging pathogenic organisms is apparent.

Similarly a chronic marginal blepharitis may contribute to the pathogenesis of a bacterial corneal ulcer. Commonly one can effect a resolution of the keratitis using a conventional therapeutic regimen without addition of any special measures directed at the infectious processes in the meibomian glands or lash follicles. Although it is virtually impossible to eliminate a chronic bacterial infection in these structures, we have found that mechanical scrubbing of the lid margins nightly using a cotton-tipped applicator and a mild shampoo (e.g., Johnson's Baby Shampoo), is highly successful in minimizing the degree of active inflammation at the lid margin and in the conjunctiva and in preventing recurrence of corneal infection (see Chapter 9).

With rare exceptions only, the patient with a presumed bacterial ulcer should be hospitalized. Initially topical antibiotics must be instilled at intervals that do not exceed 60 minutes on a continuous, 24-hour basis. The antibiotic regimen may have to be altered as culture and sensitivity data become available. Biomicroscopic evaluation of the involved eye must be performed at intervals of no more than 12 hours during the early phases of treatment to assess the clinical response to antibiotics, to decide whether or not corticosteroid therapy should be instituted, and to determine if other supportive measures are indicated. These requirements generally can be met only in a hospital.

Prolonged, careful follow-up is mandatory. Initial clinical evidence of a favorable response to treatment includes halting of the progression of a severe corneal ulcer, a decrease in the quantity of discharge, progressive clearing of a hypopyon, a decrease in the severity of anterior chamber reaction, and an increased response of the pupil to mydriatics. The appearance of the lids and conjunctiva does not accurately reflect the response to therapy; the medications may themselves be irritating, and the frequency with which they are being applied may cause the lid and conjunctiva to become more swollen and injected despite a favorable response of the keratitis. The stromal infiltrate tends to resolve slowly; its course often is hastened by instillation of corticosteroids. Corneal edema may also have a prolonged course, and its rate of resolution usually parallels that of the stromal infiltrate. So, too, does the rate of re-epithelialization; rarely will the continuity of the epithelium be restored in the presence of an active stromal infiltrate.

An eye with an active bacterial keratitis should not be patched. For practical purposes, the skin of the face will not long tolerate the application and removal of tape at hourly or more frequent intervals to permit the instillation of antibiotics. More to the point, however, patching encourages continuous closure of the lids. The temperature in the cul-de-sac increases and discharge accumulates there; both factors encourage bacterial replication, allow the organism to thrive, and render therapy less effective. We have also witnessed a case in which the eye was maintained in the open position despite the presence of a patch. Corneal sensation in the involved eye was markedly decreased, a not uncommon finding, and the patient was unaware of the contact between his cornea and the patch or the injury it produced.

REFERENCES

1. Locatcher-Khorazo, D., and Seegal, B. C.: *Microbiology of the Eye*. St. Louis, C. V. Mosby Co., 1972, pp. 15–19.
2. Khorazo, D., and Thompson, R.: The bacterial flora of the normal conjunctiva. Amer J Ophthalmol 18:1114, 1935.
3. Allansmith, M. R., Ostler, H. B., and Butterworth, M.: Concomitance of bacteria in various areas of the eye. Arch Ophthalmol 82:37, 1969.
4. DeOcampo, G., Salceda, S., and deLeon, A.: Bacterial flora of the healthy conjunctiva among Filipinos. Philipp J Surg 20:95, 1965.
5. Khristov, G.: Bacterial flora of the normal conjunctiva and in conjunctivitis. IZV Microbiol Inst (Sofia) 7:107, 1956.
6. Perkins, R. E., Kundsin, R. B., Pratt, M. V., Abrahamsen, I., and Leibowitz, H. M.: Bacteriology of normal and infected conjunctiva. J Clin Microbiol 1:147, 1975.
7. Inomata, H., and Smelser, G. K.: Fine structural alterations of corneal endothelium during experimental uveitis. Invest Ophthalmol 9:272, 1970.
8. Polack, F. M., and Kanai, A.: Electron microscopic studies of graft endothelium in corneal graft rejection. Amer J Ophthalmol 73:711, 1972.
9. Eisenstein, R., Sorgente, N., and Soble, L. W.: The resistance of certain tissues to invasion: Penetrability of explanted tissues by vascularized mesenchyme. Amer J Pathol 73:765, 1973.
10. McCulloch, C., Thompson, G. A., and Basu, P. K.: Lamellar keratoplasty using full thickness donor material. Trans Amer Ophthalmol Soc 61:154, 1963.
11. Dohlman, C. H., and Balazs, E. A.: Chemical studies on Descemet's membrane of the bovine cornea. Arch Biochem 57:445, 1955.
12. Green, W. R., and Zimmerman, L. E.: Granulomatous reaction to Descemet's membrane. Amer J Ophthalmol 64:555, 1967.
13. Naumann, G., Green, W. R., and Zimmerman, L. E.: Mycotic keratitis: A histopathologic study of 73 cases. Amer J Ophthalmol 64:668, 1967.
14. Jones, D. B.: Early diagnosis and therapy of bacterial corneal ulcers. Int Ophthal Clin 13:1, 1973.
15. Wilson, L.: Bacterial corneal ulcers. In Duane, T. D. (ed.): *Clinical Ophthalmology*. Vol. 4. Hagerstown, Md., Harper & Row, 1976, chap. 18.
16. Locatcher-Khorazo, D., and Seegal, B. C.: *Microbiology of the Eye*. St. Louis, C. V. Mosby Co., 1972, pp. 69–71.
17. Petit, T. H.: Management of bacterial corneal ulcers. In Leopold, I. H. and Burns, R. P. (eds.): *Symposium on Ocular Therapy*. Vol. 8. New York, John Wiley & Sons, 1976, pp. 57–65.
18. Davis, B. D., Dulbeco, R., Eisen, H. N., Ginsberg, H. S. and Wood, W. B., Jr. (eds.): *Microbiology*. 2nd ed. Hagerstown, Md., Harper & Row, 1973.
19. Joklik, W. K., and Willett, H. P.: *Zinsser Microbiology*. 16th ed. New York, Appleton-Century-Crofts, 1976.
20. Dubos, R. J., and Hirsch, J. G.: *Bacterial and Mycotic Infections of Man*. 4th ed. Philadelphia, J. B. Lippincott Co., 1965.
21. Jones, D. B.: A plan for antimicrobial therapy in bacterial keratitis. Trans Amer Acad Ophthalmol Otolaryngol 79:95, 1975.
22. Locatcher-Khorazo, D., Sullivan, N., and Gutierrez, E.: *Staphylococcus aureus* isolated from normal and infected eyes: Phage types and sensitivity to antibacterial agents. Arch Ophthalmol 77:370, 1967.
23. Burns, R. B.: *Pseudomonas aeruginosa* keratitis: Mixed infections of the eye. Amer J Ophthalmol 67:257, 1969.
24. Wilson, L. A.: Chelation in experimental *Pseudomonas* keratitis. Brit J Ophthalmol 54:587, 1970.
25. Fisher, E., and Allen, J. H.: Mechanism of corneal destruction by *Pseudomonas* proteases. Amer J Ophthalmol 46:249, 1958.
26. Morihara, K.: *Pseudomonas aeruginosa* protease. I. Purification and general properties. Biochim Biophys Acta 73:113, 1963.
27. Schoellmann, G., and Fisher, E.: A collagenase from *Pseudomonas aeruginosa*. Biochim Biophys Acta 122:557, 1966.
28. Brown, S. I., Bloomfield, S. E., and Tam, W. I.: The cornea-destroying enzyme of *Pseudomonas aeruginosa*. Invest Ophthalmol 13:174, 1974.
29. Okumoto, M., and Smolin, G.: Pneumococcal infections of the eye. Amer J Ophthalmol 77:346, 1974.
30. Eliot, A. J., Chamberlain, W. P., Jr., and Givner, I.: Diplobacillus of Petit in corneal ulceration. Arch Ophthalmol 25:280, 1941.
31. Fedukowicz, H., and Horwich, H.: The gram negative bacillus in hypopyon keratitis. Arch Ophthalmol 49:202, 1953.
32. McKee, H.: Ulceration of the cornea from the diplobacillus of Morax-Axenfeld. Ophthal Rec 16:183, 1907.
33. Van Bijsterveld, O. P., and Richards, R. D.: Bacillus infections of the cornea. Arch Ophthalmol 74:91, 1965.
34. Kreger, A. S., and Griffin, O. K.: Cornea-damaging proteases of *Serratia marcescens*. Invest Ophthalmol 14:190, 1975.
35. Sexton, R. R.: Unusual bacterial corneal ulcers. In Duane, T. D. (ed.): *Clinical Ophthalmology*. Vol. 4. Hagerstown, Md., Harper & Row, 1976, Chap. 20.
36. Cagle, G. D., and Abshire, R. L.: Quantitative ocular bacteriology: A method for the enumeration and identification of bacteria from the skin-lash margin and conjunctiva. Invest Ophthalmol Vis Sci 20:751, 1981.
37. Pollock, M. R.: Unsaturated fatty acids in cotton plugs. Nature 161:853, 1948.
38. Rubbo, S. D. and Benjamin, M.: Some observations on the survival of pathogenic bacteria on cotton wool swabs. Brit Med J 1:983, 1951.
39. Leibowitz, H. M., Pratt, M. V., Flagstad, I. J., Berrospi, A. R., and Kundsin, R.: Human Conjunctivitis. I. Diagnostic Evaluation. Arch Ophthalmol 94:1747, 1976.
40. Bang, F. B.: A bacterial disease of *Limulus polyphemus*. Bull Johns Hopk Hosp 98:325, 1956.
41. Levin, J., and Bang, F. B.: The role of endotoxin in the extracellular coagulation of *Limulus* blood. Bull Johns Hopk Hosp 115:265, 1964.
42. McBeath, J., Forster, R. K., and Rebell, G.: Diagnostic limulus lysate assay for endophthalmitis and keratitis. Arch Ophthalmol 96:1265, 1978.
43. Avallone, A. N., Parrett, C., Smith, R. E., Meyers, R., and Chitjian, P. A.: Rapid detection of experimental *E. coli* endophthalmitis by the limulus lysate test. Invest Ophthalmol Vis Sci 17:528, 1978.
44. Wolters, R. W., Jorgensen, J. H., Calzada, E., and Poirier, R. H.: Limulus lysate assay for early detec-

tion of certain gram negative corneal infections. Arch Ophthalmol 97:875, 1979.

45. Davis, S. D., and Chandler, J. W.: Experimental keratitis due to *Pseudomonas aeruginosa*: Model for evaluation of antimicrobial drugs. Antimicrob Agents Chemother 8:350, 1975.

46. Kupferman, A., and Leibowitz, H. M.: Quantitation of bacterial infection and antibacterial effect in the cornea. Arch Ophthalmol 94:1981, 1976.

47. Levine, R. R.: *Pharmacology: Drug Actions and Reactions.* Boston, Little, Brown, 1973, pp. 102–104.

48. Kislak, J. W., Eickhoff, T. C., and Finland, M.: Cloxacillin: activity in vitro and absorption and urinary excretion in normal young men. Amer J Med Sci 249:636, 1965.

49. Rolinson, G. N.: The significance of protein binding of penicillins. Postgrad Med J 40(Suppl):20, 1964.

50. Rolinson, G. N., and Sutherland, R.: The binding of antibiotics to serum proteins. Brit J Pharmacol 25:638, 1965.

51. Kunin, C. M.: Clinical significance of protein binding of the penicillins. Ann NY Acad Sci 145:282, 1967.

52. Rolinson, G. N.: The significance of protein binding of antibiotics in vitro and in vivo. In Waterson, A. P. (ed.): *Recent Advances In Medical Microbiology.* London, J. & A. Churchill, Ltd., 1967, p. 254.

53. Adler, F. H.: *Physiology of the Eye: Clinical Application.* 3rd ed. St. Louis, C. V. Mosby Co., 1959, pp. 46, 103.

54. Barker, B. M., and Prescott, F.: *Antimicrobial Agents in Medicine.* Oxford, Blackwell Scientific Publications, 1973, pp. 18–97.

55. Weinstein, L. S., and Perrin, T. S.: Treatment of scarlet fever with penicillin G administered orally three times a day. J Pediat 37:844, 1950.

56. Weinstein, L. S., and Daikos, G.: Treatment of scarlet fever with crystalline penicillin G administered orally or parenterally two times a day. Amer Pract Dig Treat 2:62, 1951.

57. Baum, J. L., Barza, M., Shushan, D., and Weinstein, L.: Concentration of gentamicin in experimental corneal ulcers: Topical vs. subconjunctival therapy. Arch Ophthalmol 92:315, 1974.

58. Boyle, G. L., Gwon, A. E., Zinn, K. M., and Leopold, I. H.: Intraocular penetration of carbenicillin after subconjunctival injection in man. Amer J Ophthalmol 73:754, 1972.

59. Davis, S. D., and Chandler, J. W.: Experimental keratitis due to *Pseudomonas aeruginosa*: Model for evaluation of antimicrobial drugs. Antimicrob Agents Chemother 8:350, 1975.

60. Broughton, W., and Goldman, J. N.: Intraocular penetration of chloramphenicol succinate in rabbits. Ann Ophthalmol 5:71, 1973.

61. Litwack, K., Petit, T., and Johnson, B. L., Jr.: Penetration of gentamicin administered intramuscularly and subconjunctivally into aqueous humor. Arch Ophthalmol 82:687, 1969.

62. O'Day, D. M., McKenna, T. J., and Elliott, J. H.: Ocular corticosteroid therapy: Systemic hormonal effects. Trans Amer Acad Ophthalmol Otolaryngol 79:OP71, 1975.

63. Nozik, R. A.: Periocular injection of steroids. Trans Amer Acad Ophthalmol Otolaryogol 76:OP695, 1972.

64. Schlaegel, T. F.: Essentials of uveitis. Boston, Little, Brown, 1969, p. 42.

65. Havener, W. H.: *Ocular Pharmacology.* 3rd ed. St. Louis, C. V. Mosby Co., 1974, p. 30.

66. Kupferman, A., and Leibowitz, H. M.: Topical antibiotic therapy of staphylococcal keratitis. Arch Ophthalmol 95:1634, 1977.

67. Kupferman, A., and Leibowitz, H. M.: Topical antibiotic therapy of *Pseudomonas aeruginosa* keratitis. Arch Ophthalmol 97:1699, 1979.

68. Davis, S. D., Sarff, L. D., and Hyndiuk, R.A.: Antibiotic therapy of experimental *Pseudomonas* keratitis in guinea pigs. Arch Ophthalmol 95:1638, 1977.

69. Davis, S. D., Sarff, L. D., and Hyndiuk, R. A.: Topical tobramycin therapy of experimental *Pseudomonas* keratitis. Arch Ophthalmol 96:123, 1978.

70. Davis, S. D., Sarff, L. D., and Hyndiuk, R. A.: Comparison of therapeutic routes in experimental *Pseudomonas* keratitis. Amer J Ophthalmol 87:710, 1979.

71. Leibowitz, H. M., Ryan, W. J., Jr., and Kupferman, A.: Route of antibiotic administration in bacterial keratitis. Arch Ophthalmol 99:1420, 1981.

72. Baum, J., and Barza, M.: Topical versus subconjunctival treatment of bacterial corneal ulcers. Ophthalmology 90:162, 1983.

73. Hyndiuk, R. A.: Experimental *Pseudomonas* keratitis. Trans Amer Ophthalmol Soc 79:541, 1981.

74. Leibowitz, H. M., and Kupferman, A.: Optimal frequency of topical prednisolone administration. Arch Ophthalmol 97:2154, 1979.

75. Barza, M., Baum, J., Berklay, B. and Weinstein, L.: Intraocular penetration of carbenicillin in the rabbit. Amer J Ophthalmol 75:305, 1973.

76. Leopold, I. H., and LaMotte, W. O., Jr.: Penetration of penicillin in rabbit eyes with normal, inflamed, and abraded corneas. Arch Ophthalmol 33:43, 1945.

77. Salminen, I., Jarvinen, H., and Toivanen, P.: Distribution of tritiated penicillin in the rabbit eye. Acta Ophthalmol 47:115, 1969.

78. Green, W. R., and Leopold, I. H.: Intraocular penetration of methicillin. Am J Ophthalmol 60:800, 1965.

79. Records, R. E., and Ellis, P. P.: The intraocular penetration of ampicillin, methicillin and oxacillin. Amer J Ophthalmol 64:135, 1967.

80. Records, R. E.: Intraocular penetration of dicloxacillin in experimental animals. Invest Ophthalmol 7:663, 1968.

81. Town, A. E., and Hunt, M. E.: Concentration of penicillin in the aqueous humor following systemic administration. Amer J Ophthalmol 29:171, 1946.

82. Goldman, E. E., McLain, J. H., and Smith, J. L.: Penicillins and aqueous humor. Amer J Ophthalmol 65:717, 1968.

83. Kurose, Y., and Leopold, I. H.: Intraocular penetration of ampicillin. I. Animal experiments. Arch Ophthalmol 73:361, 1965.

84. Goldman, J. N., Broughton, W., Javed, H., and Lauderdale, V.: Ampicillin, erythromycin and chloramphenicol penetration into the rabbit aqueous humor. Ann Ophthalmol 5:147, 1973.

85. Barza, M., and Baum, J.: Penetration of ocular compartments by penicillins. Surv Ophthalmol 18:71, 1973.

86. Grove, D. C., and Randall, W. A.: *Assay Methods of Antibiotics.* New York, Medical Encyclopedia, Inc. 1955, pp. 14–16.

87. Leibowitz, H. M., and Kupferman, A.: The effect of topically administered corticosteroids on antibiotic-treated bacterial keratitis. Arch Ophthalmol 98:1287, 1980.

88. Garrod, L. P., and Waterworth, P. M.: Methods of

testing combined antibiotic bactericidal action and the significance of the results. J Clin Pathol 15:328, 1962.

89. Barker, B. M., and Prescott, F.: *Antimicrobial Agents in Medicine.* Oxford, Blackwell Scientific Publications, 1973, p. 36.

90. Allison, F., and Adcock, M. H.: The influence of hydrocortisone and certain electrolyte solutions upon phagocytic and bactericidal capacities of leukocytes obtained from peritoneal exudate of rats. J Immunol 92:435, 1964.

91. Crepa, S. B., Magnin, G. E., and Seastone, C. V.: Effect of ACTH and cortisone on phagocytosis. Proc Soc Exp Biol Med 77:704, 1951.

92. Mandell, G. L., Rubin, W., and Hook, E. W.: The effect of an NADH oxidase inhibitor (hydrocortisone) on polymorphonuclear leukocyte bacterial activity. J Clin Invest 49:1381, 1970.

93. Stossel, T. P., Mason, R. J., Hartwig, J., and Vaughan, M.: Quantitative studies of phagocytosis by polymorphonuclear leukocytes: Use of emulsions to measure the initial rate of phagocytosis. J Clin Invest 51:615, 1972.

94. Aronson, S. B., and Moore, T. E., Jr.: Corticosteroid therapy in central stromal keratitis. Amer J Ophthalmol 67:873, 1969.

95. Gasset, A. R., and Kaufman, H. E.: Therapeutic uses of soft contact lenses. Amer J Ophthalmol 69:252, 1970.

96. Leibowitz, H. M., and Rosenthal, P. R.: Hydrophilic contact lenses in corneal disease. I. Superficial, sterile, indolent ulcers. Arch Ophthalmol 85:163, 1971.

97. Leibowitz, H. M., and Berrospi, A. R.: Initial treatment of descemetocoele with hydrophilic contact lenses. Ann Ophthalmol 7:1161, 1975.

Herpes Simplex Keratitis | 16

DENIS M. O'DAY, M.D.

Herpesvirus infection is a leading cause of corneal blindness and one of the most challenging problems that an ophthalmologist may face in his daily practice. Man is the only known natural host of this agent, and the complexity of his relationship with this virus is becoming apparent as mechanisms of disease are gradually unraveled. Much remains to be resolved, but what is already known is helpful in understanding both the clinical disease and its response to therapy. Up to 90 per cent of the population of the United States over the age of 15 years have antibodies to herpes simplex, indicating that they have been infected by this virus. These antibodies cross the placenta and protect most newborn infants during the first 6 months of life. Thereafter, passively transferred immunity becomes ineffective and the child becomes subject to primary infection. Premature infants, who have not had the opportunity to acquire these antibodies, and full term babies of noninfected mothers are not afforded this protection. By age 5 most children will have had a primary infection, though clinical disease will be evident in only about 10 per cent of those infected. In the remainder primary infection will be subclinical or it will go undiagnosed, but many subsequently will manifest secondary herpetic disease, most commonly in the form of benign fever blisters or gingivostomatitis.[1]

Primary herpes simplex infection tends to be mild and usually runs a self-limited course, but occasionally it has a fatal outcome. Virus can be readily isolated from primary lesions and very often from saliva, stools, and tears. Within a week of the onset of infection, neutralizing antibodies appear in the bloodstream. The titer steadily rises over the next few weeks and then falls. Ultimately the level of neutralizing antibodies tends to plateau, and, within broad limits, that level is maintained despite episodic recurrences. Complement-fixing antibodies follow a similar pattern but tend to fluctuate between recurrences. Thus, serology has distinct limitations in its diagnostic application. Only in the primary infection with herpes simplex is there a rise in serum antibodies; recurrent disease causes no significant increase. To be of value, an acute-phase serum sample must be obtained early in the course of the disease, generally within a week of its onset.

The virus is not eliminated from the body after healing of the primary infection. Instead, it persists in an almost perfect symbiotic relationship that is marred by recurrent disease, when the virus is reactivated by endogenous or exogenous stimuli from its apparently latent state. In contrast to the primary illness, recurrent episodes are not accompanied by evidence of systemic disease, presumably because immune mechanisms protect the individual. Herpesvirus has been isolated from the spinal ganglia and from the trigeminal ganglia in an animal model of chronic herpesvirus infection and from man by organ culture.[2-7] Isolation by this technique implies either that the virus is in a truly latent state or that it is replicating at a very slow rate. Significantly, this technique has so far been unsuccessful in isolating virus from sensory nerves or other nervous tissue, nor has it demonstrated virus in the lacrimal gland, conjunctiva, cornea, or iris. Presumably the virus gains access to the central nervous system during the primary infection by moving centripetally along sensory nerves to the sensory ganglion and then resides in these cells during the quiescent phase.[8-10] Under the influence of various stimuli the cycle is restarted, seemingly causing virus particles to travel centrifugally along sensory nerves to initiate a recurrent lesion, generally at the same location as the primary episode. Nothing is known of the mechanisms leading to reactivation of latent virus. However, mild trauma, exposure to strong sunlight, menstruation, psychiatric disturbance,[11] and fever often precede recurrent episodes and generally are accepted as precipitating factors.

The various strains of herpes simplex virus fall into two distinct groups based on immunologic specificity, site of isolation from the body, characteristics in cell culture, and behavior during passage in laboratory animals. Isolates from oral, facial, and ocular lesions are usually of the type I variety, whereas type II isolates are of genital origin. However, exceptions do occur. Type II herpesvirus is more virulent than type I, and ocular infections caused by the former tend to be clinically severe. Most cases of neonatal herpes are transmitted from active lesions in the maternal genital tract. An occasional case is present at birth, and presumably this results from transplacental passage of the virus. Primary herpes in infants, adolescents, and adults is usually contracted by oral or sexual contact with an infected individual, though apparently not necessarily one with an active lesion. Ophthalmologists and other physicians may be a vector of the disease through contaminated hands or instruments. Infection also may be spread by shared drops, ointments,[12] and so forth and from a nonocular site to the eye of the same individual via the hands. Lesions on the eyelid may spontaneously seed an ocular infection.

PRIMARY HERPES SIMPLEX INFECTION

Primary ocular herpes is a disease of infants and young adults, although sporadic cases may occur at all ages. The disease usually becomes overt within a week of contact, although this period may vary from 2 days to 2 weeks. Usually mild but occasionally severe symptoms of systemic illness (e.g., generalized malaise, fever) herald the onset of primary infection. Although skin, mucous membranes, and the central nervous system may be involved, in this chapter we shall be concerned only with the ocular manifestations.

Eye involvement in primary herpetic infection is frequently mild, so much so that it may be overlooked by the patient. In most cases acute unilateral redness, irritability, and a watery discharge are the principal symptoms. Typically the ipsilateral preauricular node is swollen and slightly tender. Swollen lids and a primary skin lesion may be present (Fig. 16–1), but not infrequently a careful search is needed to reveal the single or grouped vesicles or the crusted ulcers hidden among the lashes or located on the intermarginal strip (Fig. 16–2). Similar lesions may be found on the face, at the mucocutaneous junction of the mouth, in the nose, or on the trunk, but often no cutaneous lesions are present.[13]

The conjunctiva is injected and edematous. Follicles are present in the fornices and on the tarsal plate. It is not uncommon for small ecchymoses to be seen in the conjunctiva.

Corneal involvement develops within 2 weeks in about half the patients with primary herpetic conjunctivitis. The initial disease is always epithelial and presents a variety of appearances. A fine punctate keratitis may be encountered. These transient white flecks stain poorly with fluorescein and variably with rose bengal, but as they desquamate during the healing stages, fluorescein staining becomes more intense. In other patients a coarse punctate epithelial keratitis may appear and may progress to form one or several dendritic figures. These consist of closed clusters of opaque epithelial cells slightly elevated above the surface of the cornea. The swollen cells stain brilliantly with rose bengal (but poorly with fluorescein) and harbor replicating virus. Initially the disease is confined to the epithelial layer of the cornea, but within a few weeks, and independent of epithelial healing, subepithelial infiltrates appear.[13] These usually persist for several weeks, leaving small areas of focal scarring as they gradually resolve. Occasionally a disciform keratitis (Fig. 16–3) will develop with a course indistinguishable from that of recurrent stromal disease.

When typical cutaneous lid lesions or typical corneal lesions are present, the diagnosis of primary herpetic infection can usually be made on clinical grounds alone. Viral cultures from the cornea, conjunctiva, and skin lesions are helpful if the diagnosis is in doubt. Neutralizing and complement-fixing antibodies appear within a week of onset. A rising titer over a period of several weeks is useful confirmatory evidence of a herpetic infection. Adenovirus infection and TRIC agent conjunctivitis are the most important entities to be considered in the differential diagnosis.

Therapy is directed toward elimination of virus from the cornea and adjacent skin lesions.[14] It is important to treat the skin lesions since they may represent a reservoir of virus that can reinfect the cornea and conjunctiva. Idoxuridine (IDU) or vidarabine ointment is instilled five times a day into the conjunctival sac and is liberally applied to the eyelids and adjacent skin lesions. When there is no active skin involvement, IDU drops may be given hourly during the day with the ointment at bedtime. Therapy is continued until active corneal and skin lesions are healed. Trifluridine should be reserved for cases that fail to respond satisfactorily to IDU or vidarabine. If ciliary spasm or photophobia secondary to iritis occurs, a cycloplegic agent may be necessary for comfort; scopolamine

hydrobromide 0.25 per cent b.i.d. or cyclopentolate hydrochloride 1.0 per cent t.i.d. or q.i.d. is usually effective. Debridement of the corneal lesions is seldom indicated in primary herpes simplex infection but may be necessary when a resistant strain of virus is encountered or signs of antiviral agent toxicity appear. Use of an eye pad is undesirable, but sunglasses may provide symptomatic relief.

Management is usually accomplished on an outpatient basis. The patient generally is re-evaluated 2 to 3 days after the initial visit and at weekly intervals thereafter if recovery is proceeding uneventfully. Patients with severe bilateral disease or with a secondary bacterial infection should be hospitalized. The latter is treated with local antibiotics. An exception is cellulitis of the lids, which requires systemic antibiotics. Should sensitivity to the antiviral antimetabolites be encountered, careful debridement of the lesions must be relied upon. The superficial stromal infiltrates generally are transient and do not require anti-inflammatory therapy. Should more severe stromal keratitis develop, it is managed according to the same principles outlined below for recurrent herpetic keratitis. Most lesions respond rapidly and without complication to topical antimetabolite therapy, and in most adequately treated cases corneal damage tends to be minimal. Dermal involvement is superficial and heals without scarring unless bacterial infection supervenes.

RECURRENT HERPES SIMPLEX INFECTION

Resolution of the primary infection signals a new phase in the lifelong relationship between herpesvirus and its host. Although the host becomes apparently free of infection, latent virus remains present in the central nervous system and possibly in other tissues as well.[3, 7] The phenomenon of latency appears to be a mechanism by which the virus is able to maintain an existence within the host at a subviral and probably a molec-

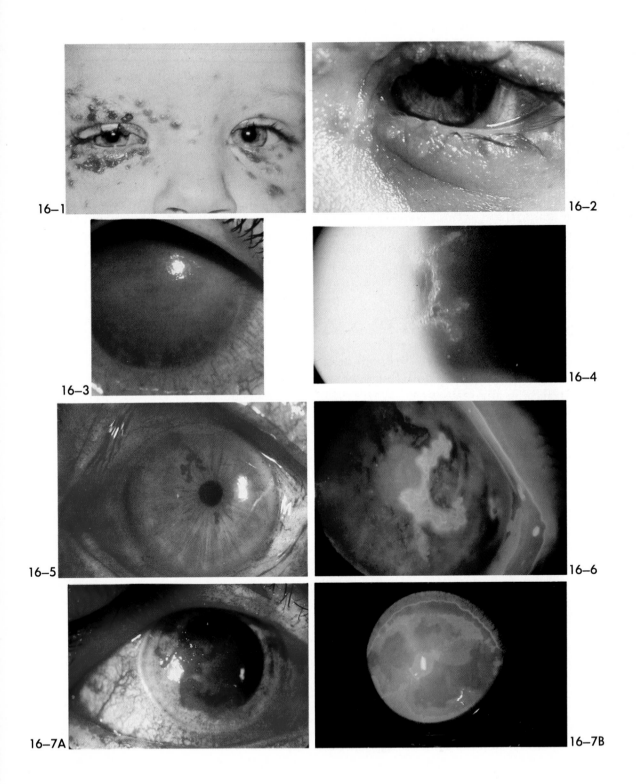

16–1

16–2

16–3

16–4

16–5

16–6

16–7A

16–7B

ular level. The essential elements for viral replication are present within the host cells but are not identifiable by electron microscopy or viral culture. However, if tissue containing these elements is submitted to organ culture, the replicative cycle is reactivated and viral particles can once again be recovered.[2] The trigeminal ganglion is a major site of latent herpes simplex virus in man and in animals.[5] Activation of latent virus, by an as yet unknown mechanism, leads to recurrent disease. Active replicating virus apparently travels via axons from ganglia to the target organ.[15] In the eye the corneal epithelium and stroma are the most common sites of recurrences.

Epithelial Disease

The initial recurrent infection of the corneal epithelium often is associated with severe pain, tearing, and photophobia. However, the intensity of these symptoms is quite variable and tends to decrease with repeated attacks as corneal hypesthesia develops. In contrast to a primary episode, recurrent disease is confined to the cornea. Ciliary injection frequently is striking and may appear out of proportion to the symptoms. In the earliest stages a plaque of opaque cells appears on the corneal surface. In most instances the dendritic shape is already discernible, but stellate or coarse punctate configurations are occasionally seen. As the disease progresses, the central cells in the plaque desquamate so that a slender linear branching ulcer is formed (Fig. 16–4). Occasionally several of these ulcers may develop on the surface of the cornea. Swollen, opaque cells laden with replicating virus line the margins of the ulcer and stain brilliantly with rose bengal (Fig. 16–5). In contrast, fluorescein stains the epithelial defect and seeps beneath the ulcer margins (Fig. 16–6). Within a few days an infiltrate appears in the superficial stroma immediately beneath the ulcer and a mild uveal reaction usually occurs. Corneal hypesthesia is focal, involving primarily the clinically affected area, but with repeated attacks it is common for marked, generalized corneal anesthesia to develop.

In some patients, particularly those treated inadvertently with topical corticosteroids or those receiving immunosuppressive therapy, segments of the lesion may broaden or an extensive area of the epithelium may desquamate so that a large epithelial ulcer develops. This lesion, known as a geographic or ameboid ulcer, can at times encompass the whole surface of the cornea (Fig. 16–7). Like the dendrite, it is the result of active viral replication in epithelial cells

---

Figure 16–1. Primary herpes in a 2-year-old with bilateral involvement of the periocular area. A conjunctivitis is present in the left eye.

Figure 16–2. Typical herpetic lesion along the lid margins in a child with primary herpes.

Figure 16–3. Disciform keratitis in a child with primary herpes. (Courtesy of Howard M. Leibowitz, M.D.)

Figure 16–4. Unstained dendritic ulcer—note ballooned cells along ulcer margin. (Courtesy of N. Brown, Moorfields Eye Hospital, London, U.K. Reprinted from O'Day, D. M., and Jones, B. R.: Herpes simplex keratitis. In Duane, T. D. (ed.): Clinical Ophthalmology. Hagerstown, Md., Loose Leaf Reference Services, 1978, vol. 4, chap. 19. Used by permission of Harper & Row.)

Figure 16–5. Dendritic ulcer stained with rose bengal.

Figure 16–6. Fluorescein stained dendritic ulcer. The margins of the ulcer are indistinct owing to seepage of the dye beneath the epithelium.

Figure 16–7. Geographic ulcer stained with A, rose bengal, and B, fluorescein. (B courtesy of Howard M. Leibowitz, M.D.)

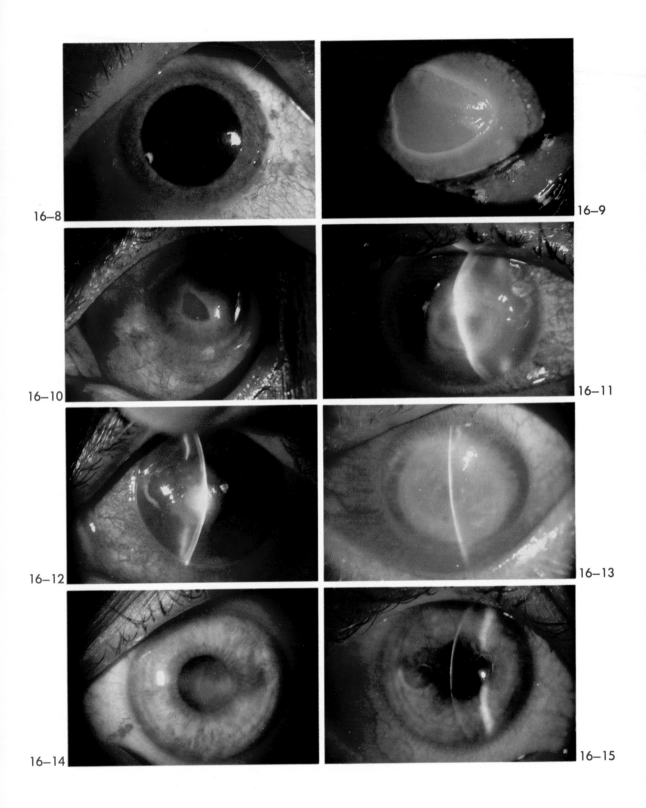

16–8

16–9

16–10

16–11

16–12

16–13

16–14

16–15

and its margins are composed of the same swollen, opaque cells. If this type of ulcer enlarges or persists, stromal involvement becomes more marked and the accompanying uveitis tends to become more intense. Rarely, a herpetic dendritic lesion may cross the limbus and encroach upon the conjunctival epithelium (Fig. 16–8).

When a dendritic ulcer is present, the diagnosis usually is obvious clinically and laboratory confirmation is seldom needed. Recognition of a geographic ulcer, however, can at times be more difficult. Despite careful observation, an equivocal appearance of the ulcer margin may not permit its differentiation from a trophic or indolent ulcer. Typically, the indolent ulcer is round or oval in shape and tends to have a smooth rolled edge composed of cells that stain poorly with rose bengal (Figs. 16–9 and 16–10). Viral replication is not a direct cause of an indolent ulceration, though it may occur after a dendritic or ameboid ulcer.[16] Rather, factors that tend to retard or block epithelial healing, particularly the excessive use of antiviral agents and underlying stromal inflammatory disease, frequently are responsible. Features of both an indolent and an active ameboid ulcer can be present in the same cornea. If the diagnosis remains in doubt, viral cultures of the ulcer margin may be helpful. However, careful sequential observation often will provide

clarification. The ameboid or geographic ulcer tends to change in configuration as a result of viral activity at its margin. In contrast, the indolent ulcer retains a remarkably constant appearance, changing little from day to day unless the precipitating cause is removed.

Management of a simple dendritic ulcer is straightforward and a number of options are available. IDU drops given hourly during the day along with the ointment at bedtime, or either IDU or vidarabine ointment administered five times a day will rapidly heal a majority of the ulcers.[17] Because they need to be instilled less frequently, the ointment formulations are most commonly used and the two drugs are equally effective.[18] Trifluridine (trifluorothymidine), the newest chemotherapeutic antiviral agent, is considerably more soluble than either IDU or vidarabine and has the advantage of being available as a 1.0 per cent drop whose instillation is recommended every 2 hours while the patient is awake (for a maximum daily dosage of nine drops). Controlled studies show that it is no more effective for the treatment of dendritic ulcers than vidarabine ointment,[19, 20] but it is considerably more expensive.

Alternatively, simple mechanical debridement of the ulcer with a cotton-tipped swab is equally effective.[14, 21] For the treatment of a simple dendritic ulcer, there is little to choose between the two

Figure 16–8. Dendritic ulceration spreading beyond limbus onto bulbar conjunctiva.

Figure 16–9. Indolent ulcer stained with fluorescein.

Figure 16–10. Indolent ulcer stained with rose bengal. Ulcer is filled with dye but edges stain poorly.

Figure 16–11. Stromal keratitis due to herpes simplex. An ulcer is present. Note confluent areas of white infiltrate.

Figure 16–12. Well-circumscribed full-thickness stromal infiltrate in a patient with active herpetic stromal keratitis.

Figure 16–13. Herpetic stromal keratitis exhibiting diffuse corneal edema with focal infiltrates.

Figure 16–14. Central corneal scarring that developed following a severe episode of herpetic stromal keratitis.

Figure 16–15. Stromal neovascularization and scarring—inactive herpetic stromal keratitis.

forms of treatment (i.e., topical medication versus debridement) in terms of cure rate and visual improvement, but the topically applied medications are generally more convenient and less traumatic for the patient. However, if one is confronted with toxicity or hypersensitivity to the available agents, or should they prove to be ineffective, debridement offers a satisfactory alternative. Photophobia and ciliary spasm may be severe and cycloplegia often is required for comfort during the first few days of treatment. Scopolamine hydrobromide 0.25 per cent b.i.d. or cyclopentolate hydrochloride 1 to 2 per cent q.i.d. usually is effective. An over-the-counter analgesic preparation may at times be helpful for the relief of pain during the initial phase of treatment. Sunglasses may also give symptomatic relief. An eye pad rarely is necessary in the treatment of dendritic keratitis except after debridement, when a pressure dressing is applied.

Virus strains resistant to idoxuridine and vidarabine are gradually emerging and can be expected to become more common. They may be recognized by a failure to heal over a 7- to 10-day period or by an increase in the size of the ulcer. When this occurs, therapy should be changed to an alternative antiviral agent or debridement should be performed. It is also important to be aware that antiviral agent toxicity may appear within a week of starting therapy[14] and may contribute to the persistence of an ulcer.

The treatment of geographic ulcers presents a somewhat more difficult problem. The patient may be receiving topical corticosteroids or a systemic immunosuppressive agent and may have significant underlying stromal disease. Antiviral agent toxicity or resistance may be present. The approaches described for the management of simple dendritic ulcers are applicable, but debridement should be performed with great care, since it is theoretically possible to inoculate the stroma during this procedure. There is evidence that trifluridine is the most effective of the antiviral antimetabolites for the treatment of geographic herpetic ulcers.[22] In general, these ulcers heal slowly and may undergo a transition to an indolent ulcer before proceeding to complete resolution.[16] Unless this observation is made, a mistaken diagnosis of treatment failure due to a resistant virus can lead to inappropriate therapy.

Stromal Keratitis

Involvement of the corneal stroma ushers in yet another phase in the relationship between herpesvirus and the host. The interaction between virus and host defenses in the cornea is complex and ill understood. Viral replication appears to occur only briefly in the stroma and is not a major factor in the persistent, deeper inflammation. However, it does produce complete virus particles, viral components, and soluble viral antigens within the corneal stroma,[23] and this mass of antigenic matter, along with antigenically altered keratocytes, is the main stimulus to inflammation.[24] This is in marked contrast to disease in the epithelium, where viral replication is the overriding concern.

Stromal keratitis usually occurs in patients who have had previous attacks of epithelial disease, though it may occur as part of the initial attack. It may also follow an episode of disciform keratitis. Interpretation of events in the cornea can be difficult, since acute inflammatory changes and reparative processes may coexist. This is particularly true when an episode has been long-standing. Structural changes from previous attacks, secondary glaucoma, and endothelial dysfunction can obscure the signs of active inflammation. At times the degree of cellular infiltration and edema will indicate that acute infiltrative inflammatory processes predominate, but at other times scarring and neovascularization will be more prominent, indicating that events in the corneal stroma are principally reparative.

Symptoms are nonspecific. Blurred vision is an almost invariable complaint and occurs early unless the lesion is markedly eccentric. Pain is variable, but the eye usually feels uncomfortable and waters. Varying degrees of photophobia and blepharospasm are encountered.

Inflammatory cells, which in the main are neutrophils, are scattered in the stroma, either diffusely or in focal collections. When inflammation is minimal, the stroma has a finely granular appearance and the opacities are stratified due to the configuration of the corneal lamellae. As the inflammation becomes more intense, the granular stratified appearance is lost and the opacities become more confluent (Fig. 16–11). In severe cases a broad, creamy, homogeneous lesion may involve the entire thickness of the cornea, justifying the diagnosis of a corneal abscess (Fig. 16–12). Histologically, such a lesion contains areas in which the corneal lamellae are necrotic. Surrounding this area of intense inflammation, a Wesselytype ring occasionally may be seen. This is a partial or complete ring of infiltrate, usually in the anterior stroma, that surrounds the main lesion and is separated from it by a relatively clear zone of cornea. It is a collection of primarily polymorphonuclear leukocytes in a region of precipitated antigen-antibody complexes.

An important sign of active stromal inflammation is an increase in thickness of the cornea due to the presence of edema fluid. In severe cases this thickening is obvious and the cornea exhibits a ground-glass appearance (Fig. 16–13). The edema commonly encompasses the infiltrate and at times may be the main feature of the disease as well as being an essential component of the stromal inflammatory reaction. It is a result of endothelial dysfunction, presumably secondary to the anterior uveitis that frequently accompanies the stromal keratitis or to the corneal inflammation per se. In mild cases the stromal thickening may not be obvious, but it can be detected by comparing the area of suspected inflammation with adjacent healthy cornea. Fine folds in Descemet's membrane invariably are present and also are indicative of active inflammation.

In a cornea that has not been subjected to previous inflammation scarring may not be present, or at least it may not be evident during the acute phase of the disease. The presence of scarring becomes more apparent with prolongation of the process, particularly as acute inflammatory events subside (Fig. 16–14). At times differentiation between edema and scar or between an infiltrate and a scar can be difficult. Nonetheless, biomicroscopic differentiation is the key to successful management of a stromal herpetic keratitis. Edema and infiltration are potentially reversible with appropriate therapy, and transparency may be restored. Scarring is unresponsive to medical therapy, and once significant stromal scarring has occurred, the clarity of the cornea is permanently impaired.

Neovascularization can occur at any stage of the disease (Fig. 16–15). Vessels enter the cornea from the limbus at all levels and progress toward a site of active inflammation. During the active stage the vessels are dilated and are cuffed by a fine granular infiltrate, but as the inflammation subsides this infiltrate disappears and the vessels may become bloodless. However, the new vessels are a permanent structural change. The first signs of reactivation of inflammation may be dilatation of these vessels along with the reappearance of blood within their lumen and a surrounding infiltrate.

An inevitable consequence of stromal keratitis is loss of corneal substance. This may not be apparent while the inflammation is active, but as edema and infiltration resolve, thinning occurs and is a predictable outcome of the inflammatory episode. Thus, an important sign of previous inflammation is the presence of focal areas of decreased corneal thickness. Such areas are known as facets. If the inflammation is sufficiently intense, the cornea may become extremely thin; a descemetocele (Fig. 16–16) may result and perforation can occur.

Examination of the corneal epithelium is an important part of the evaluation of stromal keratitis. If the epithelium is intact, the portion overlying the active stromal lesion often is edematous. This can be related both to the underlying inflammatory disease and to endothelial

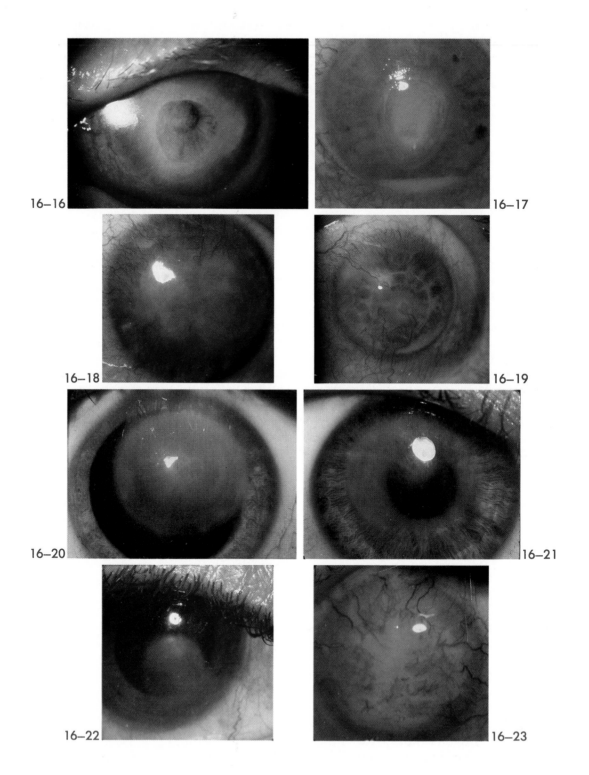

16–16

16–17

16–18

16–19

16–20

16–21

16–22

16–23

dysfunction. At times bullae occur and may secondarily break down, forming ulcers. Dendritic or geographic ulceration may coexist with stromal inflammation, or even make its first appearance subsequent to an attack of stromal keratitis.

The endothelium usually is involved in all but the most superficial lesions. Fine, white keratic precipitates may be diffusely scattered over the posterior surface of the cornea, and it is not uncommon to see large endothelial plaques develop in an area of acute stromal inflammation; secondary cornea guttata are quite common but usually disappear when the inflammation subsides. An anterior chamber reaction invariably occurs but may be difficult to evaluate in the presence of significant stromal opacification. In severe cases a hypopyon may be present (Fig. 16–17), and posterior synechiae and rubeosis occur quite commonly. The intraocular pressure may be elevated as a result of a trabeculitis.

Recurrent stromal keratitis with superimposition of acute inflammatory signs on chronic, structural changes results in a highly variable appearance on slit-lamp examination. Unless the acute changes can be separated from those due primarily to inactive disease, a successful therapeutic approach cannot be formulated. The diagnosis of herpetic stromal keratitis is presumptive and is based on the clinical information available. Only when a penetrating keratoplasty provides tissue for electron microscopy can confirmatory evidence be obtained.

It is important to be continually aware of the chronic and recurrent nature of herpetic stromal disease. Each attack inevitably causes some loss of vision, and the adverse effects of each recurrence tend to be cumulative (Fig. 16–18). The aim of therapy, therefore, is to terminate or at least suppress each episode as expeditiously as possible in order to minimize structural damage and reduce morbidity while simultaneously seeking to avoid the side effects of treatment.

Active herpetic stromal keratitis is responsive to anti-inflammatory therapy with locally administered corticosteroid preparations, and this approach is now generally advocated.[25] However, there remains a group opposed to this form of treatment.[26] Their concern is based on the apparent enhancement of viral replication by these agents, probably through suppression of local immune

---

Figure 16–16. Large central descemetocele in an area of previous stromal keratitis due to herpes.

Figure 16–17. Central herpetic stromal keratitis with hypopyon. (Courtesy of Howard M. Leibowitz, M.D.)

Figure 16–18. Residua of recurrent attacks of herpetic stromal keratitis—severe scarring, edema, and neovascularization. (Courtesy of Howard M. Leibowitz, M.D.)

Figure 16–19. Repair of a deep herpetic ulcer, presenting as bulging descemetocele with impending perforation, by lamellar keratoplasty. (Courtesy of Howard M. Leibowitz, M.D.)

Figure 16–20. Disciform keratitis. Large white keratic precipitates can be seen around the periphery of the lesion.

Figure 16–21. The same patient as in Figure 16–20 after an intensive course of topical corticosteroid. The corneal edema has resolved, leaving some central corneal scarring.

Figure 16–22. Stromal scarring resulting from repeated attacks of disciform keratitis. (Courtesy of Howard M. Leibowitz, M.D.)

Figure 16–23. Irreversible corneal changes wrought by recurrent attacks of herpes simplex keratitis—scarring, edema, and neovascularization.

defenses.[27] However, all available evidence suggests that viral replication has ceased by the time stromal inflammation has appeared and that it is an immunologic response to the deposit of viral antigens within the cornea that is responsible for stromal keratitis.[23, 24] An antiviral agent is administered concurrently with the corticosteroid in order to minimize the risk of enhancing the replication of latent virus that spontaneously reactivates in the vicinity of the eye.

In mild or transient episodes of stromal keratitis, corticosteroid therapy can sometimes be withheld with the expectation that inflammation will resolve spontaneously. Too frequently, however, without treatment the keratouveitis worsens, causing structural damage and visual loss. The therapeutic principle is to produce a clearly recognizable, progressive reduction in inflammation while minimizing the risk of enhancement of viral replication. Opinions differ concerning the way corticosteroids should be used. One method is to administer a high dose of the drug initially in order to inactivate the inflammation as rapidly as possible and then to progressively decrease the dose.[25] A second approach calls for the use of a much lower dose initially and gradually increasing the quantitiy of drug administered as required, seeking to find the minimal amount necessary to control the disease.

The response to corticosteroid varies greatly from patient to patient, making it impossible to provide more than a general indication of the dose that may be appropriate. If an insufficient dosage of corticosteroid is used, there is a real danger that the period of treatment may be unduly prolonged. The patient then is exposed to increased risk, and the goal of treatment—to minimize permanent structural change—is not realized. On the other hand, extremely high doses of corticosteroids carry a greater risk of enhancing the replication of active virus and of producing secondary glaucoma and cataract. The potential risks and benefits must be weighed for each use individually and the optimal regimen selected on the basis of clinical findings.

The selection of the appropriate corticosteroid preparation has been outlined in Chapter 13. In my experience prednisolone acetate 1.0 per cent suspension (Econopred Plus or Pred Forte) is the agent of choice. Systemic corticosteroids should not be used, and periocularly injected corticosteroids rarely, if ever, are indicated. For treatment of a moderately severe stromal keratitis, prednisolone acetate 1.0 per cent drops, given at least four times a day, would probably be needed to produce an anti-inflammatory effect. A more severe keratitis might require topical application of the corticosteroid as often as every hour. An antiviral agent should be given concurrently. While there is little to choose among the three currently available antiviral agents in terms of efficacy in this situation, the potential need for long-term therapy raises the specter of drug toxicity. For this reason I prefer to use the least toxic of the available antivirals, trifluridine. A cycloplegic may be needed for comfort and to prevent the formation of posterior synechiae if the accompanying uveitis is at all significant.

The patient must be seen frequently during the early stages to monitor the response to therapy. If the keratitis is sufficiently severe to require the hourly application of a corticosteroid, then the patient must initially be evaluated at 24-hour intervals to ensure that the clinical course is proceeding satisfactorily. As the inflammatory keratitis begins to improve, the dose of corticosteroid is gradually reduced and the interval between follow-up examinations is lengthened. When the inflammatory keratitis has resolved but the patient is still using the corticosteroid, it is important to continue to reduce the dose slowly before finally discontinuing the medication. Abrupt cessation may result in reactivation of the keratitis due to the inflammatory rebound phenomenon,[25] and it may rapidly progress to stromal ulceration and even perforation. Reduction of corticosteroid dosage with ultimate termination of its use may require several months.

Some patients will need long-term administration of corticosteroid in low dosage. To administer a lower dose, the corticosteroid can be administered less often and/or a more dilute preparation can be used (e.g., prednisolone acetate 0.125 per cent [Econopred, Pred Mild]). It may be advantageous in this instance to use an alternative corticosteroid base such as fluorometholone (FML), which is less likely to elevate the intraocular pressure. A careful watch must be kept for signs of toxicity to the concomitantly administered antiviral agent, particularly because these signs can be partially suppressed by the administration of the corticosteroid. The development of toxicity requires a change of antiviral therapy.

Manipulating the dose of corticosteroid in response to the degree of inflammation is successful in many patients and often results in a remarkable improvement in visual acuity as the inflammation subsides. However, in some instances, particularly when there have been numerous recurrences with permanent damage to the cornea and related structures, the outlook is less satisfactory. In such patients the course can become more protracted. Neovascularization and stromal necrosis may develop, recurrences may become excessively frequent and debilitating, and vision may be markedly reduced. Keratoplasty, appropriately timed, can have a dramatic effect on the course of the disease, restoring vision and reducing morbidity. Nonetheless, it should be emphasized that the decision to employ surgery for an active keratitis is a serious one, and the uncertain prognosis must be balanced against the degree of disability and disease present.

Complications of Stromal Keratitis

The course of stromal keratitis in any patient is unpredictable. Although it is true that management has been improved by a better understanding of the pathogenic mechanisms and by the intelligent use of corticosteroids and antiviral agents, there are still many patients in whom this disease remains difficult to control. It is of some value, therefore, to examine the untoward events that interfere with successful treatment in these patients.

Herpetic Epithelial Keratitis. The recurrence of a dendritic or an ameboid ulceration in a patient with active stromal keratitis who is being treated with corticosteroid is a disastrous event. It means that the antiviral agent administered concurrently with the corticosteroid to suppress viral replication in the epithelium is ineffective. Unless the epithelial disease can be arrested, stromal inflammation cannot be effectively treated. Stromal ulceration will almost certainly develop and ultimately the eye may be lost. Fortunately, with three topical antiviral agents now available, alternative therapy can be substituted. In the event that the virus appears resistant to all agents, careful debridement should be performed. At the same time it is essential that the dosage of corticosteroid be reduced until the epithelial disease is brought under control. While the corticosteroid is being reduced, the patient must be watched very carefully for signs of a rebound in inflammation. Inevitably some intensification in stromal inflammation can be anticipated, but if stromal ulceration does not develop, corticosteroid therapy can be delayed until the epithelial disease has resolved. However, should stromal inflammation progress to active ulceration, particularly if perforation appears imminent, corticosteroid therapy should be reinstituted despite active epithelial disease. A lamellar patch graft can be considered as a temporizing measure at this stage (Fig. 16–19), but penetrating keratoplasty should be avoided if at all possible. Effective treatment of this complication is facilitated by its prompt recognition during the early stages; whenever an epithelial defect develops during the course of an active stromal keratitis, the possibility of intercurrent epithelial disease should be considered in the differential diagnosis.

Indolent Ulceration. By definition, indolent ulcers are difficult to heal. Clinically it may be difficult, if not impossible, to decide whether or not the margins of the ulcer contain active replicating virus. To confuse the matter further, ulcers are encountered in which a portion of the epithelial margin appears to be of ameboid or geographic configuration (i.e., contains virus), while another portion appears to be indolent in type (i.e., contains no virus). When a diagnosis of indolent ulcer is made, it is important to decide what has precipitated the arrest of epithelial regeneration. If toxicity to the antiviral agent in the therapeutic regimen is thought to be a significant etiologic factor, then use of an alternative antiviral drug may be followed by epithelial regrowth. It must be realized that signs of toxicity may persist for weeks after the drug is discontinued, so that dramatic resolution may not occur immediately.[14] If it appears that the underlying stromal inflammation is contributing to the epithelial disease, then the correct approach is not to discontinue corticosteroid administration but, rather, to increase the dose under an umbrella of the antiviral agent. The use of patching or a therapeutic hydrophilic contact lens, combined with tear supplements, may be necessary in selected patients.[28] If all else fails, a tarsorrhaphy can be of benefit, and on occasion excisional keratoplasty may be required.

Stromal Ulceration. When infiltration of the corneal stroma is intense, it is not unusual for the epithelium to break down. At times a superficial ulcer will develop in the stroma and will subsequently erode rapidly into the deeper layers of the cornea. A descemetocele may develop and ultimately the cornea may perforate. Development of this complication is an indication for hospitalization, and in the differential diagnosis the presence of a secondary infection, of either bacterial or fungal origin, must be considered. Since the patient is usually on corticosteroid therapy, the severity of the inflammation may be masked, but any rapid increase in inflammatory signs in the cornea or anterior chamber should suggest the possibility of secondary infection. Material scraped from the ulcer margins and from its base should be cultured for bacteria and fungi, and Gram- and Giemsa-stained smears should be examined. If an infectious agent is isolated, it should be treated with appropriate specific therapy. A noninfectious ulcer should be treated by the administration of corticosteroid in increased dosage, combined with trifluridine, while the patient is maintained under careful supervision. Keratoplasty is indicated in those ulcers which worsen despite treatment, especially if perforation seems imminent. Once a cornea has perforated, the most effective management is keratoplasty, performed as expeditiously as possible to avoid complications of anterior synechiae formation. A soft contact lens or cyanoacrylate adhesives may be useful in maintaining the chamber until such surgery can be performed.

Secondary Glaucoma. It is not uncommon for the intraocular pressure to rise in the presence of a protracted stromal keratitis accompanied by an anterior uveitis. Presumably this results from an associated trabeculitis. Unless intraocular pressure is checked at each visit, this complication can be overlooked, with serious adverse effects on vision. Accurate measurement of the pressure level may be difficult or impossible unless one has access to an electronic tonometer or a pneumotonometer. If there is a doubt about the level of intraocular pressure, prophylactic therapy with an epinephrine formulation, a topical beta blocker, and/or a systemically administered carbonic anhydrase inhibitor must be considered. The possibility should always be borne in mind that the intraocular pressure elevation may have been caused by corticosteroid administration in a steroid-responsive individual. Reduction in dosage or substitution of fluorometholone for prednisolone acetate is justified when this possibility appears likely.

Secondary Cataract. Secondary cataract, from the combined effect of the disease and steroid administration, can at times complicate the management of these patients. The approach must always be conservative, although surgery may be indicated if the lens becomes intumescent. A combined keratoplasty with lens extraction ultimately may be required for visual restoration.

Disciform Keratitis

In some patients the recurrence of stromal disease will present in a rather typical form. A disc of stromal edema develops, usually in the central cornea but sometimes eccentrically, combined with signs of moderate anterior chamber inflammation and epithelial edema (Fig. 16–20). Vision is invariably reduced, and this condition is associated with usually mild but occasionally severe orbital pain, tearing, and photophobia. There may or may not be a history of dendritic or other form of epithelial ulceration, but an active epithelial herpes infection can appear subsequently.

The diagnosis of this lesion is purely clinical, and few histopathologic specimens are available. In contrast to the variable appearance of other forms of stromal herpetic keratitis, this lesion is remarkably uniform. Slit-lamp examination reveals a circumscribed area of corneal thickening, largely reflecting the presence of stromal edema. A fine granular infiltrate may be seen scattered throughout the disk of stromal edema, but typically there is a noticeable absence of leukocytic infiltration. Usually the overlying epithelium is intact but is characterized by the presence of microcystic edema. There are folds in Descemet's membrane, and the endothelium in the disciform area may be covered with keratic precipitates. Even with a history of ocular herpes, the diagnosis often is not conclusive. Herpes simplex is the most common presumed cause of disciform keratitis, but the differential diagnosis includes varicella-zoster, vaccinia, and mumps infections. Chemical agents that penetrate the cornea and damage the endothelium directly can also cause this type of corneal lesion.

Disciform keratitis usually responds well to the topical administration of corticosteroids (Fig. 16–21), and the therapeutic principles outlined above for the treatment of stromal keratitis apply here. The amount of corticosteroid required usually is less than that needed to treat other types of herpetic stromal keratitis. Similar complications must be anticipated. Vision usually is markedly affected by disciform keratitis, but necrosis of stromal lamellae seems to be an exception. In most instances recovery of normal or near normal levels of vision can be anticipated. Keratoplasty is never indicated in the acute stage and is rarely required unless repeated attacks take a cumulative toll on corneal clarity (Fig. 16–22).

Rates of Recurrence

Published studies indicate that recurrence of herpes simplex keratitis is common despite therapy.[29-31] Among patients whose first attack of dendritic keratitis was treated with idoxuridine, 26 per cent had a recurrence within the following 24 months, whereas 43 per cent of patients in whom a second or subsequent attack was treated with idoxuridine developed a further recurrence in the ensuing 24 months.[29] Among patients who took part in various clinical trials at Moorfields Eye Hospital, treatment with idoxuridine, trifluorothymidine, carbolization, photoinactivation, and placebo did not result in significantly different recurrence rates of herpetic keratitis. Fifty per cent of all patients had recurrences within 2 years. Follow-up data on these patients over a 9-year period showed a 45 per cent recurrence rate among those whose initial episode of herpetic corneal disease had been treated and an 85 per cent recurrence rate among those in whom a second or subsequent episode of herpetic corneal disease had been treated.[30, 31] The use of topical corticosteroids does not appear to increase or otherwise influence the recurrence rate of herpetic keratitis.[29]

Each recurrence of herpes simplex keratitis can produce irreversible alterations of the cornea that exact their toll on vision. Scarring, edema, and neovascularization interfere with corneal transparency, and surface changes produce irregular astigmatism (Fig. 16–23). Treatment of this disease must be aggressive, having as its goal the elimination of replicating virus and the suppression of corneal inflammation. Because herpes simplex keratitis is extremely variable and is characterized by an unpredictable course and frequent recurrences, the status of the eye must be assessed often if optimal therapy is to be maintained.

ADDENDUM

Since this chapter was written, Shimeld and associates,[32] using organ culture techniques, have reported the isolation of herpes simplex virus from two of three corneal disks of patients with chronic stromal keratitis. This finding has now been extended to five of seven corneas.[33] Although there is considerable electron microscopic and immunologic evidence that viral replication does occur in the corneal stroma, this is the first time that live virus has been demonstrated. Whether this represents truly latent virus or a proliferation of residual virus particles is still uncertain at this stage. The therapeutic implications of this finding await further study.

REFERENCES

1. Buddingh, H., Schrum, D. I., Lanier, J. C., and Guidry, D. J.: Studies of the natural history of herpes simplex infections. Pediatrics 11:595, 1953.
2. Stevens, J. G., and Cook, M.: Latent herpes simplex virus in spinal ganglia in mice. Science 173:843, 1971.
3. Nesburn, A. B., Cook M. L., and Stevens, J.: Isolation of herpes simplex virus from rabbit trigeminal ganglia between episodes of recurrent ocular infection. Arch Ophthalmol 88:412, 1972.
4. Stevens, J. G., Nesburn, A. B., and Cook, M.: Latent herpes simplex virus recovered from trigeminal ganglia of rabbits with recurrent eye infection. Nature 235:216, 1972.
5. Baringer, J., and Swoveland, P.: Recovery of herpes simplex virus from human trigeminal ganglia. N Engl J Med 288:648, 1973.
6. Bastian, F. O., Rabson, A. S., Yee, C. L., and Tralka, T. S.: Herpesvirus hominis: Isolation from human trigeminal ganglion. Science 178:306, 1972.
7. Scriba, M.: Herpes simplex virus infection in guinea pigs: An animal model for studying latent and recurrent herpes simplex virus infection. Infect Immunol 12:162, 1975.
8. Goodpasture, E. W.: Herpetic infection with special reference to involvement of the nervous system. Medicine 8:223, 1929.
9. Roizman, B.: An inquiry into the mechanism of recurrent herpes infections in man. In Pollard, M. (ed.): Perspectives in Virology. New York, Harper & Row, 1965.
10. Fenner, F.: The Biology of Animal Viruses. New York, Academic Press, 1968.
11. Cleobury, J. F., Skinner, G. R. B., Thouless, M. E., and Wildy, P.: Association between psychopathic disorder and serum antibody to herpes simplex virus (type 1). Brit Med J 1:438, 1971.
12. Sheward J. D.: Perianal herpes simplex. Lancet 1:315, 1961.
13. Jones, B. R.: The management of ocular herpes. Trans Ophthalmol Soc UK 79:245, 1959.
14. O'Day, D. M., and Jones, B. R.: Herpes simplex keratitis. In Duane, T. D. (ed.): Clinical Ophthalmology. Vol. 4. Hagerstown, Md., Harper & Row, 1978.
15. Cook, M. L., and Stevens, J. G.: Pathogenesis of herpetic neuritis and ganglionitis in mice: Evidence of intraaxonal transport of infection. Infect Immunol 7:272, 1972.
16. O'Day, D., Poirier, R. H., Jones, D. B., and Elliott, J. H.: Vidarabine therapy of complicated herpes simplex keratitis. Amer J Ophthalmol 81:642, 1976.
17. Laibson, P. R., and Krachmer, J. H.: Controlled comparison of adenine arabinoside and idoxuridine therapy of human superficial dendritic keratitis. In Pavan-Langston, D., Buchanan, R. A., and Alford, C. A., Jr. (eds.): Adenine Arabinoside: An Antiviral Agent. New York, Raven Press, 1975.
18. Pavan-Langston, D., and Dohlman, C. H.: A double blind clinical study of adenine arabinoside therapy of viral keratoconjunctivitis. Amer J Ophthalmol 74:81, 1972.
19. Coster, D. J., McKinnon, J. R., McGill, J. I., Jones, B. R., and Fraunfelder, F. T.: Clinical evaluation of adenine arabinoside and trifluorothymidine in the treatment of corneal ulcers caused by herpes simplex virus. J Infect Dis 133(Suppl):A173, 1976.
20. Van Bijsterveld, O. P., and Post, H.: Trifluorothy-

midine versus adenine arabinoside in the treatment of herpes simplex keratitis. Brit J Ophthalmol 64:33, 1980.

21. Coster, D. J., Jones, B. R., and Falcon, M. G.: Role of debridement in the treatment of herpetic keratitus. Trans Ophthalmol Soc UK 97:314, 1977.

22. Coster, D. J., Jones, B. R., and McGill, J. I.: Treatment of amoeboid herpetic ulcers with adenine arabinoside or trifluorothymidine. Brit J Ophthalmol 63:418, 1979.

23. Dawson, C., Togni, B., and Moore, T. E., Jr.: Structural changes in chronic herpetic keratitis. Arch Ophthalmol 79:740, 1968.

24. Meyers, R. L., Chitjian, P. A., and Fiorello, P.: Studies on immunopathogenesis of chronic and recurrent herpes simplex virus keratitis. XXIII International Congress of Ophthalmology. Excerpta Medica, Oxford International Congress, Series 442, 1978, p. 159.

25. Aronson, S. B., and Moore, T. E., Jr.: Corticosteroid therapy in central stromal keratitis. Amer J Ophthalmol 67:683, 1969.

26. Thygeson, P.: Historical observations on herpetic keratitis. Surv Ophthalmol 27:82, 1976.

27. Cooper, J. A., Jr., Daniels, C. A., and Trofatter, K.

F., Jr.: The effect of prednisolone on antibody-dependent cell-mediated cytotoxicity and the growth of type I herpes simplex virus in human cells. Invest Ophthalmol Vis Sci 17:381, 1978.

28. Leibowitz, H. M., and Rosenthal, P. R.: Hydrophilic contact lenses in corneal disease. I. Superficial, sterile indolent ulcers. Arch Ophthalmol 85:163, 1971.

29. Carroll, J. M., Martola, E. L., Laibson, P. R., and Dohlman, C. H.: The recurrence of herpetic keratitis following idoxuridine therapy. Amer J Ophthalmol 63:103, 1967.

30. McGill, J., Williams, H. P., McKinnon, J. R., Holt-Wilson, A. B., and Jones, B. R.: Reassessment of idoxuridine therapy of herpetic keratitis. Trans Ophthalmol Soc UK 94:542, 1974.

31. McGill, J., Fraunfelder, F. T., and Jones, B. R.: Current and proposed management of ocular herpes simplex. Surv Ophthalmol 20:358, 1976.

32. Shimeld, C., Tullo, A. B., Easty, D. L., and Thomsitt, J.: Isolation of herpes simplex virus from the cornea in chronic stromal keratitis. Brit J Ophthalmol 66:643, 1982.

33. Easty, D. L.: Personal communication.

17 Herpes Zoster Ophthalmicus

IRVING RABER, M.D.
PETER LAIBSON, M.D.

Hutchinson[1] first described a case of herpes zoster ophthalmicus in 1865. Since then numerous reports have appeared documenting the viral etiology and varied clinical manifestations of this disease complex. The disease is not yet completely understood and presents numerous problems that tax both the tolerance of the patient and the therapeutic modalities of the physician.

The virus responsible for herpes zoster is the same organism that causes varicella (chickenpox) and is referred to as the varicella-zoster virus. It consists of a DNA core embedded in a protein capsid and surrounded by a lipid envelope. This virus is morphologically identical to the herpes simplex virus but differs from it antigenically, in its culture characteristics, and in its clinical behavior.

Virus particles have been demonstrated in the trigeminal ganglion and frontal nerve, and degenerative changes have been identified in the trigeminal ganglion and in axons of the frontal and ophthalmic nerves in herpes zoster ophthalmicus.[2] Most cases of this disorder seemingly result from reactivation of latent virus in the trigeminal ganglion. The responsible organisms apparently are the residua of a previous chickenpox infection.[3] Though infectivity is low, exogenous viruses also seem able to reinfect susceptible individuals and cause disease following direct or indirect contact with a patient suffering either from chickenpox or herpes zoster.[4–6] Zoster may develop in adults after exposure to chickenpox and, conversely, varicella in children may follow exposure to zoster. The incubation period for reinfection cases ranges from 5 to 14 days.[5, 6] A droplet mode of transmission usually occurs, but rare cases have been reported that implicate contact with infected (varicella or zoster) skin surfaces.

The disease usually increases in frequency and severity with advancing age. There is a gradual disappearance of detectable antibody to the varicella-zoster virus after the age of 50,[7] suggesting a failure of the immune mechanism of the host to keep latent virus in check. Presumably this accounts for the greater prevalence of the disease among older individuals. Cases also are attributed to an inadequate immune response to the chickenpox virus following initial exposure. In any event, whether one invokes a reactivation mechanism or exogenous infection, cases often involve immunologically compromised individuals. Herpes zoster may be especially severe and may become generalized in patients with a malignant disease, particularly lymphoma, and in others whose immune mechanisms are defective.[8-12] However, the appearance of zoster should not be interpreted as definitive evidence of the presence of hidden malignant disease. In 800 patients with herpes zoster Juel-Jensen did not find a higher incidence of malignancy than in the population at large.[3] Similarly, Ragozzino and coworkers[13] examined 590 patients with herpes zoster who had been followed for many years and detected no increased incidence of malignant disease.

Among the various forms of this disease only thoracic zoster exceeds ophthalmic zoster in prevalence. The ophthalmic form comprises about 7 per cent of all cases of herpes zoster.[4] The supraorbital and supratrochlear branches of the frontal nerve, which supply the upper lid and forehead, are most frequently involved. The lacrimal and nasociliary branches of the ophthalmic nerve may also be involved, either simultaneously or later, and there may be an associated involvement of the maxillary branch of the trigeminal nerve. Actual involvement of the globe occurs in about 50 per cent of cases.[4] The nasociliary branch of the ophthalmic nerve provides the sensory nerve supply to the cornea, ciliary body, iris, and conjunctiva. Its terminal branch is the anterior ethmoidal nerve, which innervates the tip of the nose via the external nasal nerve. This is the anatomic explanation for Hutchinson's rule, which states that the occurrence of zoster lesions at the tip of the nose signals the presence of ocular inflammation (Fig. 17–1). Conversely, the eye is less

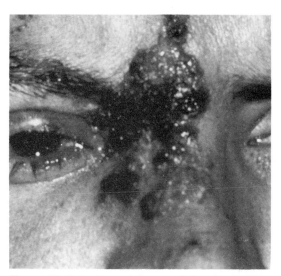

Figure 17–2. Lesions at the medial aspect of the lower lid without involvement of the maxillary nerve. This reflects involvement of the infratrochlear branch of the nasociliary nerve, which supplies the medial aspect of the lower lid and conjunctiva.

often involved when the nose is spared. Obviously there is no hard and fast relationship, and the physician must look carefully for ocular involvement whenever a zoster lesion involves any portion of the skin innervated by the first division of the fifth cranial nerve.

Another anatomic correlation worth noting is that involvement of the lower eyelid does not necessarily mean that the maxillary nerve and its infraorbital branch are involved. The infratrochlear branch of the nasociliary nerve supplies the medial aspect of the lower lid and conjunctiva. Thus, involvement of the nasociliary nerve alone can cause vesicles to erupt along the medial aspect of the lower lid margin (Fig. 17–2).

CLINICAL FEATURES

Initially the patient usually experiences the sudden onset of systemic symptoms common to most viral infections: headache, malaise, fever, and chills. This is followed in a day or two by neuralgic pain in the area of the involved dermatome. Within a few days of the onset of pain the skin becomes erythematous and hyperesthetic, and edema and the erup-

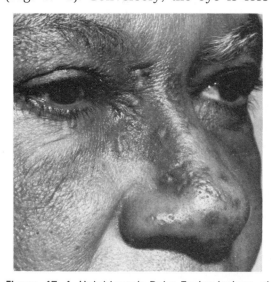

Figure 17–1. Hutchinson's Rule: Zoster lesions at the tip of the nose signal the likely presence of ocular inflammation. This reflects involvement of the nasociliary branch of the ophthalmic nerve (which innervates the cornea, ciliary body, iris, and conjunctiva) and of its terminal branch, the anterior ethmoidal nerve, which innervates the tip of the nose via the external nasal nerve.

tion of vesicles follow shortly thereafter (Fig. 17–3). The vesicles first are filled with clear fluid (from which virus can be cultured for 2 to 3 days) (Fig. 17–4), but the contents of the vesicles rapidly become turbid and yellow. The rash is almost always unilateral, rarely extends across the midline, and is usually accompanied by regional (preauricular and/or submandibular) adenopathy. Unless secondary infection intervenes, the acute inflammation subsides in 1 to 3 weeks. Although the vesicles become crusted (Fig. 17–4), the skin ulcers, which can extend deeply into the dermis (Fig. 17–5), may take weeks to heal and leave deep, pitted, permanent scars over the dermatome. In herpes zoster ophthalmicus the scarring of the eyelid (Fig. 17–6) may be sufficiently severe to cause lid retraction or ptosis, ectropion, loss of tissue, and sloughing of lashes.

OCULAR INVOLVEMENT

The ocular findings may be quite varied but can be grouped into three broad

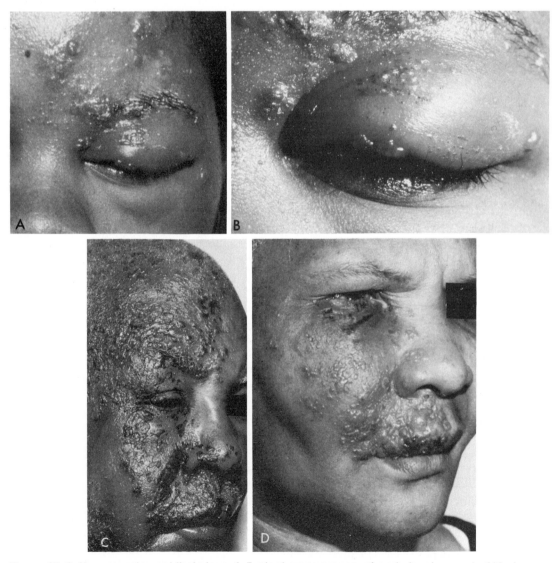

Figure 17–3. Herpes zoster ophthalmicus. *A,* Typical appearance of early involvement of V_1 dermatome. *B,* Closeup of lids. *C,* Involvement of V_1 and V_2. *D,* Involvement of V_2 only with accompanying conjunctivitis.

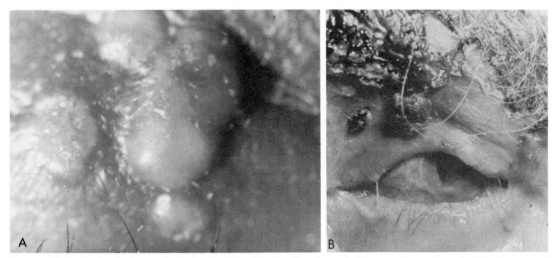

Figure 17–4. Zoster lesions. *A,* Early vesicles filled with clear fluid may be cultured. *B,* Subsequent crusting of the vesicles. (Courtesy of Howard M. Leibowitz, M.D.)

Figure 17–5. Zoster involvement of the dermis that will leave deep, permanent scars. (Courtesy of Howard M. Leibowitz, M.D.)

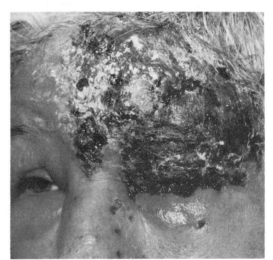

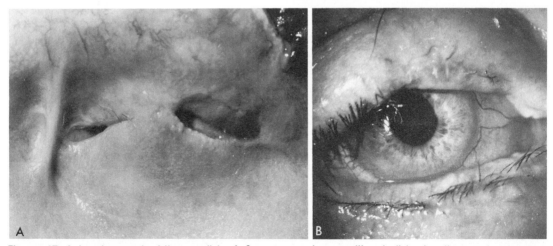

Figure 17–6. Involvement of the eyelids. *A,* Severe scarring resulting in lid retraction and ectropion. A temporary tarsorrhaphy of the skin and muscle layers, shown here, was required to protect the cornea until definitive reconstructive surgery could be performed. *B,* Chronic thickening of the lid with deformation of the lid margin. (Courtesy of Howard M. Leibowitz, M.D.)

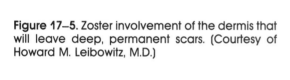

categories: those associated with inflammatory changes, those resulting from nerve damage, and those occurring secondary to tissue scarring.[14] Inflammatory changes may be direct or indirect; the direct changes include punctate keratitis, superficial stromal opacities, and disciform and mucous-plaque keratitis, and the indirect changes are the result of a vasculitis that can present an episcleritis and scleritis, iritis, papillitis, and proptosis of the globe with total third nerve palsy. Neuroparalytic keratitis, paralysis of the extraocular muscles, and postherpetic neuralgia are complications associated with nerve damage. Chronic tissue scarring (Fig. 17–7) generally is most evident in the lids, in the surrounding skin, and in the conjunctiva; it gives rise to postherpetic neuralgia, exposure keratitis, deformity of the lid margin, trichiasis, and tear film abnormalities.

The ocular complications also may be considered as occurring in three phases: acute, chronic, and relapsing.[14] Acute changes usually occur 2 to 3 days after the onset of the rash and include ocular lesions associated with inflammatory changes, extraocular muscle palsies, and some cases of neuroparalytic keratitis. Those components of ocular involvement attributed to vasculitis tend to be-

come chronic, giving rise to ischemic atrophy and a keratitis manifested by dense cellular infiltrates and lipid deposition. Finally, ocular complications have a tendency to relapse, even years after the initial rash. The stimulus responsible for the relapse generally is unknown, but the sudden withdrawal of topically administered corticosteroid is a documented cause.

Conjunctivitis

During the acute stages of the skin rash conjunctival involvement is common. Follicular or catarrhal conjunctivitis with regional adenopathy is usually seen. Petechiae may be scattered throughout the inflamed palpebral conjunctiva. In the most severe cases an inflammatory pseudomembrane or even necrotizing membranous inflammation may be observed. Vesicular lesions of the conjunctiva are rare. The conjunctivitis usually is self-limited, and unless the inflamed mucous membrane becomes secondarily infected, it tends to resolve simultaneously with the skin eruption.

Episcleritis and Scleritis

A simple episcleritis may develop at the same time as the vesicular skin eruption, and, though painful, it usually disappears without residua as the skin con-

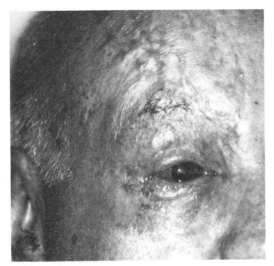

Figure 17–7. Chronic scarring of the lids and surrounding skin following an attack of herpes zoster ophthalmicus.

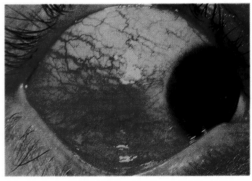

Figure 17–8. Scleritis associated with herpes zoster ophthalmicus.

dition subsides. In the acute stages there may be a coincident nodular scleritis (Fig. 17–8), which resolves with the episcleritis. However, in some cases a deep, localized nodular scleritis develops 2 to 3 months after the acute disease has cleared. This nodule is very resistant to treatment and may take months to resolve, frequently leaving an area of scleral thinning or even a staphyloma. Recurrences at the same site are not infrequent.[15]

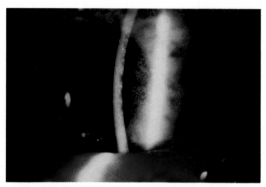

Figure 17–9. Early zoster keratitis characterized by coarse punctate intraepithelial lesions.

Keratitis

The cornea frequently is involved during the course of herpes zoster ophthalmicus, and keratitis represents one of the most serious manifestations of the disorder. All layers of the cornea may be affected as part of acute, chronic, or relapsing forms of the disease.[16]

The earliest corneal changes consist of a coarse punctate epithelial keratitis characterized by multiple fine, raised, intraepithelial lesions usually located near the limbus (Fig. 17–9).[17] At times this is accompanied by mild stromal edema and the cornea may have a ground-glass appearance. The epithelial abnormalities may assume a dendritic configuration similar to herpes simplex keratitis (Table 17–1);[18, 19] this has been described as medusa-like figures,[18] microdendrites,[16, 20] or stellate-shaped lesions (Fig. 17–10).[20] Characteristically, multiple small, fine, slightly raised lesions are encountered in the peripheral cornea. These stain well with rose bengal but only sparingly with fluorescein. The stellate or microdendritic lesions are transient, appearing within a few days of the onset of the skin rash and resolving 4 to 6 days later. Zoster virus can be isolated from these lesions,[18] but the time that the cultures are obtained appears to be critical. It is known that virus can be recovered from the early cutaneous lesions of zoster but generally during the first 72 hours only. Recovery of the virus from corneal microdendrites seems subject to the same limitation; documented positive cultures were

Table 17–1. DIFFERENCES BETWEEN HERPES SIMPLEX AND HERPES ZOSTER EPITHELIAL KERATITIS*

Herpes Simplex	Herpes Zoster (Acute)	Herpes Zoster (Delayed)
Fine, lacy, dendritic epithelial ulcerations with terminal end bulbs	Multiple, small, raised stellate areas of epithelial keratitis; usually peripheral (microdendrites)	Coarse, elevated gray-white, mucous plaques (macrodendrites)
Edges stain with rose bengal; ulcer base stains with fluorescein	Stain with rose bengal better than with fluorescein	Stain with rose bengal and alcian blue; only sparingly with fluorescein
Steroid enhancement	No apparent steroid effect	No apparent steroid effect
Normal tear film	Mucoid discharge	Unstable tear film
Removed by scraping epithelium	Removed by scraping epithelium	Removed without damage to underlying epithelium
Current or past history of cold sores	Typical zoster skin vesicles	Typical zoster scarring of the skin
Herpes simplex readily isolated from edge of ulcer	Herpes zoster may be isolated from the lesion	No virus isolated

*Modified from Marsh, R. J., Fraunfelder, F. T., and McGill, J. I.: Herpetic corneal epithelial disease. Arch Ophthalmol 94:1899, 1976.

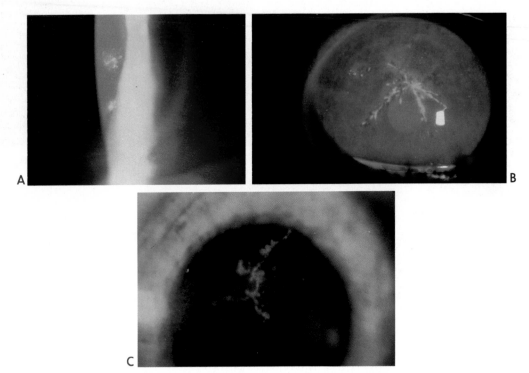

Figure 17–10. Dendritic lesions in herpes zoster keratitis. *A,* Microdendrites. *B,* Medusa-like dendrite. *C,* Branching, dendritic mucous plaque.

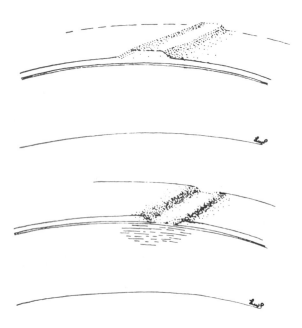

Figure 17–11. Diagrammatic representation of the epithelial characteristics of the dendritic lesions of herpes zoster (above) and herpes simplex (below). (From Piebenga, L. W., and Laibson, P. R.: Dendritic lesion in herpes zoster ophthalmicus. Arch Ophthalmol *90*:268, 1973. Copyright 1973, American Medical Association.)

taken within 48 hours of the zoster prodromata, whereas cultures taken later all have been negative. Since the corneal lesions seemingly yield a low titer of virus, culture tubes must be held for at least 4 weeks to avoid missing a slowly developing positive inoculation.[18]

Microdendrites appear early in the course of the disease; that is, they coincide with the onset of the rash or become evident shortly thereafter. They usually are multiple, small, raised, stellate lesions located in the peripheral cornea.[20] In contrast to the ulcerated dendrite of herpes simplex, the zoster microdendrite characteristically appears to be composed of swollen or heaped-up cells. The thickened edematous epithelium probably accounts for its poor, dull staining by fluorescein, contrasting it with the herpes simplex dendrite, which stains brightly because of the missing epithelial layer (Fig. 17–11). Typically the coarse, blunted appearance of the zoster dendrite contrasts with the often delicate pattern of the herpes simplex dendrite. Moreover, the terminal bulbs that frequently are a part of simplex lesions are not a feature of zoster dendrites.[20]

A second superficial lesion observed in herpes zoster ophthalmicus is the corneal mucous plaque. These were first described by Piebenga and Laibson[19] as gray, plaquelike, intermittent, linear or branching elevations on the surface of the corneal epithelium. Marsh and coworkers[20] showed that these lesions are simply mucous plaques. The majority are seen 3 to 4 months after the onset of the cutaneous lesions, but they have been noted as early as 7 days and as late as 2 years after the acute illness. Typically multiple whitish-gray plaques are observed; they overlie and are adherent to intact but edematous degenerating epithelial cells and may be located anywhere on the cornea. These plaques have sharp margins and are quite variable in size and shape, commonly appearing as linear or branching dendritiform structures. However, it has been reported that they may change in configuration, number, and size from day to day.[20] Fluorescein stains these lesions somewhat, but rose bengal stains them vividly. Since they are located on the epithelial surface, they can be removed by gentle scraping, with minimal damage to the underlying epithelium. Virus has never been isolated from these lesions, but herpes-type virus particles have been demonstrated in underlying degenerating epithelial cells by electron microscopic examination of a corneal scraping obtained from a case of varicella mucous-plaque keratitis.[21] Viral antigen also has been demonstrated by direct immunofluorescent staining of a corneal scraping from a case of varicella mucous-plaque keratitis.[22] Of the 283 patients with ophthalmic zoster examined by Marsh and colleagues, 13 per cent had acute epithelial microdendritic keratitis and 7 per cent had delayed corneal mucous plaques.[20]

There is invariably an associated ciliary injection of the bulbar conjunctiva and hyperemia of the tarsal conjunctiva. Corneal mucous plaques usually are accompanied by a mild anterior uveitis, and there also may be a profuse deposition of keratic precipitates on the endothelium (Fig. 17–12). Diffuse microcystic edema of the corneal epithelium and a faint superficial stromal haze are common. The overlying tear film tends to be unstable, resulting in the rapid formation of dry spots which not infrequently have a dendritiform shape. Results of the Schirmer test are usually

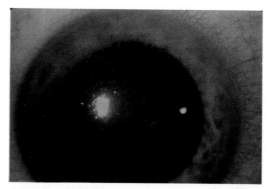

Figure 17–12. Zoster keratouveitis characterized by ciliary injection, corneal edema, and profuse deposition of keratic precipitates.

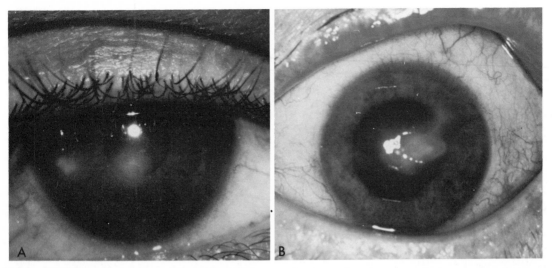

Figure 17–13. Superficial stromal opacities accompanying herpes zoster ophthalmicus: *A,* Early lesions with intact epithelium. *B,* Later, more advanced lesion with overlying epithelial defect. (*A* courtesy of Howard M. Leibowitz, M.D.)

within normal limits, but corneal sensation generally is impaired.[20] The deposition of mucous plaques may continue for several months, but ultimately they resolve and the tear film and epithelium stabilize.

Superficial stromal opacities may succeed the epithelial lesions or arise de novo (Fig. 17–13). They appear about 10 days after the onset of the rash as ill-defined granular infiltrates of varying size located just beneath Bowman's membrane. Because the opacities are often found adjacent to enlarged corneal nerves, Marsh[16] postulates that the granules may be due to the degeneration of corneal nerves secondary to viral damage. The superficial opacities usually are

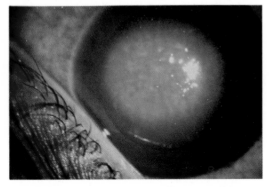

Figure 17–14. Zoster disciform keratitis.

self-limited, but occasionally they may leave some permanent scarring.

Disciform keratitis may develop weeks to months after the onset of the disease (Fig. 17–14). It frequently is located beneath a preceding superficial stromal infiltrate and may be surrounded by an immune ring (Fig. 17–15). Disciform or more diffuse stromal keratitis may arise entirely independently of epithelial involvement and most probably represents a delayed hypersensitivity reaction. If left untreated, the keratitis runs a chronic course with the development of prominent neovascularization. Lipid deposition within the stroma and irreversible scarring are frequent sequelae (Fig. 17–16).

Sclerokeratitis is an uncommon manifestation of this disease. It may present at the outset but more often occurs 1 to 3 months later. Edema and infiltration of full-thickness corneal stroma adjacent to an area of scleritis are seen and invariably there is an accompanying iritis. Marsh[16] postulates that this entity results from an immune complex vasculitis in the episcleral and scleral vessels, causing infiltration and ischemic effects in the cornea. If left untreated, the keratitis tends to run a chronic course with increasing infiltration, and subsequently neovascularization, lipid deposition,

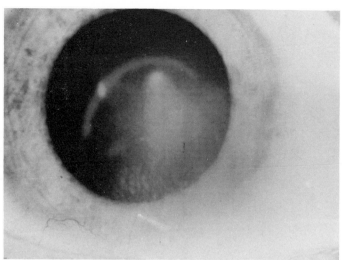

Figure 17–15. Disciform edema surrounded by an immune arc.

and scarring (Fig. 17–16). Exceptions occur and the sclerokeratitis may resolve spontaneously, but relapses months to years later can occur.

One of the most devastating corneal complications of herpes zoster ophthalmicus is neurotrophic keratitis, which can result in eventual corneal perforation (Fig. 17–17). Accompanying the acute stages of the skin rash there is often a loss of corneal sensation, but with time at least partial recovery occurs in most cases. Moreover, loss of sensory innervation to the cornea does not invariably result in neurotrophic disease; patients with an anesthetic cornea may maintain a smooth epithelial surface and a transparent cornea. Nonetheless, decreased corneal sensation combined with chronic conjunctivitis, tear film abnormalities, and lid deformities can give rise to epithelial changes with secondary stromal involvement. This usually occurs 3 to 6 months after the onset of the disease and tends to fluctuate in severity. Initially there is a loss of luster of the corneal epithelium with multiple punctate erosions in the interpalpebral area. These can progress to form indolent corneal ulcers with opaque, water-

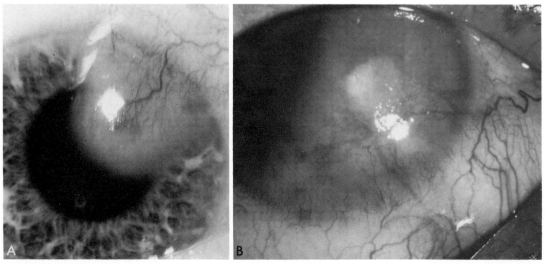

Figure 17–16. Chronic zoster stromal keratitis. *A,* Scarring and neovascularization sparing some of the pupillary area. *B,* More diffuse scarring with lipid deposition.

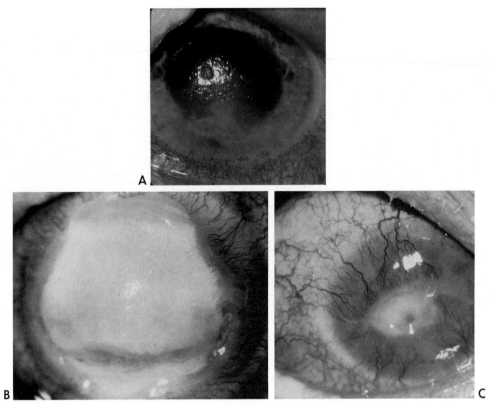

Figure 17–17. Zoster-induced neurotrophic keratitis. *A,* Early lesion characterized by epithelial degeneration and loss of luster, punctate erosions, a mucous plaque, and exfoliation of a localized area of epithelium. *B,* More prolonged involvement characterized by a large, indolent epithelial defect and edema and scarring of the underlying stroma. *C,* Interpalpebral indolent ulcer with active infiltrate and central perforation. (*A* and *C* courtesy of Howard M. Leibowitz, M.D.)

logged edges. Underlying stromal infiltration with secondary infection, thinning, and ultimately perforation may occur. These ulcers are very difficult to heal, and usually do so with some degree of stromal thinning, neovascularization, and scarring. Interestingly, the corneal anesthesia and the resultant keratitis may be confined to a sector of the cornea, while the remainder of the tissue is clear and uninvolved.

Mondino and coworkers[23] have described peripheral corneal ulcers occurring in patients with herpes zoster ophthalmicus. The ulcers had steep central edges and were associated with an anterior uveitis. The pathogenesis of these ulcers is speculative and their relationship to the herpes zoster ophthalmicus is not clear; no definite cause-and-effect relationship has been established.

Iridocyclitis

The anterior uveal tract frequently is affected by herpes zoster ophthalmicus and may be involved either early or late in the course of the disease. Iridocyclitis may be severe, with frequent recurrences. It can occur independently of corneal involvement and is manifested by ciliary injection, iridial edema and hyperemia, miosis, and cells and flare in the aqueous humor causing decreased vision, photophobia, and ocular pain. More severe cases may be accompanied by hypopyon, hyphema, anterior and posterior synechiae, and secondary glaucoma. Fine keratic precipitates frequently are deposited on the endothelium and may disrupt its dehydrating function (Fig. 17–12). The corneal endothelium is extremely vulnerable to anterior uveitis, and corneal edema may

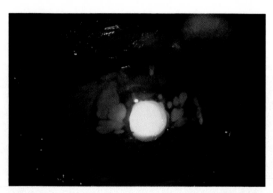

Figure 17–18. Iris atrophy following zoster kera-touveitis. (Courtesy of Howard M. Leibowitz, M.D.)

develop even in the absence of elevated intraocular pressure.

Iris atrophy is a common sequel to zoster iridocyclitis (Fig. 17–18). There is a sectorial loss of iris pigment epithelium, with ill-defined borders and adjacent sphincter atrophy. Histopathologically, zoster iritis is chiefly a vasculitis similar to periarteritis nodosa. The typical sector iris atrophy accompanying ophthalmic zoster is the result of focal ischemic necrosis caused by the occlusive vasculitis. Iris angiography demonstrates the absence of vascular filling in relation to the atrophic areas.[24] (In contrast, the iritis of herpes simplex is primarily a diffuse lymphocytic infiltration of the iris stroma, and clinically iris atrophy is characterized by well-defined scalloped edges and normal vascular filling on iris angiography.) In its most severe form the occlusive vasculitis in the anterior uvea can cause massive necrosis of the pars plicata of the ciliary body with a resultant decrease in aqueous humor production. Clinical sequelae include ocular hypotension and even phthisis bulbi.

Glaucoma

Glaucoma is commonly found sometime during the course of the disease. There are several mechanisms responsible for the elevated intraocular pressure. These include clogging of the trabeculum by pigment and/or cellular debris, inflam-mation of the meshwork (acute trabeculitis), pupillary block by posterior synechiae, and secondary angle closure by peripheral anterior synechiae. Moreover, a unilateral chronic open-angle glaucoma may develop, presumably because of irreversible damage to the trabecular meshwork.

Other Ocular Involvement

Pupillary abnormalities of purely neurologic origin occur as part of herpes zoster ophthalmicus and are not associated with inflammation of the anterior uvea. Involvement of the sympathetic nerves may result in miosis (along with the other components of a Horner's syndrome), whereas ciliary ganglion involvement apparently accounts for the tonic pupil and internal ophthalmoplegia that have been observed. The choroid and retina may be affected in the form of diffuse or focal choroiditis, hemorrhagic retinitis, vitreous opacities, central retinal artery occlusion, or retinal detachment. Papillitis and retrobulbar neuritis have been reported; at times this may indicate central nervous system involvement, but local transmission of virus from the fifth to the second cranial nerve within the orbit can occur.[4, 25]

External oculomotor palsies occur in up to 31 per cent of cases of herpes zoster ophthalmicus.[26] The third cranial nerve is most commonly involved, followed in frequency by the sixth and fourth cranial nerves, respectively. All three nerves may be affected simultaneously or in various combinations. Bilateral involvement may occur, and unilateral extraocular muscle palsies on the side opposite the skin lesions have been reported. In most cases paralysis of the extraocular muscles presents within a week of the initial appearance of the rash. Often this complication is asymptomatic because diplopia occurs only in extreme positions of gaze or because vision in the affected eye is poor. Complete spontaneous recovery is the rule, usually within a year. There seems to be a significant association between the presence of an extraocular muscle palsy and a severe skin rash, and between the muscle palsy and a subsequent severe neuralgia, iritis, and iris atrophy. Ipsilateral facial nerve palsy occasionally may be seen in conjunction with herpes zoster ophthalmicus.

Segmental cerebral arteritis and contralateral hemiplegia can occur months after the acute illness of herpes zoster ophthalmicus.[27]

PATHOLOGY

The pathology of herpes zoster ophthalmicus has been well described by Naumann and colleagues.[28] However, all but one of the 21 eyes they studied were examined months to years after the initial presentation of ophthalmic zoster. The most characteristic histologic feature was segmental lymphocytic infiltration of the long posterior ciliary nerves and vessels. Naumann and coworkers have stated that this is almost diagnostic of herpes zoster ophthalmicus. Another common finding was the extensive necrosis of the iris and the patchy necrosis of the ciliary body resulting from chronic inflammation and ischemic vasculitis. Other histopathologic features include chronic episcleritis and scleritis, scarring and vascularization of the deep corneal stroma, granulomatous reaction to Descemet's membrane,[29] nonspecific lens changes, scattered infiltrates of lymphocytes and plasma cells in the choroid, retinal vasculitis, and chronic perivascular infiltrates within the optic nerve.

LABORATORY DIAGNOSIS

The diagnosis of herpes zoster ophthalmicus is primarily a clinical one. However, there are several laboratory tests available if the diagnosis is in doubt. The varicella-zoster virus can be isolated from fresh skin vesicles or corneal "microdendrites." The virus grows only in cell line cultures of human or simian origin and will not infect any known laboratory animal. Virus particles can be observed on direct examination of infected tissue under the electron microscope and Giemsa or PAS-stained smears of scrapings from fresh vesicles can demonstrate the presence of multinucleated giant cells and eosinophilic intranuclear inclusion bodies. Immunofluorescence can also be used to identify virus in infected tissue specimens.[22, 30]

Serologic testing may be helpful in making a diagnosis. Neutralizing and complement-fixing antibodies can be demonstrated in the serum of infected individuals. Gel-diffusion precipitation and immunofluorescent techniques can also demonstrate specific antibodies to the varicella-zoster virus.

TREATMENT

The treatment of herpes zoster ophthalmicus is difficult, largely because the pathogenesis of many aspects of the disease is poorly understood. The mechanisms through which the viral infection produces many of the ocular lesions is unknown, and we can do little more here than outline basic therapeutic guidelines and our personal recommendations. During the acute stages of the rash the patient should be made as comfortable as possible with appropriate analgesics. Many authorities recommend drying of the skin lesions. Marsh[14] routinely uses an antibiotic-steroid ointment to prevent the development of large crusts and secondary infection, which tend to promote scarring. He reports no complications from the use of this regimen. Juel-Jensen,[3] on the other hand, believes that the initial eruptive phase should be treated with specific chemotherapy, and he applies 40 per cent idoxuridine (IDU) in dimethyl sulfoxide (DMSO) to the skin lesions continuously for 3 to 4 days. He claims that in the majority of patients there is improvement of the acute rash with prompt relief of pain and, perhaps of even greater importance, that late sequelae are rare. While Marsh[14] concurs that there is undoubted improvement in comfort and in the acute rash, he disagrees with the latter claim and states that the incidence of postherpetic neuralgia is not significantly altered by the topical use of 40 per cent IDU in DMSO. In either case, this preparation is not available in the United States at present, so that its use here and its effectiveness are largely of academic concern. The ophthalmologist has the choice of allowing the lesions to resolve spontaneously or with the use of saline soaks, applying a drying agent (e.g., 0.25 per cent menthol in 70 per cent isopropyl alcohol), or administering a steroid-antibiotic ointment topically to the lesions. We know of no controlled data demonstrating the superiority of a particular regimen for the eruptive dermatitis of herpes zoster ophthalmicus.

Topical corticosteroids have a well-established role in the treatment of ocular complications of herpes zoster ophthalmicus. The inflammatory stromal lesions of zoster keratitis (superficial stromal opacities, disciform keratitis, sclerokeratitis) often are sensitive to topical corticosteroids. However, topical steroids have little or no effect on acute microdendrites or delayed mucous plaques. The anterior uveitis associated with herpes zoster ophthalmicus is also very responsive to the instillation of corticosteroids.[14, 31]

As one obtains a therapeutic response from topical corticosteroids, the dosage should be decreased slowly. Too rapid withdrawal of the medication can result in a rebound keratitis and iritis. Some patients require small doses for months or even years before they can be totally weaned from topical corticosteroids. An occasional patient may require a minimal amount of medication indefinitely. One or two drops of a weak corticosteroid preparation every 3 or 4 days may control ocular inflammation. Discontinuation of this seemingly homeopathic dose may be followed by a flare-up of inflammatory activity. Long-term use of corticosteroids involves a degree of risk, and the ophthalmologist must remain alert for the various side effects of topically applied corticosteroids (see Chapter 11).

The administration of corticosteroids systemically during the acute phase of the disease is controversial. Carter and Royds,[32] Elliott,[33] Scheie,[34] and Pavan-Langston[25] are proponents of the use of high-dose systemic steroids in the acute phase of herpes zoster ophthalmicus to suppress ocular inflammation, control severe pain, and prevent postherpetic neuralgia. A starting dose of at least 60 mg. of prednisone per day is recommended, and is gradually tapered over a period of 3 to 4 weeks. The sooner treatment is initiated with systemic corticosteroids, the more likely it is to be effective, particularly with regard to postherpetic neuralgia. Systemic steroid therapy begun after the sixth week is ineffective,[33] presumably because scarring around the nerves has already begun. Similarly, low doses of corticosteroids (i.e., 15 mg. of prednisone per day) are of no value. A major drawback of the use of high-dose systemic corticosteroids to treat herpes zoster ophthalmicus is the potential danger of dissemination of the disease.[35] Most instances of zoster dissemination associated with systemic steroid administration occur in patients with immunologically crippling disease (e.g., lymphoma, leukemia). Disseminated zoster in these patients can be a life-threatening illness. Nondebilitated, otherwise healthy patients who develop dissemination of zoster suffer an illness similar to chickenpox, with little or no sequelae.

Nonsteroidal anti-inflammatory agents such as oxyphenbutazone and indomethacin have been advocated for the treatment of patients with severe scleritis and sclerokeratitis in whom corticosteroids are contraindicated.[36] These drugs are usually taken by mouth, and although they tend not to have the frequent serious side effects associated with corticosteroid use, they should not be taken lightly. They have their own side effects, which include aplastic anemia. Their effectiveness in suppressing ocular inflammation in herpes zoster ophthalmicus is quite variable and unpredictable.

Although the varicella zoster virus is susceptible to IDU in vitro, topically applied antiviral medications appear to be ineffective in ameliorating zoster keratitis. Moreover, topical antiviral agents are toxic to the epithelium and may promote epithelial breakdown. The use of systemic antiviral antimetabolites is controversial. There are reports of resolution of ophthalmic zoster following intravenous administration of cytosine arabinoside,[37–40] but a controlled trial demonstrated an adverse effect of this drug on disseminated zoster.[41] Systemic acycloguanosine (Acyclovir) may promote healing of acute zosteriform skin lesions and alleviate the pain in the early stages of herpes zoster.[42]

Topically administered artificial tears and mucolytic agents (10 to 20 per cent acetylcysteine) help stabilize the tear film and protect the cornea on a long-term basis. Corneal mucous plaques often respond to mucolytic agents but do have a tendency to recur.[14] Antibiotic drops commonly are used prophylactically during the acute stages of the disease, but there is little definitive evidence supporting this practice. However, in cases of corneal ulceration, when the epithelial barrier to bacterial invasion is no longer intact, the use of prophylactic antibiotics seems logical. Tarsorrhaphy remains the treatment of choice for a severe neurotrophic ulcer. Although therapeutic soft contact lenses have been recommended for this problem, we have found their use fraught with difficulties. The abnormal tear film causes the lenses to dry up and fall out, especially when the lids are scarred and deformed. Moreover, the absence of corneal sensation permits small foreign bodies that may lodge between the lens and the cornea to injure the cornea mechanically without causing symptoms that warn the patient something is amiss. If corneal ulceration persists or if it progresses despite conservative therapy, a conjunctival flap may be the best and safest procedure. Corneal transplantation may be required on an emergency basis for neuroparalytic ulcers that have perforated, but the visual results in these cases are poor. Penetrating keratoplasty also may be attempted to restore vision to an eye with a severely scarred and vascularized cornea. If the cornea is anesthetic, the graft generally fares poorly, particularly if tear film abnormalities and lid margin deformities aggravate the problem.

Mydriatic-cycloplegic drops are indicated in the presence of an iritis to prevent the formation of synechiae. Glaucoma often is a complication of the intraocular inflammatory response and may respond to the judicious use of topical corticosteroids. If corticosteroids alone do not control the intraocular pressure, topically applied epinephrine, timolol, or systemic carbonic anhydrase inhibitors or combinations of these agents generally are effective. The possibility that the glaucoma may be steroid-induced should not be forgotten.

Postherpetic neuralgia remains a major problem in the management of patients with zoster. The overall risk of developing this complication is approximately 10 per cent. Unfortunately, postherpetic neuralgia in the distribution of the trigeminal nerve tends to be more prolonged and severe than that encountered in other locations. Moreover, the incidence, severity, and duration of the neuralgia increase markedly with age. The role of systemically administered corticosteroids and of topical IDU in DMSO in the prevention of postherpetic neuralgia has been mentioned. Once a patient is beset by this severe, crippling problem, it is difficult to bring it under control. Hypnosis and acupuncture have been tried but have failed to produce lasting results.[43] Numerous other therapeutic regimens have been suggested. These include narcotic analgesics, minor tranquilizers, phenothiazines, antidepressants, and carbamazepine (Tegretol). Transcutaneous electrical stimulation has also been used.[44] The variety of recommended treatment modalities provides the most definitive commentary on their general lack of effectiveness.

REFERENCES

1. Hutchinson, J.: A clinical report on herpes zoster frontalis ophthalmicus (shingles affecting the forehead and nose). Roy Lond Ophthal Hosp Rep 5:191, 1865–1866.
2. Esiri, M. M., and Tomlinson, A. H.: Herpes zoster. Demonstration of virus in trigeminal nerve and ganglion by immunofluorescence and electron microscopy. J Neurol Sci 15:35, 1972.
3. Juel-Jensen, B. E.: Herpes simplex and zoster. Brit Med J 1:406, 1973.
4. Edgerton, A. E.: Herpes zoster ophthalmicus. Report of cases and review of literature. Arch Ophthalmol 34:40, 1945.
5. Klauder, J. V.: Herpes zoster appearing after trauma. JAMA 134:245, 1947.
6. Thomas, M., and Robertson, W.: Derminal transmission of a virus as a cause of shingles. Lancet 2:1349, 1968.
7. Tomlinson, A. H., and MacCallum, F. O.: The incidence of complement-fixing antibody to varicella-zoster virus in hospital patients and blood donors. J Hygiene 68:411, 1970.
8. Shanbrom, E., Miller, S., and Haar, H.: Herpes zoster in hematologic neoplasias: Some unusual manifestations. Arch Intern Med 53:522, 1960.
9. Sokal, J. E., and Firat, D.: Varicella-zoster infection in Hodgkin's disease. Amer J Med 39:452, 1965.
10. Muller, S. A.: Association of zoster and malignant disorders of children. Arch Dermatol 96:657, 1967.
11. Blodi, F. C.: Ophthalmic zoster in malignant disease. Amer J Ophthalmol 65:686, 1968.
12. Scheie, H. G.: Herpes zoster ophthalmicus. Trans Ophthalmol Soc UK 90:899, 1970.
13. Ragozzino, M. W., Melton, L. J., III, Kurland, L. T., Chu, C. P., and Perry, H. O.: Risk of cancer after herpes zoster. A population-based study. N Engl J Med 307:393, 1982.
14. Marsh, R. J.: Current management of ophthalmic herpes zoster. Trans Ophthalmol Soc UK 96:334, 1976.
15. Watson, P. G., and Hayreh, S. S.: Scleritis and episcleritis. Brit J Ophthalmol 60:163, 1976.
16. Marsh, R. J.: Herpes zoster keratitis. Trans Ophthalmol Soc UK 93:181, 1973.
17. Jones, B.: Differential diagnosis of punctate keratitis. Int Ophthalmol Clin 2:591, 1962.
18. Pavan-Langston, D., and McCulley, J. P.: Herpes zoster dendritic keratitis. Arch Ophthalmol 89:25, 1973.
19. Piebenga, L. W., and Laibson, P. R.: Dendritic lesions in herpes zoster ophthalmicus. Arch Ophthalmol 90:268, 1973.
20. Marsh, R. J., Fraunfelder, F. T., and McGill, J. I.: Herpetic corneal epithelial disease. Arch Ophthalmol 94:1899, 1976.
21. Nesburn, A. B., Borit, A., Pentelei-Molnar, J., and Lazaro, R.: Varicella dendritic keratitis. Invest Ophthalmol 13:764, 1974.
22. Uchida, Y., Kaneko, M., and Hayashi, K.: Varicella dendritic keratitis. Amer J Ophthalmol 89:259, 1980.
23. Mondino, B. J., Brown, S. I., and Mondzelewski, J. P.: Peripheral corneal ulcers with herpes zoster ophthalmicus. Amer J Ophthalmol 86:611, 1978.
24. Marsh, R. J., Easty, D. L., and Jones, B. R.: Iritis and iris atrophy in herpes zoster ophthalmicus. Amer J Ophthalmol 78:255, 1974.
25. Pavan-Langston, D.: Varicella-zoster ophthalmicus. Int Ophthalmol Clin 15:171, 1975.
26. Marsh, R. J., Dulley, B., and Kelly, V.: External ocular motor palsies in ophthalmic zoster. A review. Brit J Ophthalmol 61:677, 1977.
27. Womack, L. W., and Liesegang, T. J.: Complications of herpes zoster ophthalmicus. Arch Ophthalmol 101:42, 1983.
28. Naumann, G., Gass, J. D. M., and Font, R. L.: Histopathology of herpes zoster ophthalmicus. Amer J Ophthalmol 65:533, 1968.
29. Hedges, T. R., III, and Albert, D. M.: The progression of the ocular abnormalities of herpes zoster. Histopathologic observations of nine cases. Ophthalmology 89:165, 1982.
30. Hayashi, K., Uchida, Y., and Ohshima, M.: Fluorescent antibody study of herpes zoster keratitis. Amer J Ophthalmol 75:795, 1973.
31. Berghaust, B., and Westerby, R.: Zoster ophthalmicus—Local treatment with cortisone. Acta Ophthalmol 45:787, 1967.
32. Carter, A., and Royds, J.: Systemic steroids in herpes zoster. Brit Med J 2:746, 1957.
33. Elliott, F. A.: Treatment of herpes zoster with high doses of prednisone. Lancet 2:610, 1964.
34. Scheie, H. G.: Herpes zoster ophthalmicus. Trans Ophthalmol Soc UK 90:899, 1970.
35. Merselis, J., Kaye, D., and Hook, E.: Disseminated herpes zoster. Arch Intern Med 113:679, 1961.
36. Watson, P. G., Lobascher, D. J., Sabiston, D. W., Lewis-Fanning, E., Fowler, P. D., and Jones, B. R.: Double-blind trial of the treatment of episcleritis-scleritis with oxyphenbutazone or prednisolone. Brit J Ophthalmol 50:463, 1966.
37. Mann, J.: Cytosine arabinoside and herpes zoster. Lancet 2:166, 1971.
38. Waltruch, G., and Sachs, F.: Herpes zoster in a patient with Hodgkins disease. Arch Intern Med 121:458, 1971.
39. Fortuny, I., Weiss, R., Theologides, A., and Kennedy, B.: Cytosine arabinoside in herpes zoster. Lancet 1:38, 1973.
40. Pierce, L., and Jenkins, R.: Herpes zoster ophthalmicus treated with cytarabine. Arch Ophthalmol 89:21, 1973.
41. Stevens, D. A., Jordan, G. W., Waddell, T. F., and Merigan, T. C.: Adverse effect of cytosine arabinoside on disseminated zoster in a controlled trial. N Engl J Med 289:873, 1973.
42. Esmann, V., Ipsen, J., Peterslund, N. A., Seyer-Hansen, K., Schonheyder, H., and Juhl, H.: Therapy of acute herpes zoster with Acyclovir in the non-immunocompromised host. Amer J Med 73:320, 1982.
43. Leibowitz, H. M.: Personal communication, 1982.
44. Haas, L. F.: Postherpetic neuralgia: Treatment and prevention. Trans Ophthalmol Soc NZ 29:133, 1977.

18

Fungal Keratitis

DENIS M. O'DAY, M.D.

Although filamentous fungi and yeasts infect the cornea infrequently, the onset of a mycotic infection is still cause for grave concern. In the past treatment was generally inadequate and it was not uncommon for the eye to be lost. Recently, as a result of efforts to provide a better therapeutic approach to these infections, several new antifungal agents that can be applied topically to the eye have become available. In addition, diagnostic techniques have improved significantly. As a result, the prognosis for fungal infection of the cornea is considerably better. The majority of these infections can now be controlled and useful vision can be preserved in most cases.

PATHOGENESIS

Fungi are a part of our normal microbial environment. Although the eye is continuously exposed to these microorganisms, the normal external ocular defenses, including the lids and tear components, provide adequate protection. It would also appear that conditions necessary for attachment to corneal epithelial cells (a prerequisite for invasion) are not favorable to fungi. Thus, fungal infections, in the absence of a precipitating event, rarely occur in the human cornea.

The importance of trauma, often of a trivial nature and frequently with vegetable material, is well documented in the initiation of fungal infection.[1, 2] In the southern United States and in trop-

ical regions elsewhere in the world, trauma appears to be the most important precipitating cause of keratomycosis, a fact readily understandable in view of the ubiquitous presence of fungi in these areas. In areas with cooler climates a different spectrum of disease is seen with fungal infection. In these regions the mycotic keratitis often occurs in association with dry eyes or in corneas with extensive structural alteration.

Although almost any fungus is capable of invading the cornea, the septate filamentous molds are most frequently encountered. Infection with nonseptate fungi has been reported only rarely. The more common isolates are listed in Table 18–1. Among the yeasts, *Candida* species is by far the most frequent invader and is particularly encountered in the cooler climates. At one time it was thought that prior administration of antibiotics, and more especially corticosteroids, favored the development of a fungal infection in the cornea. However, reviews of several large series of cases have not supported this contention.[1, 2]

Table 18–1. COMMON FUNGAL ISOLATES IN CORNEAL INFECTION

Filamentous Fungi	Yeasts
Fusarium solani	*Candida* species
Aspergillus species	
Alternaria species	
Penicillium species	
Phialophora species	
Curvularia species	
Helminthosporium species	
Cladosporium species	
Acremonium species	

CLINICAL FEATURES

Filamentous Fungal Infection

The onset of a fungal infection of the cornea is almost always insidious. As has been noted, trauma, usually with vegetable matter, is frequently the precipitating event in an otherwise normal eye. Several days, or even weeks, may elapse before the presence of infection is recognized, and it is not uncommon for the traumatized epithelium to heal completely before signs of infection supervene. During this latent period the patient may experience little or no discomfort, and the eye may appear to respond to topically applied antibiotics. However, within a highly variable interval, lasting from days to sometimes weeks, the patient becomes aware of discomfort and photophobia and there may even be an accompanying discharge.

On examination during this period, the acute observer may notice a persistent infiltrate at the site of the previous superficial laceration and, as time goes by, the infiltrate gradually increases in amount (Fig. 18–1). Of some significance is the tendency of the epithelium to heal over this inflammatory focus, although there may be recurrent episodes of epithelial loss. The cornea becomes slightly thickened, and "satellite" lesions may develop peripheral to the focal area of infiltration. If the infiltrate is not overwhelmingly dense, it may be possible under high magnification to see actual fungal filaments coursing through the stroma parallel to the lamellae. In some instances a Wessely ring (Fig. 18–2) develops around the central lesion, indicative of antigen-antibody interaction with resultant chemotaxis of polymorphonuclear leukocytes. It should be cautioned that findings such as "satellite" lesions and the ring, though used as strong clinical evidence of fungal infection, may occur in other inflammatory conditions, particularly herpetic infection.

Untreated, the inflammatory signs will gradually progress, causing permanent breakdown of the epithelium, stromal ulceration (Fig. 18–3), and in some cases the formation of a descemetocele (Fig. 18–4), leading to perforation of the cornea. Neovascularization may also occur as a result of the inflammatory stimulus, and ultimately the cornea may be left severely scarred (Fig. 18–4). Associated signs, indicative of the intensity of the developing inflammation, are the presence of ciliary injection and hypopyon (Fig. 18–5). It is not uncommon to see a hypopyon develop in association with corneal infection by a filamentous fungus, even when the lesion appears quite superficial (Fig. 18–6). This does not imply that intraocular invasion has occurred.

Infection with Yeast

Yeast infections are somewhat different from filamentous fungal infections. The majority of these cases occur in structurally altered eyes, particularly in patients with collagen vascular disease or keratitis sicca, and in instances in which external ocular defenses have been altered or reduced. Most yeast infections are superficial, appearing as white raised colonies in previously ulcerated areas (Fig. 18–7) or on the surface of the eye itself. Deep invasion can occur, but most such lesions tend to remain superficial. Occasionally a more infiltrative type of yeast infection will be encountered that is indistinguishable from a filamentous fungus infection.

Although this description has emphasized the slowly progressive nature of fungal infection, an occasional case will be seen in which the infection develops rapidly with explosive signs of inflammation. In such cases, the eye can be lost rapidly unless appropriate treatment is instituted.

DIAGNOSIS

A major factor in the improved management of fungal infection has been the ability to detect the fungus at an early stage in an increasing percentage of cases, thus facilitating appropriate ther-

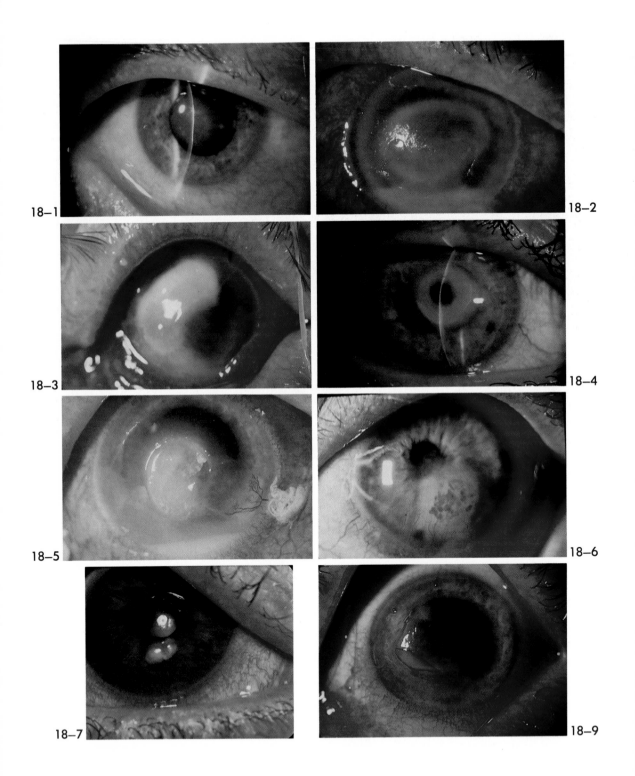

18-1

18-2

18-3

18-4

18-5

18-6

18-7

18-9

apy. A standard, general approach to the management of any suspected microbial keratitis should be followed in every case,[3] because it is impossible on clinical grounds to determine with certainty the infectious etiology of the corneal ulcer. In addition, combined infections with bacteria and fungi, or with several fungi, can occur.

Culture Media

Selection of the appropriate media for culture is based upon the need to recover the most frequently encountered bacterial and fungal pathogens. Thus, blood agar, Sabouraud's agar, thioglycolate broth, and brain-heart infusion broth should be routinely employed. When indicated (and this applies particularly to cases in children or other instances in which *Hemophilus* infection is suspected), chocolate agar may be substituted for blood agar or used as an additional plate. Fresh culture media should always be used. Media containing inhibitory compounds, such as cyclohexamide, should be avoided; they may prevent the recovery of organisms known to be pathogenic in the human cornea.

Technique

The techniques used for obtaining material from the cornea and inoculating the media have been well described and standardized.[3] It is important to remove the epithelium over the lesion, should it be intact, and to vigorously scrape the surface of the lesion, its margins, and the bed of any ulcer that is present. A Kimura spatula that has been ground down to a more slender instrument is suitable for this purpose. After the application of a topical anesthetic, the surface of the lesion and the margins are scraped vigorously. The isolate is then transferred to the culture plate by making a row of C marks, reversing the edge of the spatula with each C, so that all material on the spatula is transferred to the plate. The spatula is flamed and then allowed to cool, and the process is repeated until several rows of C streaks have been made on each solid plate. For inoculation into liquid media, the spatula is briefly immersed directly in the culture fluid. These diagnostic techniques are necessarily cumbersome and, unfortunately, they do present opportunities for contamination by airborne organisms at every step.[4]

Figure 18–1. Superficial corneal infection with *Alternaria sp.* 2 weeks following abrasion.

Figure 18–2. Well-marked Wessely ring surrounding a central corneal mycotic infection.

Figure 18–3. Corneal abscess with hypopyon. *Cladosporium sp.* was isolated in pure culture.

Figure 18–4. This central descemetocele developed following infection with *Paecilomyces lilacinus* despite therapy with natamycin.

Figure 18–5. Corneal ulcer with large hypopyon. *Aspergillus fumigatus* was isolated from the ulcer.

Figure 18–6. Corneal infection due to *Aspergillus fumigatus* with heavy neovascularization.

Figure 18–7. Colonies of *Candida albicans* in a shallow corneal ulcer. Patient had keratitis sicca and systemic lupus erythematosus.

Figure 18–9. Corneal toxicity due to topical flucytosine 1 per cent. After about 4 weeks of treatment, an epithelial ulcer accompanied by coarse superficial punctate keratopathy developed. The conjunctiva in the lower fornix was inflamed. Healing rapidly followed on withdrawal of the drug.

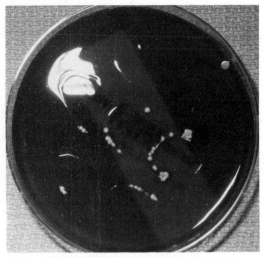

Figure 18–8. Colonies of *Candida albicans* growing in C streaks on blood agar.

Cultures

Fungal cultures may require a prolonged period of observation before an isolate is finally recovered. Although it is frequently stated that a majority of fungal isolates will be recovered within 48 hours of inoculation,[2] at least 25 per cent may require incubation for as long as 3 weeks before growth can be recognized.[4] It is, therefore, important to maintain the cultures for this length of time and to observe them repeatedly for signs of growth (Fig. 18–8). A solid plate can be maintained for only 4 or 5 days in the laboratory; hence the necessity for broth media. Sealing the plate in a plastic bag to conserve moisture will prolong its useful life. To provide optimal growth conditions, broth media should be placed on a shaker.

The temperature requirements for fungi also are quite variable, but most grow well at room temperature (25° C). However, at least one culture plate should be incubated at 37° C.

Smears

The necessity for Gram and Giemsa stains cannot be overemphasized, since this step forms the basis for selection of initial therapy. Slides should be clean and, prior to the staining procedure, the material should be fixed in methyl alcohol rather than by heat, since the latter approach can introduce artifactitious change. A Gram or Giemsa stain is all that is necessary to identify organisms in most instances, the latter being more helpful for fungal material. Occasionally a spurious organism will be identified and, in such cases, it is usually a yeast. This organism grows in Gram's iodine, so it is advisable to keep the solutions as fresh as possible. Interpretation of the slide requires some experience; to the inexperienced observer, a fibrin strand may easily be confused with fungal filaments.

MANAGEMENT

Antifungal Medications

On the basis of laborious studies with experimental models of infection and considerable human experience, an approach to the selection of antifungal therapy has been developed. Initially, heavy reliance must be placed on interpretation of the smear, since there may be a considerable delay before cultures become positive. Fortunately, experience has shown that the smear provides diagnostically useful information when carefully performed, and it is appropriate to use the smear as a starting point in the selection of therapy.

Observation of septate hyphal fragments on the smear provides strong evidence of a filamentous fungal infection. Pimaricin (natamycin) is the drug of choice in this situation. It has been shown to be effective against most filamentous organisms likely to be encountered in the cornea. The drug, available as a 5 per cent suspension, should be administered to the eye every hour during the first few days. Since there is evidence that some strains of *Aspergillus*, *Penicillium*, and *Cladosporium* are also sensitive to flucytosine, this compound is given in addition, as a 1 per cent drop instilled every 15 to 30 minutes. The same combination of flucytosine and natamycin is employed if yeast cells or pseudohyphae are seen on the smear. Flucytosine is an excellent drug against sensitive strains of *Candida*, but resistant strains do occur or may emerge during the course of treatment. Alternatively, natamycin may be used alone, since it has a good range of activity against yeast organisms.

Among the other antifungal agents that are available or are under investigation, miconazole appears to be the best agent, with the most promising efficacy for yeast infections. Unfortunately, no specific topical preparations are yet available. All of these compounds have largely supplanted the use of amphotericin B because of their efficacy and their markedly reduced local toxicity. Amphotericin methyl ester, although showing considerably less toxicity, is not available for general use. Systemic antifungal therapy is not considered necessary for most corneal infections.

During the initial treatment period, antifungal therapy should be administered on a 24-hour basis. Natamycin is given every hour and 5-flucytosine every 15 to 30 minutes. After the first few days, administration is reduced to the waking hours at a rate of 17 times a day.

Up to this point, we have considered the initial steps in management when there is positive evidence for a fungal infection. The question still remains, how should one proceed when the clinical suspicion of fungus infection is high but smears are negative and cultures have not yet incubated for a sufficient period of time to provide definite information? In general, the recommendation is to defer antifungal therapy for as long as possible while endeavoring to obtain further diagnostic information that would justify antifungal therapy. As has been pointed out by Jones,[5] the key to positive isolation of the causal organism in fungal infections is careful attention to diagnostic techniques and repeated attempts to isolate the microorganism in culture. Only in the most severe situations, when the clinical impression is strongly supportive of a fungal infection, might empirical therapy with an anti-

fungal agent be justifiable. In that circumstance, natamycin would appear to be the most appropriate agent. However, despite this justification, empirical therapy has rarely been necessary in my experience. When there is a strong clinical possibility of fungal infection in the face of a negative smear, I resort to repeated scraping and, if necessary, a biopsy in order to identify fungal material. Usually, this has been successful.

When an isolate is recovered, management is on firmer ground. Although precise identification of the microorganism may be considerably delayed, most laboratories can recognize the more common isolates. If a *Candida* or other yeast is recovered, therapy with flucytosine and natamycin should be continued.[5] If it is a filamentous infection, prompt identification of *Fusarium*, *Aspergillus*, or *Cladosporium* usually presents little difficulty and therapy with natamycin in each instance seems appropriate.[5, 6] In the case of an unidentified filamentous organism, natamycin once again should be employed. Thus, it is evident that in the initial stages of management of a fungal keratitis, natamycin and flucytosine are the mainstays of therapy. Together, they provide the broadest possible coverage for fungi likely to be isolated from the cornea.

Confirmation of the diagnosis of fungal infection is reassuring to the physician, placing his therapy on a firmer basis and providing him with some estimate of the course likely to be followed. However, several problems remain. How does one make a judgement of improvement? Is there any role for corticosteroid therapy? When should surgical intervention be employed? These are issues that continually confront the ophthalmologist in the management of each patient.

The course of recovery from a fungal keratitis is painstakingly slow. Whereas with bacterial infection one can begin to see resolution of the inflammatory changes and healing within a few days of starting antibiotic therapy, in most instances this is not the case with fungal infection. It may require *weeks* of intensive topical therapy before it becomes apparent that the keratitis is coming under control. During this period the hypopyon may wax and wane and the epithelium may periodically break down. Slowly, if topical therapy is appropriate, the keratitis will gradually resolve and it is often only in retrospect that the success of treatment becomes apparent. There is no preferred way of judging effectiveness of treatment, but careful clinical observation, supplemented by serial photography on a weekly basis, offers the best hope of detecting changes as they occur. One must largely ignore the appearance of the conjunctiva; the topically applied antifungal agents are quite irritating and, at the recommended doses, they frequently cause considerable conjunctival hyperemia, edema, and chemosis. Assessment of therapeutic efficacy is based almost entirely on the appearance of the cornea. However, the 5 per cent suspension of natamycin often forms white, ropelike strands that adhere to the surface of the corneal ulcer and collect in the inferior fornix, further complicating the evaluation. Implicit in all this is the need for prolonged topical therapy with antifungal agents. The initial intensive therapeutic regimen often can be modified, within a week to 10 days, to eight to ten drops a day, but this must be continued for at least 6 weeks.

Although natamycin, flucytosine, and miconazole are markedly less toxic than previously available antifungal agents, toxicity still occurs and may complicate therapy unless it is recognized (Fig. 18–9). If a case appears to be worsening despite what seems to be appropriate therapy, or if there is doubt that therapy is effective, then it is prudent to discontinue therapy for 24 hours and reculture the ulcer. When an infection appears to be resistant, one should consider the possibility of toxicity masking resolution of the inflammatory changes, the presence of another pathogen not yet isolated, or reinfection through contaminated ocular medications. I have also seen anterior keratitis develop as a result

of endogenous spread in intravenous drug abusers. Such patients may have recurrent infections despite apparently effective therapy.[7]

The decision to discontinue treatment on the basis of an apparent cure marks the final crucial point in management. Because these agents are fungistatic rather than fungicidal, the patient should be observed carefully for evidence of recrudescence of infection. Should reinfection occur, signs generally are forthcoming within a week. The lesion must be recultured and treated in the same manner as discussed above.

Corticosteroid Therapy

One of the most controversial aspects in the management of ocular inflammatory disease is the appropriate use of corticosteroid therapy. Very little has been published concerning the use of corticosteroids in fungal keratitis.[8-10] There is a justifiable fear that the administration of corticosteroid preparations will potentiate fungal infection and thus contribute to loss of the eye. The limited reports in the literature and my own experience suggest that, if certain principles are followed carefully, corticosteroid therapy is useful in the management of fungal infections of the cornea. These agents control the deleterious effects of the host response to the inflammatory stimulus.

There is a great deal of confusion regarding the concept of anti-inflammatory therapy in infectious disease. It is mandatory that corticosteroid treatment be administered only in combination with effective, specific antimicrobial therapy. In practical terms, this means that there must be evidence of a clinical response to a specific antifungal agent before use of the corticosteroid is considered. Since the whole purpose of corticosteroid therapy is to maintain the functional integrity of the cornea by limiting the harmful effects of the inflammatory response, their use should be restricted to situations in which vision is seriously threatened. Whereas corticosteroid therapy may be appropriate and necessary in an axially situated keratitis, lesions in the peripheral cornea generally do not require such treatment. Patients receiving this combined treatment must be under close observation so that the response can be monitored closely. Since perforation can occur in association with corticosteroid therapy, personnel with ophthalmic surgical skills must be available in case emergency corneal surgery becomes necessary. When there is definite evidence of a response to the antifungal agent and it is thought appropriate to initiate corticosteroid therapy, prednisolone acetate 1 per cent is begun at a dose of four times a day. The dose is then adjusted according to the clinical response that is observed and continued until healing occurs. Coverage with the antifungal agent is necessary, generally on at least a dose-for-dose basis, for the duration of steroid therapy. Abrupt cessation of treatment should be avoided, as this may lead to an inflammatory rebound and possible perforation.

The decision to employ corticosteroids in the treatment of fungal infection is not to be taken lightly. Unless one can comply with the conditions outlined above, it is preferable to avoid corticosteroids, though this may result in increased corneal scarring and the need for corneal transplantation at a later date. There can be no doubt that the use of corticosteroids in the presence of an ineffective antifungal agent or a partially treated fungal infection can be disastrous.

Surgery

Prior to the advent of reasonably effective antifungal therapy, aggressive surgical techniques were favored in the management of fungal keratitis.[9, 11-15] In fact, several series have been published to indicate the value of prompt therapeutic penetrating keratoplasty. At present, surgery seldom is needed during the acute phase of the infection, although it may be required later to restore vision if significant corneal scarring occurs. Occasionally, during the initial stages of infection, surgery in the form of penetrating keratoplasty or a lamellar patch graft may be required if perforation occurs. In such circumstances, a large corneal graft, encompassing the area of inflammation, is usually effective in combating the infectious process and in restoring the integrity of the globe. Only rarely has the recurrence of fungal infection been reported in the graft or in the recipient cornea peripheral to the host-graft interface; such recurrences have been due to unrecognized spread through apparently uninvolved corneas. In the past, a conjunctival flap has been advocated as a therapeutic measure in fungal keratitis, but it is rarely indicated now, except perhaps as a last resort when antifungal agents are unavailable or when there are other contraindications to continued medical treatment.

CONCLUSION

During the past 10 years, there has been a major change in the outlook for fungal infections of the cornea. Better diagnostic methods, more effective and less toxic antifungal agents, and an enhanced awareness of the pathogenic mechanisms involved in corneal inflammation have been responsible for this. There is reasonable hope that the near future will see even greater advances in the treatment of these difficult infections.

REFERENCES

1. Jones, D. B., Sexton, R., and Rebell, G.: Mycotic keratitis in South Florida: A review of thirty-nine cases. Trans Ophthalmol Soc UK 89:781, 1970.
2. Forster, R. K., and Rebell, G.: The diagnosis and management of keratomycoses. I. Cause and diagnosis. Arch Ophthalmol 93:975, 1975.
3. Jones, D. B.: Strategy for the initial management of suspected microbial keratitis. In Boswell, H. F. (ed.): Symposium on Medical and Surgical Diseases of the Cornea. St. Louis, C. V. Mosby Co., 1980, pp. 86–119.
4. O'Day, D. M., Akrabawi, P. L., Head, W. S., and Ratner, H. B.: Laboratory isolation techniques in human and experimental fungal infections. Amer J Ophthalmol 87:688, 1979.
5. Jones, B. R.: Principles in the management of oculomycoses. Trans Amer Acad Ophthalmol Otolaryngol 79:OP53, 1975.
6. Jones, D. B., Forster, R. K., and Rebell, G.: Fusarium solani keratitis treated with natamycin (pimaricin): Eighteen consecutive cases. Arch Ophthalmol 88:147, 1972.
7. Elliott, J. H., Podgorski, S. F., O'Day, D. M., and Akrabawi, P. L.: Mycotic endophthalmitis in drug abusers. Amer J Ophthalmol 88:66, 1979.
8. Aronson, S. B., and Elliott, J. H.: Ocular Inflammation. St. Louis, C. V. Mosby Co., 1972.
9. O'Day, D. M., Moore, T. E., and Aronson, S. B.: Deep fungal corneal abscess: Combined corticosteroid therapy. Arch Ophthalmol 86:414, 1971.
10. Newmark, E., Ellison, A. C., and Kaufman, H. E.: Combined pimaricin and dexamethasone therapy of keratomycosis. Amer J Ophthalmol 71:781, 1971.
11. Singh, G., and Malik, S. R. K.: Therapeutic keratoplasty in fungal corneal ulcers. Brit J Ophthalmol 65:41, 1972.
12. Polack, F. M., Kaufman, H. E., and Newmark, E.: Keratomycosis: Medical and surgical treatment. Arch Ophthalmol 85:410, 1971.
13. Sanders, N.: Penetrating keratoplasty in the treatment of fungal keratitis. Amer J Ophthalmol 70:24, 1970.
14. Jones, B. R., Jones, D. B., and Richards, A. B.: Surgery in the management of keratomycosis. Trans Ophthalmol Soc UK 89:887, 1969.
15. Forster, R. K., and Rebell, G.: Therapeutic surgery in failures of medical treatment of fungal keratitis. Brit J Ophthalmol 59:366, 1975.

Corneal Manifestations of Ocular Chlamydial Infections

19

ROBERT H. POIRIER, M.D.
SOHRAB DAROUGAR, M.D.

Ocular infections caused by *Chlamydia trachomatis* (trachoma inclusion conjunctivitis [TRIC] serotypes A to K) comprise two main groups, hyperendemic trachoma and paratrachoma.[1] The classical four stages of trachoma originally described by MacCallan (Table 19–1) outlined the changes found in this disease.[2] However, although corneal signs must be present to make a definitive clinical diagnosis of trachoma,[3] the MacCallan classification is based only on findings in the conjunctiva. Moreover, this classification fails to grade the intensity of disease and the degree of visual disability. It also tends to suggest that there is a simple, single-cycle progression of infection, whereas recent major observations have demonstrated that blinding trachoma is a multicyclic disease[1, 4] (Fig. 19–1). Trachoma remains the world's leading cause of preventable blindness, but of paramount importance is the observation that, depending on certain epidemiologic factors, trachoma is not necessarily blinding. Seemingly, amid the living conditions of industrialized areas trachoma rarely is transmitted. If the disease is acquired under these conditions, it generally is mild. Therefore, current concepts of this disease are perhaps best expressed from an epidemiologic standpoint using a system that separates ocular chlamydial infections into three distinct classes, as originally expressed by Jones.[1]

Class 1—Blinding Trachoma

The designation of class 1 trachoma is applied to infection by *Chlamydia trachomatis* serotypes A, B, Ba, and C in hyperendemic areas. Blinding trachoma occurs in eyes subjected to repeated infection by both chlamydiae and bacteria. *C. trachomatis* agent infection alone causes hyperendemic trachoma, but bacterial infection is required in addition to give rise to the complications that result in blindness.

Class 2—Nonblinding Trachoma

Class 2 trachoma includes infection by *C. trachomatis* serotypes A, B, and C in meso- or hypoendemic areas with better socioeconomic conditions. In these areas trachoma is generally mild with

Table 19–1. MacCALLAN CLASSIFICATION OF TRACHOMA

Stage 0	No signs of trachoma
Stage I	Immature follicles on upper tarsus including the central area; no conjunctival scarring
Stage IIa	Mature follicles on upper tarsus along with early papillary hypertrophy
Stage IIb	Mature follicles and advanced papillary hypertrophy of upper tarsus obscuring the tarsal vessels
Stage III	Follicles present on upper tarsus and definite scarring of the conjunctiva
Stage IV	No follicles on upper tarsus and definite scarring of the conjunctiva

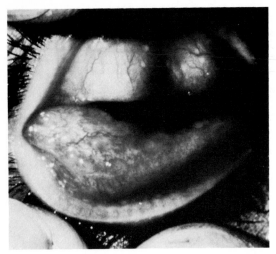

Figure 19-1. Stage 3 trachoma with reinfection from which *Chlamydia trachomatis* was isolated.

limited transmission among individuals because of improved hygiene. There is also a lower incidence of bacterial conjunctivitis.

Class 3—Paratrachoma

Class 3 trachoma includes infection by *C. trachomatis* serotypes D, E, F, G, H, I, J, and K, which commonly occurs in the urban populations of developed countries. Jones[1] uses the term paratrachoma to designate ocular and/or genital infection by *C. trachomatis* where chlamydia spread via sexual transmission from a genital reservoir with sporadic transfer to the eye. Conjunctival and corneal changes of variable severity result. Such *C. trachomatis* agent infections may present as ophthalmia neonatorum, adult inclusion conjunctivitis, *C. trachomatis* agent punctate keratoconjunctivitis, or trachoma of sexual transmission.[1]

CORNEAL MANIFESTATIONS

Blinding Trachoma

Corneal damage caused by trachoma is responsible for most of the preventable blindness in developing countries. The World Health Organization estimates that there are some 500 million people

affected by trachoma and that 2 million are blind as a result of the disease.[5] Corneal involvement by chlamydial infection can be adequately characterized only by describing the conjunctivitis that accompanies it. Indeed, trachoma basically is a chronic inflammatory process of the mucous membranes lining the posterior surface of the lids and the anterior scleral portion of the globe. It begins as a chronic follicular conjunctivitis, primarily involving the upper tarsal conjunctiva, followed in time by varying degrees of papillary hypertrophy and infiltration of the conjunctiva. As the disease progresses, conjunctival scarring occurs. Fine, linear scarring is observed in mild cases and broader confluent scars in the more severe cases. Conjunctival scarring is associated with a deficiency of tears and with distortion of the lids, particularly the upper lid, causing entropion and trichiasis. These factors are intimately linked to the pathogenesis of trachomatous keratopathy (Figs. 19–2 and 19–3). Severe corneal changes occur most often in areas where reinfections are frequent and where superimposed bacterial infections accelerate the cicatricial conjunctival response.

There is a general tendency for trachomatous corneal opacification to progress in severity with age. In villages where trachoma flourishes, the greatest number of individuals with serious visual loss is among adults.[6, 7] However, infants are nearly all infected by 3 months of age in hyperendemic areas, and superimposed bacterial corneal ulcerations with perforation are a significant reason for permanent visual loss in these children.

The continuous abrasion of the cornea by misdirected lashes in a relatively dry eye accounts for much of the destructive keratopathy. Areas of focal superficial keratitis, including punctate epithelial erosions (PEE) and punctate epithelial keratitis (PEK) are common (Fig. 19–4). The epithelial keratitis of trachoma typically involves the upper half of the cornea, but it is not uncommon to observe diffuse PEK in association with trachomatous keratoconjunctivitis sicca.

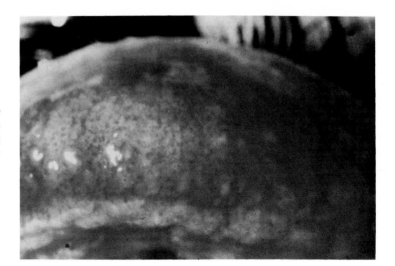

Figure 19–2. Marked papillary and follicular reaction of the upper fornix in association with early linear and stellate scarring.

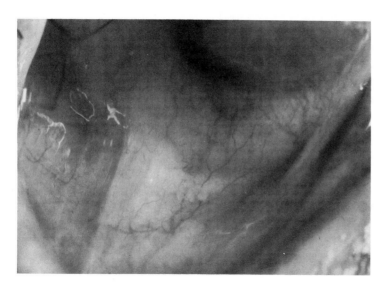

Figure 19–3. Markedly shortened lower fornix with diffuse sheet scarring and entropion.

Figure 19–4. Area of focal punctate epithelial keratitis (PEK).

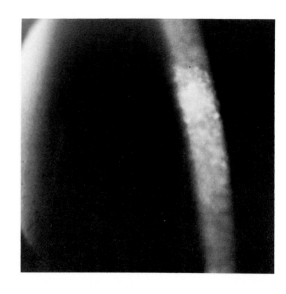

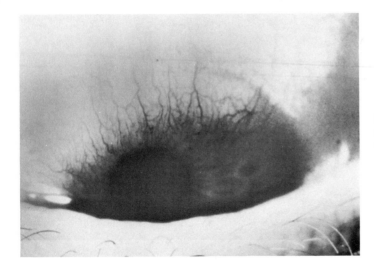

Figure 19–5. Characteristic superior pannus of severe hyperendemic trachoma.

Epithelial changes in the marginal cornea may be due either to active infection or to trichiasis. In addition, areas of punctate subepithelial keratitis (PSK) may be observed; they appear as pleomorphic, grayish opacities insinuated between vascular loops of a pannus, located at or near the corneal limbus.

A superior corneal pannus, when coupled with the characteristic conjunctival changes, is a pathognomonic sign of trachoma (Fig. 19–5). The pannus consists of a fibrovascular membrane associated with cellular infiltration and scarring. This superficial fibrovascular sheet descends from the upper limbus and covers the superior peripheral cornea, for which it has a predilection. In severe untreated cases the invading vessels may progress over the visual axis. Between the loops and branches of these uniform vessels there may be dense stromal infiltration, leaving grayish opacification. Lymphoid follicles may form at the limbus and subsequently become necrotic and scar, leaving the classic depressions known as Herbert's pits (Fig. 19–6). Occasionally, coincident marginal droplet corneal degeneration may be found in the elderly.

Diffuse opacification of the cornea (ground glass) and marked corneal thinning with vascularization are also significant forms of corneal involvement (Fig. 19–7).[6] The distribution of trachomatous corneal opacities in a large

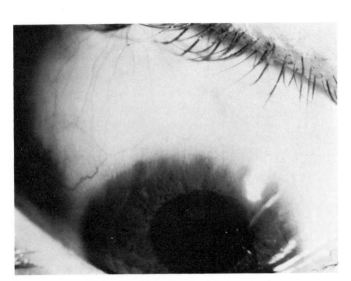

Figure 19–6. Classic Herbert's pits at superior limbus in a case of long standing trachoma.

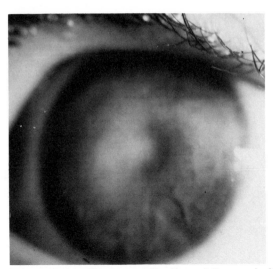

Figure 19–7. Diffuse opacification of the central cornea in a villager from Sar-Rig, Iran.

series of patients showed a predilection for the central cornea (40 per cent). Secondary bacterial ulceration frequently occurs in these compromised corneas. Superficial foreign body scars are common, and the pearllike excrescences of Salzmann's nodular dystrophy may form on the corneal surface. Descemetoceles, corneal perforation, and totally shrunken phthisic eyes complete the spectrum of severity found in areas of blinding trachoma.

Trachomatous individuals in hyperendemic areas commonly lose their eyelashes, but attempts by these individuals to remove misdirected cilia are not ef-

fective. Usually their lids are thickened, and significant ptosis, severe trichiasis, and entropion are present. The entire conjunctival architecture may be abnormal with scarring, fibrosis, calcification, and neovascularization (Figs. 19–8, 19–9, and 19–10). These severe lid changes and the chronic conjunctivitis serve as a continuous attraction for the flies that torment afflicted individuals. The flies feed on ocular discharges and also harbor ocular bacterial pathogens. Fluorescein placed in the eye of one child was transmitted by flies to the eyes of other nearby children within a 20- to 40-minute interval.[1] Thus, it is highly probable that flies act as vectors, carrying chlamydial and bacterial pathogens from the eyes of one individual to another in an affected community, thereby facilitating the spread of recurrent conjunctivitis (Figs. 19–11 and 19–12). As we have indicated, the end result includes a superior trachomatous pannus, dense corneal scarring, keratoconjunctivitis sicca, and reactive corneal neovascularization secondary to trichiasis and entropion.

According to the World Health Organization,[3] the diagnosis of trachoma requires the presence of two of the following signs: (1) lymphoid follicles on the upper tarsal conjunctiva; (2) typical conjunctival scarring; (3) vascular pannus; and (4) limbal follicles or their sequelae, Herbert's pits. The presence of at least two of these signs should be regarded

Figure 19–8. Post-trachomatous degeneration of upper tarsus.

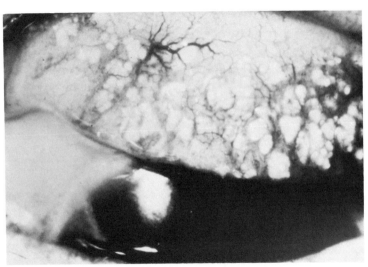

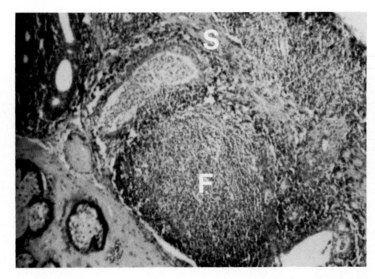

Figure 19–9. Trachoma with follicle formation (F) and scarring (S). (×450.) (Wilson Collection, Institute of Ophthalmology, London).

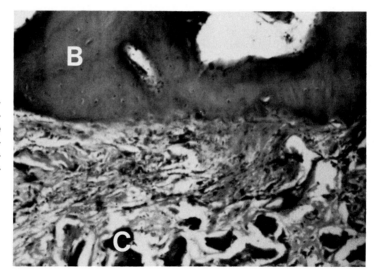

Figure 19–10. Complete disorganization of normal lid architecture with calcium (C) and bone formation (B) in patient with posttrachomatous degeneration (Wilson Collection, Institute of Ophthalmology, London).

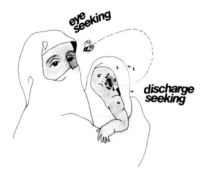

eye seeking

discharge seeking

Figure 19–11. Interpersonal transmission of ocular discharges between mother and infant.

role of flies in
COMMUNICABLE OPHTHALMIA

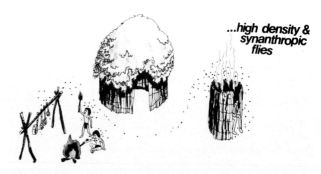

...high density & synanthropic flies

Figure 19–12. High-risk environmental factors of poverty and lack of sanitary facilities close the environmental lock in a chain of epidemiologic factors that includes synanthropic flies.

ENVIRONMENTALLY DETERMINED

only as minimal criteria upon which to base a clinical diagnosis. Their presence in a significant proportion of suspected cases in a community indicates that trachoma is endemic in the population.

Nonblinding Trachoma

In nonblinding trachoma the conjunctival changes usually are milder with fine scarring and little conjunctival degeneration (Fig. 19–13). There is minimal superior corneal pannus.

Paratrachoma

The spectrum of disease in this group includes chlamydial ophthalmia neonatorum or inclusion conjunctivitis of the newborn, adult inclusion conjunctivitis in which there is generally no corneal

involvement, TRIC agent (chlamydial) punctate keratoconjunctivitis (TPK), and cases virtually identical to typical trachoma. The causal chlamydial agent is genitally transmitted, so that the disease is most prevalent among those who come in contact with genital tract secretions, newborns and sexually active adults. The conjunctival response in adults generally is a mixed reaction with both papillary and follicular changes, whereas the follicular response in infants is absent (Fig. 19–14). This group of disorders rarely produces the blinding complications associated with true trachoma.

The incubation period of chlamydial ophthalmia neonatorum classically is said to be 5 to 12 days after birth. However, if the placental membranes rupture before delivery, infection can occur earlier and has been documented as early as the first day of life. Initially there is a

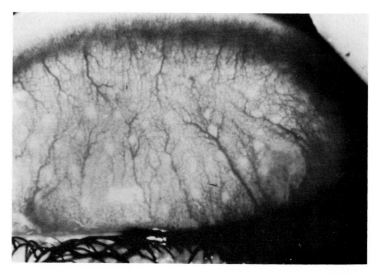

Figure 19–13. Mild trachomatous papillary and follicular response in a school-aged youngster in Minab, Iran, where a better standard of living has contributed to a reduction in the number of cases of blindness resulting from trachomatous disease.

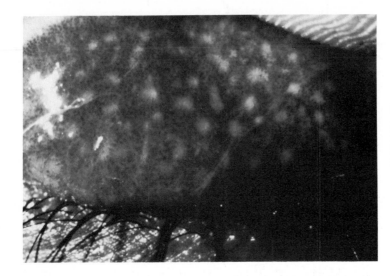

Figure 19–14. Severe mixed papillary and follicular reaction in a 24-year-old from San Antonio, Texas, with paratrachoma (TRIC agent).

slight watery discharge, which becomes progressively more copious and more purulent. The eyelids become swollen and there is moderately severe conjunctival hyperemia. The palpebral conjunctiva becomes thickened as a result of diffuse infiltration by inflammatory cells, and this is manifested as papillary hypertrophy. Pseudomembranes may develop. The conjunctivitis of chlamydial ophthalmia neonatorum occasionally produces conjunctival scarring.[8] One child in a large series was found to have scarring, follicles, and a significant pannus, and opacification of the corneal stroma and pannus, identical to trachoma, was observed in another child from whom *Chlamydia trachomatis* type E was isolated[9, 10] (Fig. 19–15).

The conjunctival response in adults is characterized by hyperemia, a mucoid discharge, and papillary hypertrophy. Small lymphoid follicles then become evident and tend to become particularly prominent in the lower conjunctiva. The patient generally is symptomatic and complains of a foreign body sensation. Ptosis of the upper lid and preauricular adenopathy frequently accompany the conjunctivitis. Corneal involvement is common and takes the form of a diffuse punctate epithelial keratitis and/or discrete subepithelial infiltrates. The latter tend to be most prevalent near the lim-

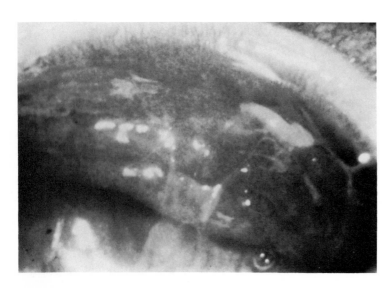

Figure 19–15. Nonfollicular papillary reaction with early synechial scarring in an infant with chlamydial ophthalmia neonatorum.

bus (marginal infiltrates) and may be accompanied by corneal neovascularization. At times the neovascularization may be extensive and a trachoma-like pannus may form. Conjunctival scarring is rare but has been reported.[1]

The corneal manifestations of TRIC agent punctate keratoconjunctivitis (TPK) consist of superficial punctate epithelial keratitis, deep punctate epithelial keratitis, and subepithelial punctate keratitis. The punctate epithelial keratitis associated with the early state of infection presents as spots that may be fine or coarse and that are opaque, slightly raised, and visible on slit-lamp examination (Fig. 19–16). They stain poorly with fluorescein but take up rose bengal. It has been suggested that those alterations are due to chlamydial invasion.[11] In deep punctate epithelial keratitis the lesions are in basal epithelium

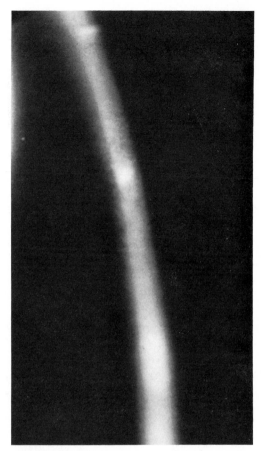

Figure 19–17. Deep punctate epithelial keratitis in TRIC agent keratoconjunctivitis.

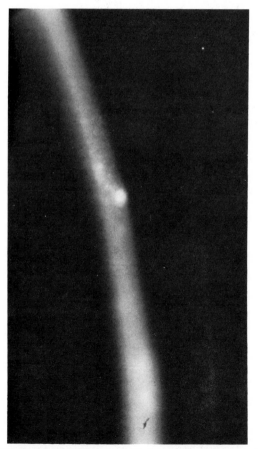

Figure 19–16. Raised PEK (punctate epithelial keratitis) in a 28-year-old female with paratrachoma (TRIC agent punctate keratoconjunctivitis).

and may invade Bowman's membrane (Fig. 19–17). When the infection continues for 3 weeks or more, subepithelial punctate lesions may appear. The lesions are large and have a dirty yellowish tinge; they may be visible to the naked eye (Fig. 19–18). The lesions are generally located in the upper half of the cornea near the limbus, but in severe corneal involvement they may appear in other areas of the cornea. As these spots become less active, they lose their contour and density and become less distinctive. The subepithelial punctate keratitis may persist for several months. In severe untreated cases a reactive micropannus may form at the upper limbus, and it may progress to a classic pannus (Fig. 19–19). When this is coupled with conjunctival scarring, it is virtually indistinguishable from trachoma as defined by the WHO Expert Committee on Trachoma (Figs. 19–20 and 19–21).

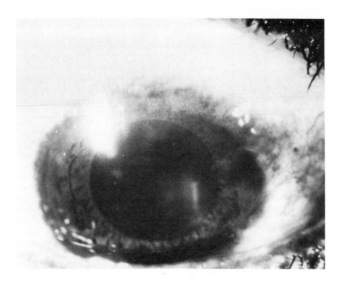

Figure 19–18. Large subepithelial lesions in TRIC agent (chlamydial) keratoconjunctivitis.

Figure 19–19. Micropannus and subepithelial keratitis in a young adult with paratrachoma.

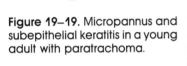
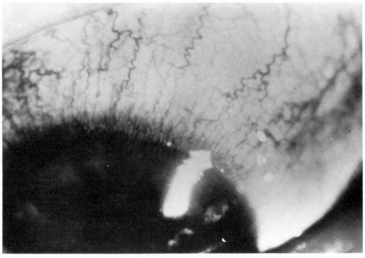

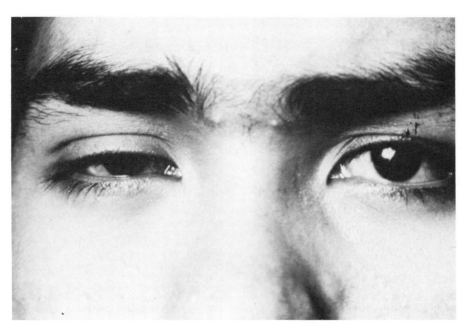

Figure 19–20. Chronic paratrachoma with pannus, conjunctival scarring, and ptosis.

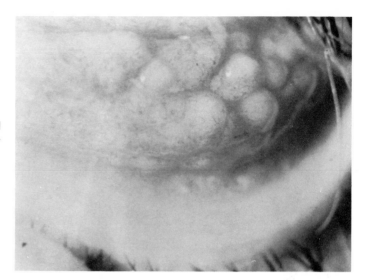

Figure 19–21. Chronic follicles and linear scars in patient with paratrachoma.

LABORATORY DIAGNOSIS

TRIC agent punctate keratoconjunctivitis (TPK) and adenovirus infection frequently are confused. Their differentiation, and indeed the diagnosis of paratrachoma, is of paramount importance since there is effective treatment for chlamydial infections (Figs. 19–22 and 19–23).[12] Several laboratory tests are available to assist in the diagnosis of chlamydial infections of the eye. In conjunctival scrapings, chlamydial inclusions can be demonstrated by Giemsa, iodine, or fluorescein-antibody staining.[13, 14] The classic Halberstaedter-Prowazek intracytoplasmic inclusion bodies are intracellular microcolonies of *Chlamydia trachomatis*. The sensitivity of these tests is poor except in cases of chlamydial ophthalmia neonatorum (Fig. 19–24). In the acute stage of infection cytologic demonstration of a mixed population of polymorphonuclear and mononuclear cells is suggestive of chlamydial ocular infection. Cultural tests for isolation of chlamydiae in irradiated McCoy cells, McCoy cells treated with IUDR or cycloheximide, and HeLa cells

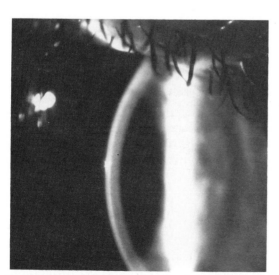

Figure 19–22. Isolated subepithelial keratitis in a patient with adenoviral keratoconjunctivitis not infrequently confused clinically with TRIC agent (chlamydial) infection.

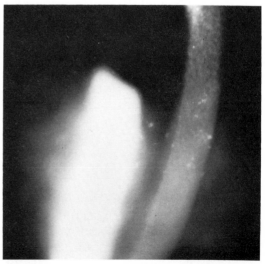

Figure 19–23. Fine and coarse epithelial keratitis in an adenoviral infection clinically indistinguishable from early TRIC agent infection.

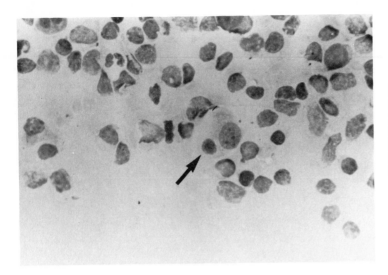

Figure 19–24. Classic Halberstaedter-Prowazek intracytoplasmic inclusion (*arrow*) stained with Giemsa in conjunctival epithelial cell from an infant with chlamydial ophthalmia neonatorum. (× 1000.)

treated with DEAE-dextran are highly sensitive methods.[15, 16, 17] Cultural isolation in irradiated McCoy cells has yielded chlamydiae in up to 90 per cent of chlamydial ophthalmia neonatorum and inclusion conjunctivitis cases and in up to 72 per cent of cases of severe hyperendemic trachoma.[18]

Cultures require specialized facilities and experienced staff; regrettably, they are not available in many centers. However, a rapid and simple serologic test for chlamydial infections has been described.[19] It is based on the detection of type-specific IgG and IgM in blood and IgG and IgA in the tears using a modified microimmunofluorescence test. Tear samples are collected by application of small sponges into the lower fornix, and finger-prick blood samples are also collected on cellulose sponges. The specimens can be sent to the laboratory without cold storage. This serologic test is as sensitive as cultural tests for diagnosis of chlamydial ocular infections.

TREATMENT

Trachoma

Treatment programs for trachoma have included evaluation of vaccines for prevention of the disease, but to date the results have been disappointing.[1, 20] At the present time there is no effective vaccine that can be recommended for use in human populations.[21]

Chemotherapy can be highly effective, though the optimal agent and route of administration are not entirely clear. Tetracycline ointment has been the mainstay of treatment and is usually given twice daily for 6 consecutive days each week for one half year.[5] Erythromycin ointment is also effective and can be substituted for tetracycline. However, topical ointments cannot be completely relied upon in individuals with thickened and scarred conjunctiva. Oral tetracyclines, particularly the long-acting preparations, are effective, but their use must be limited in children under 7 years of age and in pregnant women and nursing mothers. Continuous delivery of erythromycin estolate at a rate of 10 μg. per hour from inserts has been evaluated and the results appear promising.[1] Oral sulfonamides are effective but cause an unacceptably high incidence of side effects; they are less effective locally.

In individuals at high risk from trichiasis and entropion, surgical repair can forestall the likelihood of serious corneal involvement.[22] For those in whom corneal disease has resulted in marked visual loss, the promise of large-scale visual rehabilitation programs, including keratoplasty, remains largely unfulfilled. The expense, lack of corneal donor material, and logistics of follow-up care render the programs impractical. Economic growth of developing nations with improvement in standards of living, including those in rural areas, holds the greatest potential for reducing the number of people needlessly blinded by trachoma.

Paratrachoma

Paratrachoma infections respond well to chemotherapy. Chlamydial ophthalmia neonatorum responds to topically applied sulfonamides, tetracyclines, or erythromycin given four times daily for 2 to 3 weeks.[9] Although recent studies have shown a significant failure rate,[21] most treatment failures are thought to be the result of inadequate application of the drug by the parents of children with the disease. Ointments are difficult to apply to the eyes of children, and ophthalmic formulations of tetracycline and erythromycin are available only in this form. It has been suggested that treatment with antibiotic ointment be supplemented with sulfonamide drops instilled prior to each dose of ointment.[21]

In addition to the ocular manifestations in babies, chlamydial pneumonia has been reported.[23] Systemic treatment with tetracycline is effective but is contraindicated in the pediatric population (age 8 and under) and in the nursing mother. Erythromycin and sulfonamides are currently the most acceptable alternate drugs.[24]

Adults with paratrachoma respond promptly to oral tetracyclines. A dose of 1 gram of tetracycline per day (250 mg. four times daily) is usually prescribed, though 1.5 grams daily (500 mg. three times a day) has been recommended for those weighing more than 150 pounds.[21] In either case the drug must be taken for 3 weeks to eliminate infection and effect a cure. Oral erythromycin also is effective in the treatment of adult paratrachoma. Like the tetracyclines, erythromycin must be used in full recommended doses for 3 weeks. Oral sulfonamides similarly are effective, but their use is associated with a high incidence of undesirable side effects and appears to be merited only under unusual circumstances. Rifampicin and chloramphenicol have also been advocated.[25]

Topical tetracycline appears to have only a limited effect on adult paratrachoma. It seemingly suppresses or eliminates the agent if administered for 3 to 6 weeks, but the keratitis and follicular conjunctivitis resolve only partially.[21] Moreover, topical therapy has no effect on the genital infection that usually accompanies adult paratrachoma. The administration of topical tetracycline in conjunction with a systemic antibiotic might be of value.

The parents of infants with chlamydial ophthalmia neonatorum as well as the consorts of young adults with paratrachoma should be treated in a manner identical to that used in treating the adult with overt disease.

SUMMARY

Serious corneal disease secondary to infections caused by *Chlamydia trachomatis* is found in hyperendemic trachoma areas and accounts for the majority of the world's preventable blindness. Rural epidemiologic factors that facilitate the transmission of trachoma and contribute to its severity remain as significant problems for public health programs in developing nations.

In industrialized areas paratrachoma infections caused by *Chlamydia trachomatis* produce a spectrum of corneal and conjunctival disease. These infections range from chlamydial ophthalmia neonatorum to TRIC agent punctate keratoconjunctivitis to cases virtually identical to trachoma. These chlamydial infections may be mistaken for adenoviral keratoconjunctivitis, but recent diagnostic advances allow the clinician to make the diagnosis and ensure effective chemotherapy.

REFERENCES

1. Jones, B. R.: The prevention of blindness from trachoma. Trans Ophthalmol Soc UK 95:16, 1975.
2. MacCallan, A. F.: Epidemiology of trachoma. Brit J Ophthalmol 15:369, 1931.
3. World Health Organization Technical Report Series No. 234. Expert Committee on Trachoma. Third Report 3–48. Geneva, World Health Organization, 1962.
4. Jones, B. R., Darougar, S., Mohsenine, H., and Poirier, R. H.: Communicable ophthalmia: The blinding scourge of the Middle East. Brit J Ophthalmol 60:492, 1976.
5. Tarizzo, M. L. (ed.): Field Methods for the Control of Trachoma. Geneva, World Health Organization, 1973.
6. Hosni, F. A.: Clinical aspects of corneal trachoma. Brit J Ophthalmol 62:159, 1978.
7. Dawson, C. R., Daghfous, T., Messadi, M., Hoshiwara, I., and Schachter, J.: Severe endemic trachoma in Tunisia. Brit J Ophthalmol 60:245, 1976.
8. Forster, R. K., Dawson, C. R., and Schachter, J.: Late follow-up of patients with neonatal inclusion conjunctivitis. Amer J Ophthalmol 69:467, 1970.
9. Freedman, A., Al-Hussaini, M. K., Dunlop, E. M. C., Emarah, M. H. M., Garland, J. A., Harper, I. A., Jones, B. R., Race, J. W., duToit, M. S., Treharne, J. D., and Wright, D. J. M.: Infection by TRIC agent and other members of the Bedsonia group; with a note on Reiter's disease. Trans Ophthalmol Soc UK 86:313, 1966.
10. Markham, R. H. C., Richmond, S. J., Walshaw, N. W. D., and Easty, D. L.: Severe persistent inclusion conjunctivitis in a young child. Amer J Ophthalmol 83:414, 1977.
11. Jones, B. R.: The clinical features of viral keratitis and a concept of their pathogenesis. Proc R Soc Med 51:917, 1958.
12. Poirier, R. H.: Chlamydial infections: Diagnosis and management. Trans Amer Acad Ophthalmol Otolaryngol 79:109, 1975.
13. Jones, B. R.: Laboratory tests for chlamydial infection. Brit J Ophthalmol 58:438, 1974.
14. Gordon, F. B., Dressler, H. R., and Quan, A. L.: Relative sensitivity of cell culture and yolk sac for detection of TRIC infection. Amer J Ophthalmol 63(Suppl):1044, 1967.
15. Darougar, S., Kinnison, J. R., and Jones, B. R.: Simplified irradiated McCoy cell culture for isolation of Chlamydiae. Excerpta Medica Int Cong Ser 223:63, 1970.
16. Schachter, J.: Chlamydial infections. N Engl J Med 298:540, 1978.
17. Kuo, C. C., Wang, S. P., Wentworth, B. B., and Grayston, J. T.: Primary isolation of TRIC organisms in HeLa 229 cells treated with DEAE-dextran. J Infect Dis 125:665, 1972.
18. Darougar, S., Woodland, R. M., Forsey, T., Cubitt, S., Allami, J., and Jones, B. R.: Isolation of Chlamydia from ocular infections. In Hobson, D., and Holmes, K. K. (eds.): Nongonococcal Urethritis and Related Infections. Washington, American Society for Microbiology, 1977, pp. 295–298.
19. Darougar, S., Treharne, J. D., Minassian, D., El-Sheikh, H., Dines, R. J., and Jones, B. R.: Rapid serological test for diagnosis of chlamydial ocular infections. Brit J Ophthalmol 62:503, 1978.
20. Clements, S., Dhir, S. P., Grayston, J. T., and Wang, S. P.: Long term follow-up study of a trachoma vaccine trial in villages of northern India. Amer J Ophthalmol 87:350, 1979.
21. Schachter, J., and Dawson, C. R.: Human Chlamydial Infections. Littleton, Mass., PSG Publishing Co., 1978.
22. Sandford-Smith, J. H.: Surgical correction of trachomatous cicatricial entropion. Brit J Ophthalmol 60:253, 1976.
23. Beem, M. O., and Saxon, E. M.: Respiratory tract colonization and a distinctive pneumonia syndrome in infants infected with Chlamydia trachomatis. N Engl J Med 293:306, 1977.
24. Beem, M. O., and Saxon, E. M.: Letter to the editor. N Engl J Med 296:1124, 1977.
25. Darougar, S., Viswalingam, M., Treharne, J. D., Kinnison, J. R., and Jones, B. R.: Treatment of TRIC infection of the eye with rifampicin or chloramphenicol. Brit J Ophthalmol 61:255, 1977.

VIII

CORNEAL ABNORMALITIES RESULTING FROM LACRIMAL INSUFFICIENCY

Diagnosis and Management of Tear Film Dysfunction

20

R. DOYLE STULTING, M.D., Ph.D.
GEORGE O. WARING III, M.D.

The dry eye or, more precisely, tear film dysfunction commonly aggravates both patients and ophthalmologists. Tear film dysfunction often spurs the patient to the ophthalmologist initially, and, since the disorder is chronic, frequently drives the exasperated patient to a succession of ophthalmologists. The harried clinician can assume one of two attitudes toward this persistent problem: (1) give the patient some reassurance, a cursory explanation of "dry eyes," a handful of artificial tears, and a return appointment "in a year or so," or (2) take an orderly approach to ferret out the diagnosis and design useful management.

In this chapter we present a systematic clinical approach to the diagnosis and management of tear film dysfunction. The first section deals with diagnosis, including appreciation of the patient's psychologic stress, assessment of ocular signs, and evaluation of related systemic disease. We then outline techniques of management, beginning with satisfaction of psychologic needs, proceeding to local therapy of the eye itself, and concluding with management of associated systemic disease.

PATHOPHYSIOLOGY OF THE TEAR FILM

The preocular tear film is currently conceptualized as a three-component structure (Fig. 20–1, Table 20–1). Mucin, primarily produced by conjunctival goblet cells, spreads directly over the hydrophobic surface of the epithelium, reducing the surface tension and allowing the aqueous layer to spread uniformly over the cornea and conjunctiva. Without mucin the aqueous tears would bead up on the surface of the lipid-containing, hydrophobic epithelial cell walls like rain water on a newly waxed car. The aqueous layer produced by acinar secretory cells of the main lacrimal gland and by the accessory lacrimal glands contributes most of the volume to the tear film, carries inorganic salts, lysozyme, and immune globulin, and allows diffusion of oxygen to the avascular cornea. The surface lipid layer, produced by the meibomian glands, is thought to retard evaporation, to lubricate the lids, and to assist in preventing the tear meniscus from flowing over the lid margin. Tears are normally produced at a rate of 1 to 2 μl. per minute, maintaining an average volume of 5 to 10 μl. in the conjunctival cul-de-sac and preocular tear film.

Between blinks the surface lipid molecules diffuse through the aqueous component, contaminating the mucin layer, increasing the surface tension, and producing breakup of the tear film. The resultant focal dry spots stimulate corneal nerve endings to produce a reflex blink. As the upper lid descends like a squeegee over the ocular surface, it sweeps the contaminated mucous layer into the inferior fornix, where a fine mucous thread forms, to be removed by the lacrimal drainage system. When the lids open, aqueous and lipid spread over the surface of the globe, reconstituting the tear film (Fig. 20–2). For details of

Table 20–1. COMPONENTS OF PREOCULAR TEAR FILM

Component	Major Source	Major Components	Function	Affected Disease States
Lipid	Meibomian glands	Waxy and cholesterol esters	Lubrication ↓ Evaporation ↑ Tear film thickness	Seborrheic blepharitis
Aqueous	Main and accessory lacrimal glands	Water (98%) Lysozyme Tear-specific prealbumin Lactoferrin Immunoglobulin A Other proteins Electrolytes	Hydration Lubrication Antimicrobial Oxygenization Mechanical debris removal	Keratoconjunctivitis sicca
Mucin	Goblet cells	Glycoproteins	↓ Surface tension	Hypovitaminosis A

this model, the reader is referred to published reviews.[1,2]

Although there are disorders that primarily involve a single layer of the tear film (e.g., decreased mucus production in vitamin A deficiency, reduced aqueous production in keratoconjunctivitis sicca, and abnormal lipid production in meibomian keratoconjunctivitis), it is often difficult clinically to isolate and identify discrete dysfunction of a single tear film layer. For example, in keratoconjunctivitis sicca, a primary aqueous deficiency, corneal drying can result in epithelial irregularities that interact poorly with the mucin layer. Decreased bacteriostatic and flushing action by the tear film may allow colonization by pathogenic bacteria that produces a low-

grade conjunctivitis or blepharitis, with resultant lid deformity and meibomian gland dysfunction. Thus, although the three-component tear film concept is important, the clinician should recognize that multiple-component dysfunction is common.

The term triple S syndrome has been suggested to describe the association of seborrhea, staphylococcus, and sicca, all of which result in punctate epithelial keratopathy. The seborrheic component is manifested as meibomian gland dysfunction, commonly associated with seborrheic dermatitis, seborrhea sicca, or acne rosacea.[3] Reduced or altered meibomian secretions may destabilize the tear film or exert a toxic effect on the corneal epithelium; it has been sug-

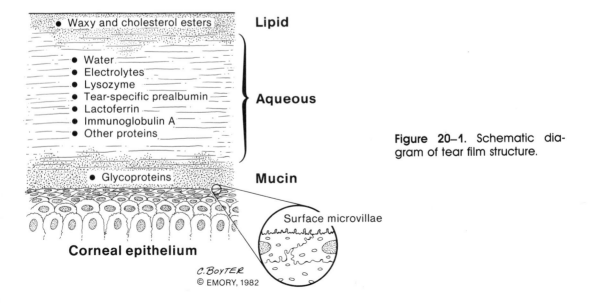

Figure 20–1. Schematic diagram of tear film structure.

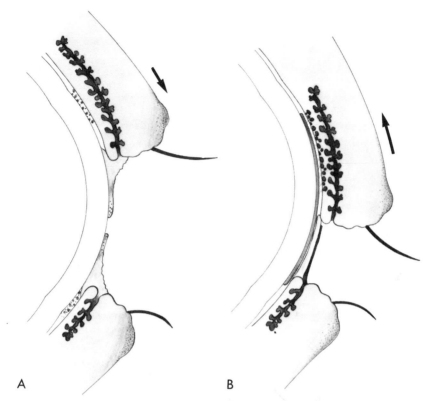

A   B

Figure 20–2. Theoretical model of tear resurfacing by blinking. *A,* As upper eyelid descends, it removes the broken-up, contaminated tear film in a squeegeelike manner. *B,* As the upper lid rises, the goblet cells deposit mucin on the corneal epithelium, aqueous tears are pulled up from the marginal tear strip, and meibomian glands lay down a superficial lipid layer. (From Waring, G. O.: Discussion of presentation by Wepman, B., and Baum, J.: Ocular findings in Bell's palsy. Ophthalmology *86:*1947, 1979. Used by permission.)

gested that this occurs when triglycerides are de-esterified to form free fatty acids, perhaps by the action of bacterial lipases. The staphylococcus and other organisms that are permitted by tear dysfunction to colonize the ocular surfaces produce exotoxins that may contribute to irritative ocular symptoms.

TERMINOLOGY

The terms used in this field are often confusing, some of them being very loosely defined and others changing their meaning from a historical usage to more contemporary usage. We discuss the terminology here in an attempt to clarify the problems for the reader and to define their use in this chapter.

Dry Eye. This colloquial nonspecific term refers to any tear film abnormality, usually with corneal epithelial abnormalities.

Tear Film Dysfunction. This more formal nonspecific term designates any tear film abnormality and specifically includes disorders of the aqueous, mucin, and lipid components of the tear film.

Keratoconjunctivitis Sicca. This is a specific deficiency of the aqueous component of the tear film. It is usually included as part of Sjögren's syndrome. Literally the term denotes inflammation of the cornea and conjunctiva secondary to drying.

Mucin Deficiency. This term denotes a specific deficiency of the mucous component of the tear film, usually associated with scarring and keratinization of the conjunctiva.

Xerophthalmia. Etymologically this term means "dry eye," but it has come to denote ocular manifestations of vitamin A deficiency and protein-calorie malnutrition, from focal conjunctival keratinization through keratomalacia.

Meibomian Keratoconjunctivitis. This term refers to inflammation of the cornea and conjunctiva resulting from excess, deficient, or abnormal meibomian gland secretions.

Sjögren's Syndrome. Definitions of this systemic disease have changed since Sjögren's studies in the 1930s and vary in different medical specialties. The disorder includes a combination of aqueous tear deficiency, salivary gland dysfunction, and a systemic inflammatory disease, usually a connective tissue disorder. Many clinicians currently recognize two types of Sjögren's syndrome: (1) inflammation of multiple exocrine glands, usually the lacrimal and salivary glands, without an associated well-defined systemic connective tissue disease; this is also called primary Sjögren's syndrome, the sicca syndrome, or sicca complex; and (2) a systemic connective tissue disorder associated with either dry eyes or dry mouth, referred to as secondary Sjögren's syndrome. In either of the two types the salivary and lacrimal glands may be enlarged.

SUBJECTIVE DIAGNOSIS

The patient with tear film dysfunction may complain of vague symptoms that to the physician, who frequently sees people going blind, may represent relatively minor complaints. However, even the most minor discomfort, when constantly present—like sand in one's shoe or the Chinese water torture—can disrupt a patient's lifestyle. Such persistent discomfort can trigger fears of glaucoma, cataracts, cancer, or blindness. It is therefore important to listen carefully and empathize as the patient describes these problems.

When the tear film fails to perform its functions of lubrication, oxygenation, and removal of debris, symptoms of foreign body sensation (grittiness, scratchiness, sandiness), fatigue, and dryness result (Table 20–2). The patient may

Table 20–2. SYMPTOMS OF TEAR FILM DYSFUNCTION

Symptoms usually worse in evening
Foreign body sensation (grittiness, sandy, scratchy feeling)
Fatigue when reading or watching television
Burning
Photophobia
Blurred vision or fluctuating acuity
Dry sensation
Tearing or excessive mucous secretions
Decreased tearing in response to irritations or emotions

experience severe pain, especially in the presence of filamentary keratopathy. Loss of the smooth refractive surface of the tear film causes blurred vision, which can vary from blink to blink, accounting for a variable manifest refraction and for complaints of variable vision throughout the day. Surface drying may produce reflex tearing and the misleading complaint of *excess* tears. Typically, symptoms of tear deficiency are worse late in the day, with prolonged use of the eyes (as when the patient reads or watches television), and in conditions of heat, wind, and low humidity (as on the beach or ski slopes). Symptoms that are worse in the morning suggest an associated chronic blepharitis, recurrent corneal epithelial erosion, or exposure keratopathy.

OCULAR SIGNS OF TEAR FILM DYSFUNCTION

Evaluation of the ocular signs of tear film dysfunction (Table 20–3) begins with observation during the interview. This is the best time to measure blink rate, to study completeness of blinks, and to look for epiphora—before the patient has been subjected to bright lights, drops, and manipulation of the eyes. The skin around the eyes should be examined for the presence of contributory dermatologic problems such as rosacea as well as for signs of topical drug toxicity (e.g., eczematoid wrinkling of the eyelid skin).

Using first a hand light and then the slit lamp, one should examine the con-

Table 20–3. SIGNS OF TEAR FILM DYSFUNCTION

Sign	Comment
Bulbar conjunctival vascular dilation	Diffuse distribution over globe without limbal accentuation
Redundancy of inferotemporal bulbar conjunctiva	Roll of conjunctiva may lie on eyelid margin
Decreased height of tear meniscus	May be influenced by factors such as lid position
Irregular corneal surface	Manifested as loss of luster and irregular light reflection
Increased tear film debris	Best seen with slit lamp as fine particles in retroillumination or stained with rose bengal
Punctate epithelial keratopathy	Best seen with slit lamp in broad tangential illumination as gray dots localized over inferior third of cornea; stain with rose bengal and fluorescein
Filaments and mucous plaques	Located anywhere on corneal surface
Marginal or paracentral thinning or perforation	Usually occurs quietly with minimal inflammation or pain
Inadequate blinking	Incomplete blinks or nocturnal lagophthalmos
Meibomian gland dysfunction	Inspissation, dilatation, cheesy discharge with lid massage, recurrent chalazion
Blepharitis	Lid margin irregularity, erythema, and edema with loss of lashes

figuration of the lid margin, its approximation to the ocular surface, and the completeness of voluntary gentle lid closure.[4] Eyelid inflammation, crusting, sparseness of lashes, trichiasis, inspissation and dilation of meibomian glands, telangiectases of the eyelid margin, and irregularity of the eyelid margin are signs of chronic blepharitis. Plaques of keratinization suggest severe drying, as in cicatricial pemphigoid.

The marginal tear strip serves as a tear reservoir; it has been suggested that estimation of its height with the slit lamp might be a useful measure of tear film volume.[1] A tear meniscus less than 0.1 mm. high occurs in only 7 per cent of a normal population;[5] however, the tear film meniscus height does not correlate well with tear flow rate as measured by the Schirmer test, possibly because meniscus height reflects other variables such as blink rate, interpalpebral fissure width, lid position, and distance of the meibomian glands from the globe.[5] We find this test (assessment of tear meniscus height) to be of questionable value in evaluating patients with tear film dysfunction.

Before manipulating the lids, the clinician should examine the precorneal tear film with the slit lamp—using direct focal illumination, broad tangential illumination, and retroillumination—searching for small gray particles of mucus and debris floating up and down against a background of focal gray epithelial dots in the interpalpebral area. These findings, easily accentuated by rose bengal stain, strongly suggest keratoconjunctivitis sicca. The reduced tear flow less efficiently washes the debris toward the lacrimal puncta, so it accumulates in the tear film and in the mucous thread that occupies the inferior conjunctival cul-de-sac. The clinician also searches for the corneal epithelial abnormalities caused by dry eyes, dry spots, and punctate epithelial keratopathy. Dry spots appear as irregular geographic patches (best seen in retroillumination) where the tear film breaks up rapidly, allowing the superficial corneal epithelium to desiccate, lose its surface microprojections, and desquamate, forming the focal gray spots of punctate epithelial keratopathy (Fig. 20–3).[6] These spots reflect the presence of abnormal epithelial cells that have keratinized, lost their desmosomal attachments, and developed breaks in their plasma membrane.[7]

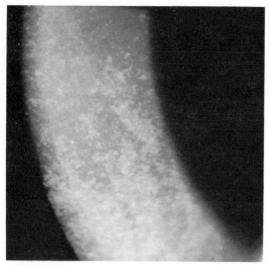

Figure 20–3. Punctate epithelial keratopathy. Multiple gray spots on the corneal surface represent abnormal epithelial cells that have keratinized, lost their desmosomal attachments, and developed breaks in their plasma membrane.

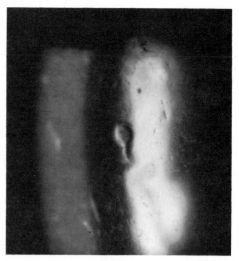

Figure 20–4. Filaments of mucus, desquamated cells, and cellular debris in keratoconjunctivitis sicca.

It has been suggested that mucus production is increased in aqueous tear deficiency. However, since the number of goblet cells is decreased in keratitis sicca, the increased mucus probably reflects a decreased rate of removal due to diminished tear flow, rather than increased production.[8] Mucus adheres to foci of degenerated corneal epithelial cells to form filaments (Fig. 20–4)[7, 9] or plaques (Fig. 20–5).[10] Filaments are discrete, translucent, bulbous strands of mucus, intertwined desquamated cells,

and cellular debris that dangle from the corneal surface and stain with fluorescein and rose bengal. They vary in length from a small stub to 1 cm. In keratoconjunctivitis sicca they are characteristically located on the inferior third of the cornea. Blinking produces severe pain because the filaments are firmly attached to the richly innervated epithelium. The flat, white, amorphous plaques consist of mucus and epithelial cells embedded in a proteinaceous matrix. Symptoms related to mucous plaques are generally less severe than those from filaments, and they often are

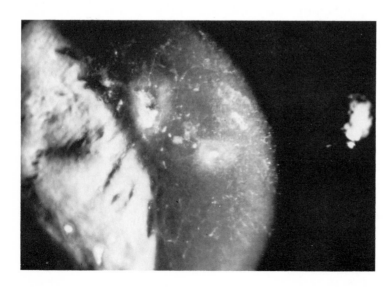

Figure 20–5. Mucous plaques in a case of severe keratoconjunctivitis sicca.

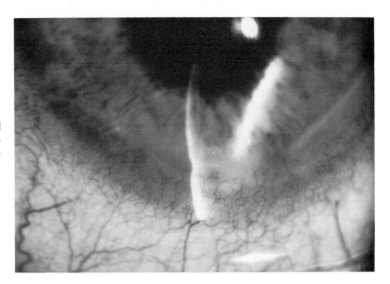

Figure 20–6. Inferior marginal furrow in a patient with keratoconjunctivitis sicca and rheumatoid arthritis.

difficult to distinguish from those of the underlying tear deficiency.

Corneal thinning and perforation can complicate keratoconjunctivitis sicca, particularly in the presence of rheumatoid arthritis.[11, 12] This keratolysis usually produces little ocular inflammation, corneal infiltration, pain, or vascularization. It can occur beneath an intact epithelium. Discrete marginal furrows or gutters appear parallel to the limbus, usually inferiorly (Fig. 20–6), and can extend 360°, producing a central island of cornea that looks like a contact lens.[11] Alternatively, a smooth-sided crater may appear centrally (Fig. 20–7).[13, 14] Either type may perforate quietly, become

sealed by iris, and heal, only to be discovered later by the ophthalmologist as an incidental finding during routine examination or when a similar process recurs in the same eye or involves the opposite eye (Fig. 20–8). Progressive corneal melting may follow cataract surgery in patients with tear deficiency.[14] The pathogenesis of this melting is unclear but probably reflects the same abnormal connective tissue destruction and poor healing ability characteristic of associated diseases like rheumatoid arthritis.

After the initial examination, several diagnostic procedures can be carried out to investigate further and to quantitate tear film function (Table 20–4).

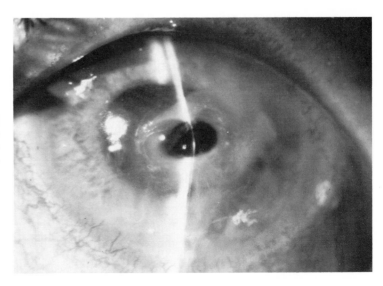

Figure 20–7. Central corneal melting with formation of a descemetocele in a case of keratoconjunctivitis sicca and rheumatoid arthritis.

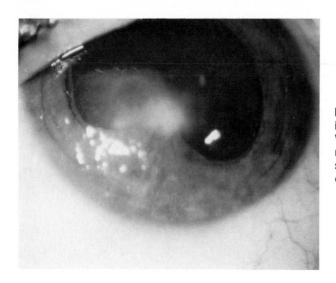

Figure 20–8. Healed corneal perforation in a patient with keratoconjunctivitis sicca. When located peripherally, a perforation may be sealed by iris and heal without symptoms, to be found later on routine examination.

Special Stains

Patients with tear film dysfunction probably become symptomatic because of dry spots on the cornea. Identification of dry areas with topically applied stains substantiates the diagnosis. Patients who complain of nonspecific itching, burning, and stinging without identifiable corneal surface pathology present a more difficult diagnostic problem. The two commonly used dyes are rose bengal and fluorescein, although alcian blue, tetrazolium, trypan blue, and bromothymol blue have also been tried.[15]

Rose bengal is a vital dye (tetraiodotetrachlorofluorescein) that stains dead and degenerating epithelial cells; it neither penetrates into the corneal stroma nor diffuses into the intercellular spaces of the epithelium as fluorescein does. Keratinization and conjunctival epithelial abnormalities are more easily visualized with rose bengal than with fluorescein, and rose bengal stains mucous particles, strands, filaments, and plaques more vividly than fluorescein. Rose ben-

Table 20–4. AIDS IN DIAGNOSIS OF TEAR FILM DYSFUNCTION

Rose bengal stain
Fluorescein stain
Schirmer test
Tear lysozyme level
Tear osmolarity
Tear breakup time

gal is, therefore, a more useful diagnostic stain in tear film deficiencies.

Only small volumes of rose bengal dye are sold. As a result, drug companies find marketing it unprofitable, and it is sometimes commercially unavailable. At the time of this writing, rose bengal is available in a 1 per cent ophthalmic solution (Smith & Nephew, England; Akorn, USA) and as dye-impregnated paper strips (Barnes-Hind).

Rose bengal produces discomfort on instillation into the conjunctival cul-de-sac and it stains facial skin and clothing; therefore, many clinicians prefer to instill only a fraction of a drop in the eye. They snap a cotton applicator handle in two, leaving a slightly ragged end on which they place part of a drop, and then transfer it to the inferior cul-de-sac, warning the patient of the discomfort prior to instillation. The discomfort is approximately proportional to the amount of staining that occurs,[16] so that it may be considerable in many patients with tear film dysfunction. Excess dye is rinsed from the eye with an irrigating solution.

Normal eyes exhibit minimal rose bengal staining of the cornea and conjunctiva, usually inferonasally and on the caruncle. In keratoconjunctivitis sicca a strip of punctate staining appears across the globe within the palpebral fissure (Figs. 20–9 and 20–10). Sjögren thought that this staining pattern was

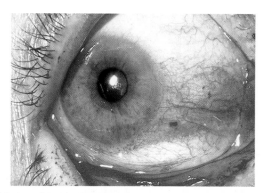

Figure 20–9. Triangular pattern of rose bengal staining of the medial bulbar conjunctiva corresponding to the palpebral fissure in a patient with keratoconjunctivitis sicca.

pathognomonic for aqueous tear deficiency.[17] Van Bijsterveld devised a scoring system to quantitate the degree of rose bengal staining.[18] He estimated the intensity of staining in three areas, the medial bulbar conjunctiva, the lateral bulbar conjunctiva, and the cornea; each area was assigned a score of 0 to 3 points, for a maximum score of 9 points. Using this system, normals were accurately distinguished from abnormals with a 4 per cent false positive and 5 per cent false negative rate, using 3.5 points as the upper limit of normal.[18]

Rose bengal highlights the small mucous particles that float in the tear film, the filaments that cling to the corneal surface, and the excessively large mucous thread in the cul-de-sac. Areas of keratinization of the conjunctiva also stain brilliantly.[15] (If rose bengal is instilled after Schirmer testing, localized artifactitious conjunctival staining will occur at the site of filter paper placement.)

Fluorescein is a water-soluble dye that is excluded from the cornea by the intact epithelium. In tear deficiency states small focal areas of degenerated corneal epithelium take up the fluorescein stain to create a diffuse stippled pattern, usually over the inferior third of the cornea (punctate epithelial keratopathy, PEK). Fluorescein fails to stain the excess mucus or conjunctival changes that accompany tear film dysfunction.

Schirmer Test

Clinical measures of tear film volume and tear flow rates would help the clinician quantitate the severity of aqueous deficiency in keratoconjunctivitis sicca. Although methods of obtaining these data are available using sophisticated apparatus such as fluorophotometry, they are not useful in daily clinical practice. These methods have documented that the tears normally are produced at a rate of about 1 to 2 μl. per minute, with an average volume in the conjunctival cul-de-sac and preocular tear film of 5 to 10 μl. However, the Schirmer test, though crude by comparison, remains the only practical clinical measurement of tear production.

The Schirmer test measures the volume of tears produced during a fixed time period. It is performed by placing the folded 5-mm. end of a standard size number 41 Whatman filter paper strip over the lower lid, between its middle third and lateral third. The patient, with eyes open in a dimly lighted room, looks straight ahead and blinks normally. After 5 minutes the strip is removed,

Figure 20–10. Diagrammatic illustration of the rose bengal staining pattern in keratoconjunctivitis sicca.

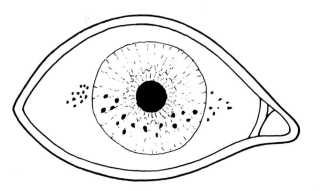

and the amount of wetting is measured from the fold. Jones modified the Schirmer test by the instillation of topical anesthetic, being careful to remove excess fluid before insertion of the filter paper.[19] He reasoned that this technique would eliminate the reflex tearing produced by irritation from the filter paper and that the resultant wetting would then represent basic tear secretion, primarily from the glands of Krause and Wolfring. The clinical value of these two techniques continues to be debated.

Although Schirmer reported 15 mm. of wetting as the lower limit of normal, lower values are common in asymptomatic subjects.[18, 20] One report indicates that even if 5.5 mm. of wetting were used as the lower limit of normal, one out of every six asymptomatic individuals would be misclassified as having a tear deficiency.[18] An individual, when tested on multiple occasions, may give extremely variable Schirmer test results.[21] Perhaps a part of the variability in Schirmer test results seen by many investigators is due to lack of careful attention to variables such as lid margin stimulation and variable time after drop instillation.[22] In spite of its imprecision, the test is simple, inexpensive, readily available, easily performed, and without side effects. As such, it remains one of the most common clinical techniques for measuring aqueous tear production.

We think the Schirmer test is especially valuable when it shows readings of only a few millimeters without anesthetic, a clear documentation of a severe decrease in tear production.

Tear Lysozyme

Lysozyme is an antibacterial enzyme, representing approximately 30 per cent of total tear protein, that cleaves the mucopeptide bacterial cell wall component N-acetyl glucosamine (β 1–4) N-acetyl-muramic acid at the β 1–4 linkage. It is secreted by the acinar and ductular epithelial cells of the lacrimal gland, and its concentration in the tears of patients with keratoconjunctivitis sicca is decreased.[23, 24] The lysozyme test is more sensitive and accurate than the Schirmer test and rose bengal staining for the diagnosis of keratoconjunctivitis sicca, with a false positive rate of 1 per cent and a false negative rate of less than 2 per cent.[18] The tear lysozyme concentration varies remarkably little with age,[18, 25] but there are small variations in normal individuals at different times of measurement and in response to environmental changes.[26, 27]

Lysozyme can be measured spectrophotometrically by its ability to clear a suspension of *Micrococcus lysodeikticus* into which a tear sample is placed.[28] Alternatively, the diameter of the zone of lysis surrounding a tear-soaked disk placed on a *Micrococcus lysodeikticus*–seeded agar plate can be determined.[29, 30] More recently, a radial immunodiffusion technique has been described.[31] Because of special laboratory requirements, the test is available at only a few centers.

Tear Osmolarity

Because of reduced aqueous secretion, the concentration of solutes in the tears is elevated in keratoconjunctivitis sicca. When 311 milliosmoles per liter is used as the upper limit of normal, elevated tear osmolarity is 95 per cent sensitive and 94 per cent specific for this disorder.[32] It is important that tear samples be obtained from the tear meniscus using a micropipette without stimulating reflex tearing and that samples be transported under oil to prevent evaporation.[33] Osmolarity is determined by freezing point depression with a commercially available osmometer capable of performing measurements on samples as small as 0.1 μl. Because special techniques are required for sample handling and special equipment needed for determination of osmolarity may not be readily available, this technique has not gained widespread use.

Tear Film Breakup Time

The development of focal corneal dry spots is the basic mechanism by which tear film dysfunction affects the cornea. A useful clinical method to detect these spots is the tear breakup time, the time between a complete blink and the appearance of the first randomly distributed corneal dry spot.[34] It is a clinical estimate of the length of time that the tear film remains stable and intact. Decreased tear film breakup time is thought to be the hallmark of mucin-deficient tears and does not necessarily correlate with aqueous tear production as measured by the Schirmer test.[35-37]

To measure the tear breakup time, a fluorescein strip moistened slightly with balanced salt solution or similar ocular irrigant is touched lightly against the inferior tarsal conjunctiva, and the patient is asked to blink several times to distribute the dye throughout the tear film. The examiner may not touch the lids, but simply encourages the patient to stare straight ahead without blinking while he observes the cornea through the slit-lamp biomicroscope using broad tangential illumination with the cobalt blue filter. The time between a complete blink and the appearance of the first defect (black spot) in the fluorescein film is measured with a stopwatch (Fig. 20–11). Several determinations are made in succession and the individual results are averaged.

Normal tear breakup time has been reported as greater than or equal to 10 seconds,[34] although the normal value may be lower and may not be closely reproducible.[38] It is susceptible to variables such as lid holding (which may stretch the tear film), topical anesthetics (which damage epithelial surface microprojections),[34] and environmental conditions (such as humidity and air flow). It therefore must be performed carefully and before any ophthalmic drops are instilled. Results may vary when individuals are measured on multiple occasions,[38] reducing the clinical usefulness of the test. Nonetheless, breakup time remains the only convenient direct clinical measurement of tear film stability and certainly has diagnostic value when it is very short (i.e., 1 to 2 seconds).

The tear breakup time is defined with respect to the appearance of *randomly* distributed dry spots and, as such, reflects the tear film stability over the normal corneal surface. The occurrence of nonrandomly distributed dry spots reflects the presence of localized corneal surface irregularities and not just tear film dysfunction.[39]

Dye Dilution Tests

An estimate of tear production can be made by observing the rate at which topically instilled dye disappears from the preocular tear film. This may be done qualitatively with the slit lamp using a mixture of fluorescein and rose bengal[40] or quantitatively using a fluorophotometer.[41] Although these tests demonstrate significantly reduced tear volumes in keratoconjunctivitis sicca, they do not correlate well with the severity of rose bengal staining or with the values of the Schirmer test.[42]

SYSTEMIC DIAGNOSIS

Although Sjögren was not the first to describe the association of chronic arthritis, keratoconjunctivitis sicca, and xerostomia, his classic monograph published in 1933[43] increased recognition of the syndrome that now bears his name. Keratoconjunctivitis sicca may also be associated with several other systemic disorders (Table 20–5), most notably systemic lupus erythematosus (SLE).

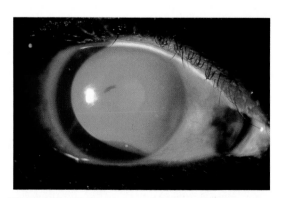

Figure 20–11. Break-up of the tear film can be observed as the appearance of a dark spot when the fluorescein-containing tear film is observed with cobalt-blue filtered light.

Table 20–5. CONDITIONS ASSOCIATED WITH TEAR FILM DYSFUNCTION*

Alterations in the Tear Film Composition

Aqueous Deficiency

Congenital

1. Aplasia or hypoplasia of the lacrimal gland (alacrima congenita, Bonnevie-Ullrich syndrome)
2. Anhidrotic ectodermal dysplasia
3. Aplasia of lacrimal nerve nucleus
4. Congenital familial sensory neuropathy with anhidrosis
5. Familial autonomic dysfunction (Riley-Day syndrome)
6. Holmes-Adie syndrome (pupillotonia, hyporeflexia, segmental hypohidrosis)
7. Multiple endocrine neoplasia

Acquired

1. Senile or idiopathic atrophy of lacrimal gland
2. Atrophy or hypofunction of the lacrimal gland associated with systemic diseases
   A. Connective tissue diseases
      Rheumatoid arthritis
      Systemic lupus erythematosus
      Periarteritis nodosa
      Scleroderma
   B. Hematopoietic and reticuloendothelial disorders
      Felty's syndrome
      Malignant lymphoma
      Lymphosarcoma
      Thrombocytopenic purpura
      Lymphoid leukemia
      Hemolytic anemia
      Hypergammaglobulinemia
      Waldenström's macroglobulinemia
      Chronic hepatitis
      Primary biliary cirrhosis
   C. Endocrine dysfunction
      Hashimoto's disease
      Climacteric in females
   D. Renal disorders
      Renal tubular acidosis
      Diabetes insipidus
   E. Skin and mucocutaneous diseases (mainly cause mucus deficiency but may reduce aqueous tear flow due to scar formation)
      Acanthosis nigricans
      Scleroderma
      Erythema multiforme (Stevens-Johnson syndrome)
      Exfoliative dermatitis
      Ocular cicatricial pemphigoid
      Dermatitis herpetiformis
      Epidermolysis bullosa
      Ichthyosiform erythroderma
      Congenital ichthyosis
   F. Miscellaneous
      Sarcoidosis
      Adult celiac disease
      Amyloidosis
      Lipodystrophy
3. Postsurgical
   Partial or total dacryoadenectomies
   After blepharoplasty
4. Traumatic, inflammatory, or neoplastic lesions of the lacrimal gland

5. Neuroparalytic
   Lesions of VII nerve and geniculate ganglion
   Lesions of greater superficial petrosal nerve
   Lesions of sphenopalatine ganglion and the lacrimal branch
   Lesions of trigeminal nerve, including gasserian ganglion
6. Toxic and iatrogenic
   Belladonna and its alkaloids
   Botulism
   Deep anesthesia
   Practolol
7. Nutritional and debilitating disorders
   Typhus
   Cholera
   Starvation
   Ascorbic acid and vitamin B_{12} deficiency (?)

Mucus Deficiency

1. Vitamin A deficiency
2. Diphtheritic keratoconjunctivitis
3. Trachoma
4. Mucocutaneous disorders enumerated above
5. Chemical, thermal, and radiational injuries of the conjunctiva
6. Topical medications: echothiophate iodide, sulfonamides, and practolol

Lipid Deficiency

1. Chronic blepharitis
2. Acne rosacea

Surface Abnormalities Causing Faulty Dispersion of Tear Film

Focal Elevations or Depressions on Corneal Surface

1. Multiple forms of punctate epithelial keratopathy
2. Salzmann's nodular degeneration
3. Nonhealing epithelial or stromal defects
4. Epithelial basement membrane dystrophy (map, dot, fingerprint)
5. Lattice corneal dystrophy
6. Reis-Bückler's corneal dystrophy
7. Epithelial edema

Elevations at Limbus Leading to Dellen Formation

1. Pterygium
2. Postoperative inflammatory reaction
3. Neoplasms

Improper Contact Lens Fit

Defective Spreading of the Tear Film

Alterations of Blink Mechanism

1. CNS disorders
2. Hyperthyroidism
3. Drug induced
4. After contact lens wear

Lagophthalmos

1. Facial palsy
2. Nocturnal lagophthalmos
3. Scars of the lids
   Traumatic
   After blepharoplasty
   After infection (e.g., zoster)

Mechanical Factors

1. Exophthalmos
2. Ectropion
3. Symblepharon

*Modified from Maudgal, P. C., and Missotten, L. (eds.): *Superficial Keratitis*. The Hague, Dr. W. Junk Publishers, 1981, p. 151.

The essential histopathologic feature of Sjögren's syndrome is lymphocytic destruction of the exocrine glands. These lymphoid infiltrates are composed of both T and B cells.[44] As the disease progresses, connective tissue replaces the normal lacrimal gland architecture. The formation of islands of myoepithelial cells is a characteristic feature of Sjögren's syndrome.

Various definitions have been given for Sjögren's syndrome. Some require the presence of keratoconjunctivitis sicca, xerostomia, and arthritis (although only 62 per cent of Sjögren's cases had arthritis).[17] Others require either clinical evidence of keratoconjunctivitis sicca or pathologic features of the disease in lacrimal or salivary gland biopsy specimens. More recently it has been suggested that *primary* Sjögren's syndrome be defined as the presence of both xerostomia and keratoconjunctivitis sicca without an associated systemic connective tissue disorder and that *secondary* Sjögren's syndrome be defined as the presence of a well-documented connective tissue disorder in addition to xerostomia or keratoconjunctivitis sicca. Stated differently, aqueous tear deficiency may occur alone (keratoconjunctivitis sicca), in association with dry mouth (primary Sjögren's syndrome), or as a manifestation of systemic connective tissue disease (secondary Sjögren's syndrome) (Fig. 20–12). There is now evidence that the clinical, laboratory, genetic, and immunologic characteristics of primary and secondary Sjögren's syndrome are different, supporting this classification (Table 20–6).[44, 45]

Nonocular exocrine gland dysfunction is common in Sjögren's syndrome. Salivary gland involvement may cause a sensation of dry mouth with fissured lips and tongue along with difficulty in chewing or swallowing. There may be severe dental caries and atrophy of the filiform papillae of the tongue. Crusts may form in the nose and there may be a chronic cough. Recurrent salivary gland enlargement has been reported in 74 to 82 per cent of patients with primary Sjögren's syndrome, but it was

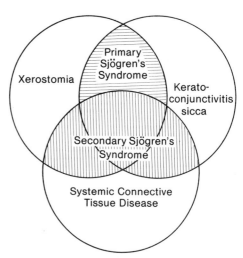

Figure 20–12. Classification of exocrine gland disorders. Aqueous tear deficiency can occur alone (keratoconjunctivitis sicca), in combination with salivary gland dysfunction (primary Sjögren's syndrome), or in association with systemic connective tissue disease (secondary Sjögren's syndrome). (Modified from Manthorpe, R., et al.: Sjögren's syndrome. A review with emphasis on immunological features. Allergy *36*:139, 1981. © 1981, Munskgaard International Publishers Ltd., Copenhagen, Denmark.)

seen in only 14 to 23 per cent of patients with secondary Sjögren's syndrome associated with rheumatoid arthritis.[47, 48] Respiratory tract involvement produces hoarseness, nonproductive cough, and increased incidence of respiratory tract infections. Dysphagia, gastric mucosal atrophy, and atrophic gastritis occur in addition to vaginal dryness with associated dyspareunia and pruritus.

Extraglandular lymphocytic infiltration involving kidney, liver, lung, or muscle occurs in about 25 per cent of patients with Sjögren's syndrome.[45] Purpura, Raynaud's phenomenon, renal involvement, and myositis are more common in primary than in secondary Sjögren's syndrome.[46] Other systemic symptoms may include fever, fatigue, arthralgias, and myalgias.

An elevated sedimentation rate appears in most patients with primary or secondary Sjögren's syndrome.[48] Leukopenia occurs in about 30 per cent of patients with primary Sjögren's syndrome and is common in secondary Sjögren's syndrome associated with SLE, but rarely appears in secondary Sjö-

Table 20–6. CLINICAL, GENETIC, AND IMMUNOLOGIC FEATURES OF PRIMARY AND SECONDARY SJÖGREN'S SYNDROME

| | | Secondary Sjögren's Syndrome | | |
Finding	Primary Sjögren's Syndrome (Per Cent)	With Rheumatoid Arthritis (Per Cent)	With Systemic Lupus Erythematosus (Per Cent)	References
Clinical				
History of parotid enlargement	74–82	14–23	1–10[1]	47, 48, 76
Parotid enlargement on examination	39	26	–	48
Purpura	45	5	9–20[1]	47, 76
Renal involvement	27	0	46–65[1]	47, 76
Myositis	23	0	48[1]	47, 76
Raynaud's phenomenon	32	5	10–26[1]	47, 76
Lymphadenopathy	50	18	29–59[1]	47, 76
Genetic				
HLA-B8	59	9	—	77
HLA-DRW3	64	9	—	77
HLA-DRW4	28	64	—	77
Immunologic				
Antinuclear antibody	56–88	56–100	90[1]	48, 76, 78, 79
LE-cell	0	20	75–80[1]	48, 76
Anti–salivary duct antibody	25	69[2]	–	45
Anti–SS-A	70–88	0–9	58	79, 80
Anti–SS-B	48–71	0–3	8	79, 80
Anti-Ha	73	6[3]	85[4]	81
Anti-DNA	0	0	55	78
Rheumatoid arthritis precipitin	5	76	7[1]	79

1. Frequencies for systemic lupus erythematosus patients not selected for Sjögren's syndrome.
2. 26% with rheumatoid arthritis alone.
3. 0% with rheumatoid arthritis alone.
4. 3% with systemic lupus erythematosus alone.

gren's syndrome associated with rheumatoid arthritis. Thrombocytosis is seen in Sjögren's syndrome associated with rheumatoid arthritis; thrombocytopenia occurs in Sjögren's syndrome associated with SLE.[46]

A variety of autoantibodies have been found in patients with Sjögren's syndrome (Table 20–6). Antinuclear antibody (ANA) is present in most patients with primary or secondary disease. Anti–salivary duct antibody is found in about 20 per cent of patients with primary Sjögren's syndrome (interestingly, it is seen in about the same proportion of patients with rheumatoid arthritis alone) and in 70 per cent of patients with Sjögren's syndrome secondary to rheumatoid arthritis. Several non–organ-specific autoantibodies against soluble nuclear antigens have also been identified. Of particular interest are the soluble nuclear antigens SS-B and Ha.

Described independently and varying slightly in physical properties, these antigens are immunologically similar or identical. Most patients with primary Sjögren's syndrome produce antibodies to SS-B and Ha; however, such antibodies are rare in patients with Sjögren's syndrome associated with rheumatoid arthritis. (Interestingly, anti-Ha has been found in most patients with Sjögren's syndrome associated with SLE, whereas anti–SS-B is reportedly uncommon in that group.) In contrast, rheumatoid arthritis precipitin is found in patients with Sjögren's syndrome associated with rheumatoid arthritis but not in primary Sjögren's syndrome or in Sjögren's syndrome associated with SLE. Thus, these non–organ-specific autoantibodies may enhance our ability to distinguish between primary and secondary Sjögren's syndrome.

Tissue typing data also suggest a genetic difference between primary and secondary Sjögren's syndrome. HLA-DRW3 and HLA-B8 are increased in frequency in primary Sjögren's syndrome. In contrast, the frequencies of HLA-DRW3 and HLA-B8 are not increased in Sjögren's syndrome with rheumatoid arthritis, whereas the frequency of HLA-DRW4 is elevated (Table 20–6).

The true incidence of Sjögren's syndrome is unknown. One might argue that the decrease in tear flow that occurs with age[20] causes many of the complaints in patients with common "dry eyes." However, postmortem examination has revealed classic parotid changes in four out of 900 cases,[16] and other clinical studies have indicated that the diagnosis of Sjögren's syndrome is commonly overlooked. In fact, it has been estimated that Sjögren's syndrome is the second most prevalent autoimmune disease, following rheumatoid arthritis.[16]

The diagnosis of Sjögren's syndrome is important because of the frequent association of Sjögren's syndrome and systemic disease. Female patients with primary or secondary Sjögren's syndrome are 44 times more likely than the normal population to develop lymphoid malignancy. If parotid enlargement has occurred sometime during the course of the disease, risk of lymphoid malignancy is increased to 67 times that of a normal population.[49] Thyroid function abnormalities also are common in Sjögren's syndrome.[48] A recent investigation of 24 patients with Sjögren's syndrome disclosed evidence of thyroid dysfunction in 16. Two of these patients had clinically evident but unrecognized hypothyroidism. Ten were already on replacement therapy at the time of the study.[50]

Thus, the ophthalmologist must attempt to identify those patients with dry eye complaints who fall into the diagnostic category of Sjögren's syndrome. This can be accomplished by seeking a history of fever, malaise, weight loss, myalgias, arthralgias, and other unexplained systemic symptoms. Laboratory evaluation should include a hemogram, sedimentation rate, antinuclear anti-body, rheumatoid factor, serum protein electrophoresis, thyroid function studies, and anti–SS-A and anti–SS-B.

Finally, when suspicion of Sjögren's syndrome is high, a labial biopsy to look for lymphoid infiltration of the minor salivary glands, diagnostic of Sjögren's syndrome, can be performed.[51] These glands are located inside the lip; the biopsy is best performed by an otolaryngologist.

When a diagnosis of Sjögren's syndrome has been made, the physician should remain alert for the appearance of new symptoms that might signify the onset of treatable systemic disease, e.g., thyroid dysfunction, lymphoid malignancy, or undiagnosed connective tissue disease.

MANAGEMENT

Tear film dysfunction is a chronic disorder that the clinician and patient can usually control but not cure. For successful management the clinician must deal effectively with three areas: psychologic, ocular, and systemic.

Psychologic Management

The cornerstone of management is an empathetic and careful explanation of dry eyes in terms that the patient can understand. Although it takes extra time and great patience to close the examining room door and give such thoughtful counseling, this will surely reduce the patient's complaints, chronic frustration, and consultation with multiple ophthalmologists. In mild tear film deficiency states unassociated with systemic disease it is important that the patient know that (1) the disease is chronic and incurable, (2) its symptoms can be controlled by careful adherence to a therapeutic regimen, (3) adherence to such a regimen may be more disruptive than the disease itself, and (4) the condition is not likely to lead to serious or permanent ocular damage.

A different approach is required for

the patient with severe tear deficiency. The physician must communicate a more urgent message, emphasizing the possible loss of sight and the potential need for minor surgical procedures like tarsorrhaphy or punctal occlusion. The patient must know that "dry eye" is an incurable disease that can lead to loss of sight and that strict adherence to a therapeutic regimen is required to keep the disease under control. Although the physician should seek symptoms of a lymphoid malignancy associated with Sjögren's syndrome (fever, fatigue, lymphadenopathy, etc.),[49] it seems unreasonable to frighten the systemically asymptomatic patient with comments about an increased risk of cancer.

Ocular Management

Ocular therapy for tear film deficiency is directed toward the following goals: (1) replacement using tear substitutes, (2) decreased tear drainage, (3) decreased tear evaporation, (4) improved surfacing by the tear film, (5) treatment of associated local problems (e.g., symptomatic mucous strands, blepharitis), and (6) increased tear production. It is important to direct management simultaneously toward both tear film abnormalities and associated disorders to achieve a maximal and sustained response to therapy. We therefore offer a step-by-step approach to the local management of tear deficiency.

Artificial Tears

Replacement with artificial tears is the cornerstone of therapy in most cases. Just as tear deficiency states rarely involve dysfunction of only one tear film component, treatment rarely involves replacement of a single component.

The ideal artificial tear is one that produces patient satisfaction because it creates a stable preocular tear film. It should be comfortable to use and have a soothing property without epithelial toxicity, based on proper selection of wetting agent and preservatives, a pH between 7.0 and 7.5 maintained by buffers, and a normal osmolarity in the range of 300 milliosmoles based on solute concentration. It should not leave a lid residue, requiring appropriate polymer chemistry and drop size (probably 25 μl. rather than the 50 to 75 μl. now used). It should require infrequent instillation, based on a long retention time created by proper viscosity and absorptive properties. It should allow clear vision, the tear creating a smooth, clear film on the cornea as a result of the proper refractive index and surfacing properties. It should be inexpensive. Table 20–7 summarizes some of the commercially available preparations.

Polymeric systems include substituted cellulose ethers (methylcellulose, hydroxypropyl methylcellulose, and hydroxymethylcellulose), polyvinyl alcohol, and proprietary formulations involving multiple components.

Methylcellulose is a relatively viscous substance that increases retention time but can produce blurred vision, crusting, and sticking of the eyelids. Hydroxypropyl methylcellulose is thought to resemble mucin somewhat in its surface properties.[52] Polyvinyl alcohol increases retention time of tear solutions in a manner that is less viscosity-dependent than that of the cellulose ethers. In addition, polyvinyl alcohol produces a thicker precorneal tear film and perhaps drags aqueous with it as it spreads over the ocular surface.[53]

Poloxamers are polymers that become more viscous in response to an increase in temperature, as occurs on instillation in the eye. They are used in some contact lens solutions and have been tried as tear substitutes.[54]

Commercially available artificial tear formulations were evaluated for their effect on the tear breakup time in normal subjects, and a remarkable variation in magnitude and duration of effect was observed. Adapt, Adapettes, Adsorbotear, and Tears Naturale increased tear breakup time for 90 to 115 minutes after instillation, but Tearisol decreased tear breakup time.[55]

One approach to artificial tear formu-

Table 20–7. ARTIFICIAL TEAR SOLUTIONS

Product	Manufacturer	Polymeric System	Preservatives	Buffer System	Osmolarity[1] (mOsm.)	pH[1]	Viscosity[2] (CPS)	Tear Breakup Time[2,3] Effect	Tear Breakup Time[2,3] Duration (min.)
Adsorbotear	Alcon	POV[4] 1.67%[5] HEC	THIM 0.004% EDTA 0.1%	Phosphate	305	7.5	25–30	Increased	100
Hypotears	Cooper	PVA[5] PEG	BAC 0.01% PEG 0.03%	None	224[6]	5.6[7]	2[8]	N.A.[9]	N.A.
IsoptoTears IsoptoPlain[10]	Alcon	HPMC 0.5%	BAC 0.01%	Phosphate	254	7.4	20–25	Increased	60
Lacril	Allergan	HPMC 0.5% GEL 0.01%	CHLOR 0.5%	Borate-citrate	373	5.8[11]	25–30	Increased	60
Liquiflm Forte	Allergan	PVA 3.0%	THIM 0.002% EDTA 0.01%	Phosphate	295[12]	5.9[12]	3–5	Increased	60
Liquiflim Tears	Allergan	PVA 1.4%	CHLOR 0.5%	None	269[6]	4.3[7]	3–5	Increased	60
Lyteers	Barnes-Hind	HEC 0.2%	BAC 0.01% EDTA 0.05%	Phosphate	414	7.3	5–10	Increased	50
Neo-Tears	Barnes-Hind	HEC[5] PVA PEG	THIM 0.004% EDTA 0.02%	Phosphate	293	7.0	5–25[8]	N.A.	N.A.
Tearisol	Cooper	HPMC 0.5%	BAC 0.01%	Borate-carbonate	283	7.6	10–15	Decreased	40
Tears Naturale	Alcon	HPMC 0.3% Dextran 0.1%	BAC 0.01% EDTA 0.05%	None	291	6.9[6]	3–5	Increased	90
Tears Plus	Allergan	PVA 1.4% POV 0.6%	CHLOR 0.5%	None	292	4.8[6]	3–4[8]	N.A.	N.A.
Ultra Tears Isopto Alkaline[10]	Alcon	HPMC 1%	BAC 0.01%	Phosphate-citrate	256	7.5	225+	Increased	70

1. Jeglum, E. L., and Laibson, P. R.: Unpublished data. Mean of five samples unless otherwise noted.
2. Lemp, M. A.: Design and development of an artificial tear. American Academy of Ophthalmology and Otolaryngology meeting, Dallas, September, 1975.
3. Lemp, M. A., Goldberg, M., and Roddy, M. R.: The effect of tear substitutes on tear film breakup time. Invest Ophthalmol 14:255, 1975.
4. Abbreviations: BAC, benzalkonium chloride; CHLOR, chlorobutanol; EDTA, ethylenediaminetetraacetic acid; GEL, gelatin A; HEC, hydroxyethyl cellulose; HPMC, hydroxypropyl methylcellulose; PEG, polyethylene glycol; POV, povidone; PVA, polyvinyl alcohol; THIM, thimerosal; CPS, centipoise.
5. Proprietary formulation.
6. Pooled data, including two additional lots tested by one of the authors (RDS).
7. Pooled data, including three additional lots tested by one of the authors (RDS).
8. Data supplied by manufacturer.
9. Not available.
10. Identical formulations.
11. Two-sample average.
12. Four-sample average.

lation is based on the theory that hypertonicity is responsible for the signs and symptoms of tear deficiency. Thus, hypotonic preparations such as Hypotears are now available. However, pretreatment osmolarity is regained in 1 to 2 minutes after instillation of the hypotonic solution,[56] and no difference in tear osmolarity or rose bengal staining was seen when long-term therapy with isotonic and hypotonic saline was compared,[33] leaving the validity of this approach in question.

Preservatives used in artificial tear preparations include thimerosal, benzalkonium chloride, chlorobutanol, and EDTA. Thimerosal has a high incidence of hypersensitivity reactions and should be considered a possible culprit in any patient who fails to respond or worsens on adequate tear replacement.[57] Benzalkonium chloride, on the other hand, has been shown to shorten tear breakup time in rabbits and humans,[58] suggesting a detrimental effect on tear film stability. For preservative-sensitive patients in whom no alternatives are available, the ophthalmologist or pharmacist can prepare cellulose ether type artificial tears directly from the commercially available powder, which contains no preservative, and dispense them in small containers that are less likely to become contaminated.

Slow-release hydroxypropyl cellulose conjunctival inserts (Lacrisert) have become available, and an initial uncontrolled, open clinical trial suggested that the patients who tolerate them enjoy freedom from frequent drop instillations.[59] Many elderly patients have difficulty placing the insert in the cul-de-sac, and other patients complain of blurred vision, gumminess, and lid crusting.

In spite of the information available on tear film physiology and the numerous types of artificial tear preparations available, there are no clear guidelines for the selection of tear replacements. In theory, patients with a relatively normal Schirmer test but a decreased breakup time might benefit most from polymers that prolong the breakup time and do not contain benzalkonium chloride, whereas patients with a very low Schirmer test might benefit most from the increased retention of a higher viscosity tear. It is not so simple in clinical practice. In fact, patient satisfaction with an artificial tear preparation is often a matter of personal preference. Rather than loading the patient down with eight or ten different tear samples or sending him off to the drugstore to "pick up some artificial tears," one might supply samples of two or three preparations of varying viscosity and composition, from which the patient can select the most efficacious. The physician lends counsel and encouragement during this process.

Frequency of instillation is also a matter of personal preference. Patients with mild disorders find that the charge to put drugs in every hour during the day makes the treatment worse than the disease, whereas those with severe dry eyes eagerly follow the admonition to use drops every 15 minutes. Tear substitutes should be used often enough to *prevent* symptoms and not be instilled only after symptoms appear. Since the severity of symptoms varies from time to time, patients learn to vary the frequency of instillation according to need. Many elderly patients require instruction in the administration of drops—a task best performed in the physician's office. If there is difficulty with this, a family member may have to assist, sustained release inserts may be used, or punctal occlusion may be instituted earlier than usual.

Ointments may prolong relief, but the resulting blurred vision usually discourages their use except at bedtime.

Mucous filaments and mucous plaques attached to the cornea can produce severe pain. The painful filaments can be removed from the anesthetized cornea with a fine forceps. Acetylcysteine (Mucomyst 10 per cent), a mucolytic agent that works by preventing or breaking disulfide bonds, effectively treats filaments and plaques when used topically five times daily. It also is available in a 20 per cent solution, which generally produces too much discomfort for patient satisfaction. It is packaged in a clumsy, rubber-topped dropper bottle, but a cooperative pharmacist may be willing to transfer it to a conventional ophthalmic dropper bottle. The patient should know that the smell of rotten eggs appears in a few days but that the medication remains effective. Although it is said that the shelf life of acetylcysteine is only a few days, it is probably effective for weeks, particularly when refrigerated. Generally, patients use it only 10 to 14 days, and once the bout of mucous attachments to the cornea has cleared, the medication can be stopped. Acetylcysteine may also reduce less severe symptoms of foreign body sensation in the absence of filaments or plaques, and the ophthalmologist should prescribe it to supplement tear substitutes in refractory cases.

A thorough history of systemic drug ingestion must be obtained. The lacrimal gland receives both sympathetic and parasympathetic innervation, and several classes of medications can decrease tear flow (Table 20–8).[60] Antimuscarinic agents and antihistamines are present in many nonprescription sedatives, antitussives, decongestants, and analgesics. These medications should be eliminated in the tear-deficient patient if possible.

When artificial tears, mucolytics, elimination of systemic medications that decrease tear production, and eyelid hygiene fail to relieve the patient's symptoms, punctal occlusion should be

Table 20–8. DRUGS THAT DECREASE TEAR PRODUCTION

Category	Drugs
Antimuscarinics	Atropine
	Scopolamine
Antihistamines	—
Beta-adrenergic blockers	Practolol
	Timolol
Ganglionic blockers	Hexamethonium
General anesthetics	Nitrous oxide
	Enflurane
	Halothane
Hypnotics	Nitrazepam
Phenothiazines	—
Psychotropics	Diazepam (Valium)
	Clomipramine
	Nialamide
Other	Phenazopyridine HCl (Pyridium)

considered. Before this procedure is performed, the Schirmer test without anesthetic should be about 3 mm. or less on repeated testing. Any time the puncta are occluded, the patient may develop epiphora. This is particularly true in keratoconjunctivitis sicca patients, since this entity has exacerbations and remissions. The patient should understand that epiphora may occur and it is prudent to perform temporary punctal occlusion with surface thermal cautery, cyanoacrylate adhesive,[61] or a punctum plug (which is not commercially available).[62]

To perform punctal occlusion, inject 0.5 ml. of local anesthetic through a 30-gauge needle (the small size diminishes discomfort considerably) just inferior to the punctum itself, insuring that it penetrates through to the conjunctiva. The patient should be warned that ecchymosis may occur. Apply a disposable cautery tip to the punctal orifice (not into the canaliculus) until the tissue whitens and constricts. This occludes the punctum for 3 to 5 days, and during this time the patient can determine whether or not comfort is increased and if epiphora occurs.[63] Some patients experience so much symptomatic relief that they will accept a degree of epiphora. If the trial is successful, close the puncta permanently with a Hyfrecator or a narrow-tipped cautery (Fig. 20–13). Insert the needle tip deeply into the canaliculus and apply the current or heat until the tissue turns white and constricts. Then apply heat or current around the surface of the orifice to further constrict and close it. Sometimes the punctum and canaliculus will recanalize, and closure must be repeated. Both puncta should be closed for maximal effect; one for moderate effect.

In patients with severe dry eyes, occlusive spectacles can provide remarkable symptomatic relief (Fig. 20–14). The ophthalmologist must elicit the aid of a talented optician to fashion a plastic occluder that bridges the space between the spectacle frame and the patient's face. The process is time-consuming (and therefore expensive), since the

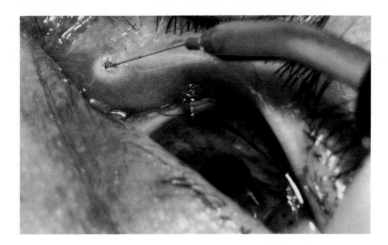

Figure 20–13. Permanent punctal occlusion using the Hyfrecator. The tip is inserted 3 to 4 mm. into the canaliculus and current is applied on a setting of 20 to 25 until a 1-mm. zone of whitening is seen surrounding the punctum.

plastic must be molded to fit facial contours. A flesh-colored plastic reduces cosmetic embarrassment, and a dark-colored plastic reduces glare. Sometimes the occlusion is so effective that the spectacle lens will fog, requiring that small holes be drilled in the plastic to provide venting. Swimmer's goggles, taped-on thin plastic kitchen wrap, or plastic occlusive bubbles (e.g., Expobandage) are available for temporary use, but few individuals will endure the inconvenience and cosmetic embarrassment very long.[64]

In our experience soft contact lenses have little role in the management of keratoconjunctivitis sicca; the lens tends to dry, resulting in rapid accumulation of deposits, curling of its edges, dislocation, and increased corneal trauma that may lead to secondary infection.

However, there are two circumstances in which soft contact lenses, particularly those with high water content, can be effective in a dry eye: persistent epithelial defects and filamentary keratopathy. When they are used, frequent instillation of artificial tears or balanced salt solution will help prevent drying of the lens.

A lateral tarsorrhaphy is important in the management of dry eye patients with severe tear deficiency and with persistent epithelial defects, stromal melting, or a penetrating keratoplasty. In these circumstances the ophthalmologist should be quick to perform a tarsorrhaphy, either in an outpatient setting or at the conclusion of surgery. It protects the ocular surface, reduces the need for frequent instillation of artificial tears, and can be taken down easily with a snip of

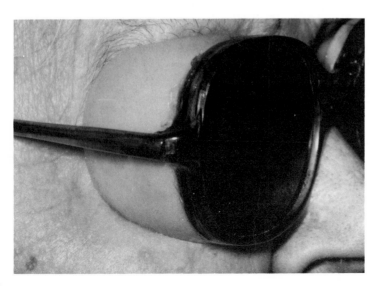

Figure 20–14. Occlusive spectacles. Flesh-colored custom-fitted plastic can be used to bridge the space between the spectacles and the patient's face, creating a moist chamber that reduces the rate of evaporation of tears.

the scissors, leaving little cosmetic residua.

Management of eyelid abnormalities includes the surgical repair of entropion, ectropion, or a lax lower lid; epilation or cryoablation of trichiasis; and taping the lids shut to reduce nocturnal lagophthalmos. Chronic blepharitis is treated by improving lid margin hygiene with warm soaks, scrubs, and massage, along with topical antibiotics (bacitracin, tetracycline) and oral tetracycline (250 mg. q.i.d. for 30 days, then once daily for 6 months).

Tarsorrhaphy may be performed by placing a 4-0 or 5-0 nonabsorbable monofilament suture through the eyelid skin, taking four or five intratarsal bites through the excised eyelid margin, and tying large knots to prevent the sutures from pulling into the skin. This technique avoids cumbersome and unsightly bolsters.[65]

Topical glucocorticoids are best avoided in keratoconjunctivitis sicca, even though they often produce symptomatic relief.[66, 67] Glucocorticoids decrease fibroblastic activity and synthesis of procollagen and proteoglycans, and they may potentiate corneal thinning and perforation.[11, 68, 69] Chronic use may be associated with posterior subcapsular cataracts, secondary elevation of intraocular pressure, and decreased resistance to infection.

Systemic Management

Since keratoconjunctivitis sicca is frequently associated with systemic connective tissue diseases, one might reason that successful management of the systemic disease, usually with glucocorticoids, nonsteroidal anti-inflammatory drugs, or immunosuppressives, would result in decreased ocular symptoms and possibly in increased tear flow. Unfortunately, there are no controlled clinical trials to document this, and the experience of most clinicians is that patients with Sjögren's syndrome do not experience improvement in their ocular symptoms when treated with systemic medications.[48, 66, 67, 70, 71] This is perhaps to be expected, since the lacrimal gland has often been irreversibly replaced by fibrous tissue resulting from chronic inflammation. In theory, anti-inflammatory medication might prevent such destruction of lacrimal tissue if used early in the course of the disease. In spite of the lack of objective improvement in tear flow, some steroid-treated patients report improvement in ocular symptoms;[48, 66, 67, 70, 71] however, the potentially dangerous side effects of long-term systemic glucocorticoid or immunosuppressive therapy contraindicate their use for the relief of ocular symptoms.

Investigators continue to search for systemic medications that might help manage keratoconjunctivitis sicca. For example, thymic factor has recently been reported to prevent autoimmune salivary gland destruction in the lupus-like syndrome of New Zealand black mice.[72] A new drug, bromhexine, is used systemically to increase pulmonary mucus secretion and has been reported to increase tear production.[73] However, these early results are currently debated,[74, 75] and further clinical trials are necessary to elucidate the drug's potential effectiveness.

EDITOR'S NOTE

At the time this material was submitted for publication, a new experimental drug—a high viscosity carboxypolymethylene gel—was being investigated clinically as a topical ophthalmic medication for the treatment of dry eyes of varying etiology. The material, referred to colloquially as Gel Tears, is a clear, semisolid gel formulation of synthetic, high-molecular-weight, cross-linked polymers of acrylic acid. Although not very different from conventional ophthalmic ointments in appearance, it differs measurably in its chemical and physical properties. Among the most dramatic of these differences is the ability of this material to persist in the conjunctival sac for many hours, slowly melting, while absorbing fluid and retaining it locally to lubricate the eye. The interval that a given dose persists varies, but residual formed gel is regularly observed in the lower fornix 8 to 12 hours after instillation.

The Gel Tears preparation produces a generous marginal tear strip and a precorneal tear film and imparts an appearance of moisture to the ocular surface that is not seen with conventional artificial tear preparations. It produces relief of foreign body sensation, burning, and other symptoms of lacrimal insufficiency that persists for hours. With time, use of Gel Tears results in a reduction of conjunctival hyperemia and superficial punctate keratopathy. It does not, as one would expect, alter basic tear secretion; the Schirmer test remains unchanged. Surprisingly, in view of the symptomatic relief and improvement in clinical signs, tear breakup time does not appear to change substantially. However, this can be difficult to assess because the presence of the gel can interfere with accurate performance of the test.

At present the gel is dispensed in the usual foil tube used for ophthalmic ointments. The optimal dose of Gel Tears is only a fraction of that of ophthalmic ointments; only an amount the size of a match head is dispensed. This small amount of material is instilled into the depths of the lower fornix, where it appears to adhere to the forniceal conjunctival surface and where it tends to remain. There have been surprisingly few complaints of the gel dislodging, smearing the cornea, and obscuring vision. However, if too great a quantity of Gel Tears is instilled, the material does obscure vision and, because of its remarkable ability to persist, vision may not clear in the 10- to 20-minute interval characteristic of conventional ointments.

Initial studies by Leibowitz of dry eye patients using conventional artificial tear preparations hourly without relief show that most such patients require Gel Tears only once or twice daily for satisfactory amelioration of their symptoms. The early experience with this agent suggests that it is superior in its effectiveness to all existing tear replacement formulations. However, only more extensive study will determine if this initial enthusiasm is justified.

REFERENCES

1. Holly, F. J., and Lemp, M. A.: Tear physiology and dry eyes. Surv Ophthalmol 22:69, 1977.
2. Holly, F. J.: Formation and rupture of the tear film. Exp Eye Res 15:515, 1973.
3. McCulley, J. P., and Sciallis, G. F.: Meibomian keratoconjunctivitis. Amer J Ophthalmol 84:788, 1977.
4. Kate, J., and Kaufman, H. E.: Corneal exposure during sleep (nocturnal lagophthalmos). Arch Ophthalmol 95:449, 1977.
5. Lamberts, D. W., Foster, C. S., and Perry, H. D.: Schirmer test after topical anesthesia and the tear meniscus height in normal eyes. Arch Ophthalmol 97:1082, 1979.
6. Pfister, R., and Renner, M.: The histopathology of experimental dry spots and dellen in the rabbit cornea: A light microscopy and scanning and transmission electron microscopy study. Invest Ophthalmol Vis Sci 16:1025, 1977.
7. Maudgal, P. C., and Missotten, L. (eds.): Superficial Keratitis. The Hague, Dr. W. Junk Publishers, 1981.
8. Ralph, R. A.: Conjunctival goblet cell density in normal subjects and in dry eye syndromes. Invest Ophthalmol Vis Sci 14:299, 1975.
9. Wright, P.: Filamentary keratitis. Trans Ophthalmol Soc UK 95:260, 1975.
10. Fraunfelder, F. T., Wright, P., and Tripathi, R.: Corneal mucus plaques. Amer J Ophthalmol 83:191, 1977.
11. Brown, S. I., and Grayson, M.: Marginal furrows: A characteristic corneal lesion of rheumatoid arthritis. Arch Ophthalmol 79:563, 1968.
12. Krachmer, J. H., and Laibson, P. R.: Corneal thinning and perforation in Sjögren's syndrome. Amer J Ophthalmol 78:917, 1974.
13. Gudas, P. P., Altman, B., Nicholson, D. H., and Green, W. R.: Corneal perforations in Sjögren syndrome. Arch Ophthalmol 90:470, 1973.

14. Radtke, N., Meyers, S., and Kaufman, H. E.: Sterile corneal ulcers after cataract surgery in keratoconjunctivitis sicca. Arch Ophthalmol 96:51, 1978.

15. Norn, M. S.: *External Eye—Methods of Examination*. Copenhagen, Scriptor, 1974.

16. Shearn, M. A.: *Sjögren's Syndrome*. Philadelphia, W. B. Saunders Co., 1971.

17. Sjögren, H.: Some problems concerning keratoconjunctivitis sicca and the sicca syndrome. Acta Ophthalmol 29:33, 1951.

18. Van Bijsterveld, O. P.: Diagnostic tests in the sicca syndrome. Arch Ophthalmol 82:10, 1969.

19. Jones, L. T.: The lacrimal secretory system and its treatment. Amer J Ophthalmol 62:47, 1966.

20. Wright, J. C., and Meger, G. E.: A review of the Schirmer test for tear production. Arch Ophthalmol 67:564, 1962.

21. Pinschmidt, N. W.: Evaluation of the Schirmer tear test. S Med J 63:1256, 1970.

22. Jordan, A. J., and Baum, J. L.: On the nature of physiologic tear flow. Invest Ophthalmol Vis Sci 18(Suppl):197, 1979.

23. Meyer, K.: Mucopolysaccharides and mucoids of ocular tissues and their enzymatic hydrolysis. In Sorsby, A. (ed.): *Modern Trends in Ophthalmology*. Vol. 2. New York, Paul B. Hoeber, Inc., 1948, p. 71.

24. McEwen, W. K., and Kimura, S. J.: Filter-paper electrophoresis of tears. I. Lysozyme and its correlation with keratoconjunctivitis sicca. Amer J Ophthalmol 39:200, 1955.

25. Avisar, R., Menache, R., Shaked, P., Rubinstein, J., Hachtey, I., and Savir, H.: Lysozyme content of tears in patients with Sjögren's syndrome and rheumatoid arthritis. Amer J Ophthalmol 87:148, 1979.

26. Erickson, O. F., Hatlen, R., and Berg, M.: Industrial tear study. Filter-paper electrophoresis of tears, with results of an industrial study from 1,000 specimens sent by mail. Amer J Ophthalmol 47:499, 1959.

27. Sapse, A. T., Bonavida, B., Stone, W., and Sercarz, E. E.: Human tear lysozyme. III. Preliminary study of lysozyme levels in subjects with smog eye irritation. Amer J Ophthalmol 66:76, 1968.

28. Ronen, D., Eylan, E., Romano, A., Stein, R., and Modan, M.: A spectrophotometric method for quantitative determination of lysozyme in human tears: Description and evaluation of the method and screening of 60 healthy subjects. Invest Ophthalmol Vis Sci 14:479, 1975.

29. Van Bijsterveld, O. P.: Standardization of the lysozyme test for a commercially available medium. Arch Ophthalmol 91:432, 1974.

30. Seal, D. V., Mackie, I. A., Coates, R. L., and Farooqi, B.: Quantitative tear lysozyme assay: A new technique for transporting specimens. Brit J Ophthalmol 64:700, 1980.

31. Sen, D., and Sarin, G. S.: Immunoassay of human tear lysozyme. Amer J Ophthalmol 90:715, 1980.

32. Gilbard, J. P., Farris, R. L., and Santamaria, J., II: Osmolarity of tear microvolumes in keratoconjunctivitis sicca. Arch Ophthalmol 96:677, 1978.

33. Gilbard, J. P., and Farris, R. L.: Tear osmolarity and ocular surface disease in keratoconjunctivitis sicca. Arch Ophthalmol 97:1642, 1979.

34. Lemp, M. A., and Hamill, J. R.: Factors affecting tear film break up in normal eyes. Arch Ophthalmol 89:103, 1978.

35. Shapiro, A., and Merin, S.: Schirmer test and break up time of tear film in normal subjects. Amer J Ophthalmol 88:752, 1979.

36. Lemp, M. A., Dohlman, C. H., and Holly, F. J.: Corneal desiccation despite normal tear volume. Ann Ophthalmol 2:258, 1970.

37. Lemp, M. A., Dohlman, C. H., Kuwabara, T., Holly, F. J., and Carroll, J. M.: Dry eye secondary to mucus deficiency. Trans Amer Acad Ophthalmol Otolaryngol 75:1223, 1971.

38. Vanley, G. T., Leopold, I. H., and Gregg, T. H.: Interpretation of tear film break up. Arch Ophthalmol 95:445, 1977.

39. Norn, M. S.: Desiccation of the precorneal film. II. Permanent discontinuity and dellen. Acta Ophthalmol 47:881, 1969.

40. Norn, M. S.: Tear secretion in diseased eyes. Acta Ophthalmol 44:25, 1966.

41. Mishima, S., Gasset, A., Klyce, S., and Baum, J.: Determination of tear volume and tear flow. Invest Ophthalmol 5:264, 1966.

42. Scherz, W., Doane, M. G., and Dohlman, C. H.: Tear volume in normal eyes and keratoconjunctivitis sicca. Albrecht von Graefes Arch Klin Ophthalmol 192:141, 1974.

43. Sjögren, H.: Zur Kenntnis der Keratoconjunctivitis sicca (Keratitis filiformis bei Hypofunction der Tränendrüsen). Acta Ophthalmol 11(Suppl 2):1, 1933.

44. Talal, N., Sylvester, R. A., Daniels, T. E., Greenspan, J. S., and Williams, R. C.: T & B lymphocytes in peripheral blood and tissue lesions in Sjögren's syndrome. J Clin Invest 53:180, 1974.

45. Moutsopoulos, H.: Sjögren's syndrome (sicca syndrome): Current issues. Ann Intern Med 92:212, 1980.

46. Manthorpe, R., Frost-Larsen, K., Isager, H., and Prause, J. U.: Sjögren's syndrome. A review with emphasis on immunological features. Allergy 36:139, 1981.

47. Moutsopoulos, H. M., Webber, B. L., Vlagopoulos, T. P., Chused, T. M., and Decker, J. L.: Differences in the clinical manifestations of sicca syndrome in the presence and absence of rheumatoid arthritis. Amer J Med 66:733, 1979.

48. Bloch, K. J., Buchanan, W. W., Wohl, M. J., and Bunim, J. J.: Sjögren's syndrome. A clinical, pathological, and serological study of sixty-two cases. Medicine 44:187, 1965.

49. Kassan, S. S., Thomas, T. L., Moutsopoulos, H. M., Hoover, R., Kimberly, R. P., Budman, D. R., Costa, J., Decker, J. L., and Chused, T. M.: Increased risk of lymphoma in sicca syndrome. Ann Intern Med 89:888, 1978.

50. Karsh, J., Pavlidis, N., Weintraub, B., and Moutsopoulos, H. M.: Thyroid disease in Sjögren's syndrome. Arth Rheum 23:1326, 1980.

51. Chisolm, D. M., and Mason, D. K.: Labial salivary gland biopsy in Sjögren's disease. J Clin Path 21:656, 1968.

52. Lemp, M. A.: Artificial tear solutions. Int Ophthalmol Clin 13:221, 1973.

53. Benedetto, D. A., Shah, D. O., and Kaufman, H. E.: The instilled fluid dynamics and surface chemistry of polymers in the preocular tear film. Invest Ophthalmol Vis Sci 14:887, 1975.

54. Waring, G. O., and Harris, R. R.: Double-masked evaluation of a poloxamer artificial tear. In Burns, R. P., and Leopold, I. H. (eds.): *Symposium on Ocular Therapy*, Vol. 10. New York, John Wiley and Sons, 1979, p. 127.

55. Lemp, M. A., Goldberg, M., and Roddy, M. R.: The effect of tear substitutes on tear film breakup time. Invest Ophthalmol Vis Sci 14:255, 1975.

56. Holly, F. J., and Lamberts, D. W.: Effect of nonisotonic solutions on tear film osmolarity. Invest Ophthalmol Vis Sci 20:236, 1981.

57. Wilson, L. A., McNatt, J., and Rietschel, R.: Delayed hypersensitivity to thimerosal in soft contact lens wearers. Ophthalmol 88:804, 1981.

58. Wilson, W. S., Duncan, A. J., and Jay, J. L.: Effect of benzalkonium chloride on the stability of the precorneal tear film in rabbit and man. Brit J Ophthalmol 59:667, 1975.

59. Werblin, T. P., Rheinstrom, S. D., and Kaufman, H. E.: The use of slow-release artificial tears in the long-term management of keratitis sicca. Ophthalmol 88:78, 1981.

60. Crandall, D. C., and Leopold, I. H.: The influence of systemic drugs on tear constituents. Trans Amer Acad Ophthalmol Otolaryngol 86:115, 1979.

61. Patten, J. T.: Punctal occlusion with N-butyl cyanoacrylate tissue adhesive. Ophthalmic Surg 7:24, 1976.

62. Freeman, J. M.: The punctum plug: Evaluation of a new treatment for the dry eye. Trans Amer Acad Ophthalmol Otolaryngol 85:874, 1975.

63. Dohlman, C. H.: Punctal occlusion in keratoconjunctivitis sicca. Ophthalmol 85:1277, 1975.

64. Poirier, R. H., Ryburn, F. M., and Israel, L. W.: Swimmer's goggles for keratoconjunctivitis sicca. Arch Ophthalmol 95:1405, 1977.

65. Grove, A. S.: Marginal tarsorrhaphy: A technique to minimize premature eyelid separation. Ophthalmic Surg 8:56, 1977.

66. Eadie, S., and Thompson, M.: Keratoconjunctivitis sicca treated with cortisone and ACTH. Brit J Ophthalmol 39:90, 1955.

67. Gaulhofer, W. K.: The effect of cortisone on Sjögren's syndrome. Acta Med Scand 149:441, 1954.

68. Brown, S. I., and Weller, C. A.: Effect of corticosteroids on corneal collagenase of rabbits. Amer J Ophthalmol 70:744, 1970.

69. Brown, S. I., and Weller, C. A.: The pathogenesis and treatment of collagenase-induced diseases of the cornea. Trans Amer Acad Ophthalmol Otolaryngol 74:375, 1970.

70. Sjögren, H.: ACTH and keratoconjunctivitis sicca. Acta Ophthalmol 30:463, 1952.

71. Gurling, K. J., Bruce-Pearson, R. S., and Pond, M. H.: Sjögren's syndrome treated with ACTH. Brit J Ophthalmol 38:619, 1954.

72. Bach, M. A., Droz, D., Noel, L. H., Blanchard, D., Dardenne, M., and Peking, A.: Effect of long-term treatment with circulating thymic factor on murine lupus. Arth Rheum 23:1351, 1980.

73. Frost-Larsen, K., Isager, H., and Manthorpe, R.: Sjögren's syndrome treated with bromhexine: A randomized clinical study. Brit Med J 1:1579, 1978.

74. Mackie, I., and Seal, D. V.: Sjögren's syndrome, bromhexine, and tear secretion. Brit Med J 2:638, 1978.

75. Manthorpe, R., Frost-Larsen, K., Isager, H., and Prause, J. U.: Sjögren's syndrome treated with bromhexine: A reassessment. Brit Med J 281:1216, 1980.

76. DuBois, E. L. (ed.): *Lupus Erythematosus. A Review of the Current Status of Discoid and Systemic Lupus Erythematosus and Their Variants.* 2nd ed. Los Angeles, University of Southern California Press, 1976.

77. Moutsopoulos, H. M., Mann, D. L., Johnson, A. H., and Chused, T. M.: Genetic differences between primary and secondary sicca syndrome. N Engl J Med 301:761, 1979.

78. Manthorpe, R., Permin, H., and Tage-Jensen, U.: Auto-antibodies in Sjögren's syndrome with special reference to liver-cell membrane antibody (LMA). Scand J Rheumatol 8:168, 1979.

79. Alspaugh, M., Talal, N., and Tan, E. M.: Differentiation and characterization of auto-antibodies and their antigens in Sjögren's syndrome. Arth Rheum 19:216, 1976.

80. Moutsopoulos, H. M., Klippel, J. H., Pavlidis, N., Wolf, R. O., Sweet, J. B., Steinberg, A. D., Chu, F. C., and Tarpley, T. M.: Correlative histologic and serologic findings of sicca syndrome in patients with systemic lupus erythematosus. Arth Rheum 23:36, 1980.

81. Akizuki, M., Boem-Truitt, M. J., Kassan, S. S., Steinberg, A. D., and Chused, T. M.: Purification of an acidic nuclear protein antigen and demonstration of its antibodies in subsets of patients with sicca syndrome. J Immunol 119:932, 1977.

IX

CORNEAL ABNORMALITIES RESULTING FROM TRAUMA

Chemical Injuries of the Eye | 21

JAMES P. McCULLEY, M.D.
THOMAS E. MOORE, M.D.

The number of chemicals that are toxic to the eye is virtually infinite. Fortunately most ocular chemical injuries are minor; they are easily treated and result only in discomfort and minor tissue damage. However, alkaline and acidic materials can cause severe ocular damage and permanent visual loss. Such injuries are relatively uncommon, but the seemingly disproportionate attention accorded them in the ophthalmic literature is justified. An increased knowledge of the mechanisms of these potentially devastating injuries has led to more effective treatment and in many cases to preservation of normal tissue structure and vision. Moreover, much of the knowledge about alkali burns is applicable to other ulcerative processes.

This chapter deals first with alkali injuries, followed in less detail by acid injuries, since the knowledge of alkali burns is greater and is applicable to other chemical injuries. For greater detail on the less common chemical injuries the reader is referred to Grant's *Toxicology of the Eye*.[1]

ALKALI INJURIES

Table 21–1 lists the clinically significant alkalies in decreasing order of ocular penetrability and tendency to produce damage to ocular tissue. First in clinical significance is ammonium hydroxide.

Ammonia is a colorless gas used in fertilizers, as a refrigerant, and in the manufacture of other chemicals. In its gaseous form ammonia stimulates protective lacrimation, which prevents injury to the eye unless there is a direct blast of the gas onto the ocular surface. The gas liquefies under pressure, and liquid ammonia combined with water forms ammonium hydroxide. The most commonly encountered concentration of ammonium hydroxide is the 7 per cent solution used in household cleaning agents,[2] but concentrations up to 29 per cent are occasionally encountered.

Ammonium hydroxide is soluble in both lipids and water and passes easily through both the lipophilic corneal epithelium and the hydrophilic stroma. Indeed, it penetrates the eye more rapidly than any other alkali and therefore tends to cause the most severe ocular injuries, which explains why iris and lens damage commonly occur after injuries with this alkali. Paradoxically, ammonium hydroxide causes less initial stromal opacification than either sodium hydroxide or calcium hydroxide.

Another alkali that rapidly penetrates the eye is sodium hydroxide, also known as lye, caustic soda, or sodium hydrate and commonly encountered as

Table 21–1. CLINICALLY SIGNIFICANT ALKALIES*

Ammonium hydroxide
Sodium hydroxide
Potassium hydroxide
Calcium hydroxide
Magnesium hydroxide

*Listed in decreasing order of ocular penetrability and tendency to produce ocular damage.

471

a drainpipe cleaner. The ocular damage produced by sodium hydroxide ranks second only to ammonium hydroxide in its severity.

Potassium hydroxide (caustic potash) enters the eye with only slightly less facility than sodium hydroxide but causes injuries similar in degree to those of sodium hydroxide. However, potassium hydroxide injuries are relatively uncommon.

Calcium hydroxide, also known as calcium hydrate and found in lime, fresh lime, quick lime, slake lime, hydrated lime, plaster, mortar, cement, and whitewash, is one of the more commonly encountered alkalies causing ocular burns. Its ocular penetration is relatively poor because of a reaction with the epithelial cell membrane that forms calcium soaps. The soaps precipitate, hindering further penetration of the calcium hydroxide and thus reducing the severity of damage. However, calcium hydroxide causes the earliest corneal opacity,[3] presumably because of a reaction with the proteoglycans that results in the formation of a precipitate that leaves the glycosaminoglycans nonextractable. The stromal opacity may cause a calcium hydroxide injury to initially appear more severe than an injury caused by one of the more rapidly penetrating alkalies.

An additional, occasionally encountered alkali of clinical significance is magnesium hydroxide, which is found in sparklers and flares. The presence of this substance accounts for the observation that ocular injury associated with these devices is more severe than would be expected on the basis of a thermal injury alone.[4]

Biochemical Changes

The mechanism by which the hydroxyl ion causes damage is the same for all of the alkaline substances in question. Therefore, the difference between one alkaline substance and another resides in the cation that determines the penetrability of the individual molecules. At a high pH all alkalies saponify the fatty components of the cell membrane, causing cell death. All layers of the eye may be affected if the alkali penetrates sufficiently. The hydroxyl ion also causes a shift of hydrogen ions, which may contribute to cellular damage. Epithelial cell death is not necessary for the penetration of ammonia because it is lipid-soluble and can pass directly through the lipophilic epithelium. Of course, it can also gain access to the stroma by destroying the epithelial barrier.

In addition to causing cellular damage, alkali adversely affects the collagen matrix of the eye. At high pH cations bind to collagen and to glycosaminoglycans (substances also referred to as mucopolysaccharides) by reacting with carboxyl groups.[3] The significance of this reaction, however, is not clear. The hydroxyl anion reacts with collagen, causing hydration (swelling) of individual fibrils, which results in thickening and shortening of these fibrils. The significance of this reaction is discussed in a later section. It is possible that partial degradation (denaturation) occurs as a result of alteration of the covalent structure of the collagen molecule and that this degradation renders the collagen more soluble. Although the reaction has not been well defined to date, there are no visible changes in the collagen molecule by electron microscopy.[5] The alkali does appear to make the collagen more susceptible to enzymatic degradation, but this may reflect only a loss of protective glycosaminoglycans rather than a direct alteration of the collagen.[6]

Corneal proteoglycans, which are glycosaminoglycans bound to protein whose exact nature has not been precisely determined, are affected adversely by alkali. The hydroxyl ion hydrolyzes the glycosaminoglycan portion with resultant loss of this substance from the tissue.[7] This leaves the collagen "naked" and therefore more susceptible to enzymatic degradation.

Alkaline substances that penetrate to the ciliary body can cause both quantitative and qualitative changes in the aqueous humor.[8] The content of glucose in aqueous humor (as well as in corneal stroma) is decreased, as is ascorbate, which is required for collagen synthesis.[7, 9, 10] The lactate levels, on the other hand, have been found to be normal. As one might expect, the aqueous humor pH increases as a result of exposure to alkaline substances. The rise in pH correlates with increased tissue damage, the sharpest relative increase occurring at a pH of 11.5.

As stated above, the speed with which alkaline substances penetrate the eye varies from one substance to another. Ammonium hydroxide causes an increase in aqueous humor pH within seconds of exposure. The increase after sodium hydroxide exposure appears at 1 minute and peaks between 3 and 5 minutes after exposure.[11] The aqueous humor pH returns to normal within 30 minutes to 3 hours after exposure to alkali; it has not been possible to expedite the return to normal by external irrigation.[12]

Collagen loss in the form of corneal stromal ulceration is a common occurrence after significant alkali burns. Stromal ulceration usually occurs 2 to 3 weeks after the initial alkali burn and is therefore not a direct effect of the chemical on the collagen. After exposure of the eye to alkali, several enzymes have been found in the cornea, which may account for the ulcerative process. These include acid glycosidases,[13] which increase the loss of glycosaminoglycans from the stroma and interfere with restoration of the normal proteoglycan composition of the cornea in the early reparative phases. Granulocyte proteases, including elastase and cathepsin G, lyse collagen by cleaving terminally through the cross-linked sections. Although collagenolytic enzymes are found in high concentrations in ulcerating corneas after alkali burns,[14-18] the relative contribution of specific enzymes to the tissue injury observed clinically is not yet known.

In discussing proteolytic enzymes, it is important to differentiate between collagenolytic activity and a true collagenase. The former refers to a broad group of enzymes that have the ability to break down collagen in a variety of ways. Included in this group of proteases is collagenase itself. True mammalian collagenase cleaves the tropocollagen molecule at a site one-fourth of the distance from the "B" end of the molecule and at no other site. It also reduces the viscosity of an undenatured collagen solution in a restricted rather than an unrestricted manner, consistent with its specific activity on the molecule.[19, 20] True mammalian collagenase has been identified in ulcerating corneas after alkali burns.[20, 21]

Collagenolytic activity has been demonstrated in corneal epithelium and most likely represents the activity of a true collagenase.[11, 22] However, it is possible that the epithelium plays its principal role in the modulation of collagenase activity by polymorphonuclear leukocytes[23] that infiltrate the stroma after alkali burns.[24] Fibroblasts in the corneal stroma after alkali burns also have been shown to produce a collagenase.[25, 26] In all cases the collagenase is a membrane-bound enzyme with a molecular weight of 40,000 in its latent form and a molecular weight of 20,000 in its active form.[27] The latent or proenzyme is produced, at least in part, by combination of the active enzyme and a product of fibroblasts (molecular weight 20,000) to which it binds. It is not clear whether there are other forms of the latent enzyme present in tissues. In the normal cornea there is no latent or active collagenase present;[21, 27] an injury creates the stimulus for de novo synthesis and activation of the enzyme.[28] Collagenolytic activity can be measured 9 hours after an alkali burn of the cornea,[11] but the activity does not peak until 14 to 21 days after the burn.

Corneal ulceration usually stops when the epithelium is intact or the cornea becomes totally vascularized. Blood vessels bring in nutrients and precursors of protein and proteoglycan synthesis, cellular precursors of fibroblasts that aid in tissue repair, and serum collagenase inhibitors. It appears that complete regeneration of the epithelium plays a major role in the cessation of the ulcerative process by eliminating the stimulus to collagenase production and activation, not by discontinuing the synthesis of collagen by the epithelium itself. However, this issue has not been completely resolved.

At least two divalent ions, calcium and zinc, are necessary for collagenase to be active.[29] Calcium stabilizes the enzyme structure, and zinc has a direct role in the enzymatic activity of hydrolysis. The importance of these ions will become more apparent when enzyme inhibitors are discussed (treatment section).

Collagen breakdown and defects in collagen synthesis after alkali burns are important in the ulcerative process. A cornea in the reparative stages after a severe alkali burn presents the picture of localized scorbutus.[6, 9, 10] Fibroblasts have poorly developed endoplasmic reticulum, a sparse polyribosomal system, intracellular electron-dense bodies, and little juxtaposed fibrillary collagen; the collagen that is present is lacking in periodicity. Aqueous humor ascorbate levels are greatly decreased. The ciliary body normally concentrates ascorbate in the aqueous humor approximately 20-fold relative to its concentration in plasma. This concentrating ability is compromised or lost if the ciliary body is damaged. Ascorbate is necessary for collagen synthesis, both in vivo and in vitro. It is required for the conversion of proline and lysine to hydroxyproline and hydroxylysine respectively, necessary steps in the synthesis of mature collagen. Ascorbate is also necessary for the development and maturation of fibroblasts; it is required for the conversion of monocytes to fibroblasts and for the formation of normal rough endoplasmic reticulum. Ascorbate is also important in the synthesis of glycosaminoglycans.

In the experimental rabbit model used to evaluate aqueous humor ascorbate concentrations,[10] it was found that if ascorbate was greater than 15 mg./100 ml., no corneal ulceration occurred. This level of ascorbic acid correlated well with an absence of the picture of localized scorbutus. Conversely, with an ascorbate level of less than 15 mg./100 ml., ulceration occurred and the picture of localized scorbutus was observed. If one artifically increased the aqueous humor ascorbate levels to greater than 15 mg./100 ml. by giving systemic or local ascorbate, no ulceration occurred (i.e., adequate collagen synthesis was attained to balance the enzymatic loss of collagen).

Grading of Burn Severity and Factors That Determine Severity

There is no ideal classification or grading system for ocular alkali burns because of the many variables associated with these injuries. However, the classification proposed by Hughes[30, 31] and modified by others does have a place. It provides a base from which to plan treatment and estimate prognosis. Unfortunately, injuries to the cornea and to the surrounding tissues are not uniformly associated, and this forms the principal weakness of the grading system. Therefore, for the individual patient one must evaluate the severity of the corneal injury as well as the severity of injury to other surfaces and to deeper tissues. From this one can determine appropriate treatment and estimate prognosis. In dealing with alkali injuries and classification systems it is wise to assume that the injury will prove to be worse than it initially appears.

The classification of alkali burns by Hughes[30, 31] divides injuries into three groups as follows:

Mild—good prognosis
    Erosion of corneal epithelium
    Faint haziness of cornea
    No ischemic necrosis of conjunctiva
        or sclera
Moderately severe—good prognosis
    Corneal opacity blurs iris details
    Minimal ischemic necrosis of conjunctiva and sclera
Very severe—poor prognosis
    Blurring of pupillary outline
    Blanching of conjunctiva and sclera

Some of the inadequacies of the Hughes classification are rectified in the Roper-Hall modification[32] of Ballen's classification,[33] which divides the injuries into four groups rather than three. It also provides a degree of quantitation of conjunctival and episcleral ischemia and implies that total loss of corneal epithelium is significant. This classification is the one preferred by the authors.

Grade I—good prognosis (Fig. 21–1)
    Corneal epithelial damage
    No ischemia
Grade II—good prognosis (Fig. 21–2)
    Cornea hazy but iris details seen
    Ischemia of less than one third at the limbus
Grade III—guarded prognosis (Figs. 21–3 and 21–4)
    Total loss of corneal epithelium
    Stromal haze obscures iris details
    Ischemia affects one third to one half at limbus
Grade IV—poor prognosis (Figs. 21–5 and 21–6)
    Cornea opaque, obscuring view of iris or pupil
    Ischemia affects more than one half at limbus

It is apparent that poor prognostic factors relate to the *area of chemical*

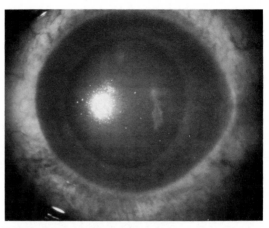

Figure 21–2. Grade II alkali injury with epithelial damage and stromal edema blurring iris details. Minimal perilimbal ischemia at 9 o'clock. Eye recovered totally in 2 weeks.

exposure (e.g., extent of corneal epithelial loss, extent of conjunctival, episcleral, and scleral ischemia) and to the degree of chemical penetration (e.g., degree of corneal clouding, presence of hypotony and/or cataracts). Total corneal anesthesia also is an indicator of a poor prognosis. However, it is important to note that in the acute phase relative corneal anesthesia occurs whenever all of the corneal epithelium is lost. It is only after the cornea has re-epithelialized and sufficient time has elasped for regrowth and establishment of the nerve endings in the epithelium that corneal anesthesia becomes a significant prognostic indicator.

Biochemical factors that govern the severity of the injury produced by exposure to an alkaline substance include the quantity of chemical to which one is exposed, the hydroxyl ion concentration (pH) of the solution, the nature of the associated cation (which affects penetrability and, in the case of ammonia, directly reacts with tissue), and the duration of exposure to the chemical. All of these factors affect the penetration of individual molecules. Most alkaline substances will penetrate into and through a cornea devoid of epithelium with approximately the same facility. Exceptions include ammonia (which penetrates more rapidly) and calcium hydroxide (which penetrates somewhat

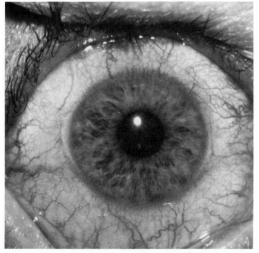

Figure 21–1. Grade I alkali injury with corneal epithelial damage and conjunctival hyperemia. No blurring of iris details. Eye recovered in 4 days with return of 20/20 vision.

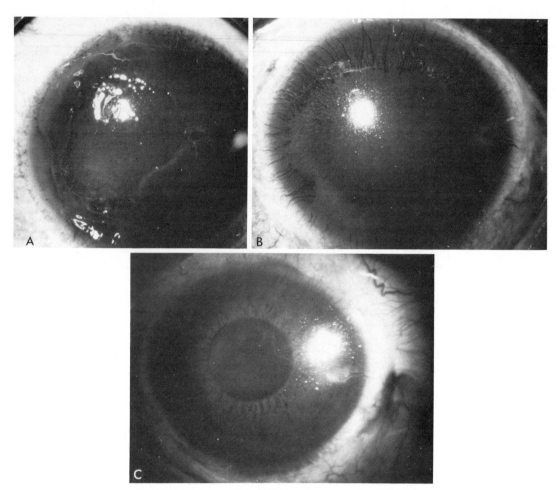

Figure 21–3. Grade III alkali injury. *A,* Loss of corneal epithelium, stromal edema, and opacity obscuring iris details. Perilimbal ischemia from 10 o'clock to 2 o'clock. *B,* Two weeks later, less ischemia and stromal haze. *C,* Seven weeks after injury, minimal scarring in peripheral cornea at 3 o'clock. Vision 20/25.

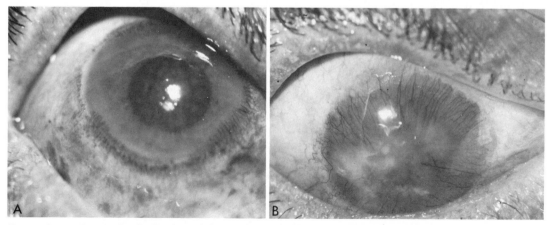

Figure 21–4. Grade III alkali injury. *A,* Injury similar to that shown in Figure 21–3*A. B,* Outcome not as good as that in the eye shown in Figure 21–3. Corneal scarring and vascularization resulted.

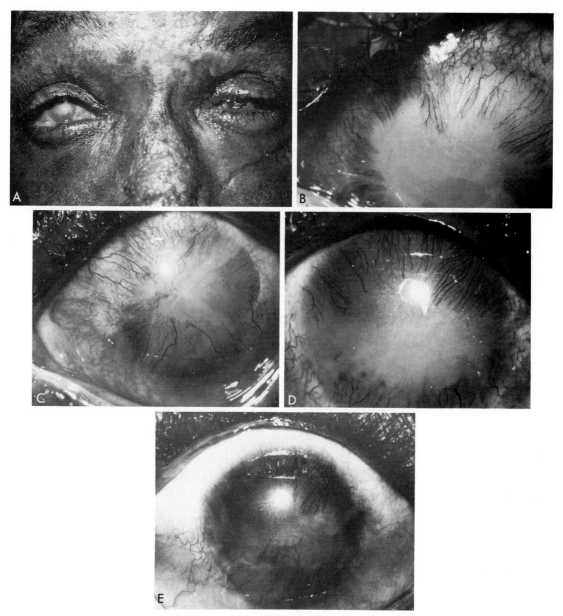

Figure 24–5. Grade IV alkali injury. *A,* Initially lid edema prevented good view of globes. Three weeks after the injury both corneas are opaque, but ischemia is less prominent than initially secondary to vessels recanalizing. *B,* Right eye—cornea vascularizing and stromal opacity persisting. *C,* Right eye—4 months after injury, the cornea is scarred and almost totally vascularized. Vision in a dark room is 20/400. *D,* Left eye—cornea vascularizing and stromal opacity persisting but less prominent than in right eye. *E,* Left eye—4 months after injury, less scarring and vascularization than in right eye. Vision in a dark room is 20/200.

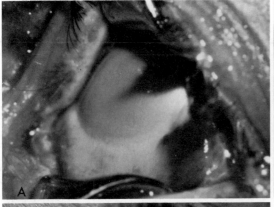

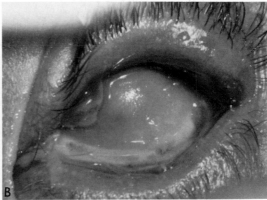

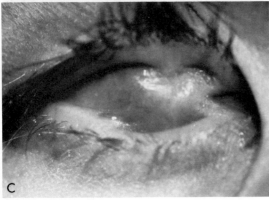

Figure 21–6. Grade IV alkali injury. *A,* Porcelainized cornea and 360 degrees of perilimbal ischemia. *B,* Three weeks after injury—ischemia and stromal opacity persist. Stromal ulceration beginning. *C,* One year after injury—surface of globe is covered with keratinized epithelium. Fornices are almost totally obliterated.

less rapidly). All alkaline substances disrupt the epithelium by saponifying cell membranes, which then allows them ready access to the stroma. Ammonium compounds, in addition to saponifying cell membranes, are lipid-soluble and can rapidly traverse the epithelium. The soaps that calcium hydroxide forms with cell membranes tend to create a relative barrier to penetration of calcium hydroxide into the stroma. However, this is not an absolute barrier, as evidenced by the significant injury to deeper tissues that often occurs after exposure to this compound.

Clinical (With Pathologic Correlation) Stages After Alkali Burn

Acute (Immediate to 1 Week After Burn)

The most significant immediate occurrence after exposure to alkaline substances is the disruption of cellular membranes. Depending upon the degree of chemical penetration, there is loss of corneal and conjunctival epithelium, keratocytes, corneal nerves, endothelium, and blood vessels, cellular and vascular components of iris and ciliary body, and lens epithelium.[30] In relatively mild injuries this is manifested clinically by defects in corneal and conjunctival epithelium. In more severe and widespread injuries there is also loss of conjunctival goblet cells. Following deeper penetration of the chemical, corneal edema (Fig. 21–7) and ischemic necrosis of perilimbal tissue (Figs. 21–3A, 21–4A, and 21–6A), ciliary body, and iris occurs. The very severe injuries caused by deep penetration are characterized by fibrinous iritis and cataract formation. In addition to the loss of various cellular components in the anterior segment of the eye and adnexa, there is often a loss of vascular perfusion (secondary to thrombosis), which contributes to ischemia and localized hemorrhage.[8]

The intraocular pressure in the early phases after an alkali burn may be in-

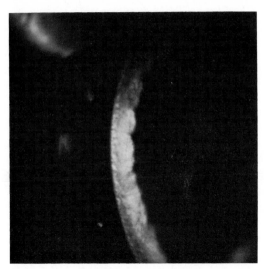

Figure 21–7. Marked stromal edema present 1 day after Grade III alkali injury.

creased in a bimodal fashion.[34-37] An initial peak occurs within seconds and is due to hydration of collagen fibrils, resulting in longitudinal shortening of the collagen fibers and resultant compression of the globe. The second peak occurs within hours and is due to the impedance of aqueous humor outflow by increased episcleral venous pressure, trabecular meshwork damage, and inflammatory debris obstructing the outflow channels. Prostaglandins partially contribute to the second phase,[35, 37] whereas alpha-adrenergic compounds such as phenylephrine partially inhibit it.

After the initial elevation intraocular pressure will be variable, depending on the balance between decreased aqueous humor production and decreased outflow. Hypotony may occur if the ciliary body is severely damaged, or severe glaucoma may be present if the outflow channels are primarily damaged. Normal intraocular pressure results from a relative balance between the two. Therefore, during this phase one cannot estimate the intraocular pressure level; it must be measured by appropriate tonometric techniques.

Corneal clouding may be seen within minutes after an alkali burn. It can be attributed partially to stromal edema and partially to changes in the proteoglycans[3] (Fig. 21–6A). The latter contributes to corneal opacification, especially after calcium hydroxide burns, which are characterized by precipitation of the glycosaminoglycans. In very severe injuries porcelainization of the stroma cannot be explained totally by these two mechanisms, and presumably there is an associated change in corneal collagen.

Within a few hours to 48 hours of an acute injury there is partial loss of stromal glycosaminoglycans with resultant decrease in stromal metachromatic staining.[7, 31] Also within a short period of time, the ocular structures are infiltrated by polymorphonuclear leukocytes, monocytes, and fibroblasts. The basal lamina of the epithelium remains intact initially but begins to show evidence of breakdown by 7 to 10 days after the injury.

Early Reparative Phase (1 to 3 Weeks)

During the early reparative phase the conjunctival and corneal epithelia begin to regenerate and in all but the more severe injuries completely cover the ocular surfaces.[30] Corneal neovascularization (Fig. 21–5B) and invasion of inflammatory cells parallel epithelial regrowth. The corneal opacity begins to clear and in mild to moderate cases may completely clear during this period. The invasion of fibroblasts and the associated synthesis of new collagen and glycosaminoglycans continues and reaches a peak by 14 days after the injury. During this time the corneal endothelium begins to regenerate in rabbits. However, in man, in whom the corneal endothelium has very little, if any, regenerative capability, one begins to see the formation of retrocorneal fibrous membranes. Iritis disappears (except in the more severe injuries) and recanalization of iris and ciliary body blood vessels occurs.[8, 30] In the more severe injuries granulation tissue replaces much of the iris and ciliary body, resulting in severe fibrosis of these structures.[8]

It is during this interval that corneal

ulceration tends to occur. Most commonly the ulceration begins 2 to 3 weeks after the injury. If ulceration becomes either progressive or recurrent, it represents a serious clinical problem, as discussed below.

Late Reparative Phase and Sequelae (3 Weeks and Longer)

During this phase the balance between collagen synthesis and collagen degradation in the cornea will determine the presence or absence of stromal ulceration. Prevention of corneal ulceration does not prevent corneal scarring and opacification after severe burns. However, if one is able to prevent ulceration, the prognosis is improved both for retention of the globe and for vision. Progressive or recurrent corneal stromal ulceration, leading to descemetocele formation or perforation, is the most severe complication of an alkali burn.[30] The onset of ulceration is most common in the second to third week after exposure to alkali. The ulcerative process presumably is mediated by collagenase and other proteolytic enzymes and is not a nonspecific dissolution of stromal collagen. It is the progressive type of corneal ulceration that most commonly leads to loss of the eye (Fig. 21–8). On the other hand, the recurrent, less severe type of stromal ulceration may cause significant visual loss by producing an irregular corneal surface and irregular astigmatism (Fig. 21–9).

Progressive corneal vascularization occurs after more severe alkali burns and often does not subside until the entire cornea is vascularized (Fig. 21–4B). In the more severe injuries this is not necessarily an undesirable end point. The cornea is not apt to perforate in areas where it is vascularized,[38] perhaps because antiproteases in blood are available to the stroma. A fibrovascular pannus may overgrow the cornea in moderately severe injuries. This may occur in conjunction with progressive corneal neovascularization as well as in association with injuries that are not severe enough to stimulate stromal vascularization. When penetration of alkali has destroyed the corneal endothelium beyond its compensatory reserve, persistent corneal edema will result. In many of these cases retrocorneal, iritic, and cyclitic fibrous membranes will also develop.[39]

Permanent loss of corneal innervation with a resultant neuroparalytic or neurotrophic keratitis may occur with more severe injuries. This, along with permanent ocular surface abnormalities (discussed below), contributes to the poor prognosis for corneal transplantation in these patients.

Abnormalities of the tear film are among the more commonly encountered sequelae of an alkali burn and can occur

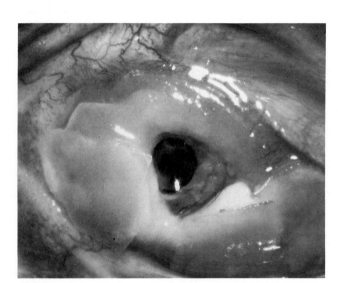

Figure 21–8. Large central stromal ulcer that has perforated 6 weeks after a neglected Grade IV injury. Ulcer surrounded by necrotic tissue. (From Smolin, G., and Thoft, R. A.: The Cornea. Boston, Little, Brown, & Company, 1983.)

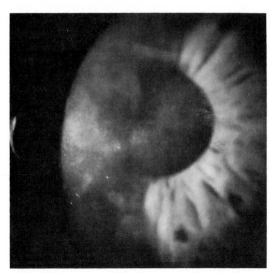

Figure 21–9. Surface faceting after recurrent epithelial breakdown with minimal superficial stromal loss.

as the result of all but the most mild burns. The aqueous and mucin components of the tear film may be adversely affected.[40] Scarring, with loss of the accessory lacrimal glands and/or the ductule openings of the major lacrimal gland, may result in an aqueous deficiency. However, this is less common than an eye with copious aqueous secretions but an unstable tear film, presumably the result of a mucin-deficient state that reflects a diffuse loss of goblet cells. A deficiency of mucin leads to keratinization of the conjunctival and corneal epithelium. The tear film abnormalities,

producing epithelial cell damage (Fig. 21–10) and keratinization, and the loss of corneal innervation remain as two major obstacles to the success of corneal transplantation and visual rehabilitation of patients with alkali burns. As the mechanisms of corneal ulceration have become better understood, these two problems have taken on relatively greater significance. Recent advances in dealing with these problems will be discussed in the section on treatment of alkali burns.

The intraocular pressure in the late phases after an alkali burn can range from a state of hypotony to glaucoma. If ciliary body damage is severe, resultant fibrosis of the ciliary body can lead to hypotony and subsequent phthisis bulbi. On the other hand, after less severe injuries or injuries primarily affecting the outflow channels, severe secondary glaucoma can develop (Fig. 21–11). Glaucoma can result from fibrous proliferation in the anterior chamber angle, extensive peripheral anterior synechiae obstructing the trabecular meshwork, or increased episcleral venous pressure. However, the latter appears to be a relatively uncommon or even nonexistent phenomenon. Synechiae and fibrous proliferation are said to be more apt to develop in eyes with fibrinous iritis or a hypopyon during the acute phase.

Symblepharon formation is variable and relates to the extent of conjunctival

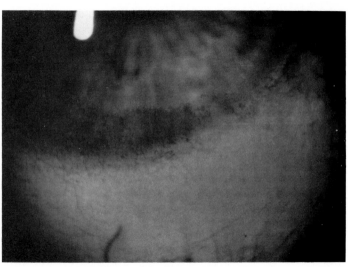

Figure 21–10. Residual mucin-deficient state with unstable tear film resulting in epithelial cell damage (stained with rose bengal).

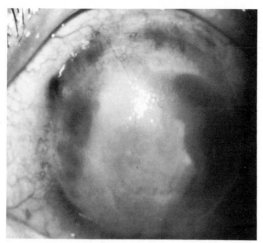

Figure 21–11. Absolute glaucoma after Grade III injury. Note perilimbal staphyloma at 10 o'clock, presumably the effect of prolonged elevation of intraocular pressure upon an area of thin tissue.

necrosis (Fig. 21–12). Symblephara are especially prone to develop where two raw surfaces devoid of epithelium come into contact with each other (e.g., raw bulbar and tarsal conjunctival surfaces in apposition). Contracture of fibrovascular tissue in the substantia propria of the conjunctiva may contribute to the progression of symblephara and to the development of entropion, trichiasis, and exposure with associated further damage to the ocular surface.

Persistent or recurrent iritis is relatively uncommon but has been described after moderately severe alkali burns. Cataracts may develop early[30] as a result of direct alkali damage to lens epithelium or later as a result of lens damage from the alkali or the inflammatory process.[41]

Treatment

General Considerations

The treatment of alkali burns must be adjusted according to the severity of the injury. Primary goals include the restoration of an intact ocular epithelium, control of the acute inflammatory reaction, support of the reparative processes, and avoidance of complications. The severity of the injury determines whether a patient with an alkali burn is treated as an inpatient or as an outpatient. Because of the complexities of treating the more severe injuries, these patients should be admitted to the hospital.

The therapeutic approach to patients with alkali burns will be dealt with in four different time frames relative to the onset of the acute injury: immediate treatment, early (acute phase) treatment, intermediate treatment, and treatment of complications and sequelae.

Immediate (Emergency) Treatment

The most important component of the treatment of ocular alkali burns is immediate irrigation with any nontoxic liquid—the sooner the better. The composition of the irrigant is less important than the speed with which it is begun.

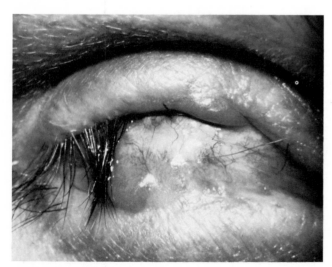

Figure 21–12. Marked symblepharon formation after a Grade IV injury.

Water, ionic solutions, and buffered solutions are equally effective; delay in mixing a buffered solution or obtaining a specific ionic solution is unwarranted. If water is the only liquid available, it should be used. However, if one has access to sterile saline, it is preferred because a small amount of cellular damage is produced by the hypotonicity of water. The use of acidic solutions to neutralize alkali is risky and not recommended.[3]

There are no absolute guidelines to the optimal length of irrigation, but too much is better than too little. As a starting point one might plan to irrigate for a minimum of 30 minutes. The adequacy of this regimen can be assessed minutes after its completion by measuring the pH of the inferior cul-de-sac to determine if it has returned to normal. When alkaline particulate matter (e.g., particles of calcium hydroxide) is embedded in the tissue, it must be removed. One must carefully evaluate both the superior and the inferior cul-de-sac for retained particulate matter. Calcium hydroxide embedded in the tissue may not irrigate out freely; one can use a 0.01 to 0.05 molar EDTA solution as an irrigant to dissolve it.[3] A Q-tip soaked in the sodium EDTA is a useful adjunct for mechanical removal.

Several methods for facilitating irrigation have been suggested, including the implantation of a "T" tube and the use of an irrigating scleral lens.[42] These have not proved to be superior to simple retraction of the lids and the manual use of intravenous tubing connected to the irrigating solution.

The place of tissue debridement in the acute management of alkali burns has not been precisely established. There are differing opinions regarding the appropriate amount of necrotic tissue to be debrided during the acute phase of the injury. The authors feel that debridement should not be a part of acute treatment except for removal of necrotic tissue containing foreign debris.

Paracentesis, either alone or in combination with irrigation of the anterior chamber with buffered solutions (e.g., phosphate buffer), has been advocated by others.[12, 43] The efficacy of these procedures has not been proved, and the authors advise that this not be done because of the inherent risks.

Early (Acute) Phase Treatment

It is in this phase of treatment that many advances have been made, but a number of traditional treatment modalities are still valid. Topical antibiotics are given to protect the eye from secondary infection. Mydriatic-cycloplegics are instilled to prevent the formation of posterior synechiae and the development of ciliary spasm with its attendant discomfort. When intraocular pressure cannot be measured or if it is elevated (usually best determined with a MacKay-Marg tonometer or a pneumotonometer), carbonic anhydrase inhibitors should be administered. Theoretically, topically applied timolol maleate should be an effective agent, but its efficacy and freedom from adverse side effects have not been established in this situation.

If the injury is minor, immediate irrigation, topical instillation of an antibiotic and a mydriatic-cycloplegic agent, and application of a pressure patch may be all that is required. With increasing severity, many of the therapeutic modalities listed below will be necessary. One should not overtreat the minor injuries, but careful examination at least daily is necessary in treating the more severe injuries.

In all but minor burns topical corticosteroids are indicated to reduce the number of inflammatory cells infiltrating the corneal stroma. These inflammatory cells are the major source of proteolytic enzymes responsible for corneal ulceration. It has been shown in rabbits that there is no deleterious effect from the use of topical steroids during the first week after an alkali burn.[44] Clinical experience in man indicates that topical steroids may be used during the first 10 days after an alkali burn even if the epithelium is not intact. It may, in fact, be true that by decreasing the inflammation with topical steroids, one may assist corneal re-epithelialization. The use of a topical steroid such as 1.0 per cent prednisolone acetate, q. 1 h. during the day, has proved both safe and effective. If the epithelium is not intact at the end of 10 days, the steroids must be tapered rapidly and discontinued, since at this point the risk of potentiating ulceration outweighs the potential benefits. (See Chapter 11 for a discussion of the role of topical corticosteroids in ischemic necrosis of the peripheral cornea.) On the other hand, if the epithelium is intact or when epithelial regeneration is complete, steroids may be given with relative safety.

The data on whether steroids inhibit or potentiate tissue collagenase are contradictory.[25, 45, 46] There seems to be no significant effect on the enzyme itself, but the intracellular systems producing the enzyme are inhibited.[46] This suggests that the adverse effects of steroids in the later phases (more than 10 days) after injury are due principally to inhibition of reparative processes while collagen breakdown is allowed to continue. Apparently this results in a potentiation of the ulcerative process.

A number of substances have been shown to be inhibitors of collagenase, but their effect in vivo is weak. As stated above, collagenase can be measured within 9 hours of an acute alkali burn. However, the basement membrane does not begin to break down until approximately 7 days after injury, and frank stromal ulceration begins, on the average, 2 to 3 weeks after injury. On the basis of these facts one could choose to delay the use of collagenase inhibitors until there is clinical evidence of collagen breakdown (7 to 14 days after injury). However, since collagenase activity begins soon after injury and since, early in the process, there undoubtedly is significant enzymatic activity underway, accounting for breakdown of the basement membrane seen after about 7 days, the authors recommend the initiation of topical application of collagenase inhibitors in the early phases of treatment. Better to be "ahead of the process than to be chasing it."

A 0.2 molar solution of sodium EDTA inhibits collagenase reversibly[47] by chelating calcium and/or zinc, both of which are necessary for enzymatic activity. However, it is relatively toxic and therefore not a suitable inhibitor for clinical use. A 0.2 molar solution of calcium EDTA has a much greater affinity for zinc ions than for calicum ions and inhibits collagenase[47-49] by exchanging the calcium ion for a zinc ion. The early ophthalmic literature stated that the inhibtion of corneal collagenase by calcium EDTA occurred as the result of its combination with a second calcium ion, but this is incorrect. This compound can combine with only one divalent ion, and it exerts its effect through the exchange of the calcium for a zinc ion. Calcium disodium EDTA, like sodium EDTA, is a reversible inhibitor of collagenase.

A 0.2 molar solution of cysteine[47, 50-52] will irreversibly inhibit collagenase; it acts by chelating divalent ions and by disrupting disulfide bonds. Unfortunately, cysteine is not commercially available, and it is both relatively difficult to prepare and relatively unstable once formulated. Therefore, from a practical standpoint there are serious impediments to the clinical use of this compound.

A 0.1 molar solution of penicillamine also inhibits collagenase by chelating divalent ions and by disrupting disulfide bonds.[53] It may also inhibit the infiltration of inflammatory cells into the stroma. However, it too is unavailable commercially.

Either 10 per cent or 20 per cent N-acetyl cysteine (0.6 to 1.2 molar) is commercially available in the form of Mucomyst. This solution given q. 2 h. while the patient is awake, although not proven effective in a double masked controlled clinical trial, has been shown to be an effective inhibitor of collagenase in man.[51] It not only chelates divalent ions, but also disrupts disulfide bonds and is an irreversible inhibitor of collagenase. Although it is a relatively unstable solution, it can be used for approximately 4 to 7 days without replacement if kept refrigerated.

There are serum inhibitors of collagenase that are proteinaceous in nature. The presence of these proteins seems to offer at least one reason why vascularized corneas do not ulcerate. Alpha-1 and alpha-2 macroglobulin and beta-1 globulin are effective natural collagenase inhibitors in the rabbit. Alpha-2 macroglobulin and beta-1 globulin are effective inhibitors in man. Alpha-1 antitrypsin seems not to be an effective inhibitor of human corneal collagenase.[54]

An alternative method of attacking the collagenase component of corneal stromal ulceration calls for inhibition not of the active enzyme, but rather of enzyme synthesis. The topical instillation of a 0.5 per cent suspension of medroxyprogesterone in 1 per cent aqueous methylcellulose b.i.d., subconjunctival injection of 10 mg. of depomedroxyprogesterone weekly, or intramuscular injection of a depopreparation inhibit the production of collagenase.[55] The exact site of inhibition is not known, but it occurs prior to the production of the active enzyme. Use of such a compound has an added advantage: it decreases the inflammatory response somewhat without being antianabolic or inhibitory to corneal vascularization. Its place in the treatment of alkali burns is not yet established, but clinical trials are in progress. Cyclic AMP is a known inhibitor of collagenase synthesis whose role and significance are not clear, and corticosteroids have an inhibitory effect on the production of the enzyme.

In severe injuries in which epithelial regeneration is a problem, soft contact lenses are of great benefit in facilitating epithelial healing. It is best to fit the soft lens as soon after the acute injury as possible. A lens with greater oxygen permeability is preferred. Lens retention may be a problem, particularly if significant chemosis is present. The soft contact lens may cause difficulty in evaluating the status of the epithelium, but use of a high-molecular-weight fluorescein that is not taken up by the lens can help alleviate this problem. Once the epithelium has healed, the therapeutic soft contact lens should be left in place for at least 6 to 8 weeks.

Given the information presented above on aqueous humor ascorbate and the scorbutic state that exists in association with more severe alkali burns, the use of ascorbate supplements may prove to be of added therapeutic benefit. This has not been established in man, but trials of oral ascorbate (2 gm. q.i.d.) and a topical 10 per cent solution made up in artificial tears (q. 1 h. for 14 doses daily) are in progress. Theoretically, if this regimen (devised by Pfister[10]) permits the maintenance of an aqueous humor ascorbate level of 15 mg./100 ml. or higher, the cornea should not ulcerate. Supplemental ascorbate should not be of therapeutic value in ulcerative conditions not associated with loss of ciliary body concentrating ability. In fact, supplemental ascorbate has been shown to potentiate the inflammatory response and the resultant stromal ulceration in the presence of normal ciliary body function.[56]

When ischemia is prominent, one of us (T.E.M.) has found subconjunctival heparin to be effective in aiding revascularization.[57] Subconjunctival injections of 0.75 ml. heparin (750 units) mixed with 0.2 ml. lidocaine 2 per cent and 0.35 ml. NaCl are given every other day. As many as ten injections are administered until revascularization occurs. It should be pointed out that a therapeutic effect may not be obvious for several weeks, accounting for the difficulty in establishing a definite cause-and-effect relationship for this form of treatment. Another factor causing skepticism about the effectiveness of this regimen results from experience with inadequate treatment (e.g., only one or two heparin injections).

The formation of symblephara can be discouraged by the use of scleral lenses or symblepharon rings, which prevent apposition of the raw tarsal and bulbar conjunctival surfaces. A simpler but effective means of decreasing symblepharon formation is to lyse the conjunctival adhesions daily as they form. An ointment-coated glass rod is an ideal instrument for this; when a glass rod is not available, a sturdy glass thermometer or a tightly spun cotton-tipped applicator is an effective substitute.

Other forms of early treatment that have fallen into disuse include the subconjunctival injection of serum or blood, topical vasodilators, lamellar keratoplasty, mucous membrane grafts, and artificial epithelium (glued-on contact lenses).

Intermediate Treatment

The nature of the alkali burn and its response to early treatment will determine appropriate therapy 3 to 4 weeks after injury until the eye has stabilized. Thereafter one must deal with the complications and sequelae of the alkali burn. Effective measures instituted during the earlier phases of treatment should be continued. The major problem during this period is the persistence of epithelial defects and associated stromal ulceration. The first step is to encourage epithelial regeneration by refitting therapeutic soft contact lenses. If this fails, one can attempt to stimulate epithelial mitosis by increasing the acetylcholine concentration available to the epithelium or by providing an artificial equivalent (e.g., phospholine iodide, carbachol).[58] It is thought that acetylcholine stimulates an increase of intracellular cyclic GMP relative to cyclic AMP, resulting in stimulation of cellular mitosis.

If these drugs are effective, epithelial healing occurs within 1 week. The drugs appear to be most effective in relatively uninflamed eyes. Once epithelial regeneration is complete, the topical agent used to increase epithelial acetylcholine should be discontinued. This allows the cell to shift from mitosis to protein synthesis with the restoration of normal formation of hemidesmosomes to anchor the epithelial cells. While mitosis is being stimulated, the corneal surface must be protected because cells in active mitosis are poorly adherent to the underlying stroma. A soft contact lens should be maintained in place during this time.

Mucomimetic tear substitutes may help to stabilize the tear film. However, in the more severe injuries they provide little added benefit during this phase. If exposure is a significant contributing problem, one should consider a tarsorrhaphy or a scleral lens. The latter is also of benefit if trichiasis is associated with exposure. Progression of symblephera may be stimulated by a tarsorrhaphy, but in a setting characterized by marked surface drying a therapeutic soft contact lens will not be retained.

Should the above fail, one may consider a conjunctival flap. It is usually best to wait until the conjunctiva has recovered from its acellular phase before attempting a flap procedure. Unfortunately, when the injury is so severe that nonsurgical maneuvers fail, the associated conjunctival abnormality generally precludes a successful conjunctival flap. In such a case it has been recommended that a mucous membrane graft of 0.4-mm. thickness be used.[59] The timing of such an operation and the size of the mucosal graft are controversial. The procedure is carried out early and as a routine by some[60] but limited to areas of severe necrosis and delayed until a later date by others.[59] This procedure has not gained broad acceptance, and one wonders if tissue unable to support its own growth is likely to support the growth of transplanted tissue. It would seem that mucosal grafts have a place only in the later restoration of an obliterated cul-de-sac.

For unilateral cases in which more conventional treatment modalities are unsuccessful, transplantation of conjunctiva from the contralateral normal ocular surface has been recommended by Thoft.[61] A conjunctival recession is first performed along with a superficial keratectomy. Four pieces of normal conjunctiva are then sutured to the ocular surface so that they bridge the corneal limbus. This has been effective in the rehabilitation of the ocular surface in later phases of treatment, and in selected circumstances it may prove to be beneficial as a component of earlier treatment.

If perforation results from the ulcerative process and the perforation site is relatively small, one may try a tissue adhesive such as butylcyanoacrylate to seal the perforation.[62] Alternatively, a patch graft[63] provides a definitive surgical closure.

Late Treatment of Complications and Sequelae

The replacement of tears after an alkali burn is still less than ideal. No completely satisfactory mucomimetic preparation is available to compensate for the loss of the normal mucin component of tears. Claims that polyvinylpyrrolidone is a more effective mucomimetic substance than other available tear substitutes[40] have not been substantiated clinically, and, from a practical standpoint, we can do little better than to have the patient instill an artificial tear preparation q. 1 h. while awake. Other approaches to the replacement of tears or protection of the ocular surface have included the use of ointments, minipumps (which are cumbersome and difficult to keep sterile), and parotid duct translocation.[64] Unfortunately, parotid secretions have not proved to be mucomimetic, and significant epiphora, especially at mealtime, has limited the use of this technique.

Other therapeutic considerations include the control of glaucoma, if it exists, protection of the ocular surface with soft contact lenses or scleral lenses if necessary, and the use of topical steroids if there is chronic inflammation. If surface problems persist despite the use of therapeutic or scleral contact lenses, a conjunctival flap may be performed. In cases in which the alkali burn is uniocular, transplantation of conjunctiva from the contralateral eye, as described above, may be considered. If distortion of the lids or fornices contributes to surface problems or if the eye is being prepared for corneal transplantation, entropion repair and reconstruction of the fornices must be undertaken. If a cataract has

formed acutely and is contributing to ocular complications (glaucoma, uveitis), it should be removed early. On the other hand, if there are no associated complications, one should defer cataract extraction until the eye has completely recovered from the injury to avoid wound healing problems.

Penetrating keratoplasty in this population is fraught with problems. Postoperative compliance is a major problem among many individuals in this group and must be seriously considered if transplantation surgery is contemplated.[65] In all cases stromal and epithelial wound healing can be major problems postoperatively. However, with newer surgical techniques and better understanding of the disease process, the prognosis is somewhat better.[66, 67] The use of conjunctival transplantation to rehabilitate the surface prior to corneal surgery in uniocular burns may be a major advance. In all cases it is best to delay penetrating keratoplasty for at least 1 year after the active process has become quiescent. This gives the tissue time to approach structural and biochemical normalcy and allows time for the inflammatory process to totally subside. Conversion of conjunctival epithelium to morphologically and biochemically normal corneal epithelium is a slow process,[68, 69] and the ability of chemically damaged, conjunctivally derived corneal epithelium to maintain its functional integrity is challenged after penetrating keratoplasty. Control of glaucoma, restoration of normal lid-globe relationships, and reconstruction of the fornices must be accomplished preoperatively if corneal transplantation is to be successful.

Several surgical considerations related to corneal transplantation in this patient population merit emphasis.[66, 67] Subconjunctival granulation tissue should be resected if it has not already been removed at the time of fornix reconstruction. One must always anticipate unusual and complicated anterior chamber abnormalities that will not become apparent until the host bed is prepared. If fibrovascular membranes are encountered in the anterior chamber, these must be resected. The epithelium should be left on the donor button if at all possible. A careful microsurgical approach is required, using fine (e.g., 10-0 nylon) suture material. All knots should be buried beneath the surface to avoid disruption of corneal epithelial integrity.

There are several important postoperative considerations to remember. A maximal effort should be made to suppress inflammation with the aggressive use of topical steroids. Often a soft contact lens and artificial tear instillation will be necessary to assist in the maintenance of an intact corneal epithelium. Glaucoma should be anticipated and controlled if it occurs.

In desperate cases that are not suitable candidates for penetrating keratoplasty, a keratoprosthesis may be considered. The nut-and-bolt and collar-button types have done poorly because of stromal melting and extrusion.[70-72] Through-and-through prostheses, with the optical post brought out through the upper lid, have had limited success[71, 73] (Fig. 21–13). The major complications associated with all types of keratoprostheses include extrusion, retroprosthetic membrane, glaucoma, retinal detachment, and infection.

ACID INJURIES

Ocular acid injuries occur only slightly less often than injuries produced by alkaline substances.[32] Despite this, little has appeared in the ophthalmic literature other than case reports describing acid injuries. Generally, one finds small sections in review articles; very few papers deal with ocular acid injuries in depth. Fortunately, most such injuries are mild because they result from contact with weak acids or dilute strong acids. Nonetheless, severe injuries can occur and are most commonly associated with exposure to heavy metal acids (e.g., chromic), other mineral acids (e.g., sulfuric or sulfurous), or hydrofluoric acid. The reasons these acids produce more severe injuries is discussed below.

The clinical picture of a severe ocular acid injury is fairly constant irrespective of the offending agent.

Acid injuries will be discussed in a manner similar to that followed for alkaline injuries, and areas in which the two types of injury are dissimilar will be emphasized.

Clinically Significant Acids (Table 21–2)

Sulfuric acid is encountered most commonly in the form of oil of vitriol or battery acid. In its pure form it is an odorless, colorless, oily liquid. However, when contaminated with slight impurities, it becomes yellowish or brown and emits a foul odor. Injuries caused by concentrated sulfuric acid are more severe than can be accounted for on the basis of the hydrogen ion alone. Additional damage results from such injuries because concentrated sulfuric acid has a great avidity for water; it combines with water, releasing heat, and therefore has a charring effect. As the concentration of sulfuric acid decreases, the substance causes injuries similar to those resulting from hydrochloric acid burns that can be explained on the basis of hydrogen ion effects alone. Therefore, sulfuric acid injuries range from mild to very severe.

The frequency of injuries caused by battery acid is increasing.[74] The majority are minor, but severe injuries with loss of vision or the globe have occurred. Most such injuries, especially the more severe ones, result from battery explosions. When sulfuric acid combines with water in the battery, hydrogen and oxygen are produced by electrolysis, especially when the battery is charging, and this gaseous mixture explodes on contact with a spark or with fire. The offending source commonly has been a spark associated with the use of jumper cables or the use of a match or cigarette lighter for illumination. Resultant injuries often represent a combination of acid burn, contusion from particulate matter, laceration, and intraocular foreign body penetration or perforation.

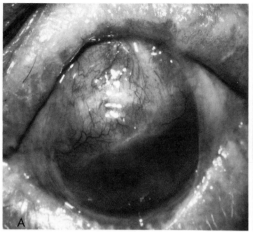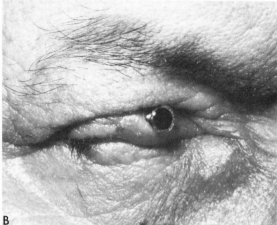

Figure 21–13. *A*, Eye 1 year after a Grade IV alkali injury (poor candidate for keratoplasty). *B*, Through-and-through prosthesis in place for 1½ years with 20/25 vision and a 20-degree field.

Sulfur dioxide may be encountered as sulfurous anhydride or sulfurous oxide. It is a colorless gas that is easily compressed to a liquid with a boiling point of −10° C. It is used as a fruit and vegetable preservative, bleach, and refrigerant. When used as a refrigerant, it is mixed with oils that permit prolonged surface contact and therefore result in more severe tissue damage. Sulfur dioxide itself is very volatile; either a direct jet of the gas or the liquid in oil is required to produce severe injury. Sulfur dioxide gas in low concentration causes only minor ocular irritation and little significant ocular damage. However, if one is exposed to a direct jet of sulfur dioxide gas for several seconds, severe ocular injuries may occur.[75] Exposure to liquid sulfur dioxide may produce a mild injury with few residua or a severe injury resulting in an opaque, vascularized cornea and marked symblepharon

Table 21–2. CLINICALLY SIGNIFICANT ACIDS*

Hydrofluoric Acid
Sulfurous Acid
Sulfuric Acid
Chromic Acid

Hydrochloric Acid
Nitric Acid

Acetic Acid

*Listed in three groups in decreasing order of tendency to produce ocular damage.

formation. Initially injuries caused by liquid sulfur dioxide are associated with little discomfort; the sulfur dioxide damages corneal nerves and causes anesthesia, but in time one sees opacification of these affected corneal nerves. The visual acuity is not severely affected at first either but worsens within a few hours to several days along with other ocular signs.

The injury produced by sulfur dioxide is not the result of its freezing effect on the tissue.[75] Combined with water, it forms sulfurous acid, and both sulfur dioxide and sulfurous acid denature proteins and inactivate numerous enzymes. The sulfurous acid is highly soluble in both lipid and water and penetrates ocular tissues well.

Hydrofluoric acid, or hydrogen fluoride, is a weak inorganic acid but a strong solvent. It is often encountered in industry either in its pure form or mixed with other agents (e.g., nitric acid, ammonium difluoride, or acetic acid). Stock solutions of hydrofluoric acid are either 49 per cent or 70 per cent, and it may be used in these concentrations or in dilutions as low as 0.5 per cent. It affects most substances but does not affect polyethylene or polypropylene. Rubber can withstand hydrofluoric acid for limited periods of time.

Hydrofluoric acid is used in the etching and polishing of glass and silicone and in frosting glass. It is also used in the pickling or chemical milling of metals; in the refining of uranium, tantalum, and beryllium; in the alkylation of high octane gasoline; and in the production of elemental fluoride, inorganic fluoride, and organic fluorocarbons. Its most frequently encountered use is in the expanding semiconductor business, where it is employed in the production of silicone products.

Much has been written on skin burns from hydrofluoric acid, but the literature on ocular injuries is sparse. Although there are no well-documented, published human cases of ocular hydrofluoric acid burns, a rabbit model has been described.[76] The tissue damage resulting from hydrofluoric acid in this model will be discussed below. Apparently hydrofluoric acid produces more severe injury than many other acids because of the activity of the fluoride ion. The damage produced by hydrofluoric acid can be partially reproduced by sodium or potassium fluoride. A possible mechanism through which fluoride damages tissue is its binding of divalent ions. Because of its small molecular weight and size, it may also penetrate tissues more readily.

Chromic acid is derived from chromic oxide and chromium trioxide. These are brown solids, soluble in water, with which they combine to form a strong caustic acid. There have been rare cases of severe ocular injury resulting from direct instillation of the liquid onto the ocular surfaces. More commonly injuries are associated with exposure to droplets in the chrome-plating industry. Repeated exposure to these droplets results in chronic conjunctival inflammation and a brown discoloration of the epithelium in the interpalpebral fissure.

Concentrated hydrochloric acid is a 38 per cent solution, but it is more common as technical muriatic acid, a 32 per cent solution. Exposure to hydrogen chloride gas is irritating and results in protective tearing, which prevents severe ocular damage. Exposure to liquid hydrochloric acid may produce mild to severe ocular damage, depending upon the factors discussed in this chapter.

Nitric acid is colorless in its pure form. However, in its commercial form it has a yellowish tint, the result of formation of nitrogen oxides. Burns produced with nitric acid are similar to those produced with hydrochloric acid. An exception is the resultant epithelial opacity, which is yellowish rather than white.

Acetic acid is encountered as ethanoic acid, ethylic acid, methane carboxylic acid, vinegar acid, and glacial acetic acid. It is a relatively weak inorganic acid and therefore produces only minor damage unless it is encountered in a concentrated form. For instance, there is only 4 to 10 per cent acetic acid in vinegar, and injuries resulting from exposure to vinegar, if not prolonged, produce only minor damage. However, "essence of vinegar" contains 80 per cent acetic acid, which may produce more severe damage. The most concentrated form of acetic acid, glacial acetic acid, causes severe ocular injury. Acetic acid vapor is irritating, producing reflex lacrimation and therefore usually only mild hyperemia. It would seem that exposure to greater than a 10 per cent solution of acetic acid is required to produce a severe injury unless the exposure is prolonged.

Biochemical Changes

All acids tend to coagulate and precipitate protein. However, the anionic portion of acids varies, and there is a differing affinity for protein among the anions. This correlates with the degree of precipitation and denaturation that results when these anions combine with tissue proteins.[77] Therefore, both the hydrogen ion and the anionic portion of the acid contribute to the adverse effects on tissue proteins. Acids also break down the intramolecular forces of proteins, such as collagen. This reaction with collagen results in a shortening of the collagen fibers and a resultant rapid increase in intraocular pressure.[34, 78] As will be discussed in greater detail below, the coagulated cells on the surface serve as a relative barrier to further penetration of acids. The tissue proteins also have a buffering effect on acids, which contributes to the localized nature of acid burns.[79]

Different acids denature corneal glycosaminoglycans differently, as measured by their effect on stromal swelling pressure.[75] This varying effect is demonstrated by studies of stromal metachromatic staining or hexosamine content. There is no loss of metachromatic staining or hexosamine in the early phases after hydrochloric acid burns; in later phases there is a loss but only in areas of scarring.[77] In contrast, there is a marked decrease in acid mucopolysaccharide content by the fifth day following a severe sulfuric acid burn.[80] Decreased stromal metachromatic staining has also been demonstrated after severe hydrofluoric acid burns.[76] It has been suggested that stromal turbidity occurring after an acid burn results not from changes in collagen, but, rather, from precipitation of the stromal mucoids.[81]

Aqueous humor changes have been less thoroughly studied after exposure to acid than after alkaline injuries. Aqueous humor pH is decreased 15 minutes after exposure to hydrochloric acid.[78] Protein content and prostaglandin activity in the aqueous humor are elevated during the first several hours after exposure to hydrochloric acid.[78]

The presence of proteolytic enzymes after acid burns has not been evaluated. However, when ulceration occurs, it seems likely that the same endogenous proteolytic enzymes that are active after alkali burns are at fault. Ulceration is rare after hydrofluoric burns unless divalent ions are made available to the cornea; divalent ions cause the ulcerative process to become prominent.[82] Possibly the fluoride ion combines with divalent ions, such as calcium and zinc, which are required for collagenase activity, in effect serving as an enzyme inhibitor. Marked subconjunctival hemorrhage is encountered after hydrofluoric acid burns; the fluoride ions bind calcium and may act as an anticoagulant.

No defect in collagen synthesis has been established after acid burns. However, in the more severe burns with associated ciliary body damage it is possible that aqueous humor and corneal ascorbate are decreased and that a localized scorbutic state exists, similar to that found after severe alkali burns.[9, 10]

Grading of Burn Severity and Factors That Determine Severity

No specific classification system has been proposed for acid burns. However, the Roper-Hall modification[32] of Ballen's scheme[33] can be used to classify acid burns. This classification is outlined in the previous section on alkalies.

Signs indicating a bad prognosis after acid injury reflect acid penetration of the tissues. They include complete corneal anesthesia, conjunctival and episcleral ischemia, severe iritis, and lens opacification.

Acids in general produce less severe injuries than alkalies. This is largely attributable to coagulation of the epithelial surface by the acid, forming a relative barrier to further penetration of the acid. The corneal stroma also has a buffering capability for solutions with a pH less than 4.[79] However, there are exceptions to this. Sulfuric acid causes increased tissue devastation because of its great avidity for water. Sulfurous acid is both water- and lipid-soluble and penetrates well into the cornea. Hydrofluoric acid also penetrates well, and its fluoride ion seems to be responsible for the additional associated tissue damage.[76]

For any acid, the degree of tissue damage will correlate with the quantity and concentration to which the eye is exposed as well as with the length of the exposure. Generally speaking, fumes containing hydrogen ions and droplets of acidic solutions cause only minor injury; the more severe injuries are the result of a direct splash of acidic chemical onto the ocular surface. Acids also tend to cause severe tissue damage only if their pH is less than 2.5, providing the epithelium is intact. If the epithelium is removed prior to exposure, severe damage can occur at a higher pH.

The lipid solubility of acids varies and has a significant effect on the tissue-penetrating capabilities of individual acids. Sulfurous acid is more lipid-soluble than hydrochloric acid, which is more soluble than phosphoric acid, which in turn is more soluble than sulfuric acid.[75] However, if the concentration is increased (with a resultant decrease in pH), there is less of an apparent difference in penetration among these acids because they destroy the epithelial barrier.

The severity of surface damage produced by acids partially depends on their anionic affinity for protein. The greater the protein affinity, the greater the degree of protein precipitation and denaturation. Increased protein affinity results in increased surface damage but decreased penetration. The protein affinity for a number of acids has been determined and is listed in order of increasing protein affinity: hydrochloric, trichloracetic, metaphosphoric, sulfosalicylic, picric, tungstic, and tannic.[77] All cause the pattern of tissue damage expected from their protein affinity with the exception of hydrochloric acid, which produces a more severe injury than one would anticipate from its protein affinity. The severity of injury after hydrochloric acid exposure may partially relate to its relatively high lipid solubility.

Clinical Stages (with Pathologic Correlation) After Acid Burn

Acute (Immediate to 1 Week After Burn)

Many types of acids can produce ocular injury, so the outcome is variable. Acids tend to penetrate more slowly than alkalies,[77] explaining the sharper demarcation of the injury. Acids tend to be poorly lipid-soluble; they bind to protein and coagulate tissue, the latter forming a relative barrier to penetration. The involved tissues also have a natural buffering capacity for acids. As outlined above, however, exceptions exist; sulfuric acid, sulfurous acid, hydrofluoric acid, and heavy-metal acids, such as

chromic acid, cause more severe ocular damage and tend to penetrate more readily.

Exposure of surface epithelium to acid results in coagulation of the cells with varying degrees of opacification. This is true for both conjunctival and corneal epithelium. The opacification is apparent within a few seconds after exposure (Fig. 21–14). It is more pronounced if the acid is concentrated or has a high protein affinity, causing the epithelium to turn white.[77] However, epithelium injured by either nitric or chromic acid will be yellow or brown. Following even severe hydrofluoric acid injury, the epithelium is only minimally opaque (Fig. 21–15).

The opacity is generally limited to the area of direct contact with the acid, and the affected epithelial cells begin to slough within hours after the injury. In severe injuries the entire epithelial surface of the cornea may slough as a single sheet (Fig. 21–15), but often the underlying stroma is clear. However, if the acid has penetrated to deeper layers, other structures will be affected, including keratocytes and endothelial cells. The depth of cell death will depend on the degree of penetration of the acid. Clinical manifestations indicative of acid penetration include stromal granularity, stromal edema, ischemia (Fig. 21–16), severe iritis, and cataract formation. Except in the most severe cases, one does not encounter significant ischemia on the basis of vascular endothelial necrosis or vascular thrombosis.

If the injury is mild, the epithelium will regenerate within a few days and the eye will totally recover. Following more severe injuries the underlying stroma may have a grayish, ground-glass appearance secondary to the direct action of the acid and to infiltration by inflammatory cells. On occasion, even after a severe sulfuric acid burn, an opaque stroma may be associated with minimal endothelial or deeper structure damage.[80] Moreover, the stroma occasionally may be severely damaged but not appear cloudy. This is especially

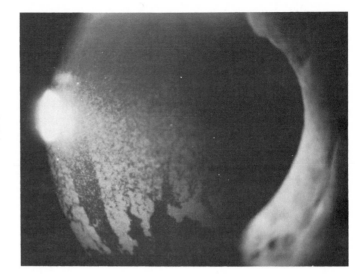

Figure 21–14. Whitened epithelium after hydrochloric acid injury. Area of opacity is limited to cells that came into direct contact with acid. Eye recovered totally in 4 days.

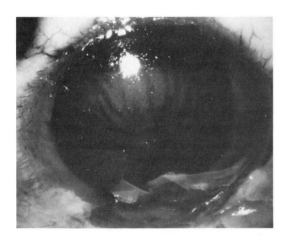

Figure 21–15. Two days after a severe hydrofluoric acid injury. Epithelium is minimally opaque but exfoliating in a sheet. Underlying stroma is relatively clear but edematous.

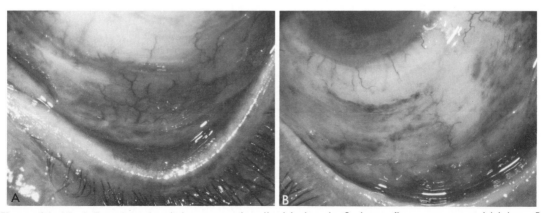

Figure 21–16. *A,* Tarsal and cul-de-sac conjunctival ischemia 2 days after a severe acid injury. *B,* Marked diffuse bulbar ischemia at same time.

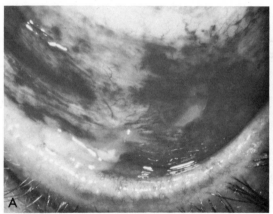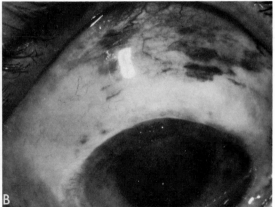

Figure 21–17. Subconjunctival hemorrhage 5 days after severe acid injury. *A,* Tarsal and cul-de-sac hemorrhage. *B,* Bulbar hemorrhage.

true after sulfur dioxide or hydrofluoric acid burns (Fig. 21–15).

Within minutes to hours of an acid burn, the conjunctiva will become hyperemic and chemotic. Subconjunctival hemorrhage is not uncommon (Fig. 21–17). Edema of the corneal stroma also may occur but does not necessarily indicate penetration of the acid deeply into the stroma or to the endothelium; stromal edema can result from loss of the epithelial barrier to water flow. In the early phases after an acid burn, a mild, reflex iritis often is present. This will clear in a few days to weeks after a mild injury, as will the conjunctival and even the stromal abnormality.

Inflammatory cells begin to infiltrate the corneal stroma, both from the limbus and through the disrupted anterior surface, during the first 24 hours after an acid injury. The intensity of the infiltrate is generally far less than that seen after alkali burns. In addition, within minutes after exposure to acid, the intraocular pressure may increase in a manner similar to that seen after alkali burns. Most likely this is secondary to shrinkage of the collagen fibers.[34, 78] The intraocular pressure then remains high for more than 3 hours with less of a biphasic pattern than is encountered after alkali burns. A sustained increase in intraocular pressure occurs only if the hydrogen ion reaches the anterior chamber[3] and is at least partially mediated by prostaglandin.[78] After the early increase the intra-

ocular pressure may be normal, elevated, or decreased depending upon the relative involvement of ciliary body and outflow channels.

Early Reparative Phase (1 to 3 Weeks)

Since most acid burns are mild, most recover by this stage. Moderate burns generally are followed by gradual repair of the tissue damage and resolution of the inflammatory response during this period. Vessels begin to invade the stroma approximately 1 week after the burn and then begin to regress during the second or third week; the regression is accompanied by a decrease in stromal edema. In these cases the only sequela is apt to be a minimal stromal opacity.[77] The more severe acid burns are characterized by stromal ulceration and progressive corneal vascularization (Fig. 21–18) at approximately 2 weeks after injury. The latter may take the form of deep stromal vascularization or surface vascular overgrowth.

Late Reparative Phase and Sequelae (3 Weeks and Longer)

All but the most severe injuries will have recovered by 3 weeks after the burn. In those that have not, one is apt to observe persistent and progressive opacification and/or vascularization of the stroma or corneal ulceration.

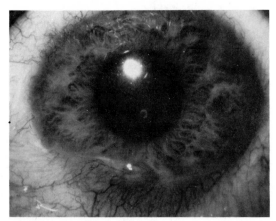

Figure 21-18. Pannus formation over inferior cornea 6 months after moderately severe acid injury. Pannus progressed over next 12 months but spared the visual axis.

Stromal ulceration is relatively uncommon after acid burns. In the rabbit model of ocular hydrofluoric acid burns, ulcers rarely occur in the absence of treatment. When the eye is irrigated promptly with water, normal saline, or magnesium chloride, there is a 6 per cent ulceration rate. However, early irrigation with calcium chloride is followed by a 50 per cent incidence of ulceration. If a mixture of the divalent ions normally found in the cornea is used as an irrigant, there is a 25 per cent ulceration rate.[82] This phenomenon presumably reflects the fact that the fluoride ion binds divalent ions, which are necessary cofactors for proteolytic enzyme activity. By replacing the divalent ions, one replaces these cofactors and allows stromal ulceration to proceed.

The rabbit model is characterized by a dense calcific band keratopathy in the interpalpebral fissure[76] (Fig. 21–19). It is not clear why this occurs or whether it will occur after severe hydrofluoric acid burns in man.

Retrocorneal fibrous membranes appear during the late reparative phase if the endothelium has been severely damaged. Other sequelae characteristic of this phase include recurrent epithelial erosions (Fig. 21–20), delayed cataract formation, glaucoma, and hypotony with subsequent phthisis bulbi. Tear film abnormalities, persistent or recurrent iritis, entropion with trichiasis, and

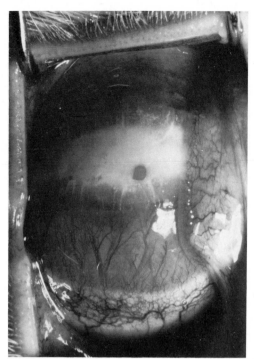

Figure 21-19. Calcific band keratopathy in hydrofluoric acid rabbit model.

symblepharon formation also may occur. The mechanism of each of these problems is the same as described for alkali burns.

Treatment

General Considerations

The treatment of acid burns must be adjusted to the severity of the injury. Primary therapeutic goals include the restoration of an intact epithelial surface, the support of the reparative process, and the avoidance of complications. Although treatment is similar to that recommended for alkali burns of equal severity, most acid burns are mild and do not require extensive therapy. Severe acid burns are treated in a manner similar to severe alkali burns.

Immediate (Emergency) Treatment

The most important factor is the speed with which one begins irrigation. What one uses for irrigation is less important, and it is inadvisable to attempt to neutralize the acid solution with either al-

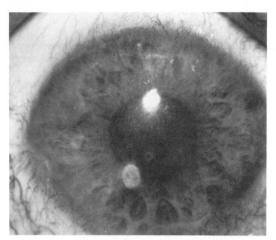

Figure 21–20. Superficial stromal faceted scar at 7 o'clock between visual axis and limbus resulting from recurrent epithelial breakdown after a moderately severe acid injury.

kali or a buffer solution. Water and saline are the most commonly used irrigants. If both are equally available, normal saline is preferred to avoid the damage caused by the hypotonicity of water. However, the damage caused by water is minimal and is more than compensated for by the beneficial effect of rapid irrigation when saline is not immediately available.

A measure of the pH in the inferior cul-de-sac prior to beginning irrigation is helpful. There are no absolute guidelines regarding the optimal interval for irrigation. In general, the irrigation period needed to return the pH to normal is shorter after acid burns than after alkali burns. In any case initial irrigation for 20 to 30 minutes is not excessive. After a delay of approximately 5 minutes to allow for equilibration, one should remeasure the cul-de-sac pH; further irrigation is required only if the pH is still abnormally low.

It has been recommended that 0.03 per cent benzalkonium chloride be used as the irrigant after ocular hydrofluoric acid burns.[83] However, in the rabbit model of hydrofluoric acid burn,[76] use of 0.03 per cent benzalkonium chloride caused additional ocular damage and had no beneficial therapeutic effect.[82] It is therefore recommended that this solution not be used after ocular hydrofluoric acid burns. Topical pastes of 25 to 50 per cent magnesium sulfate or magnesium oxide have been recommended on the basis of extrapolation from the treatment of skin burns, but they are too toxic for use in the eye.[82] Irrigation with isotonic calcium chloride, calcium gluconate, or 0.2 per cent hyamine has also been found to be toxic to the normal eye and to produce an additive toxic effect when used as an irrigant for ocular hydrofluoric acid burns.[82] Subconjunctival injection of 10 per cent calcium chloride or calcium gluconate, as well as isotonic lanthanum chloride, has been found to be significantly toxic to the normal as well as to the hydrofluoric acid–burned eye.[82] Subconjunctival injection of isotonic magnesium chloride appears to have no therapeutic benefit.[82] Water, normal saline, and isotonic magnesium chloride have been found to be equally effective as irrigants in the emergency treatment of ocular hydrofluoric acid burns.[82] Therefore, to re-emphasize the basic therapeutic principle, the speed with which one irrigates is more important than the material with which one irrigates. The remainder of the considerations in the treatment of acid burns are the same as those recommended for alkali burns whether the injury is mild or severe.

REFERENCES

1. Grant, W. M.: *Toxicology of the Eye.* 2nd ed. Springfield, Ill., Charles C Thomas, 1974.
2. Stanley, J. A.: Strong alkali burns of the eye. N Engl J Med 273:1265, 1965.
3. Grant, W. M., and Kern, H. L.: Action of alkalies on the corneal stroma. Arch Ophthalmol 54:931, 1955.
4. Harris, L. S., Cohn, K., and Galin, M. A.: Alkali injury from fireworks. Ann Ophthalmol 3:849, 1971.
5. Henriquez, A. S., Pihlaja, D. J., and Dohlman, C. H.: Surface ultrastructure in alkali-burned rabbit corneas. Amer J Ophthalmol 81:324, 1976.
6. Gnadinger, M. C., Itoi, M., Slansky, H. H., and

Dohlman, C. H.: The role of collagenase in the alkali-burned cornea. Amer J Ophthalmol 68:478, 1969.

7. Cejkova, J., Lojda, Z., Obenberger, J., and Havrankova, E.: Alkali burns of the rabbit cornea. II. A histochemical study of glycosaminoglycans. Histochemistry 45:71, 1975.

8. Pfister, R. R., Friend, J., and Dohlman, C. H.: The anterior segments of rabbits after alkali burns. Arch Ophthalmol 86:189, 1971.

9. Levinson, R. A., Paterson, C. A., and Pfister, R. R.: Ascorbic acid prevents corneal ulceration and perforation following experimental alkali burns. Invest Ophthalmol 15:986, 1976.

10. Pfister, R. R., and Paterson, C. A.: Additional clinical and morphological observations on the favorable effect of ascorbate in experimental ocular alkali burns. Invest Ophthalmol Vis Sci 16:478, 1977.

11. Pfister, R. R., McCulley, J. P., Friend, J., and Dohlman, C. H.: Collagenase activity of intact corneal epithelium in peripheral alkali burns. Arch Ophthalmol 86:308, 1971.

12. Paterson, C. A., Pfister, R. R., and Levinson, R. A.: Aqueous humor pH changes after experimental alkali burns. Amer J Ophthalmol 79:414, 1975.

13. Cejkova, J., Lojda, Z., Obenberger, J., and Havrankova, E.: Alkali burns of the rabbit cornea. I. A histochemical study of β-glucuronidase, β-galactosidase and N-acetyl-β-D-glucosaminidase. Histochemistry 45:65, 1975.

14. Slansky, H. H., Freeman, M. I., and Itoi, M.: Collagenolytic activity in bovine corneal epithelium. Arch Ophthalmol 80:496, 1968.

15. Brown, S. I., Weller, C. A., and Wassermann, H. E.: Collagenolytic activity of alkali-burned corneas. Arch Ophthalmol 81:370, 1969.

16. Itoi, M., Gnadinger, M. C., Slansky, H. H., Freeman, M. I., and Dohlman, C. H.: Collagenase in the cornea. Exp Eye Res 8:369, 1969.

17. Brown, S. I., Weller, C. A., and Akiya, S.: Pathogenesis of ulcers of the alkali-burned cornea. Arch Ophthalmol 83:205, 1970.

18. Brown, S. I., and Weller, C. A.: The pathogenesis and treatment of collagenase-induced diseases of the cornea. Trans Amer Acad Ophthalmol Otolaryngol 74:375, 1970.

19. Eisen, A. Z., Jeffrey, J. J., and Gross, J.: Human skin collagenase. Isolation and mechanism of attack on the collagen molecule. Biochim Biophys Acta 151:637, 1968.

20. Berman, M., Dohlman, C. H., Gnadinger, M., and Davison, P.: Characterization of collagenolytic activity in the ulcerating cornea. Exp Eye Res 11:255, 1971.

21. Gordon, J. M., Bauer, E. A., and Eisen, A. Z.: Collagenase in human cornea. Immunologic localization. Arch Ophthalmol 98:341, 1980.

22. Brown, S. I., and Weller, C. A.: Cell origin of collagenase in normal and wounded corneas. Arch Ophthalmol 83:74, 1970.

23. Lazarus, G. S., Brown, R. S., Daniels, J. R., and Fullmer, H. M.: Human granulocyte collagenase. Science 159:1483, 1968.

24. Kenyon, K. R., Berman, M., Rose, J., and Gage, J.: Prevention of stromal ulceration in the alkali-burned rabbit cornea by glued-on contact lens. Evidence for the role of polymorphonuclear leukocytes in collagen degradation. Invest Ophthalmol Vis Sci 18:570, 1979.

25. Hook, R. M., Hook, C. W., and Brown, S. I.: Fibroblast collagenase partial purification and characterization. Invest Ophthalmol 12:771, 1973.

26. Newsome, D. A., and Gross, J.: Regulation of corneal collagenase production: Stimulation of serially passaged stromal cells by blood mononuclear cells. Cell 16:895, 1979.

27. Berman, M. B., Leary, R., and Gage, J.: Latent collagenase in the ulcerating rabbit cornea. Exp Eye Res 25:435, 1977.

28. Berman, M. B., Leary, R., and Gage, J.: Evidence for a role of the plasminogen activator–plasmin system in corneal ulceration. Invest Ophthalmol Vis Sci 19:1204, 1980.

29. Berman, M. B., and Manabe, R.: Corneal collagenase—evidence for zinc metalloenzymes. Ann Ophthalmol 5:1193, 1973.

30. Hughes, W. F., Jr.: Alkali burns of the eye. II. Clinical and pathologic course. Arch Ophthalmol 36:189, 1946.

31. Hughes, W. F., Jr.: Alkali burns of the eye. I. Review of the literature and summary of present knowledge. Arch Ophthalmol 35:423, 1946.

32. Roper-Hall, M. J.: Thermal and chemical burns. Trans Ophthalmol Soc UK 85:631, 1965.

33. Ballen, P. H.: Treatment of chemical burns of the eye. Eye Ear Nose Throat Monthly 43:57, 1964.

34. Chiang, T. S., Moorman, L. R., and Thomas, R. P.: Ocular hypertensive response following acid and alkali burns in rabbits. Invest Ophthalmol 10:270, 1971.

35. Paterson, C. A., and Pfister, R. R.: Ocular hypertensive response to alkali burns in the monkey. Exp Eye Res 17:449, 1973.

36. Stein, M. R., Naidoff, M. A., and Dawson, C. R.: Intraocular pressure response to experimental alkali burns. Amer J Ophthalmol 75:99, 1973.

37. Paterson, C. A., and Pfister, R. R.: Intraocular pressure changes after alkali burns. Arch Ophthalmol 91:211, 1974.

38. Brown, S. I., Wassermann, H. E., and Dunn, M. W.: Alkali burns of the cornea. Arch Ophthalmol 82:91, 1969.

39. Matsuda, H., and Smelser, G. K.: Endothelial cells in alkali-burned corneas. Arch Ophthalmol 89:402, 1973.

40. Lemp, M. A.: Cornea and sclera. Arch Ophthalmol 92:158, 1974.

41. Awan, K. J.: Delayed cataract formation after alkali burn. Canad J Ophthalmol 10:423, 1975.

42. Morgan, L. B.: A new drug delivery system for the eye. Indus Med 40:11, 1971.

43. Bennett, T. O., Peyman, G. A., and Rutgard, J.: Intracameral phosphate buffer in alkali burns. Canad J Ophthalmol 13:93, 1978.

44. Donshik, P. C., Berman, M. B., Dohlman, C. H., Gage, J., and Rose, J.: Effect of topical corticosteroids on ulceration in alkali-burned corneas. Arch Ophthalmol 96:2117, 1978.

45. Brown, S. I., Weller, C. A., and Vidrich, A. M.: Effect of corticosteroids on corneal collagenase of rabbits. Amer J Ophthalmol 70:744, 1970.

46. Koob, T. J., Jeffrey, J. J., and Eisen, A. Z.: Regulation of human skin collagenase activity by hydrocortisone and dexamethasone in organ culture. Biochem Biophys Res Comm 61:1083, 1974.

47. Brown, S. I., and Weller, C. A.: Collagenase inhibitors in prevention of ulcers of alkali-burned cornea. Arch Ophthalmol 83:352, 1970.

48. Itoi, M., Gnadinger, M. C., Slansky, H. H., and Dohlman, C. H.: Prévention d'ulcères du stroma de

la cornée grâce à l'utilisation d'un sel de calcium d'E.D.T.A. Arch. Ophthalmol (Paris) 29:389, 1969.

49. Slansky, H. H., Dohlman, C. H., and Berman, M. B.: Prevention of corneal ulcers. Trans Amer Acad Ophthalmol Otolaryngol 75:1208, 1971.

50. Brown, S. I., Akiya, S., and Weller, C. A.: Prevention of the ulcers of the alkali-burned cornea. Preliminary studies with collagenase inhibitors. Arch Ophthalmol 82:95, 1969.

51. Slansky, H. H., Berman, M. B., Dohlman, C. H., and Rose, J.: Cysteine and acetylcysteine in the prevention of corneal ulcerations. Ann Ophthalmol 2:488, 1970.

52. Brown, S. I., Tragakis, M. P., and Pearce, D. B.: Treatment of the alkali-burned cornea. Amer J Ophthalmol 74:316, 1972.

53. Francois, J., Cambie, E., Feher, J., and Van Den Eeckhout, E.: Collagenase inhibitors (penicillamine). Ann Ophthalmol 5:391, 1973.

54. Berman, M. B., Barber, J., Talamo, R. C., and Langley, C. E.: Corneal ulceration and the serum antiproteases. I. Alpha-1 antitrypsin. Invest Ophthalmol 12:759, 1973.

55. Newsome, D. A., and Gross, J.: Prevention by medroxyprogesterone of perforation in the alkali-burned rabbit cornea: Inhibition of collagenolytic activity. Invest Ophthalmol Vis Sci 16:21, 1977.

56. Foster, C. S., Zelt, R., Kenyon, K. R., and Chakraborti, B.: Ascorbate therapy for experimental corneal burns. Invest Ophthalmol Vis Sci 19(Arvo Suppl):227, 1980.

57. Aronson, S. B., Elliot, J. H., Moore, T. E., Jr., and O'Day, D. M.: Pathogenetic approach to therapy of peripheral corneal inflammatory disease. Amer J Ophthalmol 70:65, 1970.

58. Cavanagh, H. D.: Herpetic ocular disease: Therapy of persistent epithelial defects. Int Ophthalmol Clin 15:67, 1975.

59. Ballen, P. H.: Mucous membrane grafts in chemical (lye) burns. Amer J Ophthalmol 55:302, 1963.

60. Denig, R.: Transplantation of mucous membrane of mouth for various diseases and burns of the cornea. New York Med J 57:1074, 1918.

61. Thoft, R. A.: Conjunctival transplantation. Arch Ophthalmol 95:1425, 1977.

62. Webster, R. G., Jr., Slansky, H. H., Refojo, M. F., Boruchoff, S. A., and Dohlman, C. H.: The use of adhesives for the closure of perforations: A report of two cases. Arch Ophthalmol 80:705, 1968.

63. Dohlman, C. H., Boruchoff, S. A., and Sullivan, G. L.: A technique for the repair of perforated corneal ulcers. Arch Ophthalmol 77:519, 1967.

64. Bennett, J. E.: The management of total xerophthalmia. Arch Ophthalmol 81:667, 1969.

65. Klein, R., and Lobes, L. A., Jr.: Ocular alkali burns in a large urban area. Ann Ophthalmol 8:1185, 1976.

66. Brown, S. I., Tragakis, M. P., and Pearce, D. B.: Corneal transplantation for severe alkali burns. Trans Amer Acad Ophthalmol Otolaryngol 76:1266, 1972.

67. Brown, S. I., Bloomfield, S. E., and Pearce, D. B.: A follow-up report on transplantation of the alkali-burned cornea. Amer J Ophthalmol 77:538, 1974.

68. Thoft, R. A., and Friend, J.: Biochemical transformation of regenerating ocular surface epithelium. Invest Ophthalmol Vis Sci 16:14, 1977.

69. Friend, J., and Thoft, R. A.: Functional competence of regenerating ocular surface epithelium. Invest Ophthalmol Vis Sci 17:134, 1978.

70. Girard, L. J., Hawkins, R. S., Nieves, R., Borodofsky, T., and Grant, C.: Keratoprosthesis: A 12-year follow-up. Trans Amer Acad Ophthalmol Otolaryngol 83:OP252, 1977.

71. Cardona, H., and DeVoe, A. G.: Prosthokeratoplasty. Trans Amer Acad Ophthalmol Otolaryngol 83:OP271, 1977.

72. Dohlman, C. H., Schneider, H. A., and Doane, M. G.: Prosthokeratoplasty. Amer J Ophthalmol 77:694, 1974.

73. Rao, G. N., Blatt, H. L., and Aquavella, J. V. Results of keratoprosthesis. Amer J Ophthalmol 88:190, 1979.

74. Holekamp, T. I. R., and Becker, B.: Ocular injuries from automobile batteries. Trans Amer Acad Ophthalmol Otolaryngol 83:805, 1977.

75. Grant, W. M.: Ocular injury due to sulfur dioxide. II. Experimental study and comparison with ocular effects of freezing. Arch Ophthalmol 38:762, 1947.

76. McCulley, J. P., Whiting, D. W., and Lauber, S.: Experimental ocular hydrofluoric acid burns. Invest Ophthalmol Vis Sci 18(Arvo Suppl):195, 1979.

77. Friedenwald, J. S., Hughes, W. F., Jr., and Herrmann, H.: Acid burns of the eye. Arch Ophthalmol 35:98, 1946.

78. Paterson, C. A., Eakins, K. E., Paterson, E., Jenkins, R. M., II, and Ishakawa, R.: The ocular hypertensive response following experimental acid burns in the rabbit eye. Invest Ophthalmol Vis Sci 18:67, 1979.

79. Friedenwald, J. S., Hughes, W. F., Jr., and Herrmann, H.: Acid-base tolerance of the cornea. Arch Ophthalmol 31:279, 1944.

80. Schultz, G., Henkind, P., and Gross, E. M.: Acid burns of the eye. Amer J Ophthalmol 66:654, 1968.

81. Lewin, L., and Guillery, H.: *Die Wirkurgen von Arzneimitteln und Giften auf das Auge.* 2nd ed. Berlin, August Huishwald, 1913.

82. McCulley, J. P., Pettit, M., and Lauber, S.: Treatment of experimental ocular hydrofluoric acid burns. Invest Ophthalmol Vis Sci 19(Arvo Suppl):228, 1980.

83. de Treville, R. T. P.: Hydrofluoric acid burns management. Medical Series Bulletin. No. 17–70, 1970. Industrial Hygiene Foundation of America.

Epithelial Downgrowth

22

RICHARD S. SMITH, M.D.

Invasion of the anterior chamber by corneal or conjunctival epithelium is one of the most serious complications of accidental or surgical penetration of the eye. Collins[1] is credited with the first description of epithelial invasion of the globe with his report of an implantation cyst that occurred many years after traumatic perforation. The early literature was reviewed by Perera,[2] who described three types of epithelial invasion based on histopathology and prognosis. These included "pearl" tumors of the iris, post-traumatic iris cysts, and epithelialization of the anterior chamber.

Epithelial pearl tumors of the iris are rarely seen and probably represent implantation of a small fragment of skin, conjunctiva, or a hair follicle during penetrating injury from trauma or surgery. Epithelial pearl tumors grow slowly, rarely reach a large size, and seldom cause secondary inflammatory complications.

Post-traumatic epithelial cysts of the anterior chamber are generally grouped with epithelial downgrowth, making it difficult to ascertain their true incidence. Epithelial cysts present as translucent structures usually connected either to the surgical wound or to the site of accidental trauma (Fig. 22–1). Cases have been described in which the cyst expands into the posterior chamber either through an iridectomy or, in aphakic patients, through the pupil. An epithelial cyst may be present for many years before it reaches a size that requires treatment. The term epithelialization of the anterior chamber refers to a membranelike growth of epithelial cells that lines the interior surfaces of the eye (Fig. 22–2). Despite its name, the entity is not confined to the anterior chamber. It is not known why epithelial cyst formation occurs in some instances and true epithelialization occurs in others. Although epithelial pearl tumors and epithelial cysts have an excellent prognosis, quite the opposite is true of epithelialization. The true incidence of this problem is difficult to ascertain. Published series suggest that the overall occurrence of this complication is infrequent.[3-7] A better perspective perhaps is given by those authors who report the incidence as a function of the total number of eyes removed following cataract extraction.[2, 4, 8-10] These latter figures sug-

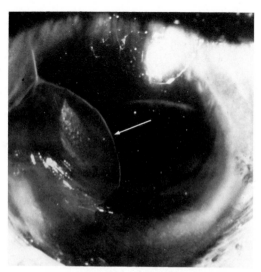

Figure 22–1. Epithelial cyst of the anterior chamber (arrow). (Courtesy of Howard M. Leibowitz, M.D.)

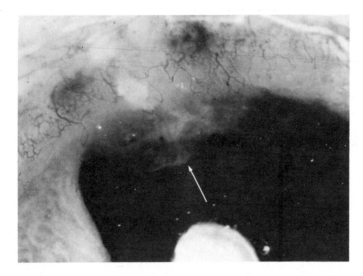

Figure 22–2. Epithelialization of the anterior chamber—a membrane-like growth of epithelial cells on the posterior corneal surface (arrow). (Courtesy of Howard M. Leibowitz, M.D.)

gest that nearly one out of every five globes enucleated after cataract surgery is removed because of epithelial invasion of the anterior chamber.

GENERAL CHARACTERISTICS OF EPITHELIALIZATION OF THE ANTERIOR CHAMBER

Epithelialization may occur following an uncomplicated cataract extraction with a benign postoperative course. More frequently, however, the patient has clinical findings indicative of surgical complications. These findings include iris incarceration, entrapment of lens or vitreous in the wound, delayed formation of the anterior chamber, prolonged hypotony, and the presence of a filtering fistula. The patient may present with ocular pain or irritability, tearing, and a gradual but relentless decrease in postoperative visual acuity.

By use of the slit-lamp biomicroscope, a gray, relatively transparent membrane may be seen on the posterior corneal surface (Fig. 22–3).[11] In the early stages of development the membrane often has a convex, slightly thickened edge that points to the location of a leaking wound. The rate of growth on the posterior corneal surface is variable, but in time the membrane often extends somewhat below the visual axis. It is rare for the advancing epithelium to progress all the way to the inferior chamber angle.

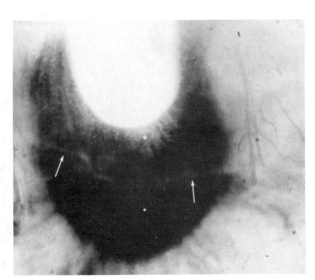

Figure 22–3. Epithelialization of the anterior chamber—a relatively transparent membrane with a thickened convex edge on the posterior corneal surface (right arrow). Note the presence of deep corneal neovascularization (left arrow). (Courtesy of Howard M. Leibowitz, M.D.)

In addition to the sheet of proliferating epithelium on the posterior cornea, the iris often is involved. The epithelium may cover much of the anterior iris surface and advance over the anterior surface of the vitreous (Fig. 22–4) or through the pupil or iridectomy site onto the posterior surface of the iris, spreading over the ciliary body and peripheral retina. The growth of epithelium on the iris is usually more rapid than its growth on the cornea.[12-15]

Since there is considerable variation in the rate of growth of the epithelium, the extent of involvement is not necessarily a reliable indication of the duration of activity. Some cases have demonstrated considerable coverage of the iris and cornea within the first week after surgery, but others have failed to produce clinical signs until several months or years after surgery. In many instances deep corneal vascularization accompanies growth of the epithelial sheet on the posterior cornea; stromal and epithelial edema become evident as the corneal endothelium is destroyed (Fig. 22–5). Although the iris may not be pulled into the wound initially, the proliferation of epithelium on both the posterior corneal and anterior iris surfaces often produces broad anterior synechiae. Some authors have reported a

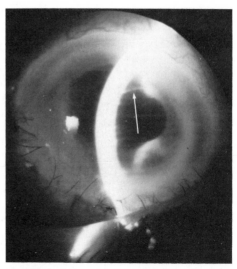

Figure 22–5. Corneal edema present well below the visible edge (arrow) of the epithelial membrane on the posterior corneal surface, presumably reflecting endothelial damage below the advancing epithelial membrane.

decrease in corneal sensation, but this is not a constant finding.

In the absence of spontaneous arrest or successful treatment, affected eyes exhibit a chronic iritis of variable activity. Ultimately many eyes develop an intractible secondary glaucoma. The mechanism of the glaucoma may relate directly to the development of anterior synechiae, or it may be due to blockade of the trabecular meshwork by epithelium. The intraocular growth of epithelium also may block the site of iridectomy and the pupil, producing seclusion or occlusion of the pupil.

DIFFERENTIAL DIAGNOSIS

A number of conditions must be considered in the differential diagnosis of epithelialization.[12] A shelving corneal incision may suggest the growth of a membrane adjacent to the incision. This is particularly likely to occur if Descemet's membrane is accidentally detached during surgery. In some instances Descemet's membrane may be reduplicated after surgery or it may proliferate across the iris surface. The latter phenomenon also occurs following trauma,

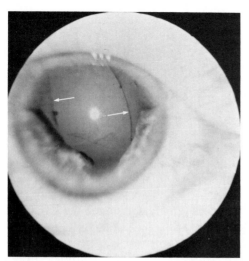

Figure 22–4. Epithelial membrane has grown over the anterior surface of the vitreous humor (arrows indicate edge of membrane). (Courtesy of Howard M. Leibowitz, M.D.)

following chronic inflammation, in Chandler's syndrome, or in the iris-nevus (Cogan-Reese) syndrome.

A thickened vitreous face in contact with the posterior cornea following cataract surgery can mimic the presence of a corneal epithelial membrane. Careful slit-lamp examination should demonstrate continuity between this structure and the adjacent vitreous humor extending through the pupil or the site of iridectomy. Many of the same factors that lead to epithelial invasion of the anterior chamber cause fibrovascular tissue to form and proliferate on the posterior corneal surface and on the anterior surface of the iris. This can produce a clinical picture similar to epithelial invasion. The formation of fibrous or vascular retrocorneal membranes following anterior segment surgery probably occurs much more frequently than it is diagnosed; such tissue growth is particularly likely to occur after penetrating keratoplasty.[16] Thus, when there is a strong clinical suspicion of epithelial invasion of the anterior chamber, the diagnosis should, if possible, be confirmed by specular microscopy and proved by biopsy before the radical treatment discussed later in this chapter is undertaken.

ETIOLOGY

It is useful to consider some of the probable reasons for the occurrence of epithelial invasion. Theobald[4] pointed out that there are two factors essential for occurrence of epithelialization: (1) delayed wound healing, and (2) proximity to the wound of an area of proliferating corneal or conjunctival epithelium. Many factors can contribute to poor healing of a corneoscleral incision. It is obvious that entrapment of iris, fragments of lens capsule and/or cortex, or vitreous humor in the wound will produce a delay in healing and often an abnormal scar or fistula. Since surface epithelium proliferates following injury and has a tendency to migrate along free surfaces, any irregularity or interruption

of wound apposition could permit abnormal extension of this normal healing process. An incision of irregular shape as well as buckling or overriding of the edge of the wound can also result in a leaking incision. Incorrect placement or inappropriate tightness of sutures can add to the problem.[5] It has been shown both clinically and experimentally that penetration of a corneoscleral suture into the anterior chamber, even 10-0 nylon, can cause epithelial invasion along the suture track.[17] If such a problem is compounded by tying the suture too tightly, resulting tissue necrosis facilitates epithelial invasion. Some surgeons have begun to return to the use of nonabsorbable sutures left permanently in place following cataract surgery. It is interesting to note the old observation of Christensen[5] that epithelial invasion is more likely to take place along a silk suture than along absorbable sutures. The high incidence of fistulas demonstrated either by a positive Seidel test or on histopathologic examination of eyes with epithelial invasion also suggests strongly that errors in wound closure with prolonged hypotony and incarceration of material in the wound play a major role in allowing epithelium to pass through the incision and enter the eye. The literature contains numerous illustrations of the migration of epithelium along the wound, and, in almost all enucleated globes, careful serial sectioning will demonstrate an area of continuity between the surface of the eye and the intraocular epithelium.

In the case of cataract extraction, the importance of placement of the conjunctival flap and its influence on the occurrence of epithelial invasion is an issue that has been debated for many years. Unfortunately, reliable statistics on the incidence of epithelial ingrowth after cataract extraction performed with a limbus-based versus a fornix-based flap are not available. Since epithelium has a strong tendency to proliferate and migrate following injury,[5] logic dictates that it might be best to avoid placement of the conjunctival incision directly above the corneoscleral incision. Unfortunately there is no firm evidence to support this thesis. Indeed, epithelialization of the anterior chamber can occur in the absence of a conjunctival incision (e.g., after penetrating keratoplasty[18-22]), demonstrating that the cornea also can serve as the source of the invading epithelium. This suggests that the importance placed on the type of conjunctival flap used in cataract surgery as a factor in the etiology of this disorder should be limited.

Unlike neoplastic tissue, normal epithelium, even in its proliferative phase, cannot infiltrate or erode normal tissue. Injured epithelium proliferates and migrates along free surfaces, and this property presumably accounts for its ability to invade the anterior chamber in the face of faulty or delayed wound closure. Numerous efforts have been made in experimental animals to duplicate the type of anterior chamber epithelial invasion seen in human patients;[2, 4, 11, 23] for the most part these efforts have not been successful. It has proved very difficult to produce epithelialization, even by the intentional inclusion of conjunctival tissue in experimental animals. However, a picture resembling that in humans has been produced from time to time.[14, 15, 24] These experimental results may not be very different from the clinical situation. Many eyes with inclusion of iris, lens, or vitreous in the wound, with delayed anterior chamber formation, or with filtering fistulas that are free of epithelial invasion, are seen in every ophthalmic pathology laboratory. This suggests that the production of this complication in humans may be as difficult as it is in experimental animals.

More than 40 years ago Terry suggested that endothelial damage might contribute to epithelial growth on the posterior corneal surface.[3] Ultrastructural studies of this condition, though infrequent, tend to confirm this hypothesis.[25] Endothelial cells have not been identified beneath or within the invading epithelial sheet. Furthermore, the epithelium is separated from Descemet's membrane by a fibrous connective tissue sheet of variable thickness. Experimental studies have still not answered the questions of whether endothelial destruction is a prerequisite for the growth of epithelium, whether the invading epithelium destroys endothelium, or whether the presence of viable endothelium always inhibits the proliferation and extension of invading epithelium.

In recent years Folkman[26] and other workers have proposed the existence of an angiogenic factor secreted by tumors that is capable of inciting the growth of blood vessels in normally avascular tissues such as the cornea. The same group has also noted that free-floating tumor cells proliferating in the anterior chamber of the eye produce a spherical structure that ceases growth when it reaches a certain size. Although the cells appear viable, further growth occurs only if the tumor cells attach themselves to a vascular surface such as the iris. If such an event occurs, rapid proliferation takes place.[27] It is interesting to speculate that the invading epithelium, although not neoplastic, may respond in a similar manner to the presence of a vascular supply on the iris and may be inhibited from growing in more vigorous fashion on the posterior corneal surface because of the absence of some essential factor.

PATHOLOGY

Poor wound healing is a precursor of epithelial downgrowth. In the case illustrated by Figure 22–6, perforation of a scarred, vascularized cornea occurred several days before the patient sought medical attention. The keratoplasty specimen shows growth of an epithelial sheet around the wound edge and for a short distance over Descemet's membrane. With healthy endothelium the ingrowth of epithelium is unlikely because of the phenomenon of contact inhibition.[3, 28] In this case no endothelial cells are seen and epithelial invasion has begun.

Inadequate coaption of an anterior segment wound provides a route for epithelial invasion. After cataract surgery the patient shown in Figure 22–7 devel-

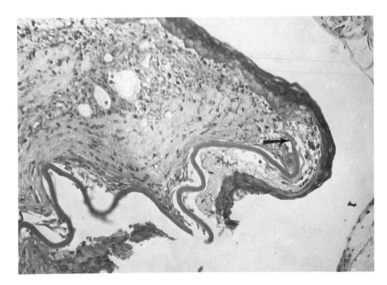

Figure 22–6. Epithelium has grown around the disrupted Descemet's membrane (arrow) at the site of perforation.

oped total anterior synechiae and secondary glaucoma. The enucleated globe revealed a wide gap between the cut edges of Descemet's membrane and sheets of epithelium binding the iris to the posterior corneal surface. Although it is unusual for the entire cornea to be covered with epithelium, large areas may be involved (Figs. 22–8 and 22–9).

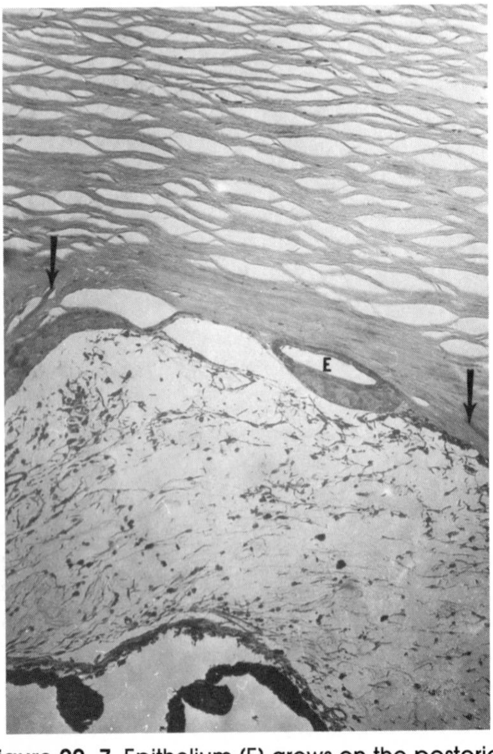

Figure 22–7. Epithelium (E) grows on the posterior corneal surface. There is a wide gap (arrows) between the cut ends of Descemet's membrane.

The epithelium tends to grow more rapidly when in contact with the iris.

Once epithelium gains access to the anterior chamber, involvement may extend beyond the iris and cornea. Following one penetrating anterior segment wound, epithelium grew over the atrophic ciliary body (Fig. 22–10), across a fibrovascular cyclitic membrane (Fig. 22–11), and even across the retina (Fig. 22–12). Such a case illustrates the need for prompt surgical intervention as well as the necessity for determining the extent of involvement.

TREATMENT

Treatment of epithelial invasion of the anterior chamber depends on the form this invasion takes. Epithelial pearl tumors of the anterior chamber usually remain small and grow slowly if at all. If such a tumor presents a problem, simple excision is usually satisfactory. Epithelial cysts have been aspirated, coagulated with diathermy (Fig. 22–13), and treated with corrosive solutions, with local radiation, and by partial or complete surgical removal. The limited number of cases treated by a single individual makes it difficult to evaluate the relative success and the merits of each approach. Despite the variety of treatment modalities for epithelial cysts, Maumenee reported that none seems to

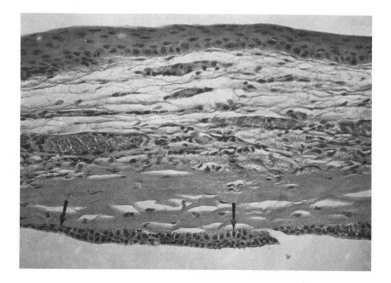

Figure 22–8. An epithelial sheet (arrows) covers the posterior surface of a scarred, vascularized cornea.

have resulted in the appearance of a typical epithelial downgrowth syndrome.[29] Even partial removal of a cyst is rarely accompanied by recurrence of the cyst.

The treatment of epithelial invasion of the anterior chamber is a far more difficult problem. In the past numerous authors advocated, with variable enthusiasm, the use of radiation therapy to destroy the epithelium. At times "good" results seemingly occurred after low-dosage radiation, but more frequently poor results followed the administration of even a much higher total radiation dose. In the best of series no more than 50 per cent favorable results were reported.[11, 30-32] Evaluation of the efficacy of radiation treatment is difficult because of the variability of epithelial growth, especially on the posterior corneal surface. In many cases growth of the retrocorneal epithelium ceases after it has passed below the visual axis. Since this occurs without radiation, it is difficult to be certain what effect radiation has. Furthermore, histopathologic examination of eyes that have received considerable doses of radiation has revealed healthy, vigorous, apparently proliferating epithelium. There seems to be little supportive evidence that radiation treatment of eyes with diffuse epithelial invasion of the anterior segment is of any value, and its use has largely been abandoned.

Radical surgical intervention, as originally described by Maumenee,[12] may at times be successful. Before undertaking such drastic surgery, a positive diagnosis is essential. The clinical appearance of this entity through the specular microscope is described in Chapter 5. Iris epithelialization can be identified by application of photocoagulation; epithe-

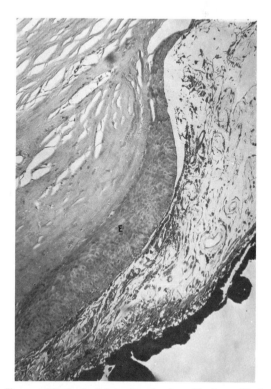

Figure 22–9. A thick sheet of epithelium (E) is sandwiched between the iris and the posterior corneal surface.

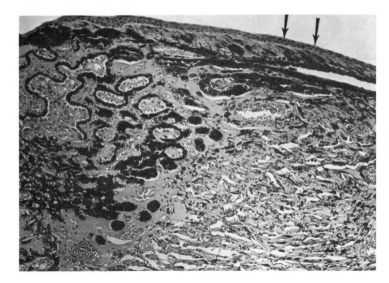

Figure 22–10. A sheet of epithelium (arrows) extends over the atrophic ciliary body.

Figure 22–11. A sheet of epithelium (arrows) covers the anterior surface of a fibrovascular cyclitic membrane.

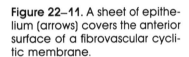
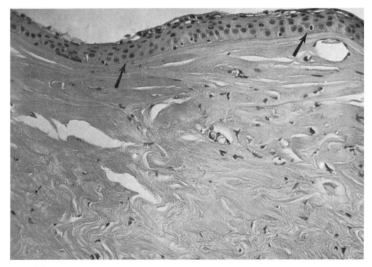

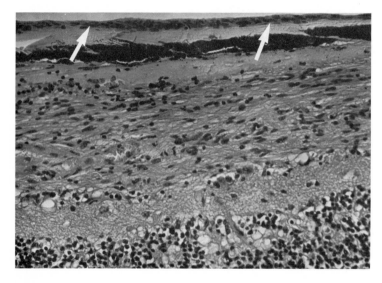

Figure 22–12. A thin layer of epithelium (arrows) covers an atrophic retina.

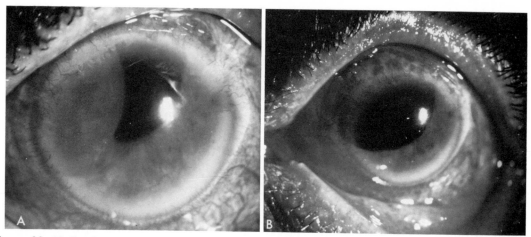

Figure 22–13. Treatment of an epithelial cyst in the anterior chamber. *A,* Preoperative appearance. *B,* Appearance after surgical excision. No recurrence 5 years postoperatively. Corrected visual acuity 20/25. (Courtesy of Howard M. Leibowitz, M.D.)

lium covering the iris immediately thickens and turns white, whereas uninvolved iris turns brown.[9, 33] A diagnostic biopsy should be performed, either by iridectomy or by the removal of a small portion of membrane from the peripheral cornea.

Surgical management of epithelialization of the anterior chamber requires exquisite attention to detail and includes several steps. Attention must be directed to proper closure of any existing fistula; epithelium lining the fistula must be removed prior to closure and the opening closed by direct suturing or with the aid of a scleral flap. All involved iris tissue should be excised; as indicated, identification of the extent of iris epithelialization by the preoperative placement of photocoagulation spots may at times be helpful in delineating the area of iris to be excised. Epithelial membranes on the vitreous face as well as the anterior half of the vitreous gel itself can be removed with a vitrectomy instrument (e.g., Ocutome); the same instrument can be used to excise the involved iris. If corneal transparency is insufficient to permit a closed procedure with a vitrectomy instrument, iridectomy, excision of pupillary membranes, and anterior vitrectomy are performed through a limbal incision. The globe is reformed by instillation of balanced salt solution and/or air. Cryotherapy then is applied externally to all corneal and

scleral areas whose posterior surface is covered by epithelium. Both the application of a single full-thickness transcorneal and transscleral freeze and multiple external freeze-refreeze applications have been advocated. Neither technique is ideal and both have met with failure. The use of an intraocular bubble of air in conjunction with transcorneal-transscleral freezing is said to provide a thermal insulating effect that provides improved control of the size of each cryoapplication and causes each freeze to persist longer.[34] When external freezing techniques are employed, the frozen epithelium on the posterior corneal surface often can be observed, through the slit-lamp biomicroscope, to turn white. The cells slough and disappear, generally within a week.

Alternative methods for the destruction of the retrocorneal epithelium include the direct application of cryotherapy to or the mechanical debridement of the involved area of the posterior cornea.[35, 36] Though more effective, both of the latter procedures are more traumatic to the cornea and result in a higher incidence of irreversible corneal edema. There is no practical means of identifying the extent of involvement of the ciliary processes once the epithelium has progressed behind the iris. Such eyes do not respond favorably to surgery, and most ultimately become phthisical.

Reports of the results of treatment using the most modern of microsurgical techniques indicate that epithelial downgrowth remains a devastating disease.[34, 36] The majority of eyes have a visual acuity of 20/200 or less postoperatively. Many of the therapeutic failures result from clouding of the cornea, a not surprising complication given the nature of the disease and the trauma of radical surgery. Penetrating corneal grafts appear to have an excellent prognosis for optical transparency, but visual results are usually disappointing. The visual failures result from glaucomatous damage to the optic nerve, macular disorders, or retinal detachment.

Since opacification of the cornea is most likely to occur following radical surgery, early treatment of epithelial invasion (i.e., before the invading epithelium reaches the visual axis) is indicated. Opacification of the superior third of the cornea is compatible with good vision. The prognosis of cases in which epithelium has passed below the visual axis is very poor with any sort of treatment. The recommended surgical therapy is radical and the results are far from optimal, but surgery is justifiable because the great majority of untreated eyes eventually lose useful vision as a result of bullous keratopathy, iritis, intractible glaucoma, or phthisis.

CONCLUSIONS

Epithelial pearl tumors and epithelial cysts of the anterior chamber may occur after surgery or trauma but generally have a good prognosis. By far the most serious complication of epithelial invasion of the eye is diffuse downgrowth covering the iris, posterior surface of the cornea, and other portions of the eye. Although the latter complication has a low incidence when one considers all surgical and traumatic perforations of the globe, it is nevertheless an important cause of enucleation following cataract surgery. Attention is often drawn to the possible diagnosis by observation of a transparent gray-white membrane, usually progressing down the posterior corneal surface from the superior wound. The typical patient has a history of delayed reformation of the anterior chamber, may show incarceration of iris, lens, or vitreous in the wound, and frequently has a filtering fistula. Faulty closure of the wound, related to tissue incarceration or to an irregular incision, poor apposition, or faulty suture technique, contributes to the possibility of epithelial invasion. Chronic iritis, intractible glaucoma, and decompensation of the corneal endothelium are frequent complications of untreated cases. Radiation has little role in the management of this problem. Although the results of radical surgical intervention are relatively poor, this approach remains the only effective way of salvaging eyes affected by epithelial invasion.

REFERENCES

1. Collins, E. T.: Epithelial implantation cyst in a shrunken globe. Trans Ophthalmol Soc UK 11:133, 1891.
2. Perera, C. A.: Epithelium in the anterior chamber of the eye after operation and injury. Trans Amer Acad Ophthalmol Otolarygnol 42:142, 1937.
3. Terry, T. L., Chisholm, J. F., and Schonberg, A. L.: Studies on surface epithelium invasion of the anterior segment of the eye. Amer J Ophthalmol 22:1083, 1939.
4. Theobald, G. D., and Hass, J. S.: Epithelial invasion of the anterior chamber following cataract extraction. Trans Amer Acad Ophthalmol Otolaryngol 52:470, 1948.
5. Christensen, L.: Epithelization of the anterior chamber. Trans Amer Ophthalmol Soc 58:284, 1960.

6. Allen, M. C., and Duehr, P. A.: Sutures and epithelial downgrowth. Amer J Ophthalmol 66:293, 1968.

7. Bernardino, V. B., Kim, J. C., and Smith, T. R.: Epithelialization of the anterior chamber following cataract extraction. Arch Ophthalmol 82:742, 1969.

8. Blodi, F. C.: Failures of cataract extractions and their pathologic explanation. J Iowa State Med Soc 44:514, 1954.

9. Maumenee, A. E.: Treatment of epithelial downgrowth and intraocular fistula following cataract extraction. Trans Amer Ophthalmol Soc 62:153, 1964.

10. Payne, B. F.: Epithelization of the anterior segment. Amer J Ophthalmol 45:182, 1958.

11. Calhoun, F. P., Jr.: The clinical recognition and treatment of epithelialization of the anterior chamber following cataract extraction. Trans Amer Ophthalmol Soc 47:498, 1949.

12. Maumenee, A. E.: Epithelial invasion of the anterior chamber. Trans Amer Acad Ophthalmol Otolaryngol 61:51, 1957.

13. Dunnington, J. H.: Some modern concepts of ocular wound healing. Arch Ophthalmol 59:315, 1958.

14. Regan, E. F.: Epithelial invasion of the anterior chamber. Arch Ophthalmol 60:907, 1958.

15. Cogan, D. G.: Experimental implants of conjunctiva into the anterior chamber. Amer J Ophthalmol 39:163, 1955.

16. Werb, A.: The postgraft membrane. Int Ophthalmol Clin 2:771, 1962.

17. Abbott, R. L., and Spencer, W. H.: Epithelialization of the anterior chamber after transcorneal (McCannel) suture. Arch Ophthalmol 96:482, 1978.

18. Mazow, M. L., and Stephens, R. W.: An unusual complication after keratoplasty. Surv Ophthalmol 11:205, 1966.

19. Leibowitz, H. M., Elliott, J. H., and Boruchoff, S. A.: Epithelialization of the anterior chamber following penetrating keratoplasty. Arch Ophthalmol 78:613, 1967.

20. Kurz, G. W., and D'Amico, R. A.: Histopathology of corneal graft failures. Amer J Ophthalmol 66:184, 1968.

21. Arentsen, J. J., Morgan, B., and Green, W. R.: Changing indications for keratoplasty. Amer J Ophthalmol 81:313, 1976.

22. Sugar, A., Meyer, R. F., and Hood, C. I.: Epithelial downgrowth following penetrating keratoplasty in the aphake. Arch Ophthalmol 95:464, 1977.

23. Hilding, A. C.: Corneal epithelium and penetrating corneal defect in cats. Amer J Ophthalmol 48:787, 1959.

24. Patz, A., Wulff, L., and Rogers, S.: Experimental production of epithelial invasion of the anterior chamber. Amer J Ophthalmol 47:815, 1959.

25. Iwamoto, T., Srinivasan, D., and DeVoe, A. G.: Electron microscopy of epithelial downgrowth. Ann Ophthalmol 9:1095, 1977.

26. Folkman, J., Merler, E., Abernathy, C., and Williams, G.: Isolation of a tumor factor responsible for angiogenesis. J Exp Med 133:275, 1971.

27. Gimbrone, M. A., Jr., Leapman, S. B., Cotran, R. S., and Folkman, J.: Tumor dormancy in vivo by prevention of neovascularization. J Exp Med 136:261, 1972.

28. Cameron, J. D., Flaxman, B. A., and Yanoff, M.: In vitro studies of corneal wound healing: Epithelial-endothelial interactions. Invest Ophthalmol 13:575, 1974.

29. Maumenee, A. E., and Shannon, C. R.: Epithelial invasion of the anterior chamber. Amer J Ophthalmol 41:929, 1956.

30. Vail, D.: Epithelial downgrowth into the anterior chamber following cataract extraction: Arrest by radium treatment. Arch Ophthalmol 15:270, 1936.

31. Reese, A. B.: The treatment of complications of ocular surgery. Amer J Ophthalmol 35:719, 1952.

32. Pincus, M. H.: Epithelial invasion of the anterior chamber following cataract extraction. Effect of radiation therapy. Arch Ophthalmol 43:509, 1950.

33. Meyer-Schwickerath, G.: Light Coagulation. St. Louis, C. V. Mosby Co., 1960.

34. Stark, W. J., Michels, R. G., Maumenee, A. E., and Cupples, H.: Surgical management of epithelial ingrowth. Amer J Ophthalmol 85:772, 1978.

35. Maumenee, A. E., Paton, D., Morse, P. H., and Butner, R.: Review of 40 histologically proven cases of epithelial downgrowth following cataract extraction and suggested surgical management. Amer J Ophthalmol 69:598, 1970.

36. Brown, S. I.: Results of excision of advanced epithelial downgrowth. Ophthalmology 86:321, 1979.

X

CORNEAL SURGERY

THOMAS E. MOORE, JR., M.D.

INDICATIONS FOR KERATOPLASTY

Historically, indications for keratoplasty have focused on the reasons for keratoplasty, i.e., optical, preparatory, tectonic, therapeutic, exploratory, cosmetic, and refractive.[1] These reasons served as a classification for the type of keratoplasty to be performed in order to achieve a certain defined result, which might or might not be an optimal visual result. Even then, however, it was recognized that reasons frequently overlapped and that one operation could satisfy several reasons. In the past two decades, however, attitudes toward indications for keratoplasty have become oriented more toward the preservation or restoration of optimal visual acuity. This change in attitude has been a product of better understanding of the host response and structural alteration of the cornea; corneal physiology, particularly of the corneal endothelium, precorneal tear film, and epithelium; the availability and increased knowledge of the therapeutic uses of synthetic adrenal corticosteroids; increased availability, choice, and specificity of antimicrobial agents; and marked improvement in instrumentation, especially fine surgical instruments, fine monofilament nylon suture material, and the operating microscope.

General Considerations

Corneal transplantation in humans is not a simple problem of making a wound, closing it, subsequently removing the sutures, and sending the patient on his way. Rather, it is a comprehensive undertaking that involves evaluating a patient, his eye, his cornea, and the donor cornea, performing meticulous surgery, and performing careful, daily postoperative inpatient slit-lamp examination. Frequent, intensive outpatient follow-up must continue for 6 months to a year, and less frequent ophthalmic care must be provided for the remainder of the patient's life (unless the project is abandoned or the eye is lost). Optical correction by spectacles or contact lenses usually must be provided. Nothing less than this total approach will suffice. The surgeon must understand this, and the referring ophthalmologist must understand this. More than one keratoplasty has been lost because the referring ophthalmologist misinterpreted clinical signs, for example, mistaking the corneal edema of an allograft reaction for the corneal edema of glaucoma.

The patient and his family *must* know that the onset of photophobia and decreased vision requires immediate treatment to prevent graft failure, and that pain always means something is awry. Viable tissue has been transplanted and it requires maintenance.

Patients

Patients with corneal disease must be evaluated in terms of their visual handicap, rather than a specific Snellen measurement. The very old and the very young pose special problems. An old patient with one good eye and a second eye afflicted with corneal blindness who is able to feed, clothe, and bathe himself and to indulge in the activities he enjoys should usually be left alone. If the eye is painful as a result of bullous keratopathy or ulcerating owing to herpes zoster, less substantial procedures may be performed (e.g., conjunctival flap or tarsorrhaphy). The old patient with arthritis or parkinsonism must be taught and be able to instill eye drops, and he must be able to remember to do so, or someone else must be available to do it.

The very young are totally at the mercy of their parent(s) or surrogate parent(s). They cannot understand the complexity of the surgical procedure, understand that they are not to rub the operated eye, instill drops on a prescribed regimen, keep bath or shampoo water out of their eyes, or transport themselves for postoperative visits. In cases in which amblyopia is a problem they will not patch the unoperated eye. Indeed, it requires a motivated and informed parent to enforce the discipline of patching.

In cases of monocular congenital corneal opacity with a normal fellow eye, keratoplasty is probably not indicated. If it should be performed, then it must be performed in the first 2 to 3 months of life to prevent amblyopia. In older children keratoplasty, when otherwise indicated, must be performed early to prevent the onset of acquired irreversible amblyopia. In school-age children the parents must be particularly informed of the danger of schoolyard trauma, which, in our experience, has destroyed several corneal grafts.

All our patients undergo a preoperative examination by an internist to make certain that they are acceptable candidates for general anesthesia and to determine the need for assistance in the management of concurrent systemic disease and in the diagnosis and treatment of occult disease. Cardiovascular diseases and diabetes mellitus are frequently initially diagnosed as a consequence of this procedure.

Patients with neoplastic disease may pose a problem. Ordinarily one would not subject such a patient to elective keratoplasty, but in the case of severe visual handicap and a reasonable prognosis surgery may be performed to improve the quality of life. Sensory deprivation has a profound effect on patients, and restoration of sight can have dramatic consequences. Keratoplasty is not indicated in agonal patients.

Cases of senility, mental retardation, and mental illness must be approached with great caution. For example, in Down's syndrome with keratoconus or keratoglobus, keratoplasty should not be considered until severe bilateral visual loss is present; unilateral surgery is indicated only when navigational ability is lost and the patient collides with furniture in the home or institutional environment. These patients are unable or unwilling to take care of themselves, and regardless of the consequences they will not subject themselves to any discipline. Managing these patients often requires all the cognitive and intuitive powers of the surgeon. Previous social, economic, and medical history will often reveal these individuals, and corneal surgery should rarely be performed in such patients. If surgery is to be performed, some responsible person must be available to provide the care the patient cannot give himself.

In our experience, chronic alcoholics, regardless of socioeconomic level, all end up with a failed graft given enough time. "Hard drug" addicts (e.g., heroin or amphetamine users) are seldom seen after hospital discharge and are therapeutic disasters.

A certain number of patients have no family to look after them, so available social services must be enlisted. Along with the patient, these services must also understand the *long-term* nature of keratoplasty and must be able to provide early postoperative home care as needed. They also must either provide or bear the cost of providing transportation for the many postoperative visits to the surgeon's office.

In the same vein, patients who live a

considerable distance from the surgeon's office need to have assured, dependable, and affordable transportation. A relationship must be established with a local ophthalmologist in order that immediate and appropriate care can be provided if necessary. There is practically no chance of achieving a clear keratoplasty 1 or 2 years postoperatively in a patient who lives in a location where no appropriately skilled ophthalmologist is available and who, for whatever reason, is unable to return rapidly to the operating surgeon's office on short notice when necessary.

Eyes

Lid function must be normal or nearly so. Any defect in adequate lid closure must be repaired prior to keratoplasty. In addition, entropion and trichiasis require preoperative repair. Symblepharon involving more than one quadrant should also be repaired, and sufficient time must be allowed to elapse to determine whether the lid abnormality will recur. Blepharitis must be rendered culture-negative.

The presence of a normal precorneal tear film is virtually mandatory; its compromise or inadequacy may contribute substantially to the keratopathy. Careful slit-lamp examination of the precorneal tear film and the marginal tear strip must be carried out. However, deficiencies may not be readily apparent, and clinical measurement of inadequacy is not accurate. Tear breakup time should be measured and the average for three trials calculated. The result should be in the range of 10 to 45 seconds; tear breakup time of less than 10 seconds is considered abnormal and probably represents mucin deficiency. Fluorescein staining will define true defects in the corneal epithelial layer, and rose bengal staining will reveal degenerating corneal and conjunctival epithelium that may otherwise appear normal. An assessment of tear volume can be made by the Schirmer test with and without topical anesthesia, but the results are unreliable except at extremes. Lysozyme determinations may be performed if testing materials are available. In short, a certain integrity of the accessory lacrimal apparatus is essential for successful keratoplasty. In the severe dry-eye syndromes associated with major alkali burns, Stevens-Johnson syndrome, ocular pemphigoid, or Riley-Day syndrome, the prognosis for keratoplasty varies from very poor to nil.

The role of the deep scleral plexus in supplying blood to the peripheral cornea remains poorly defined, but in inflammatory or ischemic syndromes involving this supply, appropriate pretreatment with anti-inflammatory agents and heparin is essential; otherwise the same pathogenetic mechanism will doom a keratoplasty.

Glaucoma must be controlled preoperatively by the various topical drops available (e.g., pilocarpine, carbachol, echothiophate, epinephrine, or timolol) without the use of carbonic anhydrase inhibitors. If this is not possible, a trabeculectomy should be performed before keratoplasty if there is sufficient open angle, or cyclocryotherapy may be employed if the open angle is not sufficient. Carbonic anhydrase inhibitors must be kept in therapeutic reserve since postoperative glaucoma is nearly always more difficult to treat, particularly in aphakic eyes.[2]

If a preoperative cataract is present, as determined by slit-lamp examination or B-scan ultrasonography, it should be removed at the time of keratoplasty without the use of alpha-chymotrypsin (which is employed experimentally to remove endothelial cells from Descemet's membrane). Cataract extraction performed prior to keratoplasty involves an extra operation, and after keratoplasty it is a source of further insult to the donor endothelium.

Eyes with known retinal disease, especially macular disease, are not generally candidates for keratoplasty, but exceptions are encountered, particularly among one-eyed individuals. Visual acuity and indirect ophthalmoscopy of the posterior eye may provide sufficient information about its integrity. Light fields, color perception, and two-point discrimination also are useful. However, in dense keratopathy or dense cataract other methods must be employed. The most useful is B-scan ultrasonography, which provides a view of the structural architecture of the iris, the sonic clarity of the vitreous, the presence of retinal detachment, and marked cupping of the optic nerve. This procedure should be routinely employed in all eyes that are being evaluated for keratoplasty in which the intraocular structures and posterior segment cannot be adequately visualized. In addition, electroretinography and visual evoked response testing will provide electrophysiologic indices of the visual pathways. In our experience, entoptic phenomena are unreliable. Unfortunately, there is no test that defines a normal macula through opaque media, although laser interferometry is currently being evaluated experimentally.

Successful keratoplasty involves much more than the status of the cornea and the technical details of surgery; the ocular adnexae also must be functioning adequately.

Corneas

Patients with corneal distortions and opacification producing visual handicap uncorrectable by spectacles or contact lenses are potential candidates for penetrating keratoplasty. The concept of handicap is more useful than any particular Snellen recording because patients' visual requirements vary considerably. In considering keratoplasty, it is more useful to view the cornea in prognostic categories based primarily on morphologic criteria rather than on specific etiologic diagnoses (Table 23–1). Our morphologic criteria are as follows: 0+, corneal distortion and/or opacification free of neovascularization (e.g., keratoconus, Fuchs' dystrophy, the familial dystrophies) (Fig. 23–1A); 1+A, corneal scarring free of neovascularization (e.g., perforating corneal trauma) (Fig. 23–1B); 1+B, corneal scarring or edema associated with intraocular disease (e.g., aphakic bullous keratopathy) (Fig. 23–1C); 2+, corneal scarring with superficial neovascularization (e.g., anterior microbial disease) (Fig. 23–1D); 3+, deep corneal scarring and neovascularization free of intraocular disease (e.g., deep microbial infection, interstitial keratitis, moderate chemical burn) (Fig. 23–2A); 4+, deep corneal scarring and neovascularization accompanied by intraocular inflammation (e.g., microbial keratouveitis) (Fig. 23–2B); 5+, corneal ischemia, severe fibrovascular replacement of corneal tissue and conjunctival epithelium, and/or anterior chamber obliteration with nonresponsive glaucoma (e.g., severe chemical burn, massive trauma) (Fig. 23–3).

Table 23–1. PROGNOSTIC CATEGORIES OF CORNEAL DISEASE FOR PENETRATING KERATOPLASTY

Good Prognosis	
0+:	Corneal distortion and/or opacification free of scarring or neovascularization (Fig. 23–1A)
1+A:	Corneal scarring free of neovascularization (Fig. 23–1B)
1+B:	Corneal scarring or edema, free of neovascularization, associated with intraocular disease (Fig. 23–1C)
2+:	Corneal scarring with superficial neovascularization (Fig. 23–1D)
Reasonable Prognosis	
3+:	Deep corneal scarring and neovascularization free of intraocular disease (Fig. 23–2A)
4+:	Deep corneal scarring and neovascularization accompanied by intraocular inflammation (Fig. 23–2B)
Poor Prognosis	
5+:	Corneal ischemia, severe fibrovascular replacement of corneal and conjunctival tissue, and/or anterior chamber obliteration with nonresponsive glaucoma (Fig. 23–3)

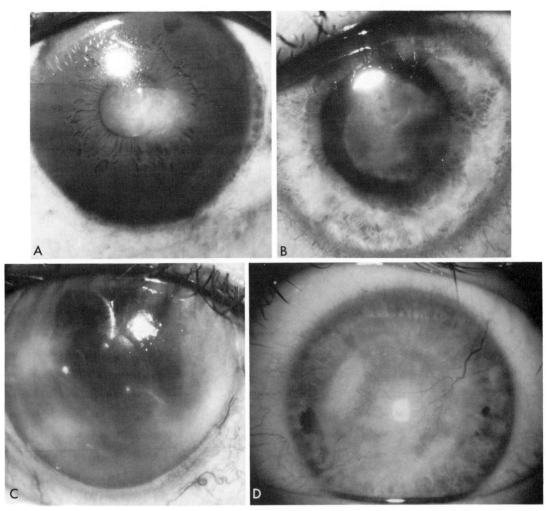

Figure 23–1. Corneal disorders with a good prognosis for penetrating keratoplasty. *A,* Central corneal edema (Fuchs' dystrophy). *B,* Central scarring without neovascularization. *C,* Stromal edema secondary to dislocated intraocular lens implant. *D,* Corneal scarring with superficial neovascularization. (Courtesy of Howard M. Leibowitz, M.D.)

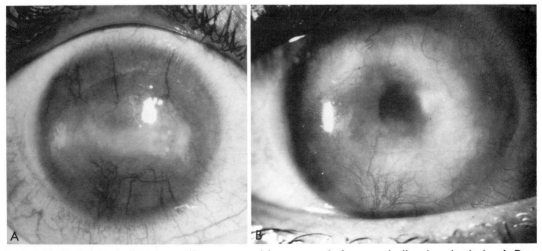

Figure 23–2. Corneal disorders with a reasonable prognosis for penetrating keratoplasty. *A,* Deep corneal scarring and neovascularization. *B,* Deep corneal scarring and neovascularization accompanied by anterior uveitis.

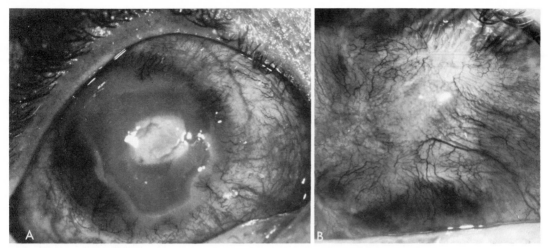

Figure 23–3. Corneal disorders with a poor prognosis for penetrating keratoplasty. *A,* Deep corneal scarring and neovascularization, stromal necrosis, indolent corneal ulcer, anterior uveitis, peripheral anterior synechiae, and glaucoma (lye burn). *B,* Fibrovascular replacement of corneal tissue, anterior chamber obliteration, and glaucoma (ammonium hydroxide burn).

These seven categories obviously represent increasing severity of inflammatory and morphologic change. However, in terms of statistically significant differences in the results of penetrating keratoplasty there are only three categories: 0 +, 1 + A, 1 + B, and 2 + have a good prognosis; 3 + and 4 + have a reasonable prognosis; and 5 + has a poor prognosis.[3]

In considering when to operate, visual loss, the degree of structural alteration (e.g., excessive thinning), and pain constitute the important factors in groups 0 +, 1 + A, and 1 + B (e.g., bullous keratopathy). In acute inflammatory disease, i.e., groups 2 +, 3 +, 4 +, and 5 +, maximal inflammatory quiescence and etiologic control should be achieved first unless perforation is imminent or actual. If this is not possible, then a tectonic graft, that is, the use of keratoplasty as replacement of an abscess (e.g., in fungal keratitis) or for restoration of the integrity of the globe (e.g., in severe "dry-eye" syndromes), may be performed with an uncertain outcome. In chronic inflammatory disease keratoplasty is indicated at any time after maximal inflammatory quiescence to abort the inflammatory process and to restore vision. In inactive inflammatory disease keratoplasty may be performed at any time providing the general surgical criteria are satisfied.

The presence of a descemetocele or a small corneal perforation may provoke too hasty surgery; often there is no need for immediate surgical intervention. In most cases the anterior chamber can be maintained or restored with a hydrophilic contact lens,[4] acetazolamide 1000 mg. per day, and absolute bed rest. Anterior synechiae will not form readily if prednisolone acetate 1 per cent suspension is used on an hourly basis, and often the pupil may be retracted from the area of perforation with 0.25 per cent scopolamine and 10 per cent phenylephrine drops instilled three to four times a day. Cultures should be taken for specific antimicrobial action. The patient may be adequately prepared for general anesthesia, and suitable donor tissue may be obtained as described later in the chapter. Cyanoacrylate adhesives, while popular, should not be used, because they are toxic and produce sterile abscesses (and they are disapproved by the FDA).

The effect of corneal anesthesia on keratoplasty prognosis is poorly defined. The transplanted cornea itself is anesthetic. Patients operated upon for herpes simplex and herpes zoster are in a reasonable to good category. Nevertheless, patients with neuroparalytic keratopathy and lesions of the central and peripheral fifth nerve can be severe management problems, not unlike patients with moderate to advanced keratitis sicca. Some even have to be reminded to blink! A combined V and VII palsy is generally considered to represent a contraindication to keratoplasty.

Finally, unless a central corneal leukoma is very dense, refraction with a hard corneal contact lens should be performed. Results of this procedure occasionally are dramatic and obviate the need for surgical intervention.

SURGICAL TECHNIQUES WITH FRESH EYES

Preparation of the Patient

Patients are usually admitted to the hospital the day before surgery. Preoperative orders are as follows:

1. Systemic medications per internist.
2. Preoperative medications per anesthesiologist.
3. Neomycin–polymyxin B–gramicidin drops (Neosporin), q. 1 h., 6 a.m. to 10 p.m.
4. Clip eyelashes.
5. Neomycin–polymyxin B–bacitracin ointment (Neosporin Ointment) lid scrub.
6. 1 per cent pilocarpine drops q.i.d. in phakic eyes.
7. Operative permit.

1. The attending physician must be notified of the patient's hospitalization so that he can assume or continue management of any intercurrent systemic disease. The physician should also order any nonroutine tests that he considers advisable. In addition, the physician should render an opinion of the anesthetic risk. Hospital staff regulations vary, but in general the surgeon is responsible for routine preoperative tests such as chest film, EKG, and blood and urine tests.
2. The anesthesiologist should order the preanesthetic medications so that he can select the drugs and dosages with which he is familiar and comfortable. The anesthesiologist should be informed of the type of anesthesia required for intraocular surgery, i.e., equivalent to

that for intracranial surgery, but should not be told how to administer it. Many anesthesiologists employ succinylcholine for anesthetic induction; therefore, a special note should be in the chart if the patient has been on a strong anticholinesterase agent, for example, echothiophate iodide. Since both the surgeon and the anesthesiologist are responsible for the patient's well-being from the time of preanesthetic medication to discharge from the recovery room, it is very important that the surgeon be confident of the anesthesiologist's skills with anesthesia for intraocular surgery so that they can perform effectively as a team. The anesthesiologist must also write a preanesthetic note in the chart concerning suitability for anesthesia.
3. Neomycin–polymyxin B–gramicidin drops (Neosporin) are employed as broad-spectrum antibiotic prophylaxis; this particular combination is used because of its effectiveness and the necessity to avoid sensitization to drugs that might subsequently be indicated for parenteral use. The usefulness of prophylactic preoperative antibiotics is still controversial; we feel that this combination and dosage may help and will not harm the patient. We do not use systemic prophylaxis. Eyes that have been affected by infectious external disease must be culture-negative prior to surgery except in emergencies.
4. Eyelashes generally are clipped by nurses before the patient is brought to the operating room, but if adequate personnel are not available, the lashes can be trimmed in the operating room prior to surgery. This is done to remove the lashes, along with the microorganisms and seborrheic detritus that cling to them, from the operative field.
5. Eyelid margins are then scrubbed with Neosporin ointment to further remove detritus and to force drug into the ducts on the lid margin.
6. Pilocarpine 1 per cent drops are used in phakic eyes four times per day to produce miosis so that the iris will "protect" the anterior lens capsule. (Nothing will protect the anterior lens capsule from inadequate surgical tech-

nique.) The dosage is limited to this strength and frequency in order to spare the patient the pain of ciliary spasm, since maximal miosis is unnecessary. In addition, the miosis produced by 1 per cent pilocarpine can be reversed during surgery if the surgeon desires mydriasis. In aphakic eyes the pupil is not altered preoperatively because it serves no purpose; aphakic miosis per se will not prevent vitreous loss, and mydriasis encourages inadvertent iridotomies.

7. An operative permit that completely describes the contemplated surgery (including photography) on the *correct* eye must be signed by the patient *before* any preanesthetic medications are given. In addition to the legalities involved, this procedure once again draws the attention of the patient and the ward personnel to the nature of the surgery and to the correct eye.

Donor Corneas

Unless the surgeon himself supervises the procurement of the corneas and their subsequent handling, it is incumbent upon him to familiarize himself with the techniques employed by his eye bank.

There is no general agreement about most aspects of donor tissue suitability, and it is beyond the scope of this discussion to consider any but fresh tissue. (Even given this limitation I shall rely mostly on personal experience.)

There is little disagreement that corneas from healthy eyes of individuals between the ages of 5 and 60 are suitable as donors. Corneas from donors much younger than 5 are thin and soft and difficult to handle. In general, over the age of 5, the younger the donor the more ideal the tissue because younger corneas have a larger number of endothelial cells. Corneas from donors much older than 60 tend to have fewer endothelial cells than tissue from younger individuals, and they are less apt to withstand the trauma of transplantation surgery. Exceptions exist, however, and corneas free of pathology from older individuals have provided excellent donor tissue.[5]

The presence of arcus senilis is not a contraindication to the use of the cornea as a donor, but for aesthetic reasons it may limit the size of the graft.

The eyes should be removed promptly postmortem and cooled to 4° C in a moist chamber. If there is a delay before enucleation, the eyelids of the deceased should be taped to ensure that they remain closed and the body should be refrigerated. Pollack and coworkers[6] have shown that thimerosal (Merthiolate) is ineffective in reducing the bacterial flora of donor eyes. They along with others[7-9] recommend irrigation of the donor eyes with saline solution immediately after enucleation and subsequently copious instillation of neomycin–polymyxin B ophthalmic solution over the cornea of the enucleated globe.

Eyes should not be taken from patients with active anterior segment disease or with a history of anterior segment or intraocular surgery. Anterior segment neoplasms should be excluded. Culture-positive bacteremia, suspected viremia, and a history of infectious hepatitis are also considered contraindications. More recently the slow virus of Jakob-Creutzfeldt disease has emerged as a definite contraindication;[10] since this is a postmortem diagnosis, cadavers in whom it is even *suspected* should be excluded. Whether this also applies to the lymphomas and leukemia is unclear. Cryptococcus transfer has also occurred in a patient who received tissue from a donor who had undergone prolonged immunosuppression, which presents another area of concern.[11] The passive transfer of rabies from a donor to the recipient of corneal tissue has been documented, and the diagnosis of rabies constitutes an absolute contraindication.[12]

Once in the operating room, the donor eye (not the anterior segment) should be immersed in Neosporin solution in a sterile medicine glass after being transferred to the scrub nurse. On a separate table the surgeon may prepare the donor eye by *very gently* removing the corneal epithelium with a moist cotton-tipped applicator or Elschnig cyclodialysis spatula. Care must be taken not to damage the basement membrane or Bowman's membrane. (If the recipient has any degree of dry eye syndrome, the donor epithelium should be left intact.)

A Graefe knife or similar knife is then used to make a scleral paracentesis wound so that the knife enters the anterior chamber on the iris surface (Fig. 23–4A). The donor aqueous is then replaced with air through a 27-gauge cannula (Fig. 23–4B) so that a large air bubble lies between the donor endothelium and the iris stroma (Fig. 23–4C), a so-called hovergraft. The purpose of this maneuver is to prevent iris stroma from abrading the endothelium.

A corneal trephine with the obturator set at 0.8 mm. is then centrally and vertically placed over the cornea (Fig. 23–4D) and the cornea is cut by *rotating* the trephine, not pressing down, against slight counter pressure from the surgeon's other hand around the globe. As soon as anterior chamber penetration has occurred, the counter pressure is instantly relaxed and the trephine is removed. It is important not to continue trephining after the anterior chamber has been entered because the donor button may tilt down, causing the trephine blade to "scalp" Descemet's membrane from the stroma. Alternatively, a 360-degree perforating wound may be completed so that, if trephination is continued, the circumscribed corneal button will rotate, causing the endothelium to rub against the iris.

The eye is then gently transferred to the assistant surgeon without squeezing the globe and pressing iris against endothelium. Air is maintained in the anterior chamber, and fine scissors are then used to complete the trephination incision (Fig. 23–4E). Because of the elasticity of Descemet's membrane, the scissors cut should be vertical to the cornea and along the outer wall of the wound. The donor button may then be left in situ or tilted slightly so that it will not fall into the anterior chamber. The eye is then replaced in the medicine glass, and the medicine glass is placed in a stainless steel basin.

Some surgeons prefer to punch rather than to cut the donor cornea. In this circumstance the anterior segment must first be removed from the globe. This is done by making a transscleral perforation over the ciliary body approximately 2 to 3 mm. posterior to the limbus and circumferentially completing the incision with scissors. The scleral lip is then elevated and the ciliary body is gently teased free from the scleral spur circumferentially. The entire cornea with its scleral rim is then transferred to a specially shaped Teflon block with the epithelial surface down (Fig. 23–5A). A trephine with the obturator backed out or without an obturator is then punched through the endothelial surface centrally and vertically (Fig. 23–5B). ("Hesitation marks" are not permissible!) The corneoscleral rim is removed, and the donor button may be left on the Teflon block or transferred to a safe container, endothelial surface up, with care being taken not to let the endothelium dry out. (Several drops of balanced salt solution are gently dropped onto the endothelium.) The donor button must not be left where it can easily be knocked over or caught on a surgical gown.

Trephination and cutting of the donor button from the external aspect of the intact eye has been a standard technique for many years. Although evidence has been presented that cutting with scissors produces more crushing damage to the peripheral endothelium of the donor button than does sharp-edge punching,[13] removal of the cornea with a scleral rim to permit punching is not necessarily a benign procedure that is devoid of endothelial trauma. It also adds a technical step to keratoplasty that often is outside the control of the surgeon and eliminates the use of preplaced sutures for those who prefer that technique.

Refinements of specular microscopy ultimately may allow the surgeon to view the morphologic integrity of the endothelium in the operating room, but this technique is not presently available for routine use. Physiologic integrity of the endothelium is still best demonstrated by the temperature reversal phenomenon,[14, 15] but testing for this cannot

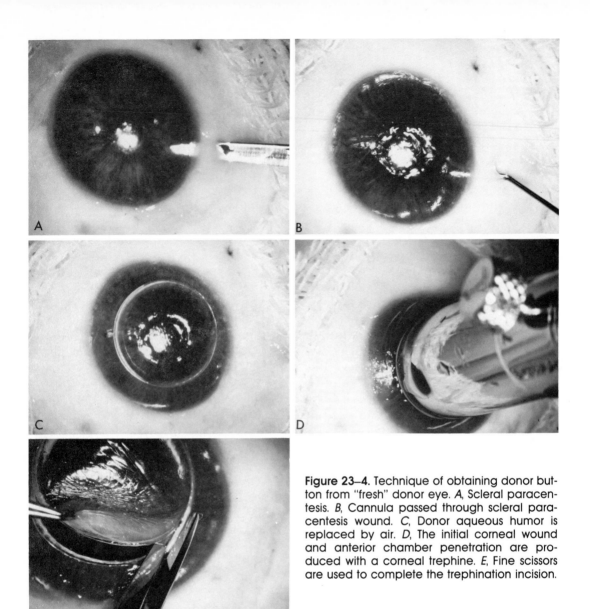

Figure 23–4. Technique of obtaining donor button from "fresh" donor eye. *A,* Scleral paracentesis. *B,* Cannula passed through scleral paracentesis wound. *C,* Donor aqueous humor is replaced by air. *D,* The initial corneal wound and anterior chamber penetration are produced with a corneal trephine. *E,* Fine scissors are used to complete the trephination incision.

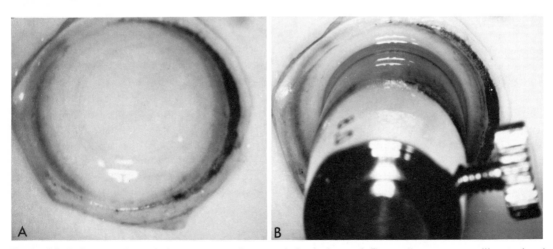

Figure 23–5. Preparation of donor cornea by punch technique. *A,* The entire cornea, with a scleral rim, has been removed from the donor eye and transferred to a Teflon block. *B,* A trephine is vertically punched through the central position of the endothelial surface.

be performed preoperatively in a practical manner. Having obtained the donor button, the corneal surgeon using current techniques is unable to assess the functional capability of its endothelium objectively prior to securing it in place in the recipient corneal bed.

Recipient Eyes

For safety, no surgical procedures should be performed on the recipient eye until *after* the donor button is prepared for use, so that inadvertent damage to the donor will not compromise the entire operation.

The recipient lids and adjacent skin are prepared using various combinations of soap, detergent, and antibacterial agents. Our preference is a 5-minute scrub with pHisoHex followed by painting of the area with povidone-iodine (Betadine). The lids are then opened and the fornices copiously irrigated with balanced salt solution (BSS). If the cornea contains a descemetocele or is perforated, the prep is limited to Betadine painting alone and the surgeon subsequently irrigates the fornices himself.

There is considerable variation among surgeons in the technique used to drape the recipient eye, but two principles are important: (1) the drape should not press against the orbit, and (2) the eye should be isolated from the field by a plastic drape adherent to the skin. A lateral canthotomy is routinely performed to offer wider exposure and to reduce postoperative lid squeezing. Lid sutures, rather than a lid speculum, are routinely used for lid retraction because much of the speculum is outside the surgeon's field of vision through the operating microscope and could be inadvertently depressed with unhappy consequences. The blades of the speculum may interfere with suturing, and a fine nylon suture may foul itself on the speculum.

Bridle sutures are inserted beneath the tendon of the superior and inferior rectus muscles so that the eye can be stabilized by the assistant during trephination, and so that it can be rotated

slightly during suturing to provide a uniform focal plane.

There is no general agreement on the use of devices to support the anterior segment during intraocular surgery, although many surgeons prefer their use in cases of high myopia and aphakia. The single ring of Flieringa, the double-connected ring of Legrand, and the "scleral expander" of Girard are the devices commonly used. It is important that these rings be properly secured. They must be sutured under direct vision to scleral tissue with a spatula-needle, because conjunctival tissue will not support the anterior segment and needle perforation into the choroid can produce a massive choroidal hemorrhage once the intraocular pressure is reduced to zero. The sclera should just fit the ring; if it is forced to do so by sutures, the anterior segment will be squeezed with consequences opposite those desired and, in addition, high astigmatism will result postoperatively. If the ring is too small, it will hinder suturing; if it is too large, it will produce severe chemosis, which will also hinder suturing. If a ring is used, there is no reason to place bridle sutures beneath the tendons of the recti. Stabilizing sutures can be secured to the ring at the 12 o'clock and 6 o'clock positions.

A corneal limbal paracentesis wound should be performed with a von Graefe or Wheeler knife, avoiding hemorrhage or aqueous loss (Fig. 23–6). The sole purpose of this incision is to provide easy access to the anterior chamber at the end of the procedure without disrupting the keratoplasty wound, in order to deepen the chamber, irrigate hemorrhage, lyse anterior synechiae, and so forth.

The identical trephine used to cut the donor should also be used to cut the recipient (Fig. 23–7A). The obturator in the trephine should be set at 0.5 mm. or less and every effort made to avoid entering the anterior chamber, which eliminates the risk of cutting the iris or lens capsule (Fig. 23–7B). The anterior chamber is then entered with a razor blade

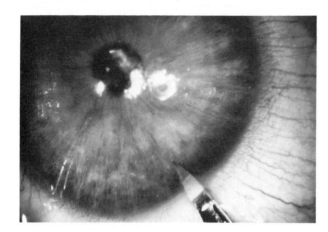

Figure 23–6. A corneal limbal paracentesis is performed on the recipient eye at the outset of the transplantation procedure to provide easy access to the anterior chamber without disrupting the keratoplasty wound.

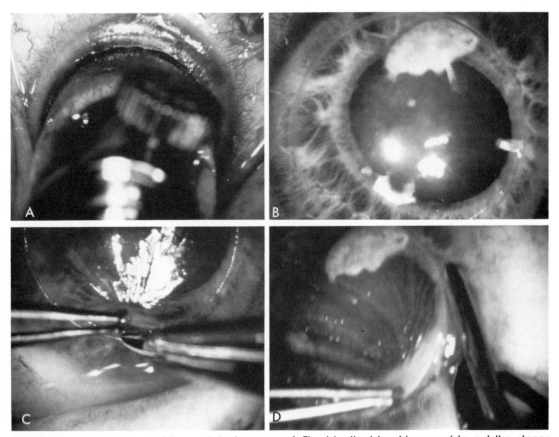

Figure 23–7. Trephination of the recipient cornea. *A,* The identical trephine used to cut the donor cornea is used on the recipient cornea. *B,* The trephine wound in the recipient cornea is partial thickness only. *C,* The anterior chamber is entered with a razor blade knife. *D,* The wound is completed with scissors.

(Fig. 23–7C) or other fine knife and the wound is completed with fine scissors (Fig. 23–7D).

Some surgeons[16] have suggested using a button that is larger than the opening in the recipient cornea in order to create a deeper anterior chamber at the end of the procedure along with a lower incidence of postoperative elevation of the intraocular pressure. However, inserting a button larger than the one removed produces a slight "dome" in the recipient cornea, which will cause refractive myopia. Moreover, the use of an oversized graft in aphakic eyes often results in a marginal graft "gully" that creates a problem in the subsequent fitting of a hard contact lens.[17]

In a phakic eye with a normal iris there is no reason to perform an iridectomy. However, if the iris has been compromised by previous iritis with or without posterior synechiae, an iridectomy should be performed. An iridectomy usually will have been performed in aphakic eyes, but the site of an earlier iridectomy may require alteration owing to membranes, an updrawn pupil, anterior synechiae, and so forth. It is more important to avoid postoperative pupillary block mechanisms than it is to protect the cosmetic appearance of the pupil.

Some years ago, when a visually disabling corneal disorder and a cataract were both present, most authorities recommended that the keratoplasty be performed prior to cataract extraction to protect the transplanted cornea from the vitreous humor. Cataract extraction was performed subsequently.[1, 7] However, keratoplasty failure after cataract extraction was high (19 to 61 per cent),[3, 18-22] and when aphakic keratoplasty began to carry an increasingly good prognosis, combined keratoplasty–cataract extraction became a generally accepted procedure. A cataractous lens may be extracted intracapsularly through a keratoplasty wound 7.5 mm. or larger (larger is easier). A large area of anterior capsule is exposed through a dilated pupil so that extracapsular extraction, if desired, also poses no particular technical problem, although postoperative inflammation is greater and there is the risk of after-cataract formation, lens reaction, and additional surgery. Intracapsular cataract extraction is performed most easily with a cryophake by the "open sky" technique (Fig. 23–8), performing lysis of any phacovitreal adhesions with the Barraquer brush. Alpha-chymotrypsin should be avoided as a precaution to safeguard the recipient and donor endothelium. Miosis may then be achieved with 1 per cent acetylcholine chloride.

Vitreous loss and vitrectomy are constant problems in aphakia and in combined procedures. In aphakic bullous keratopathy, with the anterior chamber occupied by liquid vitreous, there is no way to avoid vitreous loss. Otherwise, except for choroidal hemorrhage, one or a combination of three circumstances must be present to cause vitreous loss: (1) external pressure against an open eye, (2) inadequate anesthesia, and (3) rapid choroidal detachment and formation of suprachoroidal fluid. The first two are potentially preventable; if they are not prevented, the problem converts to one of management.

Vitrectomy may be performed prior to surgical corneal perforation with a needle inserted intraocularly through a cauterized area over the pars plana. The advantage of this maneuver is the maintenance of the hyaloid face; the disadvantages are that it is a blind maneuver, that there is risk of vitreous hemorrhage, and that a vitreoretinal adhesion will be created at the vitreous base. The aspirated volume of vitreous humor is replaced with balanced salt solution introduced into the anterior chamber before trephination is completed. This technique is certainly indicated if a keratoplasty over an intraocular lens implant with retention of the implant is to be performed.

Vitrectomy may otherwise be performed through the pupil under direct visualization and without perforation of other ocular tissue. Vitreous humor may be aspirated through a short, beveled 20-gauge or larger needle, absorbed onto cellulose sponges, and cut with scissors or aspirated and cut by the guillotine-

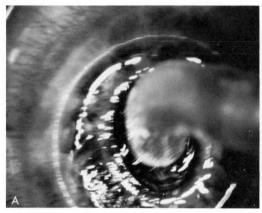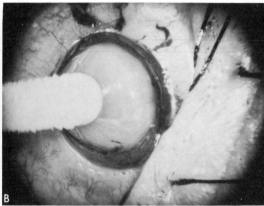

Figure 23–8. Combined penetrating keratoplasty and intracapsular cataract extraction. *A,* Tip of cryoprobe is placed in contact with the central anterior capsule through the dilated pupil. *B,* The lens is delivered by the "open sky" technique through the keratoplasty wound.

type Kaufman vitrector or by one of the more sophisticated instruments designed for "closed" vitrectomy, such as the Ocutome or VISC. Of these choices we prefer the Kaufman vitrector because it is easy to use and is disposable. The O'Malley Ocutome is a finer, more controllable instrument, but it is very expensive and elaborate to set up.

Each of these methods ruptures the anterior hyaloid face, and vitreous humor must then be aspirated until the remaining face is concave and well posterior to the plane of the iris. If only a small puncture in the hyaloid face has been made, it should be enlarged; otherwise air may become entrapped and be extremely difficult to remove. The lost volume should not be replaced until the eye is closed. If balanced salt solution is instilled, the vitreous base "floats" up and will become adherent to or incarcerated in the wound. If air is instilled, it usually goes posterior to the iris, producing iris bombé and further complicating the procedure. Sodium hyaluronate (Healon) may be used, but it usually will cause transient postoperative glaucoma.

Ideally, it would be desirable to have an intact hyaloid face well posterior to the iris, but in aphakia as well as in phakia malignant glaucoma can develop even in the presence of a sector iridectomy. This requires a return to the operating room for posterior aspiration and incision of the hyaloid face. Similarly,

after vitreous aspiration through the pupil and lysis of the hyaloid face, careful sweeping of the wound edge with a Barraquer brush, careful suturing of the button, careful reformation and examination of the anterior chamber, and careful sweeping of the anterior chamber with a Barraquer synechialysis spatula, it is not optically possible to be certain there are no strands of vitreous adherent to the wound.

Once the donor button is set in place, it should be anchored in position with four interrupted quadrant sutures of 10-0 monofilament nylon (Fig. 23–9A). If correctly placed, the donor limbs of these four sutures should wrinkle the cornea slightly and produce a perfect square of even depth. Some surgeons prefer to use a larger suture (8-0 or 9-0) for placement of the first four cardinal sutures.

A continuous suture of 10-0 monofilament nylon should begin and end at the 12 o'clock meridian so that the knot will be placed under the upper lid. Alternatively, if both needles of a double-armed suture are to be used, a mattress suture is first placed at the 6 o'clock meridian; then one needle is used to close the nasal half of the wound, the other to close the temporal half. Again, the knot is secured on the conjunctival side at the 12 o'clock meridan to improve comfort and to maintain the integrity of the corneal epithelium. Knots may be buried in corneal stroma, but even with the best technique they ultimately may be extremely difficult to remove.

Four to five loops of continuous suture should be placed in each quadrant, depending on the size of the graft. The sutures should be placed radially (Fig. 23–9B) even though they will subsequently shift to being tangential. The spatula needle through the donor edge should emerge immediately anterior to Descemet's membrane and should then be inserted immediately anterior to Descemet's membrane on the recipient edge. The length of the bite should be determined by the curve of the needle, one-half curve for a shorter bite and three-eighths curve for a longer bite. A longer bite is taken on the recipient side, since the recipient tissue is usually compromised by disease. Superficial suturing must be avoided because the sutures tend to pull through and the posterior aspect of the wound tends to gape. The wound then is initially filled by a fibrin plug,[1] allowing fibroblasts direct access to the anterior chamber and resulting in unnecessarily prolonged imbibition of aqueous humor at the wound margins.

When the continuous suture is completed, it should be secured with a four- or five-loop surgeon's knot. Individual loops should then be tightened sequentially to equal tension until the donor edge just begins to wrinkle. Too loose suturing will result in loops that move with blinking, interfering with epithelial integrity and perhaps causing a leaking wound. Too tight suturing will lead to excessive thickening of the wound margins, flattening of the anterior chamber, and sutures that pull through.

When the surgeon is satisfied with the tension of the continuous suture and with the watertight integrity of the wound, a granny knot may then be applied and the knot "slipped" onto the conjunctiva. This is followed by a square knot for security. The original interrupted sutures are then removed since they serve no further purpose and are usually rather loose.

Should a continuous loop appear too loose after the knot is tied, it can be

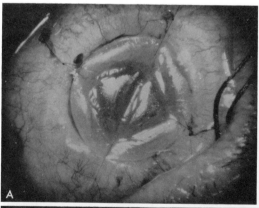
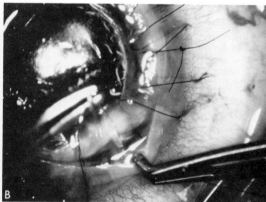
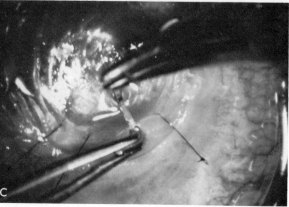

Figure 23–9. Suturing of the donor button into the recipient bed. *A,* Initial anchoring of the donor button with four interrupted quadrant sutures of 10-0 monofilament nylon. *B,* A continuous suture of 10-0 monofilament nylon generally is used to secure the graft; each bite is placed deeply and radially. *C,* Interrupted sutures of 10-0 monofilament nylon offer an alternative to a continuous suture.

tightened by passing a horizontal mattress suture beneath it and anchoring it in sclera. The plasticity of monofilament nylon usually compensates for slightly tight loops. Techniques for dealing with broken continuous suture are described by Harms and Mackensen.[23]

When the recipient tissue is of reasonably consistent density and inflammatory change (e.g., the dystrophies, central leukomas, or bullous keratopathy), we prefer a continuous suture. It results in a relatively equal distribution of tension around the circumferential wound and relative ease of maintaining the integrity of the epithelial sheet. However, compared with interrupted sutures, it is technically more difficult and, in experimental animals at least, heals more slowly.[24] If it is desirable to avoid having "all one's eggs in one basket," it is preferable to use interrupted sutures (Fig. 23–9C). This particularly applies to children and patients with Down's syndrome, in whom unexpected trauma is more likely, and to recipient corneas that are extremely variable in thickness, tissue density, and inflammatory change, such as those affected by chemical burns.

Except for extremes in graft size, 12 or 16 interrupted sutures are sufficient. The sutures should be placed 180 degrees apart, i.e., 12 and 6 o'clock, etc., avoiding the tendency to tie each suture slightly more tightly than the previous one. At the end, sutures that are too tight or too loose must be replaced. An alternative is to tie each suture with a granny knot and, after all sutures have been placed, adjust the tension of questionable sutures by slipping the knots. When the surgeon is satisfied with the tension of all sutures and the integrity of the wound, each suture can be secured with a square knot. The knot may be slipped into corneal stroma, although this may make it difficult to remove.

There is really no purpose served by using a combination of continuous and interrupted sutures except when a corneoscleral graft is employed; then interrupted, buried sutures are placed on the scleral side and a continuous suture on the corneal side. When a very fine continuous suture of uncertain tensile strength is used, more than four interrupted sutures should be placed.[25]

While sutures are being placed in a phakic eye with a miotic pupil, especially if an iridectomy has not been performed, there is sometimes a tendency for the iris to prolapse through the wound (it *seems* to occur more frequently in keratoconus), making adequate suturing impossible. Barraquer[26] has named this aqueous block and described its mechanism. The solution to this problem is *not* to follow one's impulse to do multiple iridectomies but to concentrate one's efforts on prevention. Our experience indicates that presurgical intravenous administration of 500 mg. acetazolamide in the operating room combined with prompt suturing and *reformation* of the anterior chamber prevents this complication. If it occurs nonetheless, the aqueous humor should be milked from the posterior chamber through the pupil (avoiding trauma to the anterior lens capsule) with a spatula and mydriasis should be initiated. The surgeon must bear in mind that the pupil will not dilate if the iris is trapped between the recipient corneal edge and the anterior lens capsule. With the help of an experienced assistant the prolapsed iris may be repositioned with a Barraquer synechialysis spatula and the suture passed over the spatula.

When the suturing phase of keratoplasty is completed, the anterior chamber should be reformed. Attempts should be made to dilate the pupil beyond the wound margin so that in the event of a trivial postanesthetic wound leak, the iris will not seal the leak. If the anterior chamber has not reformed spontaneously, it should be reformed with BSS introduced through a 30-gauge cannula via the preplaced limbal paracentesis (Fig. 23–10). There should be no anterior synechiae present. If this is not a certainty in a phakic eye, the anterior chamber may be filled with a large air bubble to provide appropriate contrast. If a synechia is present, it can be lysed with a synechialysis spatula via the par-

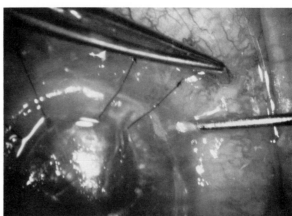

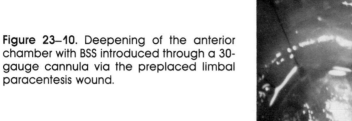

Figure 23–10. Deepening of the anterior chamber with BSS introduced through a 30-gauge cannula via the preplaced limbal paracentesis wound.

acentesis (avoiding the endothelium) (Fig. 23–11). The air bubble is then replaced with BSS. In an aphakic eye air should not be used, tempting as it is, because of its propensity to lodge posterior to the iris. The anterior chamber should be reformed with BSS; if there is uncertainty about iris or vitreous adhesions to the wound, the anterior chamber should be carefully swept with a synechialysis spatula.

If the anterior chamber will not reform, possible causes of this difficulty must be explored. The first possibility is, of course, a gross wound leak that requires resuturing. The second is air lodged posterior to the iris (in either a phakic or aphakic eye, although the latter is more common), which must be carefully aspirated through the paracentesis wound or, if need be, through the keratoplasty wound.

Pupillary block mechanisms can exist in either phakic or aphakic cases. In the former an iridectomy can be performed through the corneal limbus, and in the latter, which resembles the mechanism found in malignant glaucoma, vitreous aspiration and rupture of the hyaloid face via a posterior sclerotomy must be performed. Finally, an anterior chamber will not reform if choroidal detachment has displaced the ciliary body and iris anteriorly against the chamber angle. The choroidal detachment often can be visualized in aphakic eyes, but in any case it must be drained and the chamber must be reformed. The patient must never leave the operating room with a flat anterior chamber or with known iris or vitreous adhesions to the wound.

At the end of the operative procedure the eye is flushed with Neosporin solution, and the identical ointment is applied to the lid margins. Systemic antibiotics are not administered, although there is disagreement on this subject and that of antibiotic prophylaxis. In more than 15 years we have encountered only one case of Group A hemolytic streptococcal endophthalmitis in the early period and two cases of delayed endophthalmitis due to *Staphylococcus epidermidis* in eyes that were not known to be infected at the time of surgery. Two cotton patches along with a protective shield are taped firmly over the eye so that the lids will not open in the postanesthetic phases. Routine postanesthetic orders are written, and a minimum of analgesia, e.g., meperidine, 25

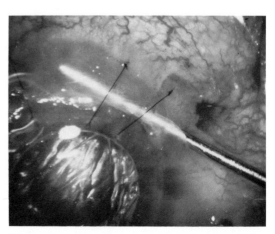

Figure 23–11. Lysis of anterior synechiae via the paracentesis wound.

mg., IM, q. 4 h., p.r.n. is provided. Keratoplasty is a relatively painless procedure, and painful events like glaucoma or infection must not be masked by narcotics.

Lamellar Keratoplasty

A central, disk-shaped penetrating keratoplasty is technically the easiest to perform and is the most frequent form of corneal transplantation. However, the variety of corneal diseases encountered by the ophthalmic surgeon requires treatment with a variety of procedures. Lamellar keratoplasty was the principal corneal procedure for keratopathy until perhaps 25 years ago. However, successful lamellar keratoplasty does not usually provide as good an optical result as penetrating keratoplasty because of opacification and distortion of the corneal lamellae at the donor-recipient interface. Nevertheless, lamellar keratoplasty retains the cardinal advantage of nonperforation of an intact eye; removal of the requirement for intrusion into the anterior chamber permits the surgeon to avoid such complications as anterior synechiae, glaucoma, and cataract formation and allows a large (i.e., greater than 8.5 mm.) lamellar keratoplasty to be performed safely. At present this procedure is used principally to increase the thickness of abnormally thinned corneal tissue rather than for visual improvement.

The possible indications for a tectonic lamellar graft include an eccentric descemetocele, a marginal ectasia or severe furrow dystrophy, or a chemical burn of the cornea and sclera. Often the procedure is a preparatory one for a later penetrating keratoplasty necessary to restore vision. Lamellar keratoplasty is especially useful in the management of recurrent pterygium that has been unresponsive to more conservative therapy (Fig. 23–12). In cases in which the recurrent pterygium extends across the visual axis, the pterygium should be excised by the "bare sclera" technique to expose the corneal limbus along the

length of involvement. This will also expose the thinness of the underlying cornea for the lamellar dissection. The distance from the corneal limbus to a point sufficiently beyond the visual axis (into normal cornea) then is measured, including a suitable allowance of 0.5 to 1.0 mm. so that suture tracts are well away from the visual axis, and a suitable trephine is selected. The recipient cornea should be dissected *before* the donor so that variations in thickness can be reproduced in the donor. The obturator in the trephine should be at a very shallow setting, less than that of the thinnest area of the recipient cornea, in order to avoid unintended perforation. The depth of the trephine incision may then be adjusted with a Paufique knife, and an appropriate dissection plane is selected before dissection is begun.

There are various techniques for dissection, but we prefer to use a 4-mm. Desmarres scarifier. This instrument will cut an even cleavage plane and is not too sharp, thus avoiding the easy formation of new planes. The cleavage should be carried past the trephination incision so that a sharp, rather than a sloped, mortice will be found.

The donor cornea is cut by the same technique. If a significant portion of the cornea has been removed, the recipient area will appear larger than the donor button when it is initially set into the lamellar bed. This discrepancy will disappear as the donor cornea is sutured into place, but the eye may be softened by the usual techniques if necessary. The interface *must* be kept free of blood, which can lead to subsequent opacification and/or neovascularization. Wound edges should be apposed with a slight tautening to compensate for imbibition edema, but the edges should not be crushed together. Choice of suturing technique is the same as for penetrating keratoplasty, except that the needle on the donor edge should emerge at the corner of the mortice or slightly on the interface side and it should be inserted into the deepest layer of the exposed recipient wound.

In cases in which a recurrent ptery-

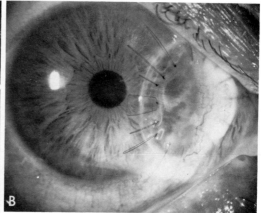

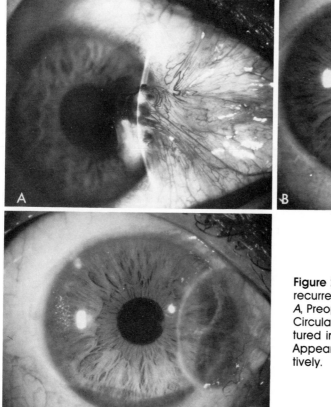

Figure 23–12. Management of unresponsive recurrent pterygium by lamellar keratoplasty. *A,* Preoperative appearance of the lesion. *B,* Circular donor, obtained by trephination, sutured in place 3 months postoperatively. *C,* Appearance of graft 1.5 years postoperatively.

gium is approaching the pupillary zone but the pupillary zone is itself normal, some form of freehand or modified free-hand lamellar keratoplasty is indicated (Fig. 23–13). Templates of simple, trimmable material may be fashioned, or a combination of Graefe-knife straight lines and trephine curves can be employed. The goal is to ensure that the donor cornea matches the tissue removed. Suture tracts must avoid the pupillary zone.

Lesions that are at or near the limbus and require removal for diagnostic or therapeutic reasons (e.g., neoplasms or dermoids) can be treated by lamellar or penetrating sclerokeratoplasty. However, at the time of surgery the surgeon *must be prepared* to perform either procedure because it may not be possible to dissect beneath the lesion. The conjunctiva in the operative area should be excised to allow adequate dissection and suturing. In our experience the dissection, either lamellar or penetrating, is

more easily performed from cornea to sclera. This is particularly true for a penetrating procedure. It is relatively easy to transect cornea to the scleral spur, perform a local cyclodialysis with a spatula, and complete the transection. However, when the dissection is being continued from sclera to cornea, the ciliary body and iris tend to herniate through the wound and complicate the operation. At the end of the procedure particular care should be taken to lyse any peripheral anterior synechiae.

Peripheral corneal lesions, such as a descemetocele, may accompany more central corneal disease and require repair or excision to ensure success of the keratoplasty. It is preferable to decenter to the limbus an 8.0- or 8.5-mm. penetrating keratoplasty if possible rather than attempt a 10- or 11-mm. lamellar keratoplasty. One edge of the keratoplasty must be sutured to limbal sclera (and its anatomic vascular plexus), and the far edge, along with suture tracts,

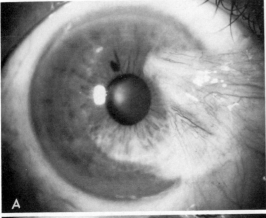

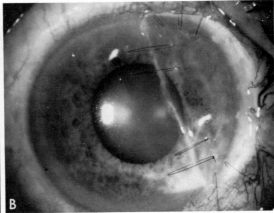

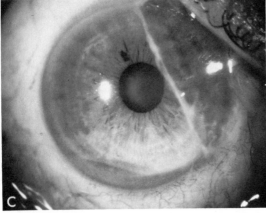

Figure 23–13. Unresponsive recurrent pterygium. A, Preoperative appearance approaching the visual axis. B, Free-hand lamellar keratoplasty sutured in place 3 months postoperatively, C, Appearance of graft 1 year postoperatively.

must be free of the pupillary zone for an optimal visual result. A peripheral iridotomy or iridectomy is required to prevent any anterior displacement of the iris against a fresh "sticky" wound.

Corneal Perforations

The optimal method for management of a corneal perforation is dictated by a number of factors including its cause, its size and location, the condition of the adjacent corneal tissue, the depth of the anterior chamber, the status of the intraocular structures, the presence or absence of concurrent ocular disease, and the state of the patient's general health. Unless a significant portion of central corneal tissue is actually avulsed, central perforating trauma should be treated by primary repair, not by keratoplasty. A healed corneal laceration frequently provides a surprisingly good visual result when a hard corneal

contact lens is fitted over the scar. Should the visual axis ultimately be too compromised to allow adequate vision, penetrating keratoplasty is indicated if the posterior pole is uncompromised.

A corneal perforation with flat anterior chamber and hypotony tends to impel the surgeon to hasty action, which often is unnecessary (Fig. 23–14). Appropriate microbiologic cultures should be obtained, antibiotic sensitivities determined, and the indicated antimicrobial or antiviral agents employed. The cornea should have a therapeutic hydrophilic contact lens placed on it in an effort to check the flow of aqueous humor through the perforation site,[27] and the patient should be put at bed rest. A hyperosmolar agent administered intravenously (if administered orally it may induce nausea and vomiting) may be helpful by reducing the volume of the posterior chamber and vitreous cavity. This regimen often will reform the anterior chamber but not relieve the hypotony. Mydriatic-cycloplegic drops should be instilled to move the iris from the perforation site and to promote the flow of aqueous humor from the posterior to the anterior chamber, reducing the potential for relative pupillary block. Intensive topical anti-inflammatory agents should be employed to prevent anterior and posterior synechiae. Cyanoacrylate adhesives should not be used; they produce sterile abscesses and have been removed from clinical investigation by the FDA because of their toxicity and possible carcinogenic activity.

At surgery, manipulation of the eye should be minimal to prevent extrusion of its contents. Only a mark should be made with the trephine, and the incision

should be completed with knife and scissors. The pathologic changes that are present determine whether repair of the perforation is best accomplished by lamellar or penetrating keratoplasty. If circumstances favor conservative measures, including the avoidance of more extensive invasion of the anterior chamber, then a lamellar bed is dissected in normal cornea around the perforation site, removing as much necrotic tissue as possible (Fig. 23–15). Frozen or preserved donor cornea can be used, and this is directly sutured into the lamellar bed with 10-0 monofilament nylon sutures. When healing is complete and the eye is free of active inflammation, a penetrating keratoplasty is performed for visual rehabilitation. If penetrating

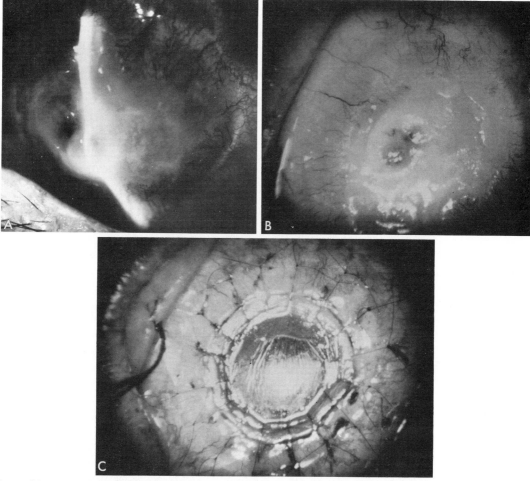

Figure 23–14. Corneal perforation (herpes simplex keratitis). *A,* Inflamed eye with perforated, necrotic corneal ulcer and flat anterior chamber. *B,* Appearance after 2 days of therapy with a hydrophilic contact lens and intensive topical corticosteroids. *C,* Penetrating keratoplasty performed as the primary mode of definitive treatment. Appearance during the latter stages of surgery.

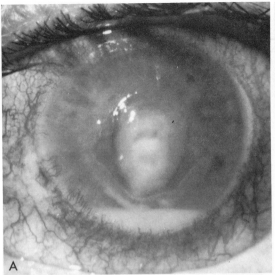

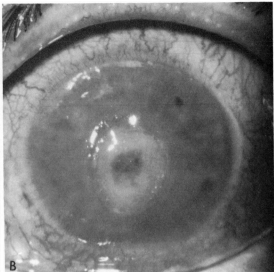

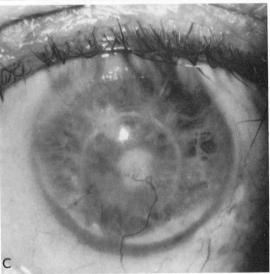

Figure 23–15. Corneal perforation (herpes simplex keratitis). *A,* Inflamed eye with perforated, necrotic corneal ulcer, shallow anterior chamber, and hypopyon. *B,* Appearance after 3 days of therapy with a hydrophilic contact lens and intensive topical corticosteroids. *C,* Lamellar keratoplasty, using frozen donor tissue, performed as the primary mode of definitive treatment. (Courtesy Howard M. Leibowitz, M.D.)

keratoplasty is undertaken as the primary mode of treatment (Fig. 23–14), it may not be possible to reform the anterior chamber at the end of the surgical procedure because of the formation of a choroidal detachment. As stated previously, this will require drainage via a sclerotomy.

Oversized Grafts

On rare occasions a patient will present with anterior segment pathology that involves more area than can be encompassed by a 10.0-mm. trephine but requires surgical therapy for the preservation of sight or the integrity of

the eye (e.g., epithelial ingrowth or the "megakeratoglobus" of Ehlers-Danlos syndrome) (Fig. 23–16). To obtain an oversized trephine, we have used sharpened laboratory cork-borers. A Flieringa ring also can be used as a template to outline the bed for a large corneoscleral graft.[28] A complete peritomy should be performed and the conjunctiva retracted by means of quadrant relaxing incisions. Bridle sutures should be placed beneath all four rectus muscles under direct visualization. Interrupted sutures should be used in all areas that will be subconjunctival, and a continuous suture may be used in corneal areas. Great care should be taken with hemostasis because by definition large areas of vas-

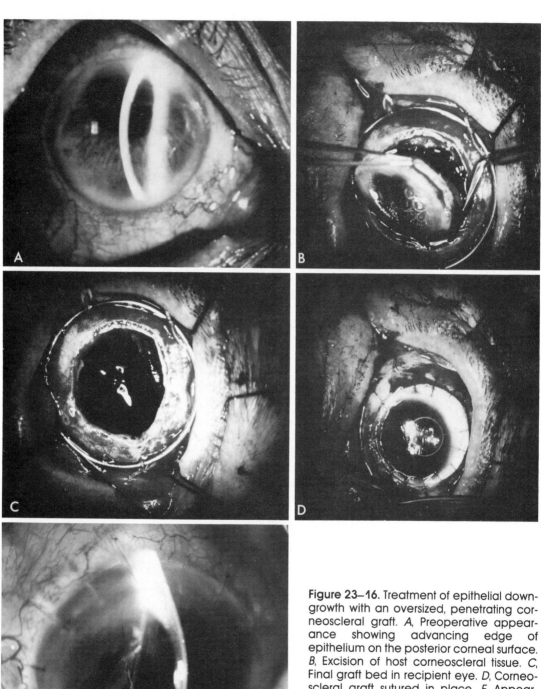

Figure 23–16. Treatment of epithelial downgrowth with an oversized, penetrating corneoscleral graft. *A,* Preoperative appearance showing advancing edge of epithelium on the posterior corneal surface. *B,* Excision of host corneoscleral tissue. *C,* Final graft bed in recipient eye. *D,* Corneoscleral graft sutured in place. *E,* Appearance of graft 4 months postoperatively.

cularized tissue will be involved. In the case of epithelial ingrowth, epithelium that cannot be removed en bloc can be frozen with the cryoprobe.[29, 30]

Postoperative Management

In the operating room the corneal surgeon can only hope to perform rational, meticulous surgery. He cannot assure graft success; that can only be achieved by careful continual postoperative management.

In addition to the usual postoperative orders for the maintenance of life and health, we routinely prescribe the following:

1. Neosporin drops q.i.d.

2. Prednisolone acetate 1 per cent suspension q. 1 h., 6 a.m. to 10 p.m.

3. Scopolamine hydrobromide 0.25 per cent b.i.d.

The first is given as broad-spectrum antibiotic prophylaxis, since it must be presumed that some microorganisms have been introduced during surgery. If drug sensitivity is a problem, then another broad-spectrum agent should be used, preferably one that is not used systemically. If bacterial, viral, or fungal infection was a problem preoperatively, then the appropriate drug must be used in therapeutic doses until cultures and clinical signs are negative. If at the end of 5 days infection is not a postoperative problem, the antibacterial regimen is altered and a less sensitizing agent (e.g., sulfisoxazole drops 3 per cent b.i.d.) is used. This regimen is maintained until the sutures are removed and the epithelium is intact.

With the use of a continuous monofilament nylon suture, the problem of stitch abscesses has virtually ceased to exist. However, if knots are exposed and are disrupting the integrity of the epithelium, a stitch abscess becomes more likely and must be treated accordingly. Superficial knots will frequently attract superficial neovascuvariztion, but if the epithelium is intact and there is no perivascular infiltrate, this is not a problem.

Intensive topical corticosteroid drops are begun immediately to suppress the anterior segment inflammatory response due to surgery and hopefully to suppress the "affector arc" of the immune response. An ancillary benefit is patient comfort. In the absence of an anterior segment inflammatory response, the corticosteroid is tapered rapidly after 3 or 4 days so that at the end of 1 week the medication is applied four times a day, after 2 weeks twice a day, and after 4 weeks once a day. This dosage then is maintained until suture removal, when it is reduced to alternate day instillation, and subsequently to two times per week. If steroid-induced glaucoma is a problem, the amount of medication must be further reduced to prednisolone acetate 0.125 per cent suspension; and, if the patient is fitted with a contact lens, to prednisolone phosphate 0.125 per cent solution.

Mydriatic-cycloplegic agents are instilled in the operating room and are continued at a therapeutic level for 2 to 3 weeks. These medications are used primarily to prevent synechiae and to enhance patient comfort by reducing contraction of the ciliary muscle. Atropine is not used because its effect is difficult to reverse in a short time. If postoperative glaucoma is a problem in the early postoperative phase, i.e., before inflammatory quiescence, we prefer to control it with topically administered epinephrine derivatives or beta-adrenergic blockers or systemically administered carbonic anhydrase inhibitors; these drugs may be used alone or in combination. However, carbonic anhydrase inhibitors may be extremely debilitating to elderly patients and miotic agents may be required. Miotic agents also are used whenever the intraocular pressure cannot be maintained under 20 mm. Hg in their absence. Later in the postoperative course, after inflammatory quiescence, miotic agents may be initiated or resumed without fear of synechia formation, and they may be used to create a pinhole effect. Mydriatics are contraindicated in the presence of some types of pseudophakia.

The patient must be examined at the bedside on the first postoperative day for evidence of wound integrity, gross graft and anterior chamber clarity, and signs of infection. If there is any doubt of the eye's status, slit-lamp examination should be performed. Thereafter slit-lamp examination, including tonometry, should be performed daily for the remainder of the hospital stay. Electronic tonometry may be preferable (and expensive), but with patience and perseverance applanation tonometry can be performed on keratoplasties 7.0 mm. or larger.

In general, after discharge from the hospital a patient with a keratoplasty should be examined once or twice a week for the first 3 to 4 weeks, then every 2 weeks for 2 to 3 months, and then every 3 weeks or monthly until sutures are removed. This outline is for the majority of good-prognosis patients—some eyes have remarkably peaceful courses and others remarkably difficult ones. During this period the surgeon will be continually adjusting drugs and dosages for the optimal result.

As a further generality, children heal faster than adults, younger adults faster than the elderly, vascularized corneas faster than nonvascularized corneas, and corneal grafts with interrupted sutures faster than corneal grafts with continuous sutures. Corticosteroids and antimetabolites delay wound healing (but no nonexperimental drug selectively accelerates wound healing). Overall, the rate of wound healing varies widely. For example, we have successfully removed a continuous suture from an atopic patient 3 weeks postoperatively but have seen poor cicatrix formation 12 and 14 months postoperatively. As a result, some surgeons recommend leaving very fine continuous sutures in place indefinitely.[25] Unfortunately, this can result in other problems; opacification of the corneal graft around the suture loops may occur and at times involve the visual portion of the graft,[34] and suture-induced astigmatism will persist.

Interrupted sutures may be removed at 10 to 12 weeks; initially every other suture is taken out with a razor-blade knife and jeweler's forceps. If the wound remains secure, the rest of the sutures are removed during a subsequent visit. Individual sutures may be removed earlier if they are loose or if they are associated with an infiltrative inflammatory reaction or a neovascular response. If possible, all sutures should be cut on the recipient side to avoid disrupting the graft epithelium. Suture fragments remaining buried in the stroma may be ignored.

Continuous sutures are usually removed at 5 to 7 months postoperatively, and, again, the recipient loop should be cut. The continuous suture is removed at one sitting. Individual loops of continuous suture may be removed at 10 to 12 weeks if they are loose or if there is an isolated infiltrative reaction; in this event the loop should be cut at its entrance into the stroma so that the cut end will retract into the stroma. Whether interrupted or continuous, the suture should not be removed until the surgeon can observe cicatrix formation or, even better, cicatrix formation and contraction throughout the stroma and Descemet's membrane. Regardless of the suture technique used, the patient must return to the office on the day after suture removal for evaluation of the integrity of the wound.

If the wound and epithelium are intact, then antimicrobial drugs are discontinued and steroid drops reduced to twice a week. Usually at this point the eye is being examined on a monthly basis until either the refractive error or the keratometric mires are stable. Depending upon the degree of aniseikonia, the degree of regular and irregular astigmatism, and the presence of other factors such as a dry-eye syndrome, an appropriate optical correction is provided.

If during the postoperative period there has been cataract formation that requires extraction for a good visual result, cataract extraction should be delayed until the keratometric mires stabilize, presumably indicating the end of collagen shortening and the completion of wound healing. We prefer a rather large cataract section, 170 degrees, and extraction by the intracapsular route and, except for minimal amounts of BSS, the avoidance of all intracameral solutions, especially alpha-chymotrypsin, in order to minimize any further damage to endothelium. The section is closed with 10-0 monofilament nylon sutures, and postoperative medications are the same as those used for keratoplasty. Any adhesions to the wound may be lysed during the cataract procedure as long as excessive manipulation and hemorrhage are avoided. We have not used any of the extracapsular techniques because of the marked increase in irrigation of the anterior chamber that is required and because of the greater inflammatory response postoperatively.

Almost all pathogenic bacterial infections occur during the early postoperative period while the patient is hospitalized, but exceptions occur (Fig. 23–17). Emphasis must be placed on prompt diagnosis by external and intracameral smear and culture and by the immediate institution of broad-spectrum antibiotics, both topically and subconjunctivally, until the laboratory studies identify the optimal drugs.[35-38] Corticosteroids must be maintained or increased, not reduced or discontinued, in order to suppress the massive inflammatory re-

sponse with its proteolytic enzyme release. The goal of combined therapy, which is still controversial,[36, 37] is to kill the microorganisms with antibiotics and concurrently to suppress the inflammatory response with corticosteroids. A further point is to preserve the eye; there may be very little hope of preserving the corneal graft, but the transplantation procedure can be repeated if the eye survives in suitable condition. Viral (e.g., herpes simplex, (Fig. 23–18), low-virulent bacterial (e.g., *Staphylococcus epidermidis*, Fig. 23–17B), and mycotic infections may occur later in the postoperative course after the patient has been discharged from the hospital. These infections should be diagnosed and treated as in any other eye, but with continuing attention to inflammatory suppression once the specific diagnosis and appropriate antimicrobial agents have been utilized.

Allogeneic tissue reactions have been known since the time of John Hunter. However, "graft rejection" (at least insofar as corneal grafts were concerned) remained a "waste-basket diagnosis" even after Maumenee[38] began focusing direct clinical attention on the subject. In 1973 Jones[39] could write, "An unequivocal clinical diagnosis of allograft reaction can be made when at least ten days after a first transplantation, a pre-

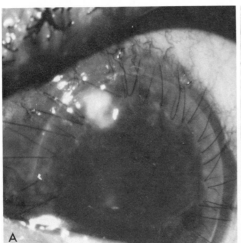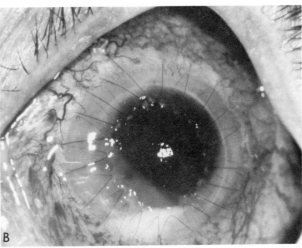

Figure 23–17. Late bacterial infection of the graft. *A, Streptococcus pneumoniae* infiltrate 6 weeks after penetrating keratoplasty for keratoglobus. *B, Staphylococcus epidermidis* keratitis and endophthalmitis following penetrating keratoplasty for aphakic bullous keratopathy. (*A* courtesy of Howard M. Leibowitz, M.D.)

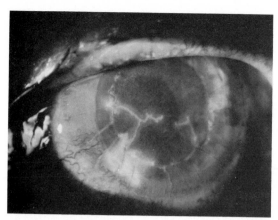

Figure 23–18. Recurrence of dendritic herpes simplex virus lesion in a corneal graft.

viously clear graft in a quiet eye rapidly develops edema, with signs of inflammation in the anterior segment including ciliary flush, with cells and usually slight flare in the anterior chamber, and when the area of edema in the graft moves across the cornea in the wake of an endothelial line—a Khodadoust line—typically commencing at and moving away from a focus of vascularization in the vicinity of the graft. Similar lines of advancing rejection may be seen in the stroma or in the epithelium, in which case the latter may be shed behind the line." (Figs. 23–19 to 23–22.) Though less common, allogeneic rejection can also occur in lamellar grafts (Fig. 23–23).

Khodadoust and Silverstein[40] have demonstrated immune corneal allograft rejection in rabbits and, although the "Khodadoust line" (Fig. 23–19) has its analogue in the human graft, its presence in the human situation is by no means necessary. In 1971 we[3] described rejection reactions morphologically as being limbal, uveal, or both. Corneal neovascularization and cellular infiltration can occur without signs of anterior uveitis, and conversely, anterior uveal inflammatory changes with graft edema can occur without visible limbal involvement. However, a combination of the two types of response is most common. A spectrum of graft rejection reactions exhibiting varying changes occurs. What is visible to the clinician depends on the anatomic status of the anterior segment at the onset of the reaction and the stage at which the graft is initially examined.

In a clear graft with intact epithelium the appearance of keratic precipitates (KP) on the endothelium (Fig. 23–20) or an increase in peripheral neovascularization and cellular infiltration (Fig. 23–21) must always be taken as an ominous sign and treated accordingly. It has been our experience that "chasing" inflammatory reactions with steroids (i.e., starting with a low dose and gradually increasing it until a response is obtained) has not resulted in satisfactory recovery of corneal graft transparency. It is more effective to initiate submaximal medication immediately, i.e., prednisolone acetate 1 per cent suspension hourly. If dramatic improvement is not present within 24 hours, daily or even

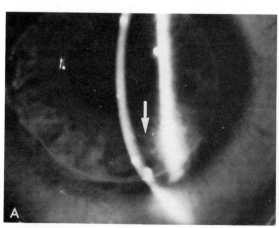
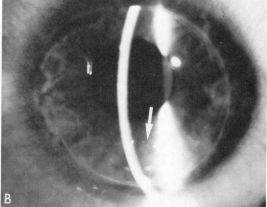

Figure 23–19. A and B, A Khodadoust line on the endothelium of a graft in acute rejection.

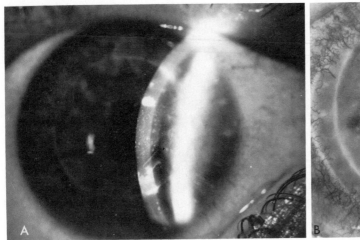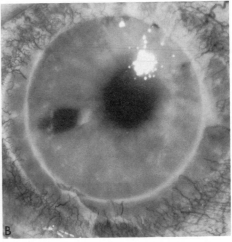

Figure 23–20. Signs of allogeneic corneal graft rejection. *A*, Keratic precipitates. *B*, Acute onset of conjunctival injection, ciliary flush, and edema of the graft.

Figure 23–21. Acute increase in peripheral neovascularization of a corneal graft, producing a "salmon patch" accompanied by edema and infiltration—signs of graft rejection.

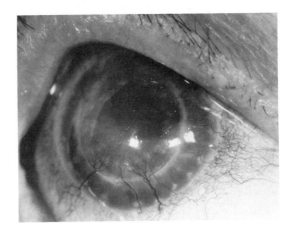

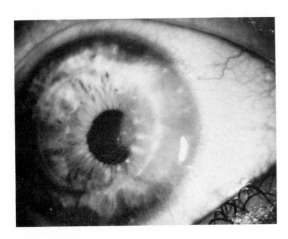

Figure 23–22. Early allogeneic corneal graft rejection showing interface between rejecting and clear portions of graft (Khodadoust line) with keratic precipitates on the endothelium of the rejecting segment.

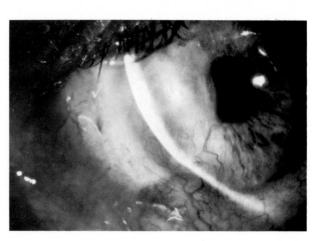

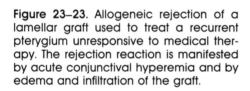

Figure 23–23. Allogeneic rejection of a lamellar graft used to treat a recurrent pterygium unresponsive to medical therapy. The rejection reaction is manifested by acute conjunctival hyperemia and by edema and infiltration of the graft.

twice daily subconjunctival injections of 4 mg. of dexamethasone phosphate must also be given until definite evidence of reversal of the corneal inflammatory response is observed. Topical therapy must be continued for 10 to 14 days after complete quiescence of anterior segment inflammatory activity and then slowly tapered by halving the dosage on a weekly basis. The graft must be followed very closely to detect any early signs of exacerbation of the reaction. Should this occur, increased corticosteroid therapy must be reinstituted promptly. Attentive patients will frequently notice the onset of photophobia before clinical signs are apparent and should be treated accordingly. A relatively high maintenance dose of steroid drops (i.e., q.i.d.) may be required for several months.

We do not use oral steroids at all because of the potentially serious side effects of this route of administration and because of the superior penetration and anti-inflammatory activity of prednisolone acetate drops.[41] The use of systemic cytotoxic agents, e.g., methotrexate or chlorambucil, must be approached by an oncologist with extreme caution; fully informed patient consent must be obtained, since the patient's life is being threatened in an attempt to save a corneal transplant, and such agents should be considered only in cases of multiple keratoplasty failures.

When high-dose local steroid regimens are employed, steroid-induced glaucoma may occur. Therefore, intraocular pressure must be checked at every examination and appropriate medications instituted when the intraocular pressure passes 20 mm. Hg. False low recordings may be obtained on edematous corneas. In phakic eyes without previous glaucoma the rise in intraocular pressure may also be a sign that anterior uveitis has been inactivated (by corticosteroid therapy). The sudden appearance of vesicular edema in a graft must be presumed to represent an immunologic graft reaction (Fig. 23–20B), not the sudden onset of glaucoma, unless the intraocular pressure is above 35 mm. Hg. In too many instances clinicians have presumed that glaucoma was at fault and discontinued all steroids, thereby guaranteeing graft failure.

In general it has been our experience that an immunologic graft reaction first diagnosed and treated more than 5 to 7 days after its onset is irreversible as far as a return of optical clarity to the graft is concerned.[3] Similarly, grafts whose optical clarity has not improved after 10 to 14 days of maximal steroid therapy usually have failed irreversibly, and the corticosteroid regimen should be tapered and discontinued. Reoperation can then be considered depending on the clinician's judgment and the patient's needs and desires. In general, after two immunologic failures that we have been unable to control we discourage further surgery. Further understanding of the HLA system and better data on "matching" may well alter this circumstance, as may such newer drugs as cyclosporin A.

As noted earlier in this chapter, glaucoma must be controlled preoperatively by medical and, if necessary, surgical means without the use of carbonic anhydrase inhibitors. Nevertheless, postoperative glaucoma is still a significant complication following penetrating keratoplasty, especially in aphakic eyes. Intraocular pressure should be determined at every postoperative visit and maintained under 20 mm. Hg. The usual antiglaucomatous drops may be used, though the clinician should note the caveats concerning echothiophate and epinephrine in aphakia. Considerable reliance must be placed on the carbonic anhydrase inhibitors, with selection of the one that is best tolerated by the patient. For short- to medium-term use, i.e., a few weeks to 3 to 4 months, we will use double the usual adult doses, for example, 500 mg. acetazolamide by mouth q.i.d. along with supplementary potassium, in an attempt to avoid glaucoma surgery. The reason for this approach is that some portion of the elevated intraocular pressure response may be induced, and as steroids are reduced to maintenance levels, the glaucoma may become easier to control. When glaucoma cannot be controlled (and is not a consequence of pupillary block or a malignant mechanism), we recommend a trabeculectomy in an area of open angle, if possible, along with an iridectomy and generous anterior vitrectomy. If this fails, we repeat the procedure. If both trabeculectomies fail, we turn to cyclocryotherapy. In spite of reports of the safety and efficacy of this procedure,[42, 43] we are unable to sufficiently quantitate cyclocryotherapy in inflamed edematous eyes to avoid with certainty the risk of irreversible hypotony and phthisis.

Postoperative management of keratoplasty may be greatly complicated by problems of the precorneal tear film or the epithelium. If fresh donor tissue is used without damage to the epithelial basement membrane, re-epithelialization should be complete by 48 to 72 hours. When preserved donor tissue is used by the punch technique, epithelium is not deliberately removed and survives on the donor for 4 to 8 weeks. The donor epithelium does not desquamate as a slough but is gradually replaced by host epithelium moving centrally from the wound edge from one or several sites. This "advancing edge" may be identified by slit-lamp examination as a line of very fine superficial vesicles that lightly stain. Replacement is probably complete when the graft epithelium acquires the normal, smooth optical luster.

If the integrity of the epithelial sheet is not intact 4 days postoperatively, then 48 hours of nonstop patching should be instituted. In the 48-hour period there will be very little inflammatory rebound from the abrupt cessation of steroids and minimal time for the incubation of unsuspected microorganisms. At the end of 48 hours the previous therapeutic regimen should be reinstituted for 48 to 72 hours, and then nonstop patching may be resumed if necessary, alternating with therapy until the epithelium is intact. Inpatients should not be discharged until epithelial integrity is restored. If patching by itself is insufficient, artificial tears and bedtime ointments may be added to the regimen. Careful attention must be focused on inflammatory change during this period, because normal epithelium will not adhere over areas of neovascularization and infiltrate. In addition, when the epithelial barrier is not intact, there is the constant risk of infection.

If re-epithelialization remains a problem (Fig. 23–24) or if a dry-eye syndrome is present, closure of the lacrimal puncta and placement of a "bandage" soft contact lens may be necessary. Failure of re-epithelialization will certainly lead to keratoplasty failure sooner or later. If this should occur in spite of the best efforts of the surgeon, re-evaluation of the entire prospect for keratoplasty must be considered, including alternative options such as conjunctival flap and keratoprosthesis. (Unfortunately, when the prognosis for keratoplasty is worst, so too is the prognosis for keratoprosthesis.)

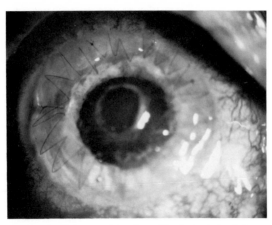

Figure 23–24. Persistent epithelial defect in a corneal graft.

Occasionally 6 to 12 weeks after surgery an epithelial defect will suddenly occur on a graft. Clinically these defects resemble recurrent erosions; presumably there is an underlying defect in the basement membrane, and the epithelial defect should be treated accordingly. If during surgery sutures are drawn too tightly or they are drawn up with uneven tension so that the wound margin is compressed and elevated, the upper lid will not pass properly over the central indentation and a dellen (Fig. 23–25) will form in the early postoperative period. The dellen can be treated with artificial tears, ointments, or patching until the anatomic malformation resolves. Epithelialization of the corneal graft may perhaps be enhanced by stimulation of epithelial mitoses with phospholine iodide or carbacholamine,[44] but the clinical effectiveness of this treatment is not certain.

Wound leaks in the early postoperative period must be terminated by either medical or surgical management while the patient is still hospitalized. Wound leaks in the intermediate period are due to direct trauma (Fig. 23–26) or to exuberant physical activity on the part of the patient. If the leak is not apparent (i.e., if normal anterior chamber depth persists), its existence will be heralded by the sudden appearance of stromal and epithelial edema in the periphery of the donor or by a sudden reduction in intraocular pressure and can be confirmed by aqueous humor dilution of applied fluorescein (Seidel's test). These leaks should be treated by patching or a soft contact lens along with mydriatic-cycloplegics and oral acetazolamide 1000 mg. per day. If this regimen is unsuccessful after 4 to 5 days, the wound must be resutured. In cooperative patients this can be performed under topical anesthesia as long as the iris is uninvolved. If interrupted sutures have been used, they may be reinforced or replaced by additional interrupted sutures. If a continuous suture is involved, it must be reinforced with interrupted (direct or horizontal mattress) sutures. Great care should be exercised not to divide the continuous suture with

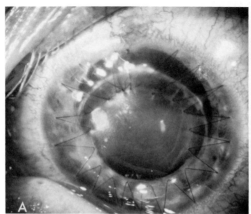
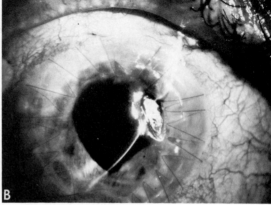

Figure 23–25. A dellen in a corneal graft. *A,* Desiccated epithelium is gray and degenerate-appearing but intact. *B,* More pronounced drying resulting in desquamation of the desiccated epithelium and in dehydration and thinning of the underlying stroma.

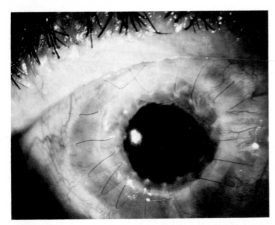

Figure 23–26. Traumatic rupture of continuous suture and wound leak 5 months postoperatively. Anterior chamber is still formed.

the cutting needle. Alternatively, loops of continuous suture may be tightened and anchored to interrupted sutures placed in the episclera; the disadvantage of this maneuver is that the anchoring suture will kink, and thus weaken, the continuous suture.

Broken interrupted sutures must be replaced if a wound leak occurs. If a continuous suture is broken and the wound is intact, the broken ends must be trimmed to the level of the anterior stroma so that surface epithelialization will occur. (Similarly, if a continuous suture has loose loops causing epithelial defects, and the wound appears secure, the loops may be removed and the cut ends allowed to retract into the stroma (Fig. 23–27). If the continuous suture is broken and the wound is leaking, one or two loops of each broken end must be freed to provide sufficient suture to allow each broken end to be tied to an interrupted suture placed at the site. The gap (Fig. 23–28) is then closed by interrupted sutures unless it is sufficiently large to permit another continuous suture to be placed. In any event the knots must be buried to prevent epithelial defects and consequent neovascularization. (If, in spite of proper burying, the knots are later impossible to remove from the corneal stroma, they should be left in place.)

If iris becomes incarcerated in a wound leak, immediate surgery should

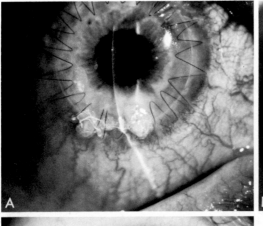

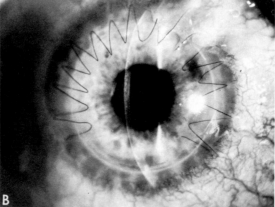

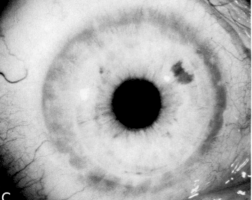

Figure 23–27. Loosening of a continuous suture. *A*, Loose loops (with adherent mucus) inferiorly in a continuous suture; wound is intact. *B*, Loose inferior loops removed; wound remains intact. Superior loops subsequently loosen and are removed. *C*, Final result.

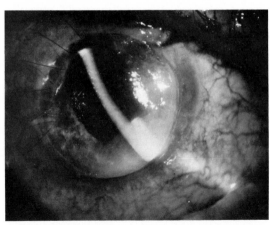

Figure 23–28. Marked dehiscence in penetrating keratoplasty wound; anterior chamber is flat. Subsequently repaired with interrupted sutures.

be performed to reposition the iris either directly through the wound or indirectly via a paracentesis incision 90 degrees away. If this is not possible, the incarcerated knuckle of iris should be pulled through the wound with forceps and an iridectomy performed flush with the wound, allowing the remaining iris to retract into the anterior chamber.

When vitreous humor is incarcerated in a leaking wound, it is generally not seen at the time. Vitreous strands may be visible by contrast if an air bubble is introduced into the anterior chamber, but great care must be taken or the bubble will move posterior to the iris, greatly complicating the procedure. Wound ruptures with prolapse of iris and/or vitreous must be cleared of both iris and vitreous. If necessary, an iridectomy and/or a vitrectomy must be per-

formed as soon as possible and the wound must be resutured. Delay will increase the potential for infection, epithelial ingrowth, and choroidal detachment.

When the surgeon decides that the wound is secure and that the cicatrix is well formed, he will remove the sutures. This procedure can be done with a razor-blade knife and jeweler's forceps. If interrupted sutures are present, alternate sutures should be removed initially and the remainder at a subsequent visit if the wound has remained secure. A continuous suture should be cut at the peripheral elbow of each loop to avoid damage to the graft epithelium.

Occasionally within a few days of suture removal a portion of the graft edge may move anteriorly. If this involves no more than 25 to 30 per cent of the circumference of the graft without marked edema and without a leak, this complication may be treated by simple patching. In 4 to 8 weeks continuing cicatrization will retract the override and produce a smooth anterior surface (with high astigmatism).

If the slippage is actually leaking, as determined by fluorescein, the patient should be put on bedrest, a soft contact lens applied, the pupil widely dilated, and carbonic anhydrase inhibitors employed. If the leak persists after 48 hours, the wound should be resutured. If the dehiscence is more complicated, it should be managed as described above.

REFERENCES

1. Leigh, A. G.: *Corneal Transplantation.* Oxford, Blackwell Scientific Publications, 1966.
2. Irvine, A. R., and Kaufman, H. E.: Intraocular pressure following penetrating keratoplasty. Amer J Ophthalmol 68:835, 1969.
3. Moore, T. E., Jr., and Aronson, S. B.: The corneal graft. A multiple variable analysis of the penetrating keratoplasty. Amer J Ophthalmol 72:205, 1971.
4. Leibowitz, H. M., and Berrospi, A. R.: Initial treatment of descemetocele with hydrophilic contact lenses. Ann Ophthalmol 7:1161, 1975.
5. Forster, R. K., and Fine, M.: Relation of donor age to success in penetrating keratoplasty. Arch Ophthalmol 85:42, 1971.
6. Pollack, F. M., Locatcher-Khorazo, D., and Gutier-

rez, E.: Bacteriologic study of "donor" eyes: Evaluation of antibacterial treatments prior to corneal grafting. Arch Ophthalmol 78:219, 1967.
7. Paton, R. T.: *Keratoplasty.* New York, McGraw-Hill, 1955.
8. Doctor, D., and Hughes, I.: Prophylactic use of Neosporin for donor eyes. Amer J Ophthalmol 46:351, 1958.
9. Rollins, H. J., and Stocker, F. W.: Bacterial flora and preoperative treatment of donor corneas. Amer J Ophthalmol 59:247, 1965.
10. Duffy, P., Wolf, J., Collins, G., DeVoe, A. G., Streeten, B., and Cowen, D.: Possible person-to-person transmission of Creutzfeldt-Jakob disease. N Engl J Med 290:692, 1974.

11. Beyt, B. E., Jr., and Waltman, S. R.: Cryptococcal endophthalmitis after corneal transplantation. N Engl J Med 298:825, 1978.
12. Houff, S. A., Burton, R. C., Wilson, R. W., Henson, T. E., London, W. T., Baer, G. M., Anderson, L. J., Winkler, W. G., Madden, D. L., and Sever, J. L.: Human-to-human transmission of rabies virus by corneal transplant. N Engl J Med 300:603, 1979.
13. Brightbill, F. S., Polack, F. M., and Slappey, T.: A comparison of two methods for cutting donor corneal buttons. Amer J Ophthalmol 75:500, 1973.
14. Davson, H.: The hydration of the cornea. Biochem J 59:24, 1955.
15. Harris, J. E., and Nordquist, L. T.: The hydration of the cornea. I. The transport of water from the cornea. Amer J Ophthalmol 40:100, 1955.
16. Zimmerman, T., Olson, R., Waltman, S., and Kaufman, H.: Transplant size and elevated intraocular pressure. Arch Ophthalmol 96:2231, 1978.
17. Paton, D.: The principal problems of penetrating keratoplasty: Graft failure and craft astigmatism. In Symposium on Medical and Surgical Diseases of the Cornea. New Orleans Academy of Ophthalmology. St. Louis, C. V. Mosby Co., 1980, p. 217.
18. Paton, R. T., and Swartz, G.: Keratoplasty for Fuchs' dystrophy. Arch Ophthalmol 61:366, 1959.
19. Hughes, W. F.: The treatment of corneal dystrophies by keratoplasty. Amer J Ophthalmol 50:1100, 1960.
20. Fine, M.: Therapeutic keratoplasty in Fuchs' dystrophy. Amer J Ophthalmol 57:371, 1964.
21. Buxton, J. N., and Chamber, F.: Indications for surgery. Int Ophthalmol Clin 10:197, 1970.
22. Lemp, M. A., Pfister, R. R., and Dohlman, C. H.: The effect of intraocular surgery on clear corneal grafts. Amer J Ophthalmol 70:719, 1970.
23. Harms, H., and Mackensen, G.: Ocular Surgery Under the Microscope. Chicago, Year Book Medical Publishers, 1967, pp. 98–99.
24. McCulley, J. P., and Eliason, J. A.: A comparison of interrupted and continuous suturing in keratoplasty (abstract). Invest Ophthalmol Vis Sci 17(Arvo Suppl):120, 1978.
25. Kaufman, H. E.: Combined keratoplasty and cataract extraction. Amer J Ophthalmol 77:824, 1974.
26. Barraquer, J., and Rutllan, J.: Corneal Surgery. Vol. 2. Surgery of the Anterior Segment of the Eye. Barcelona, Instituto Barraquer, 1971.
27. Leibowitz, H. M.: Hydrophilic contact lenses in corneal disease. IV. Penetrating corneal wounds. Arch Ophthalmol 88:602, 1972.
28. Waring, G. O., III, and Beernink, D. H.: Scleral ring as template for corneoscleral graft. Amer J Ophthalmol 85:258, 1978.
29. Stark, W. J., Michels, R. G., Maumenee, A. E., and Cupples, H.: Surgical management of epithelial ingrowth. Amer J Ophthalmol 85:772, 1978.
30. Brown, S. I.: Results of excision of advanced epithelial downgrowth. Ophthalmology 86:321, 1979.
31. Fine, M.: Postoperative management of corneal grafts. In Symposium on Medical and Surgical Diseases of the Cornea. New Orleans Academy of Ophthalmology. St. Louis, C. V. Mosby Co., 1980, p. 182.
32. Jones, D. B.: Early diagnosis and therapy of bacterial corneal ulcers. Int Ophthalmol Clin 13:1, 1973.
33. Jones, D. B.: A plan for antimicrobial therapy in bacterial keratitis. Trans Amer Acad Ophthalmol Otolaryngol 79:OP79, 1975.
34. Forster, R. K.: Etiology and diagnosis of bacterial postoperative endophthalmitis. Ophthalmology 85:320, 1978.
35. Baum, J. L.: The treatment of bacterial endophthalmitis. Ophthalmology 85:350, 1978.
36. Leibowitz, H. M., and Kupferman, A.: The effect of topically administered corticosteroids on antibiotic-treated bacterial keratitis. Arch Ophthalmol 98:1287, 1980.
37. Leibowitz, H. M.: Management of inflammation in cornea and conjunctiva. Ophthalmology 87:753, 1980.
38. Maumenee, A. E.: The influence of donor-recipient sensitization on corneal grafts. Amer J Ophthalmol 34:142, 1951.
39. Jones, B. R.: Corneal Graft Failure. Amsterdam, Elsevier–Excerpta Medica, 1973, p. 350.
40. Khodadoust, A. A., and Silverstein, A. M.: Transplantation and rejection of individual cell layers of the cornea. Invest Ophthalmol 8:180, 1969.
41. Leibowitz, H. M., and Kupferman, A. E.: Bioavailability and therapeutic effectiveness of topically administered corticosteroids. Trans Amer Acad Ophthalmol Otolaryngol 79:OP78, 1975.
42. Bellows, A. R., and Grant, W. M.: Cyclocryotherapy in advanced, inadequately controlled glaucoma. Amer J Ophthalmol 75:679, 1973.
43. Binder, P. S., Abel, R., and Kaufman, H. E.: Cyclocryotherapy for glaucoma after penetrating keratoplasty. Amer J Ophthalmol 79:489, 1975.
44. Cavanagh, H. D., Pihlaga, D., Thoft, R. A., and Dohlman, C. H.: The pathogenesis and treatment of persistent epithelial defects. Ophthalmology 81:754, 1976.

Rationale for Selection of Suturing Technique in Penetrating Keratoplasty

24

JAMES P. MCCULLEY, M.D.
JOSEPH A. ELIASON, M.D.

Although it is often stated that one technique is preferable to another, the actual choice of suturing technique in penetrating keratoplasty would appear to be based largely on the subjective preference of the surgeon. Nonetheless, recent texts on microsurgery seem to favor a continuous suture for penetrating keratoplasty.[1-3] The reasons given in support of this choice include easy removal, fewer knots with less resultant irritation, and self-adjustment of sutures placed in a less than optimal fashion.

On the other hand, there are those who prefer interrupted sutures. The proponents of this technique claim that penetrating corneal grafts secured by interrupted sutures, with or without the knots buried in the suture tract, heal more rapidly. However, there was no scientific evidence to support this claim, prompting us to investigate the matter in an experimental animal model.[4] We found that in penetrating keratoplasty wounds, use of either interrupted sutures whose knots were buried or a continuous suture provided an equally secure and watertight closure. However, wounds closed with interrupted sutures healed more rapidly and were characterized by a greater inflammatory response in the corneal stroma. Wounds closed with a continuous suture healed less rapidly but more uniformly around the entire circumference of the wound. The continuous suture incited significantly less stromal inflammation. It was not possible to determine whether these differences in wound healing were attributable solely to the difference in inflammatory response or whether additional factors were involved.

There was an apparent relative mechanical barrier within the stroma encompassed by a continuous suture. This was most evident at the wound itself and was characterized by a zone of relative impedance to vascular growth. In contrast, blood vessels grew across the stroma encompassed by interrupted sutures in an unimpeded fashion; their progress was slowed to a significantly lesser degree at the wound itself.[4] It is not known if this differential response is an independent one, related to vascular growth alone, or, alternatively, if it is in some way also related to wound healing.

These findings, along with basic suturing principles and clinical experience, permit an analysis of the relative advantages and disadvantages of the three most commonly employed suturing techniques of penetrating keratoplasty, a continuous suture, multiple interrupted sutures with knots buried in the suture tract, and multiple interrupted sutures with the knots left exposed, to ascertain the technique most appropriate for use in a given transplantation procedure. In any event, there appears to be agreement that a fine suture of 22 microns or less, made of a relatively nonreactive substance such as monofilament nylon or polypropylene, is highly desirable.

THE CONTINUOUS SUTURE

There are a number of advantages of the use of a continuous suture (Table 24–1). A continuous suture incites the least amount of inflammation of the three suturing techniques under consideration. This and the fact that wound healing is the most uniform are two major advantages of a continuous suture. More uniform wound healing theoretically should result in less corneal astigmatism. Since the growth of blood vessels is impeded within the corneal stroma encompassed by a continuous suture, particularly at the wound, this technique serves to decrease the likelihood of vascularization of the donor. This advantage would be of particular importance in recipient eyes in which the cornea is vascularized, with vessels extending a significant distance into the stroma toward the trephination site. It would also be important when factors in the recipient eye indicate a high probability for the development of excessive postoperative inflammation, a situation that encourages corneal neovascularization.

If at the time of surgery each loop of a continuous suture is drawn appropriately taut, then the elasticity of presently available materials ensures a very low incidence of problems with subsequent suture loosening. This may represent a particular advantage in patients who the surgeon suspects may not adhere rigidly to the schedule of frequent postoperative examinations. Use of a continuous suture often enables the patient to be fitted with glasses or contact lenses while the suture is still in place. Although this potential advantage cannot always be realized, it does permit early postoperative visual rehabilitation in some patients. A continuous suture is relatively easy to remove postoperatively, unless the suture is tightened excessively during surgery, causing it to cut deeply into the stroma postoperatively.

There are, however, several disadvantages of the use of a continuous suture (Table 24–1). It is technically more difficult to perform and, therefore, probably not a technique to be recommended to the surgeon who performs corneal operations only occasionally. When a continuous suture is used, a single misplaced loop cannot be readily removed and replaced, unlike individual loops

Table 24–1. SUTURING TECHNIQUES IN PENETRATING KERATOPLASTY

Advantages	Disadvantages
Continuous Suture	
1. Incites the least inflammation	1. Technically more difficult than interrupted sutures
2. Impedes vascular ingrowth at host suture line and at wound	2. Longer postoperative interval required before suture can be removed
3. Often can fit glasses or contact lens while suture is in place	3. If suture breaks or pulls free in one area, the entire suture may be affected
4. Little problem with suture loosening	
5. Easy to remove	
6. Uniform wound healing	
Interrupted Sutures with Knots Buried	
1. Able to adjust individual bites in tissue more readily	1. Stimulates more inflammation and vascularization
2. If suture pulls free in one area, remaining sutures are not significantly affected	2. Blood vessels readily bridge host suture line and wound
3. Rapid wound healing	3. Requires more frequent observation than continuous suture—if individual suture loosens, epithelium is disrupted and microorganisms may invade the stroma
4. Technically less difficult than continuous suture	4. Difficult to remove sutures—fragments may be retained
Interrupted Sutures with Knots Exposed	
1. Same as those listed for interrupted sutures with knots buried	1. Stimulates the most inflammation and neovascularization
2. Less difficult to remove than interrupted sutures with knots buried	2. Most patient discomfort
	3. Interferes with maintenance of intact epithelium, allowing microorganisms to invade the stroma

placed with the interrupted suture technique. Because a continuous suture incites less inflammation than multiple interrupted sutures (and possibly because of mechanical differences produced by the two suture techniques), wound healing is considerably slower when a continuous suture is in place. This makes it necessary to delay suture removal for a considerably longer period postoperatively. If it is not possible to correct the grafted eye visually while the continuous suture is in place, the interval prior to visual rehabilitation will be a prolonged one. There are reports of wound dehiscence after removal of a continuous suture up to 8 months postoperatively in one series[5] and 12 months postoperatively in another[6] (Fig. 24–1). There is uniform agreement that a continuous nylon suture should be left in place for a minimum of 6 months, and, depending on the circumstances of an individual case, it may be desirable to leave continuous sutures in place for a minimum of 9 to 12 months.

An additional disadvantage of the use of a continuous suture lies in the potential for a widespread effect should any disruption in its continuity be encountered. If a single loop breaks or if the suture pulls free even in a limited area, the entire suture may loosen and much or all of the wound may be adversely

Table 24–2. SUTURING TECHNIQUES IN PENETRATING KERATOPLASTY: INDICATIONS

Continuous Suture
1. Eyes with propensity for excessive postoperative inflammation
2. Sporadic or difficult patient follow-up anticipated
3. Vascularization at or near the trephine site

Interrupted Sutures with Knots Buried
1. Tenuous host bed—irregular in thickness or there is a question of the ability of the tissue to retain the sutures
2. Necessity for earlier suture removal

Interrupted Sutures With Knots Exposed
1. Fulfills indications for interrupted sutures and anticipate difficulty with suture removal if the knots are buried (e.g., uncooperative patient, patient with Parkinson's disease)

affected. Therefore, if the healing properties of the pathologic host cornea are in question, there is an added risk involved in the use of a continuous suture.

In view of these advantages and disadvantages of a continuous suture, there are several situations in which this technique would appear to be indicated (Table 24–2). They include recipient eyes that are apt to develop excessive or prolonged inflammation postoperatively, patients in whom follow-up is apt to be difficult or sporadic, and possibly vascularized host corneas in which blood vessels will be present at or near the site of trephination.

INTERRUPTED SUTURES WITH BURIED KNOTS

There are several advantages of the use of interrupted sutures with burial of the knots in the suture tract (Table 24–1). Wound healing is more rapid, and it is therefore possible to remove sutures earlier in the postoperative period than can be done safely with a continuous suture. As a result, visual rehabilitation is likely to be achieved at an earlier date. It is also technically less difficult to place interrupted sutures; individual tissue bites, if not optimally placed, can easily be removed and replaced without adversely affecting other sutures. Individual bites in the tissue can be adjusted independently of other sutures, a desirable advantage for the surgeon confronted by an irregular host bed. If a

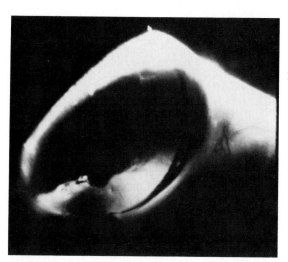

Figure 24–1. Wound dehiscence 1 day after removal of a continuous suture 12 months postoperatively.

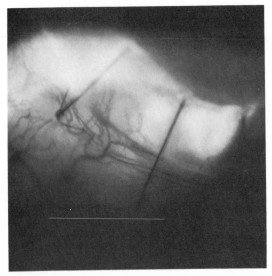

Figure 24–2. Invasion of vessels in mid-donor stroma from the vascular host bed 7 days after penetrating keratoplasty that involved use of interrupted sutures with knots buried in suture tract.

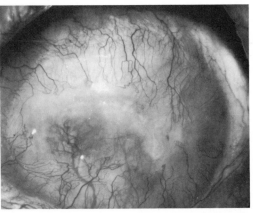

Figure 24–4. Conjunctival flap in place over a cornea known to have had an uncontrolled herpes simplex ulcerative process prior to its placement.

suture should pull free in one area, the remaining sutures are not adversely affected. Even if wound closure becomes inadequate, the problem usually can be corrected by replacing only an individual suture.

Disadvantages of the use of interrupted sutures with buried knots are also listed in Table 24–1. As stated above, this technique stimulates a greater inflammatory response in the corneal stroma than does a continuous suture. Blood vessels readily invade the host tissue encompassed by the sutures and tend to bridge the wound with ease (Fig. 24–2). Interrupted sutures are more likely to loosen than a continuous suture, causing disruption of the overlying protective epithelial layer that prevents access of microorganisms to the stroma. Consequently, interrupted sutures require more frequent observation. It is also more difficult to remove interrupted sutures whose knots have been buried. Fragments of suture material may be left behind in the suture tract, although this

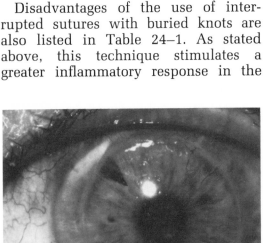

Figure 24–3. Suture fragments retained in the suture tract at 1 and 2 o'clock. No abnormality has developed as a result of retention of the suture fragment, and none should so long as the overlying epithelium remains intact.

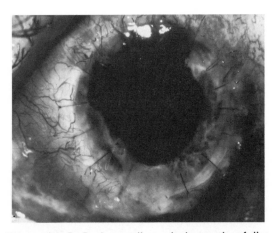

Figure 24–5. Postoperative photograph of the cornea shown in Figure 24–4 after penetrating keratoplasty was done through the conjunctival flap. The donor cornea is secured by interrupted sutures whose knots have been left exposed to facilitate subsequent suture removal.

appears to cause no difficulty as long as the overlying epithelium is intact (Fig. 24–3).

The principal indication for interrupted sutures with knots buried in the suture tract is a pathologic cornea that is thin and irregular or in which healing is expected to be irregular or questionable. This technique is also indicated whenever rapid removal of sutures postoperatively is required (Table 24–2).

INTERRUPTED SUTURES WITH EXPOSED KNOTS

This type of suture is less difficult to remove than interrupted sutures whose knots have been buried. Otherwise the advantages of the two techniques are identical (Table 24–1). The major disadvantages of interrupted sutures with exposed knots are a direct result of the exposed knots. The corneal epithelium is unable to heal over the knots and suture ends, giving microorganisms direct access to the stroma. Concurrently, the exposed suture material causes more inflammation and patient discomfort. In addition, in patients with basement membrane disorders, who are prone to the development of persistent or recurrent epithelial defects, this added disruption of the epithelial layer, along with the increased inflammation, makes this complication much more likely to occur.

The principal indication for the use of interrupted sutures with exposed knots is a patient who meets the general requirements for interrupted sutures (e.g., a pathologic cornea that is markedly irregular in thickness), and in whom one also anticipates difficulty in removing the sutures postoperatively (e.g., penetrating keratoplasty in which trephination was performed through a conjunctival flap) (Figs. 24–4 and 24–5). Use of this suturing technique might also be considered in uncooperative patients, particularly if the lack of cooperation is involuntary, such as in a patient with Parkinson's disease (Table 24–2).

CONCLUSIONS

By applying the simple principles outlined above, it should be possible in some cases to select the optimal suturing technique for penetrating keratoplasty. In such cases the nature of the corneal pathology and any concomitant ocular disturbance, along with the requirements of the patient, will dictate the choice of suturing technique. Unfortunately, in many other cases, despite our best efforts to define the optimal suturing method, the choice will not be clear-cut and is best left to the preference of the individual surgeon.

REFERENCES

1. Harms, H., and Mackensen, G.: *Ocular Surgery Under the Microscope.* Chicago, Year Book Medical Publishers, 1967, pp. 86–87.
2. Paufique, L., and Charleux, J.: Lamellar keratoplasty. In Casey, T. A. (ed.): *Corneal Grafting.* New York, Appleton-Century-Crofts, 1972, pp. 150–154.
3. Troutman, R. C.: *Microsurgery of the Anterior Segment of the Eye.* Vol. II. *The Cornea: Optics and Surgery.* St. Louis, C. V. Mosby Co., 1977, pp. 54–55.
4. McCulley, J. P., and Eliason, J. A.: A comparison of interrupted and continuous suturing in keratoplasty (abstract). Invest Ophthalmol Vis Sci 17(Arvo Suppl):120, 1978.
5. Brown, S. I., and Tragakis, M. P.: Wound dehiscence with keratoplasty: Complication of the continuous-suture technique. Amer J Ophthalmol 72:115, 1971.
6. Binder, P. S., Abel, R., Polack, F. M., and Kaufman, H. E.: Keratoplasty wound separations. Amer J Ophthalmol 80:109, 1975.

25 Donor Material for Penetrating Keratoplasty: Short-Term and Intermediate-Term Preservation

JAMES V. AQUAVELLA, M.D.
GULLAPALLI N. RAO, M.D.

The ultimate goal of a corneal preservation or storage system is to ensure the quality of the donor cornea and to extend the maximum period of endothelial viability. Ideally, the procedure must be relatively simple and inexpensive to permit utilization by a large number of eye banks, most of which have limited technical and fiscal resources. The system should also minimize the possibility of contamination and allow the preserved tissue to be easily transported. It must be practical and facilitate the entire process of bringing together the surgical team, the patient, and the donor tissue so that transplantation can be completed before postmortem changes have significantly reduced the viability of the donor endothelium. In most institutions throughout the world corneal transplantation is routinely performed after the intact donor eye has been stored in a moist chamber at 4° C from the time of enucleation.[1] Intermediate-term storage of the donor cornea in tissue culture medium, as described by McCarey and Kaufman, also is widely employed, especially in the United States.[2, 3]

SUITABILITY OF POTENTIAL DONOR TISSUE

In some instances an eye bank will be notified of the death or impending death of a potential donor before the consent for the removal of eye tissue has been obtained. In other instances the decedent will already have been identified as a donor before the eye bank is noti-

fied. In either case this represents the point at which the first screening process should be initiated to distinguish between potential "surgical" and "nonsurgical" tissue.

One of the principal criteria used is the age of the decedent. Forster and Fine[4] have presented data indicating that there is no relationship between donor age and the outcome of a corneal graft. Many eye banks in the United States place no limit on the age of acceptable tissue, but presumably this reflects a policy to accept all donations rather than an endorsement for the surgical use of older tissue. While there is little consensus about what age, if any, should be established as the upper limit for potential donor material, many surgeons use 65 years of age as the maximum acceptable based solely on clinical experience. Selection of donor tissue on the basis of age is supported by histologic and specular microscopic studies that show a general decrease in the endothelial cell population with advancing age.[5-7] Since a sufficient number of viable endothelial cells are necessary to obtain a clear graft, the use of young tissue would seem to be advantageous.

In practice an eye bank must use the age guidelines of the surgeons to whom the tissue will be directed. Although there is general agreement that younger donor tissue is preferable to older tissue, there is no clear consensus on the lower limit of acceptable donor corneal material. Many corneal surgeons set a lower limit somewhere between 5 and 10 years

Table 25–1. SUITABILITY OF DONOR CORNEAL TISSUE FOR TRANSPLANTATION

Tissue That May Represent a Health-Threatening Condition for the Recipient or Be Contraindicated Because of Endothelial Dysfunction
1. Death of unknown cause
2. Death from central nervous system disease of unknown etiology
3. Creutzfeldt-Jakob disease
4. Rabies
5. Subacute sclerosing panencephalitis
6. Congenital rubella
7. Progressive multifocal leukoencephalopathy
8. Reye's syndrome
9. Subacute encephalitis (cytomegalovirus brain infection)
10. Septicemia
11. Hepatitis
12. Intrinsic eye disease—retinoblastoma, conjunctivitis, iritis, glaucoma, corneal disease, malignant tumors of the anterior segment
13. Blast form leukemia
14. Hodgkin's disease
15. Lymphosarcoma

Tissue Whose Use Requires Caution
1. Multiple sclerosis
2. Parkinson's disease
3. Amyotrophic lateral sclerosis
4. Jaundice
5. Chronic lymphocytic leukemia
6. Diabetes
7. Surgically induced ocular abnormality (e.g., aphakia)
8. Syphilis

of age, whereas others will use tissue from donors as young as 6 months of age. The objections cited against using donor corneas from the very young include the small diameter, increased pliability, and thinness of the tissue. The authors accept donor corneal tissue without any lower age limitation.[8]

Another factor of concern is the degree of debility and the cause of death of the donor (Table 25–1). This requires a review of the hospital chart and at times an interview of hospital personnel familiar with the case. The object is to eliminate from the surgical category donors with long-term severe reductions in metabolic functions or systemic diseases that can be transmitted by the graft to the recipient. Disorders in which the recipient has developed the same disease that was present in the donor include bacterial infection,[9, 10] fungal infection,[11, 12] Creutzfeldt-Jakob disease,[13] rabies,[14] and retinoblastoma;[15] there seems to be general agreement among eye banks and corneal surgeons that the presence of these diseases precludes use of a donor cornea for penetrating keratoplasty. Corneas from donors with syphilis, tuberculosis, or hepatitis also

are generally excluded. Systemic cancer without ocular involvement usually is not a cause for rejection by most eye banks and corneal surgeons. Because of the documented transmission of Creutzfeldt-Jakob disease and rabies, it is now often recommended that any patient with dementia or a chronic atraumatic neurologic disorder not be used as a donor.

REMOVAL OF CORNEAL TISSUE

Once the decedent has been identified as a donor, the eyes are thoroughly irrigated with sterile saline solution. Several drops of a neomycin–polymyxin B–gramicidin solution then are instilled into each eye, and a liberal amount of erythromycin ointment is placed in the inferior fornix. The eyelids are taped closed and ice packs are placed over the closed lids to decrease endothelial metabolism. The cadaver should be refrigerated promptly and enucleation should be performed with 6 hours of death.

Removal of corneal tissue from a cadaver can be accomplished by enucleation of the whole eye or by excision of the cornea and a rim of sclera in situ. Enucleation is a relatively simple procedure that does not involve handling of the delicate isolated cornea. It has the advantage of preventing exposure of the corneal endothelium to trauma or exogenous contaminants and of maintaining an intact globe, which facilitates postmortem examination of the cornea. The enucleation should be performed under sterile conditions after the eyes are flushed with topical antibiotics. Following enucleation each eye is placed in a sterile moist-chamber container, which is refrigerated at 4° C and is transported to the eye bank laboratory for examination, processing, and distribution to the surgeon.

Excision of the cornea in situ has the advantage of being a time-saving, one-step process that reduces potential cosmetic damage to the cadaver and thus may be more acceptable to families contemplating postmortem tissue donation. The technique for excision is much the same as that used to remove the cornea from the enucleated eye. It may be accomplished either with a large trephine or with an ab-externo razor-blade incision through sclera 2 mm. behind the limbus. The incision, which penetrates only the sclera, is continued with small scissors around the entire perilimbal area. It is important to maintain the anterior chamber throughout this process in order to prevent compromise of the endothelium.[16]

A small forceps is used gently to lift the cornea and separate it from its attachment to the ciliary body. The cornea, along with its scleral rim, is then placed in a sterile vial containing preserving medium for shipment to the eye bank. Disadvantages of this technique are the potential for contamination of or physical damage to the endothelium and the necessity for a highly trained technician to remove the cornea from the donor.

EVALUATION OF DONOR TISSUE

All donor tissue must be evaluated to assess its suitability for transplantation. Initially, simple visual inspection is performed by directing a small lamp or light source at the cornea from the level of the limbus. This will reveal gross epithelial defects as well as stromal opacities that may be overlooked during microscopic examination. The slit-lamp biomicroscope remains the principal means for evaluating donor corneas at the present time. It allows an assessment of corneal clarity and thickness as well as observation of Descemet's membrane and the endothelium. This portion of the examination is best done with the eye intact, but it can also be performed on an excised cornea by properly positioning the fluid-filled vial containing the cornea in the beam of the slit lamp. Donor corneas in which the endothelium cannot be visualized because of extreme edema, which contain stromal infiltrates or extensive scars, or in which central cornea guttata or keratic precipitates are observed should be rejected. An epithelial defect generally does not preclude use of the tissue for penetrating keratoplasty.

Specular microscopy, using epi-illumination and an applanation cone, allows a direct view of the endothelial surface of the cornea at 100 × magnification. Cell morphology, pattern, and density may be observed and assessed. In addition, a precise measurement of corneal thickness may be obtained, although postmortem thickness measurements have not been generally useful as an indicator of the endothelial viability of donor tissue. This technique can be applied to evaluation of both the intact enucleated eye and the excised cornea. Although it permits a far superior view of the corneal endothelium than does slit-lamp biomicroscopy and is employed in some eye banks as a screening procedure, specular microscopy is not yet in routine use. However, as the equipment becomes less complex, easier to use, and less expensive, and as additional knowledge of the precise relationship between endothelial cell morphology and viability evolves, this instrument seems destined to become a standard part of the eye-banking procedure.

Additional techniques for evaluating the viability and physiologic function of the corneal endothelium have been described. They include measurement of the temperature reversal phenomenon, histochemical staining, and assessment of endothelial permeability by fluorophotometry. All subject the endothelium to additional trauma and risk of contamination and some (e.g., vital staining with nitro blue tetrazolium) interfere with the viability of the endothelium. These techniques are all experimental at the present time; none are in routine clinical use and none are recommended.

An integral part of any preservation system consists of thorough irrigation of the epithelial surface and treatment with prophylactic antibiotics. Some surgeons advocate immersing the enucleated globe in antibiotics prior to removing the cornea from the enucleated eye.[17] In spite of efforts to maintain sterility by utilizing optimal aseptic techniques, the potential for microbial contamination exists. Routine cultures should be obtained at appropriate points in the tissue harvesting and preservation procedure. If a cornea is to be excised in situ, bacterial and fungal cultures are prepared from the limbal area prior to treatment with antibiotics. When the cornea is removed from an enucleated eye, a small piece of sclera from the remainder of the eye should be cultured. If the cornea is maintained or preserved in a tissue culture solution, the solution should also be cultured. One relatively simple procedure is to pass the solution through a Millipore filter and to culture the filter. Although these procedures will not in most cases prevent the use of contaminated tissue, they may allow early identification of the organism in an immediate postoperative infection.

MOIST-CHAMBER STORAGE (SHORT-TERM PRESERVATION)

The entire enucleated eyeball is placed on a moist cotton pad and stored in a sterile glass jar at 4° C until surgery. Practically speaking, this usually involves storing the glass jar in a refrigerator. For purposes of transportation, refrigerated canisters or simple styrofoam containers containing a sufficient supply of ice can be utilized. This technique was originally described by Filatov[18] and Castroviejo.[19] It is effective, and because of its primary advantages of simplicity and low cost, it remains in wide use today.

Most corneal surgeons who use donor tissue stored by this method prefer, whenever possible, to utilize it within 24 hours after the death of the donor. In a questionnaire study conducted by Binder[20] the majority of eye banks stated that eyes refrigerated at 4° C in a moist chamber should not be utilized for transplantation after 48 hours of storage; all responding corneal surgeons agreed. There is evidence that shortened death-to-enucleation and enucleation-to-storage times allow for a period of moist chamber storage greater than 48 hours; a maximum death-to-enucleation time of 3 hours may allow a moist-chamber storage time of up to 90 hours. This, of course, is difficult to accomplish, and there seem to be few corneal surgeons willing to transplant this tissue beyond 48 hours of storage.

INTERMEDIATE-TERM STORAGE (PRESERVATION IN M-K MEDIUM)

M-K medium, described by McCarey and Kaufman,[2] is a mixture of tissue culture medium 199 (TC-199) and 5 per cent dextran (molecular weight 40,000). TC-199 uses a bicarbonate-buffered system to maintain a pH of 7.4; the pH of the medium is controlled by dissolved CO_2, which can escape, causing unwanted changes in the pH of the solution that in turn can damage the corneal endothelium. The use of an alternative buffer system with a pH indicator has been suggested,[21] but this system is not commercially available. The dextran is a colloidal osmotic agent that reduces the imbibition of fluid by the stored cornea. Antibiotics are added to the M-K medium after the cornea has been introduced. Initially penicillin and streptomycin were recommended; currently most eye banks substitute gentamicin for streptomycin.

Temperature reversal studies suggest that M-K medium maintains endothelial viability up to 5 days,[22] and reported results of clinical cases indicate that the tissue can be preserved satisfactorily for up to 96 hours postmortem.[3, 23] In Binder's study[20] two thirds of the reporting eye banks were using M-K medium–preserved donor corneas. Most eye banks and corneal surgeons preferred to transplant M-K medium–stored corneas within 72 hours after the death of the donor.

Use of this tissue storage technique requires that the cornea and a rim of adjacent sclera be excised, generally from the enucleated globe. Under sterile conditions an ab-externo incision is made into the sclera approximately 3 mm. posterior to the limbus with a No. 15 scalpel blade or similar knife. The incision is carried down to the choroid and must be sufficiently large to admit the tip of a fine, curved, round-tipped scissor blade into the suprachoroidal space. A full-thickness scleral incision parallel and 3 mm. posterior to the limbus is carried around the entire circumference of the globe with scissors, and great care is taken not to penetrate the choroid. The anterior chamber should remain intact while these maneuvers are carried out. The scleral rim then is grasped with fine-toothed forceps and elevated, gently separating the cornea and scleral rim from the uveal tissue and severing the attachment to the scleral spur. The cornea should not be folded while these steps are carried out, and, upon their completion, it is immediately placed in a sterile vial of M-K medium to which has been added 0.05 ml. of injectable gentamicin (40 mg./ml.), bringing the final concentration of the antibiotic in the storage vial to 100 mg./ml. The vial is tightly capped, appropriately labeled, and stored at 4° C.

REFERENCES

1. Van Horn, D. L., and Schultz, R. O.: Corneal preservation: Recent advances. Surv Ophthalmol 21:301, 1973.
2. McCarey, B. E., and Kaufman, H. E.: Improved corneal storage. Invest Ophthalmol 13:165, 1974.
3. McCarey, B. E., Meyer, R. F., and Kaufman, H. E.: Improved corneal storage for penetrating keratoplasty in humans. Ann Ophthalmol 8:1488, 1976.
4. Forster, R. K., and Fine, M. F.: Relation of donor age to success in penetrating keratoplasty. Arch Ophthalmol 85:42, 1971.
5. Stocker, F. W.: The Endothelium of the Cornea and Its Clinical Implications. Springfield, Ill., Charles C Thomas, 1971, p. 16.
6. Kaufman, H. E., Capella, J. A., and Robbins, J. E.: The human corneal endothelium. Amer J Ophthalmol 61:835, 1966.
7. Laing, R. A., Sandstrom, M. M., Berrospi, A. R., and Leibowitz, H. M.: Changes in corneal endothelium as a function of age. Exp Eye Res 22:587, 1976.
8. Rao, G. N., Waldron, W. R., and Aquavella, J. V.: Fate of endothelium in a corneal graft. Ann Ophthalmol 10:645, 1978.
9. Le Francois, M., and Baum, J. L.: Flavobacterium endophthalmitis following keratoplasty. Use of a tissue culture medium–stored cornea. Arch Ophthalmol 94:1907, 1976.
10. Shaw, E. L., and Aquavella, J. V.: Pneumococcal endophthalmitis following grafting of corneal tissue from a (cadaver) kidney donor. Ann Ophthalmol 9:435, 1977.
11. Beyt, B. E., and Waltman, S. R.: Cryptococcal endophthalmitis after corneal transplantation. N Engl J Med 298:825, 1978.
12. Larsen, P. A., Lindstrom, R. L., and Doughman, D. J.: Torulopsis glabrata endophthalmitis after keratoplasty with an organ-cultured cornea. Arch Ophthalmol 96:1019, 1978.
13. Duffy, P., Wolf, J., Collins, G., DeVoe, A. G., Streeten, B., and Cowen, D.: Possible person-to-person transmission of Creutzfeldt-Jakob disease. N Engl J Med 290:692, 1974.
14. Houff, R. A., Burton, R. C., Wilson, R. W., Henson, T. E., London, W. T., Baer, G. M., Anderson, L. J., Winkler, W. G., Madden, D. L., and Sever, J. L.: Human-to-human transmission of rabies virus by corneal transplant. N Engl J Med 300:603, 1979.
15. Dohlman, C. H., and Boruchoff, S. A.: Penetrating keratoplasty. Int Ophthalmol Clin 8:655, 1968.
16. Aquavella, J. V., Van Horn, D. L., and Haggerty, C. J.: Corneal preservation using M-K medium. Amer J Ophthalmol 80:719, 1975.
17. Brightbill, F. S., Terrones, C., and Gould, S.: Experimental studies with Staphylococcus aureus in M-K media. Invest Ophthalmol 15:32, 1976.
18. Filatov, V. P.: Transplantation of the cornea. Arch Ophthalmol 13:321, 1935.

19. Castroviejo, R.: Keratoplasty: Comments on the technique of corneal transplantation; source and preservation of donor material; report on new instruments. Amer J Ophthalmol 24:139, 1941.

20. Binder, P. S.: Eye banking and corneal preservation. In *Symposium on Medical and Surgical Diseases of the Cornea*. New Orleans Academy of Ophthalmology. St. Louis, C. V. Mosby Co., 1980, pp. 320–354.

21. Waltman, S. R., and Palmberg, P. F.: Human penetrating keratoplasty using modified M-K medium. Ophthalmic Surg 9:48, 1978.

22. McCarey, B. E.: In vitro specular microscope perfusion of M-K and moist chamber–stored human corneas. Invest Ophthalmol Vis Sci 16:743, 1977.

23. Bigar, F., Kaufman, H. E., McCarey, B. E., and Binder, P. S.: Improved corneal storage for penetrating keratoplasties in man. Amer J Ophthalmol 79:115, 1975.

Appendix I

ROCHESTER EYE BANK LABORATORY
TISSUE EXAMINATION PROCEDURE

A. PURPOSE:

Evaluation of donor corneas to determine surgical quality.

EQUIPMENT:

1. Pen light
2. Slit lamp
3. Specular microscope

PROCEDURE:

1. Gross Examination (Pen Light)

Corneas are grossly examined in respect to their folds, transparency, epithelial defects, and arcus. The degree of existence of all of these factors determine the tissue quality and its suitability for surgery.

2. Biomicroscopy Examination (Whole Eye)

The cornea is carefully examined for epithelial and stromal pathology, endothelial disease, and folds.

3. Specular Microscope Examination

The endothelium is examined for cell density, cell morphology, and endothelial changes, e.g., guttata. Ten photographs are taken of each surgical eye at various points along the cornea.

4. Reporting System

A. Specific gross, biomicroscopic, and specular microscopic positive features are graded on a scale of 0 to +3 (0 representing absence of the post mortem feature).

B. Final evaluation will be made according to the following criteria: Acceptable (Excellent Good Fair) or Unacceptable (unacceptable for human corneal transplantation).

B. PURPOSE:

The technical evaluation of the quality of donor corneas and the subsequent storage of those surgically acceptable in M-K Media.

EQUIPMENT:

1. (1) pen light
2. (1) slit lamp microscope
3. (1) specular microscope
4. (1) corneal prep set
5. (2) bottles M-K Media
6. (1) pair surgical gloves
7. (1) Barrier sterile field
8. (2) bottles Dacriose
9. (2) bottles Neosporin
10. (1) bottle Garamycin
11. (1) sterile syringe
12. (2) soaking bottles
13. (1) surgical mask

PROCEDURE:

1. The work surface is cleaned with septisol.
2. Assemble equipment on work surface.
3. Open Barrier sterile field and corneal prep set.
4. Place the eyes on 4″ × 4″ gauze sponges.

5. Trim away excess conjunctiva around limbus and irrigate eyes with Dacriose (1 bottle per pair of eyes).

6. Pour 10 cc of gentamicin solution into each of the sterile soaking bottles.

7. Suspend the eyes in the soaking bottles allowing the anterior segment to hang down into the gentamicin. Soak for 5 minutes.

8. Transfer the eyes from the soaking bottles to the sterile gauze sponges.

9. Rinse the anterior segment of the eye with a steady stream of Dacriose (10 cc per eye).

10. Excise the corneas with a 2 mm scleral rim using standard technique.

11. Place one cornea per bottle of M-K Media and add 0.05 cc gentamicin per bottle using tuberculin syringe.

12. Label the M-K Media. All labels to contain Eye Bank #, name of donor, time of death, time of evaluation, and time of processing.

13. Place vials in the refrigerator at 4° C.

Appendix II

EYE BANK ASSOCIATION OF AMERICA MEDICAL STANDARDS FOR MEMBER EYE BANKS
JUNE, 1980

INDEX

PURPOSES

These standards have been developed to increase the levels of quality and efficiency in dealing with eye tissue for transplantation and to standardize what, in the medical community, are considered to be proper procedures in the procurement, preservation, storage and use of eye tissue for transplantation.

No effort has been made here to deal with the procedures for transplanting corneas, since Eye Banks exist solely for the purpose of obtaining eye tissue, preserving it where necessary, and transmitting it to ophthalmologists for use.

I. MEMBERSHIP AND CERTIFICATION

Member Eye Banks must be equipped to perform functions which further the goals of the EBAA. Each Eye Bank must be certified by the Standards Committee in order to operate as an Eye Bank.

Eye Banks will be certified by the committee to perform only those functions which the committee certifies the Eye Bank is equipped to perform in accordance with these standards. Each Eye Bank must apply in writing for certification to perform any or all of the following functions:

1. Identify eye donors
2. Act as liaison between donors, physicians and recipients
3. Procure and enucleate eye tissues
4. Inspect and evaluate eye tissue
5. Conduct laboratory analysis of eye tissue
6. Preserve eye tissue
7. Store eye tissue
8. Distribute eye tissue

The Standards Committee will issue a letter of certification confirming those functions the Eye Bank is equipped to perform. Eye Banks desirous of upgrading their certification may do so at anytime by applying in writing to the Standards Committee. To be certified to conduct activities in Section I, 3–8, Eye Banks must comply with the following minimum requirements:

II. PERSONNEL

The Eye Bank must have a Medical Director.

A. Medical Director

The Medical Director must be an ophthalmologist who has completed post residency training or who has demonstrated an interest in external eye disease, corneal surgery, research or teaching.

The Medical Director shall be responsible for the day-to-day operation of the Eye Bank laboratory, the function of all Eye Bank technicians, the removal, evaluation, processing, and distribution of whole eyes and corneas, and the preparation of the annual laboratory budget. The Medical Director, in order to maintain his position, must document continuing ophthalmic and Eye Bank education every 3 years.

B. Technician

The Eye Bank must have a technician unless the Medical Director performs the technician's function. Eye Bank technicians must receive certification as an Eye Bank technician by the EBAA Technician's Certification Committee within one year of commencing work. During that one year period, they must be under the direct supervision of the Medical Director or a certified technician. A candidate for certification must complete a two part course—a didactic session and a practical session given at one of several regional centers. Proof of completion of both parts will be followed by the awarding of a certificate from the EBAA. Technicians working at the time this document is approved will have two years for certification.

a) Certification

To maintain certification all Eye Bank technicians must attend an EBAA scientific session at least once every three years.

Termination of work with a member Eye Bank will automatically void a technician's certification unless the technician becomes employed by a member Eye Bank within one year of his or her termination of previous employment. Any exception to these requirements must be approved by the Technician's Certification Committee.

b) Duties

The Eye Bank technician must:

1) Be familiar with the methods and techniques of eye enucleation (but does not necessarily have to perform enucleation).

2) Review the history and medical record surrounding the cause of death of potential eye donors to insure donor tissue suitability.

3) Have thorough knowledge of methods for inspecting and evaluating corneal tissue including the technique of slit lamp biomicroscopy.

4) Be responsible for culturing Eye Bank eyes and inoculating media; be knowledgeable about corneoscleral segment removal technics; media preparation; ability to use sterile technique and corneal and scleral preservation technics.

5) Care for the enucleation instruments and kits.

6) Assure sterility of enucleation materials.

7) Assure laboratory cleanliness.

8) Document by carefully kept records, donor information, preservation times, data obtained from tissue evaluation, and information, relating to distribution of eye tissue.

III. FACILITIES

Eye Bank Laboratory

The laboratory must be a separate area with limited access in which activities directly related to Eye Banking are carried out. It should contain a refrigerator with a mechanism for recording temperature variations and a sink with a drain and running water. There should be adequate table space for preparation of donor material. Sterility control may be aided by the use of a laminar flow hood. The room including walls, floor, and sink must be kept clean at all times. Environmental control of the room must be established on a local basis with periodic culturing of air, drains, and water faucets. This must be documented.

IV. PRE-ENUCLEATION SCREENING FOR SURGICAL TISSUE

A. Screening of Tissue Must Be Conducted for the Following:

1. Penetrating Keratoplasty

The basis for rejection of donor corneal material is divided into two categories.

a. Tissue which may represent a *health threatening* condition for the recipient or be contra-indicated because of endothelial dysfunction.
  1. Death of unknown cause
  2. Death from central nervous system diseases of unknown etiology
  3. Jakob-Creutzfeldt disease
  4. Subacute sclerosing panencephalitis
  5. Congenital rubella
  6. Progressive multifocal leukoencephalopathy
  7. Reye's syndrome
  8. Subacute encephalitis, cytomegalovirus brain infection
  9. Septicemia
  10. Hepatitis
  11. Rabies
  12. Intrinsic eye disease—retinoblastoma, conjunctivitis, iritis, glaucoma, corneal disease (e.g., keratoconus or pterygium) and malignant tumors of the anterior segment
  13. Blast form leukemia
  14. Hodgkin's disease
  15. Lymphosarcoma

b. Tissue which may require caution with regard to donor selection.
  1. Multiple sclerosis
  2. Parkinson's disease
  3. Amyotrophic lateral sclerosis
  4. Jaundice, r/o hepatitis
  5. Chronic lymphocytic leukemia
  6. Diabetes
  7. Surgically induced eye abnormality, e.g., aphakia
  8. Syphilis

2. Lamellar or Patch Grafts

Criteria are the same as listed for penetrating keratoplasty except local eye disease affecting corneal endothelium (e.g., aphakia, iritis) is acceptable for use.

B. Documentation of Donor Information

Donor screening forms must be completed and retained on all Eye Bank eyes. A sample is attached—See Section XI.

C. Method of Consent

Documentation of legal consent for enucleation is essential for medical-legal reasons. Consent for enucleation must conform with state law and documentation for consent must be retained.

D. Age and Time Limitation

Since no definite relationship has been established between the quality of donor tissue and age, the upper age limit is left to the discretion of the Medical Director. The lower limit is full term birth. It is recognized, however, that endothelial abnormalities and decreased cell density increase with age.

E. Interval Between Death and Enucleation

The time interval from death to enucleation may vary according to the circumstances of death and interim means of storage of the body. The maximum allowable interval from death to enucleation will be at the discretion of the Medical Director. However, it is generally recommended that enucleation occur within six hours of death.

F. Eye Maintenance Prior to Enucleation

The corneal integrity should be maintained following the death of an eye donor or with the identification of a prospective donor. Lid closure upon death and the application of ice packs may limit epithelial deterioration. Sterile lubricating solution or drops may be instilled in prospective donor eyes prior to death. Instillation of antibiotic into eyes prior to enucleation is left to the discretion of the Medical Director.

V.   ENUCLEATION PROCEDURE

The interval between death and enucleation should be as short as possible. Ultimate responsibility for personnel to perform enucleation and enucleation technique rests with approval of the Medical Director and existing state law. A model for this is as follows:

A.   Preparation of Donor

The donor is prepped in the usual operating room manner using pHisoHex or Betadine, taking care not to allow these preparations to run into the eyes. The area is surgically draped with sterile towels.

B.   Equipment (All in Sterile Pack)

eye speculum
two small-toothed forceps
small scissors (iris scissors)
muscle hook(s)
hemostat
enucleating spoon
enucleating scissors, medium curve
sterile drapes
surgical gloves
Betadine prep swabs or sponges
sterile normal saline
gauze 2 × 2 squares
sterile pins
two sterile moist chambers
sterile saline

C.   Procedure

Examples:

1. Total Eye Enucleation

The speculum is used to hold the lids apart, and the conjunctival sac is vigorously irrigated with sterile saline to remove all foreign body debris. A peritomy of the conjunctiva is done as close to the limbus as possible. Tenon's capsule is pushed back by invading each of the four quadrants with the small scissors. The four rectus and two oblique muscles are successively looped with the muscle hook and cut close to the eye ball. The eye is then raised sufficiently, using the encleating spoon, to locate and cut the optic nerve with the encleating scissors. The eye is removed and placed immediately into the sterile moist chamber. The eye is secured in the chamber by inserting a pin through the optic nerve where it projects through the underside of the stainless steel cage. The eye is irrigated again with sterile saline or antibiotic solution. The cage rests on a cotton roll saturated with normal saline. The eye *is not* immersed in solution. Excess solution is decanted from the bottle. After the enucleation is completed, a ball of cotton or gauze pad is placed under the eyelid and the lid is closed. The bottle is placed in the provided styrofoam case. Ice should be placed in the plastic container prior to closing the styrofoam case. If a styrofoam case is not available, the glass bottles containing the eyes should be kept in a refrigerator at 4°C until collected by the Eye Bank.

Modification of this procedure or any similar procedure is the Medical Director's responsibility.

2. Corneal-Scleral Rim Removal Only

Removal of only the corneal-scleral rim requires rigid sterile technique employing all of the usual accepted standards—skin preparation, absolute instrument sterility, and scrubbing and glove care required in live patient surgery. The potential for endothelial cell damage, contamination, and infection are greatly increased and this procedure therefore should be performed by people specially trained in the retrieval of corneal-scleral segment.

VI. TISSUE EVALUATION

In those circumstances where donor eyes go directly to the surgeon, the surgeon assumes responsibility for quality control of the eye tissue.

As soon as possible after arrival at the Eye Bank laboratory the whole eye should be vigorously irrigated with sterile saline and immersed or irrigated with broad spectrum antibiotics. The eyes should then be stored at 4°C until further evaluated.

TISSUE EXAMINATION:

A. Gross Examination

The cornea is first examined grossly for clarity, epithelial defects, foreign objects, contamination, and scleral color (e.g., jaundice).

B. Slit-Lamp Examination

The cornea is examined for epithelial and stromal pathology and in particular endothelial disease. The following eye evaluation form is recommended for use:

	Present or Yes	Absent or No
1. Is there evidence of scleral jaundice?	____	____
2. Is the epithelium intact?	____	____
3. Are there stromal opacities?	____	____
4. Grade the amount of stromal edema?	1 2	3 4
5. Folds in Descemet's membrane?	____	____
6. Guttata?	____	____
7. Evidence of ocular surgery, (e.g., aphakia, pterygium)	____	____

C. Specular Microscopy

Eye Banks are encouraged to use other methods for examining donor corneal tissue. Specular microscopy data may add useful information.

D. Cultures

Culturing of Eye Bank donor eyes should be performed despite the recognition by many that bacteriologic contamination of donor eyes does not necessarily lead to infection. Cultures may be performed either presurgically or at the time of surgery.

1. Presurgical Cultures

A moistened cotton tip applicator should be rolled over the limbal area (before excision of the corneal scleral rim for media stored corneas) and before antibiotic drops are applied. The swab should then be placed into liquid microbiologic media and sent to the microbiology laboratory.

2. Surgical Culturing

Following excision or punching of the donor button, the corneal-scleral rim should be cultured in a liquid microbiologic culture media such as trypticase soy broth or its equivalent and delivered to the laboratory. The importance of laboratory communication with the surgeon is stressed so he may be informed at the first sign of growth and so that organism identification and antibiotic sensitivities can be performed.

VII. STORAGE

Any or all of the following methods of storage may be used by an Eye Bank:

A. Whole Refrigerated Eye at 4°C (Moist Chamber)

Recommended time of tissue utilization is prior to 48 hours or at the discretion of the Medical Director.

B. Nonviable Storage

The globe may be frozen in the freezer compartment or preserved utilizing glycerin for use in emergency or lamellar grafts.

C. Stored Media Preservation

D. Organ Culture

E. Cryopreservation

VIII. DISTRIBUTION OF TISSUE

Only Ophthalmologists licensed to practice in his or her state or country, and approved for performing corneal transplant surgery by the hospital chief of staff, chief of ophthalmology or appropriate hospital surgical section head may qualify to receive Eye Bank corneal tissue. Distribution of tissue is left to the individual Eye Bank at the discretion of the Medical Director. The system of distribution must be just, equitable and fair to all patients served by the Eye Bank. Any person failing to receive satisfaction with respect to the distribution of tissue from the local Eye Bank may appeal to the Standards Committee of the EBAA for review and action. Documentation (time and date of requests for, offers of and delivery of eye tissue) should be available for inspection by this Committee. Distribution of tissue shall be made without regard to sex, age, religion, race, creed, color or national origin.

IX. EYE BANK INSPECTION

The Medical Standards Committee of the EBAA shall be responsible for establishing inspection of member Eye Banks. All member banks shall have an inspection performed by June 30, 1981. Only those storage methods listed under Section VI practiced by the Eye Bank will be inspected and certified. New Eye Bank applications after Nov., 1980, will not be acted upon until all criteria established by this Committee are met and an inspection is satisfactorily completed. An Eye Bank which fails to comply with these standards shall be given one year to comply. A program of on site inspection will be implemented.

X. AMENDMENTS

These standards may be amended as required.

The Medical Standards Committee shall be charged with proposing amendments to these standards as new medical technology, techniques and information require.

The Committee shall draft proposals and submit them to the Board of Directors. All proposed amendments must be mailed to member Eye Banks and all Eye Bank Medical Directors and Legal Counsel at least 30 days before they become effective. If the amendment is deemed required for a medical emergency, then the amendment will become effective immediately.

XI. DATA COLLECTIONS AND FORMS

Information regarding the circumstances surrounding the death of the donor must be obtained by the Eye Bank so that the suitability of the tissue for transplantation may be judged. A sample eye screening donor form below is suggested:

Donor Screening Form

Donor's Name _____   Date of Death _____

Next of Kin _____   Time of Death _____

Address of Next of Kin _____   Time of Enucleation _____

_____   Enucleation Performed by: _____

Hospital Phone Number _____

	Yes or No	Information Unavailable
1. Was the patient on a life supporting respirator? If so, how long?	_____	_____
2. During hospitalization was there any suspicion of septicemia?	_____	_____
a. Any blood cultures drawn?	_____	_____
b. Positive blood cultures found?	_____	_____
c. Unexplained fever?	_____	_____
3. Were there sites of infection in the body, e.g.?	_____	_____
a. Burns	_____	_____
b. Tracheostomies	_____	_____
c. Abscess formation	_____	_____
d. Pneumonia	_____	_____
4. Was there any progressive neurologic disease, dementia or symptoms suggesting systemic disease of viral etiology?	_____	_____
a. Creutzfeldt-Jakob	_____	_____
b. Rabies	_____	_____
c. Reye's Syndrome	_____	_____
d. Subacute sclerosing panencephalitis	_____	_____
e. Progressive multifocal leukoencephalopathy	_____	_____
f. Others	_____	_____
5. Was there evidence of prior eye disease?	_____	_____
a. Eye surgery	_____	_____
b. Recent conjunctivitis	_____	_____
c. Glaucoma, uveitis	_____	_____
d. Intraocular tumors	_____	_____
e. Diabetic eye disease	_____	_____
f. Others	_____	_____
6. Any systemic diseases such as:		
a. Leukemia	_____	_____
b. Hepatitis	_____	_____
c. Syphilis	_____	_____
d. Lymphosarcoma	_____	_____
e. Diabetes	_____	_____

7. Was cause of death known? _____

8. The primary cause of death was? _____

9. Secondary causes of death were? _____

XII.   RECORD KEEPING

A standard form for retaining donor and recipient information is suggested:

Record Form

Eye Bank Number
Name of Eye Bank
Location of Eye Bank
Phone Number
Type (media stored or NP—Not preserved or whole eye)
Age of Donor
Cause of Death
Death Date and Time
Enucleation Date and Time
Slit Lamp Report
Preservation Date and Time
Specular Microscopy (if done)
Name of surgeon receiving tissue
Date, time and method of transportation

REFERENCES

1. The Cornea World Congress: Edited by John Harry King, Jr., M.D. and John W. McTigue, M.D., Butterworths Inc., p. 402, 1965.
2. The McCarey-Kaufman Corneal Eye Bank Technique: Booklet prepared by Bernard E. McCarey, Ph.D., Thomas E. Slappey, and Herbert E. Kaufman, M.D.
3. Penetrating Keratoplasty using 37°C Organ Cultured Cornea: Donald J. Doughman, John E. Harris, Mary K. Schmitt. Trans Amer Acad Ophthalmol and Otolaryngol 81:778–793, 1976.
4. Corneal Preservation: Edited by Joseph A. Capella, M. S., Henry F. Edelhauser, Ph.D., and Diane L. Van Horn, Ph.D., Charles C Thomas Publishing Co., Springfield, IL, p. 308, 1973.

Donor Material for Penetrating Keratoplasty: Long-Term Corneal Preservation in 37° C Organ Culture

26

DONALD J. DOUGHMAN, M.D.
JOHN E. HARRIS, Ph.D., M.D.

Since the early days of corneal transplantation, the standard method for interim storage of donor eyes has been to place the intact globe in a moist chamber at 4° C.[1] Although the exact time limits of endothelial viability at 4° C have never been determined, most surgeons prefer to use tissue stored in this manner within 24 to 48 hours postmortem.[2] Since there is a shortage of fresh tissue in most eye banks, this often means that emergency surgery must be performed when eyes become available, creating at minimum an inconvenience for the patient, the surgeon, and the hospital. At times donor eyes are not used because either the patient or the surgeon is unavailable. Any method that prolongs donor storage (i.e., prolongs donor cornea endothelial viability) and allows elective scheduling of surgery provides the obvious advantages of better patient preparation and improved utilization of donor eyes, hospital beds, and operating rooms. In addition, it ensures that the surgeon will be well rested and able to operate with experienced personnel.

HISTORICAL BACKGROUND

The use of media in which to store the cornea is not a new idea. In 1947 Burki immersed corneas in liquid paraffin at 3° to 6° C and obtained 43.5 per cent clear grafts after 3 days' storage.[3, 4] Using the same technique, Rycroft extended this to 10 days.[5] However, an unacceptable amount of endothelial damage occurred with this method and it was abandoned. Blood was used as a storage medium as early as 1911.[6] Stocker reported the use of corneas stored in autologous serum for as long as 101 hours and obtained as high as 77.3 per cent clear grafts.[7] Geeraets also reported the successful use of serum for short-term storage.[8] Other media used for corneal storage have included artificial aqueous humor for up to 7 days,[9] "nutrient" medium for 14 days,[10] and various saline solutions for up to 10 days.[11]

Tissue culture was initially used in 1936 as a test of viability of the various cell layers of the cornea.[12] Archer and Trevor-Roper suspended whole eyes in tissue culture medium and noted clear corneas after 96 hours' storage, but they did not report any transplants using these eyes.[13] Until 1973 the literature on tissue culture and the cornea described the former as a measure of viability or as a procedure in experimental pathology but not as a method of donor cornea storage.[14-16] For example, lamellar grafts using tissue-cultured donor corneas were used by Messier and Haufman in 1949 in their studies of experimental wound healing of corneal grafts.[17]

At the University of Minnesota we

have been using a long-term storage technique in which we place the donor cornea in tissue culture media at 37° C, thereby maintaining corneal architecture and cellular metabolism. We call this method organ culture since during culture the cornea maintains its normal five-layer architecture and each cell type maintains its histology. The cornea remains an "organ," justifying the term organ culture. In 1973 our laboratory reported histopathologic studies of organ-cultured human corneas, demonstrating maintenance of viability during organ culture.[18] Further ultrastructural, physiologic, and metabolic studies in our laboratory indicated that corneas remained viable during organ culture. We began using organ-cultured corneas for clinical transplantation in January of 1974.

LABORATORY STUDIES

Ultrastructural Studies

Using transmission and scanning electron microscopy, we reported mainte-

nance of normal endothelial ultrastructure for up to 35 days of organ culture.[19-21] We have seen intact endothelial ultrastructure in human corneas incubated 120 days (Fig. 26–1). Although reduced to four cell layers, epithelial ultrastructure is also maintained for at least 35 days of organ culture.[21, 22] Accumulation of glycogen in the epithelium is often seen after 11 days.[21] There is degeneration of central stromal keratocytes as well as stromal swelling to about twice normal thickness during organ culture.[21, 22]

Endothelial Wound Healing Studies

A dynamic process of endothelial repair occurs during organ-culture incubation. We have observed areas of endothelial cell destruction in paired human corneas. This increased with the length of storage under standard eye bank conditions (4° C moist chamber). In contrast, the endothelial layer was intact in fellow corneas stored at 4° C in a moist chamber for the same length of time and then

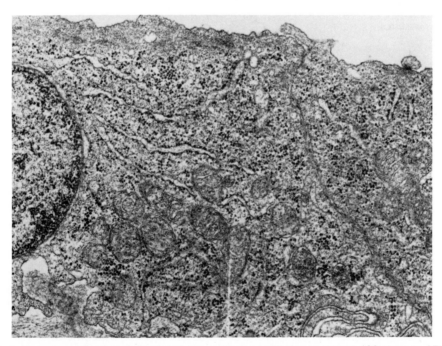

Figure 26–1. Human corneal endothelium from a 69-year-old donor stored 120 days in 37° C organ culture. Cells contain rough endoplasmic reticulum, abundant mitochondria, and ribosomes. Note normal nuclear and posterior plasma membranes. (× 20,510.) (From Doughman, D. J.: Prolonged donor cornea preservation in organ culture: Long term clinical evaluation. Trans Amer Ophthalmol Soc *78:*574, 1980.)

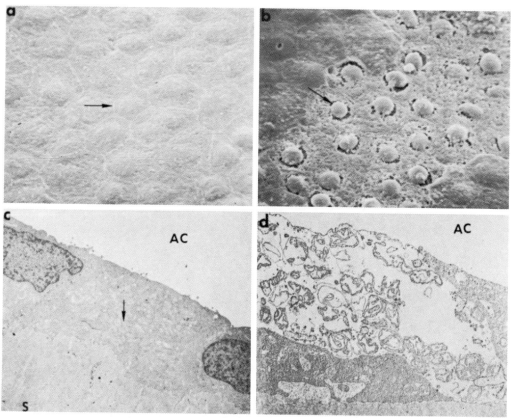

Figure 26–2. Human cornea 58 years old. Organ stored in moist chamber at 4° C for 24 hours prior to culture. *a,* Scanning electron micrograph of 21-day organ cultured cornea. Note flat irregular hexagonal cells 10 to 25 microns in diameter with well defined borders (arrow). (× 635.) *b,* Scanning electron micrograph of the moist chamber control. Note patch of lysed cells with rounded nuclei. *c,* Transmission electron micrograph of cornea in *a*. The endothelial cell layer is intact, 3 to 4 microns thick with mitochondria (arrow), endoplasmic reticulum, and ribosomes present. (AC = anterior chamber.) (× 3880.) *d,* Transmission electron micrograph of degenerating cells seen in *b*. (× 3800) (From Doughman, D. J., et al.: Endothelium of the organ cultured cornea: An electron microscopic study. Trans Amer Ophthalmol Soc *71*:313, 1973.)

placed in organ culture at 37° C for 10 to 21 days (Fig. 26–2).[19, 20] To confirm this observation we inflicted a central 4-mm. endothelial wound in human eye bank corneas and incubated these wounded corneas.[23] After as little as 24 hours of organ culture the wounded corneas demonstrated ultrastructurally intact endothelial cells at the margin of the wound, elongating and sliding toward the center of the wound (Fig. 26–3). All wounded corneas were completely covered by ultrastructurally intact and actively deturgescing endothelial cells after 7 days of organ culture, confirming that endothelial wound healing occurs during organ culture (Fig. 26–3).

Metabolic Studies

Since the cornea derives its energy from metabolism of glucose, we studied glucose metabolism by measuring the pH and glucose and lactate concentrations in the media after up to 35 days of organ culture.[21] When changing the medium twice a week, we found that the glucose concentrations fell from 110 to 30 mg./100 ml. and the lactic acid concentrations rose from 7 to 84 mg./100 ml. between changes. Because of these wide swings in glucose and lactate concentrations, we now change the medium three times a week. We have found that glucose metabolism is adequately maintained for the duration of the study (35

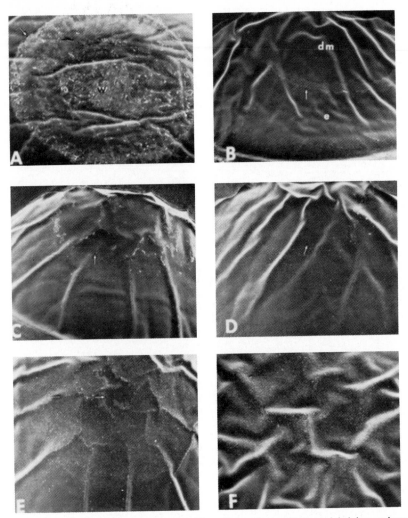

Figure 26–3. *A,* Circular endothelial wound (w). All cells in area of wound (w) have been destroyed. (× 20.) *B,* Wounded area after 24 hours' organ culture. Endothelial cells (e) outside area of wound are normal. Cells at the margin of wound (arrow) are degenerated cells. (dm = Descemet's membrane.) (× 20.) *C,* Endothelial wound after 24 hours' organ culture. Endothelial cells at margin of wound are moving centrally. Arrow indicates edge of migrating cells. (× 20.) *D,* Endothelial wound healing after 72 hours' organ culture. Arrow indicates leading edge of migrating cells advancing centrally as in *C.* (× 20). *E,* Endothelial wound after 4 days' organ culture. It is almost completely covered by endothelial cells. Arrow indicates small area of Descemet's membrane that remains uncovered (× 20). *F,* Completely healed wound after 7 days' organ culture. (× 20.) (From Doughman, D. J.: Prolonged donor cornea preservation in organ culture: Long term clinical evaluation. Trans Amer Ophthalmol Soc *78*:576, 1980.)

days). The pH remains stable at about 7.2, indicating adequate buffering of the medium even when lactic acid concentrations are elevated. We have also studied various lysosomal and cytoplasmic enzyme activities for up to 21 days in organ culture and have found no significant reduction in these enzyme activities.

Temperature Studies

In an attempt to find the ideal storage temperature for organ-cultured corneas, we compared 37° C with 4° C and with room temperature (24 to 27° C). We found that 4° C was associated with ultrastructural damage as early as 48 hours using minimal essential medium alone, minimal essential medium with 5 per cent Dextran, or McCarey-Kaufman (M-K) medium. However, human corneas can be left at room temperature in minimal essential medium for as long as 7 days without medium change and remain ultrastructurally and physiologically normal.[24] We have performed successful corneal transplants using corneas initially stored at 37° C and then reduced to room temperature for as long as 72 hours prior to transplantation. We have transported organ-cultured corneas to other surgeons in the United States under conditions in which the corneas remained at room temperature for up to 48 hours with successful results. Therefore, room temperature is well tolerated and allows transport of organ-cultured corneas without a special cooling or heating apparatus.

Immunologic Studies

Immunologic modification occurring after organ culture has been reported in a variety of other tissues,[25] such as lymphocytes[26] and thyroid allografts.[27] We have observed immunologic modification of experimental organ-cultured xenografts in rabbits.[28] Chicken and guinea pig xenograft reactions either were delayed or did not result in rejection after donor tissue was stored in organ culture for at least 3 weeks prior to transplantation. Storage in organ culture for less than 3 weeks did not result in modification of the response. Human-to-rabbit xenografts were not modified regardless of duration of storage in organ culture. Although the mechanism of this modification is not known, these data suggested that organ-cultured corneal xenograft modification is species-specific and dependent upon duration of incubation.

In an in vitro study of organ-cultured bovine corneas we demonstrated an absence after 3 weeks of strong antigenic proteins that are present in normal corneas.[29] Although this was due in part to loss of epithelium during incubation, the antigen was absent from the stroma as well, probably representing loss of soluble antigen.

Summary

Our laboratory investigation indicates that the human organ-cultured cornea maintains ultrastructural and metabolic integrity for at least 35 days at 37° C and 7 days at ambient room temperature. At 37° C the human organ-cultured cornea "heals" defects in the endothelial cell layer, probably as a result of the adjacent normal endothelial cells enlarging and sliding to cover defects left by the injured cells. Experimental chicken and guinea pig xenografts are prolonged after 3 weeks of organ culture, representing a form of immunologic modification.

CLINICAL STUDIES

Introduction

We have been using 37° C organ culture as a method of interim corneal storage for keratoplasty in humans since January, 1974, and have reported our results.[30, 31] Before discussing these results, we will review our method of organ-culture incubation with special emphasis on our procedure for sterility control to protect against bacterial or fungal contamination.

Method

After death the eyes should be cooled to 4° C as soon as possible. This can be accomplished by placing ice packs over the orbits. After enucleation, the eye is placed in a moist chamber at 4° C and flooded with gentamicin ophthalmic solution. The interval between death and placement of the cornea in organ culture should be 12 hours or less.

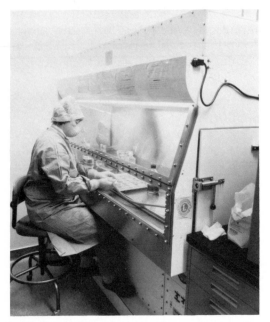

Figure 26–4. Technician working at laminar flow hood.

Table 26–1. ORGAN CULTURE MEDIA

Minimum essential media (Eagle's)
Earle's salts without L-glutamine
L-glutamine—1% final concentration
Decomplemented calf serum—10% final concentration
Penicillin 100 units/ml.
Amphotericin B 0.25% μg./ml.
Gentamicin 100 μg./ml.

utes. The cornea with a 2- to 3-mm. scleral rim is then carefully excised without loss of the anterior chamber.[32] Should the anterior chamber collapse, endothelial damage may occur owing to lens-iris diaphragm touch, and these corneas should not be used for transplantation. The cornea is placed epithelial side down in a sterile Falcon tissue culture dish containing fresh medium (see Table 26–1 for constituents of the medium) and incubated for 45 minutes at 37° C (Fig. 26–5). The cornea is then transferred into three separate washes of medium and gently dipped five times in each Petri dish, with medium completely covering both the scleral rim and the cornea. This dish is placed in the incubator (Fig. 26–6). We use a water-jacketed tissue culture incubator at 37° C and an atmosphere of 5 per cent CO_2, 95 per cent filtered air, and 100 per cent humidity. The medium is changed three times a week.

All organ-culture procedures, including preparation of the globe, preparation of the media, changing of the media, and so forth, are performed utilizing sterile technique in a vertical laminar flow hood by a technician wearing a face mask, cap, gown, and sterile gloves (Fig. 26–4). The globes are removed from the moist chamber and are immersed in 0.3 per cent gentamicin solution for 5 min-

Sterility Control

In a previously reported study of 230 eyes that were cultured upon receipt at our Eye Bank,[31] 152 (66 per cent) were contaminated with 176 organisms. Neosporin treatment (immersion of the globe for 3 minutes) sterilized only 36 per cent of eyes, whereas gentamicin sterilized 78 per cent. Although gentamicin was more effective in decontaminating donor eyes, it did not totally eliminate pathogenic microorganisms. *Pseudomonas aeruginosa* and *Proteus mirabilis* organisms were still present on a significant percentage of globes following gentamicin immersion. Four of the corneoscleral segments contaminated after the anti-

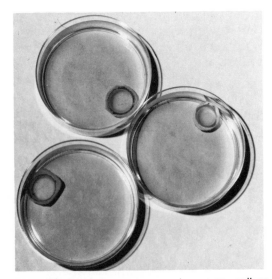

Figure 26–5. Human corneas in organ culture media.

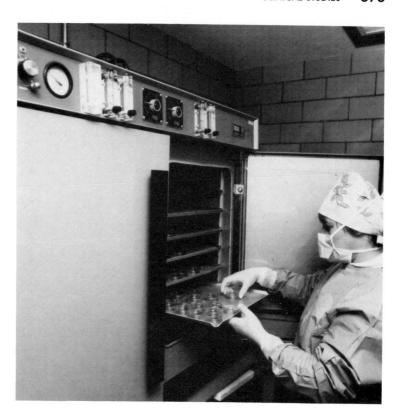

Figure 26–6. Technician placing tray of human corneas in incubator.

biotic immersion subsequently became contaminated with the same organism during organ culture in spite of the presence of penicillin, gentamicin, and amphotericin B in the culture medium. Presumably these organisms were carried over from the donor eye. There were seven additional cases of contamination with organisms not identified on the donor prior to organ culture. Presumably these cases represent environmental contamination or contamination by laboratory personnel. Thus, in this series of 230 eyes obtained from nonseptic donors 4.8 per cent became contaminated during prolonged organ-culture storage.

Therefore, since we began using organ-cultured donor corneas for clinical keratoplasty we have employed a terminal quarantine procedure to detect contaminated corneas. Initially we use a 2-day quarantine; that is, 48 hours prior to transplantation a final change of medium was performed. Samples of medium from that final change were then streaked on blood agar and Sabouraud's media, and the Petri dish with the donor cornea was closed until opened by the

surgeon at the time of surgery. If the diagnostic microbiologic media grew organisms or the Petri dish containing the donor cornea became turbid or there was a change in pH as evidenced by the phenol red indicator, the cornea was discarded. In January, 1976, we modified our routine by placing the corneas in M-K medium at the time of the terminal change and continued incubation at room temperature or 37° C for 48 more hours. This was done to thin the thickened organ-cultured donor corneas. Quarantine procedures were carried out as described above. However, the M-K medium contains no indicator, so turbidity of the M-K medium was the only check of the container holding the donor cornea. In all cases samples of the medium and the scleral rims were frozen for future recall after surgery.

In May, 1976, we transplanted an organ-cultured cornea to a 76-year-old diabetic female. The diagnostic microbiologic media showed no growth, and the M-K medium containing the donor cornea appeared clear. The postoperative course was complicated by smoldering

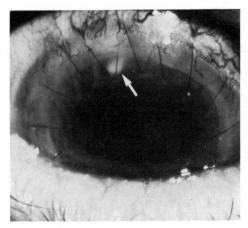

Figure 26–7. Round, white fluffy mass (arrow) on endothelium at host-graft junction 2 months postoperatively. Anterior chamber tap showed *Torulopsis glabrata*. (From Doughman, D. J.: Prolonged donor cornea preservation in organ culture: Long term clinical evaluation. Trans Amer Ophthalmol Soc *78*:605, 1980.)

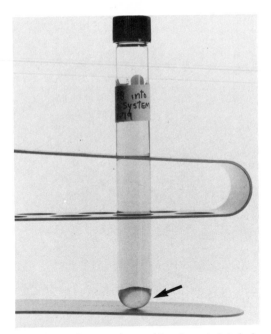

Figure 26–8. Cornea (arrow) in closed vial during terminal sterility check.

inflammation. Two months postoperatively a fluff-ball mass was noted on the posterior cornea at 12 o'clock (Fig. 26–7). An aqueous tap revealed abundant growth of *Torulopsis glabrata*. The frozen donor rim and the medium were then cultured in Sabouraud's medium, and this also revealed abundant growth of *Torulopsis glabrata*. (We have reported the details of this case.[33]). We stopped using organ-cultured donor corneas and closely observed other patients who had organ-culture transplants for signs of infection. None occurred. Random sterility checks of frozen donor rims and medium from other organ-cultured corneal cases showed no evidence of contamination.

After a 3-month moratorium organ-cultured donor corneas were again used. However, because of this one case of fungal endophthalmitis, we changed our terminal quarantine procedure. Based upon Lindstrom's findings that organ-cultured corneas remain metabolically active and intact in a closed system (i.e., no medium changes) for 14 days at 24° C and 10 days at 37° C,[24] we now place the donor cornea in 60 ml. of medium without antibiotic or amphotericin B in a closed system at 37° C for 14 days prior to surgery (Fig. 26–8). In addition, at least one medium change prior to terminal storage the antibiotics and amphotericin B are removed from the medium to avoid antibiotic carryover that could inhibit microbial growth and mask contamination. Samples from the last medium change as well as 10 ml. of medium from the terminal medium are placed on solid and liquid media for detection of anaerobic and aerobic bacteria as well as of fungi and yeast by the diagnostic microbiologic laboratories at the University of Minnesota Hospitals. If any of the diagnostic media show growth of organisms or if the medium in which the donor cornea is placed shows evidence of turbidity or change in pH, the donor cornea is discarded. We feel that this scrutiny in the terminal quarantine procedure should assure as sterile tissue as possible for transplantation. Because of the risk of microbial contamination, we no longer recommend final transfer of the cornea to M-K medium in order to thin the tissue prior to transplantation.

Clinical Results

From May 20, 1974, to July 30, 1979, the senior author performed 124 penetrating keratoplasties in 116 patients using donor corneas stored by the 37° C organ-culture method. Ten patients were lost to follow-up or died and were removed from the series, leaving 114 penetrating keratoplasties in 104 patients. These were not consecutive cases. Because of the 3-month moratorium placed on organ-cultured grafts following the case of *Torulopsis glabrata* endophthalmitis, only 4° C refrigeration (four cases) or M-K medium (13 cases) stored corneas were used during that time. In addition, five M-K–stored corneas were used during this 5-year period when operating room time became available within 24 to 48 hours, a time too short for the terminal sterility check procedure needed to use organ-cultured corneas. With these exceptions, the 114 grafts were consecutive, not selected, cases.

Standard microsurgical technique was employed, using 10-0 monofilament nylon running or interrupted sutures. Donor epithelium that remained after culture was left in place. Postoperatively all patients received topical steroids, antibiotics, and cycloplegics. When indicated, systemic steroids were also given. Suture removal was performed when the vessels reached the edge of the graft, when the sutures loosened, or when wound healing appeared complete as judged by the density of the surgical scar.

Diagnoses of recipients are listed in Tables 26–2 and 26–3. All recipients

Table 26–2. ORGAN-CULTURED CORNEAL TRANSPLANTS: SUCCESSFUL RECIPIENT DATA

Preoperative Diagnosis	Prognosis*		
	Favorable	*Intermediate*	*Unfavorable*
Keratoconus			
Uncomplicated	18		
Vascularized recipient cornea		1	
Regraft: irregular astigmatism		1	
Aphakic bullous keratopathy			
Uncomplicated	17		
Failed graft, etiology unknown		1	
Thick with band keratopathy		1	
3 immune rejections in fellow eye		1	
Fuchs' dystrophy			
Localized	5		
Generalized		14	
Generalized with dry eye			1
Pseudophakos bullous keratopathy			
Intraocular lens removed		3	
Intraocular lens retained or replaced		3	
Herpes simplex keratitis			
Active thinning or perforated			3
Inactive scar	4		
Failed keratoplasty			
Immune rejection			2
Persistent epithelial defect		1	
Etiology unknown		1	
Familial dystrophy	7		
Leukoma			
Thin—vascularized cornea			2
Traumatic—scarred and vascularized		2	
Miscellaneous			
Fungal ulcer, healed and quiet	1		
Corneal cyst	1		
Neuroparalytic keratitis			1
Chemical burn			1
Total	53	29	10
	(58%)	(31%)	(11%)

*Polack's classification.[34]

Table 26–3. ORGAN-CULTURED CORNEAL TRANSPLANTS: FAILED RECIPIENT DATA

Preoperative Diagnosis	Prognosis*		
	Favorable	Intermediate	Unfavorable
Aphakic bullous keratopathy			
Generalized		5	
Postoperative silicone replacement of vitreous with corneal touch			1
Shallow anterior chamber, 2 prior penetrating keratoplasties			1
Chemical burn			2
Previous immune rejection			5
Leukoma			
Traumatic with shallow anterior chamber			2
Anterior cleavage syndrome			1
Herpes simplex			
Perforation			1
Vascularized cornea		2	
Radiation keratitis			1
Epithelial downgrowth			1
Total	0	7 (32%)	15 (68%)

*Polack's classification.[34]

were assigned to a prognostic group according to Polack's classification.[34] All patients were seen by the author or by another ophthalmologist with a follow-up time of not less than 6 months. Donor data are shown in Table 26–4. The time interval between death of the donor and placement of the corneoscleral segment into organ culture has been divided into enucleation time (e.g., time from death of donor to enucleation) and postenucleation time (i.e., time between enucleation and placement in organ culture). All donor corneas came from eyes donated to the eye bank and were removed by resident ophthalmologists or trained morticians.

In this series of 114 penetrating keratoplasties donor corneas were stored by organ-culture incubation at 37° C for an average of 16.5 days with a range from 3 to 35 days (Table 26–4). Of the 114 transplants, 92 (81 per cent) remain clear and 22 (19 per cent) have failed. There is a statistically significant difference in the length of follow-up time; the successful group was followed for an average of 28.8 months and the failed group for an average of 40.5 months. All unsuccessful grafts were clear for at least 4 weeks before failing. Therefore, in this series, no cases of primary graft failure occurred.

Donor age, enucleation time, postenucleation time, and duration of organ-culture storage did not differ between the successful and the unsuccessful grafts, which indicates that in this study these factors were not important to the success of penetrating keratoplasty. Of the 92 clear grafts, 53 (58 per cent) were in a favorable, 29 (31 per cent) were in an intermediate, and 10 (11 per cent) were in an unfavorable preoperative prognostic category (Table 26–2). Of the 22 failed grafts, 15 (68 per cent) were thought to have an unfavorable prognosis, whereas an intermediate prognosis comprised 7 (32 per cent) of the failed grafts (Table 26–3). There were no favorable prognosis cases in the failed group.

Specular microscopic examination showed a mean endothelial cell count of 1,598 cells per mm.[2] (Fig. 26–9). This is almost identical to the mean cell count of 1,548 cells per mm.[2] found by Bourne and coworkers in an earlier study of 14 organ-cultured transplants,[35] and it compares favorably with the results of other studies of transplanted corneas stored by M-K, cryopreservation, or 4° C refrigeration.[36] These findings support the conclusion that the endothelium of organ-cultured corneas survives storage and transplantation and

Table 26–4. ORGAN-CULTURED CORNEAL TRANSPLANTS: DONOR CORNEA DATA

	Total Series (N=114)			Successful (N=92)			Failed (N=22)		
	Average	SD	Range	Average	SD	Range	Average	SD	Range
Duration in organ culture (days)	16.5	6.5	3–35	16.5	5.8	3–29	16.6	8.9	3–35
Donor age (yr.)	35.3	17.7	5–71	35.4	17.1	5–68	32.4	20.9	5–71
Enucleation time (hr.)	3.8	3.8	1–26	3.5	3.8	1–20	4.9	4.1	1–26
Postenucleation time (hr.)	6.4	5.0	0–24	6.2	4.5	0–24	7.4	6.6	0–16
Follow-up time (mo.)	31.0	19.0	6–63	28.8	18.8	6–62	40.5	17.6	6–63

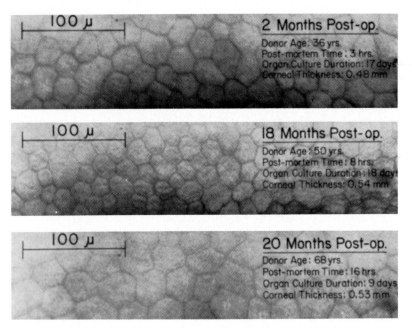

Figure 26–9. Central corneal endothelium of three clear organ-cultured grafts as photographed with a clinical specular microscope. (Courtesy of William M. Bourne, M.D. From Doughman, D. J.: Prolonged donor cornea preservation in organ culture: Long term clinical evaluation. Trans Amer Ophthalmol Soc 78:605, 1980.)

maintains endothelial cell density postoperatively as well as that of corneas preserved by other methods.

Immune rejection was the leading cause (8 cases [36 per cent]) of graft rejection (Table 26–5). An additional 25 cases of reversed immune rejection occurred. The diagnosis of immune rejection was made when the sudden onset of inflammatory signs (aqueous cells, flare, ciliary flush) appeared at least 3 weeks postoperatively in a previously quiet eye with a clear graft and no other cause of inflammation could be identified. Based upon the best comparative estimates we are able to make with published series of corneal grafts using donor material stored by other methods, it appears that organ-culture storage fails

to modify immune graft rejection. Certainly organ-culture storage of donor cornea does not provide absolute protection from immune graft rejection.

Donor corneas stored by the organ-culture technique swell considerably. They can be used directly, but the surgeon must deal with a thick donor that is stained pink by the phenol red indicator (Fig. 26–10). Suturing is not a problem, nor do the sutures loosen as the graft thins, but visualization of the anterior chamber is impeded. The donor cornea loses its pink color within 24 hours. Phakic grafts are usually thin by 48 hours postoperatively, but aphakic grafts remain thick for a much longer interval. By the second postoperative week, however, the clarity and thickness of phakic and aphakic grafts are the same (Fig. 26–11). Placement of organ-cultured donor corneas in M-K medium 16 hours prior to surgery causes the donor tissue to thin considerably and improves visualization of the anterior chamber during surgery. Postoperatively phakic grafts are thin and clear within 24 to 48 hours, but there is still a delay in the deturgescence of aphakic grafts. Phakic transplants are thinner than

Table 26–5. ORGAN-CULTURED CORNEA: CAUSES OF FAILED KERATOPLASTIES

Cause	Number (Per Cent)
Immune rejection	8 (36.4)
Uncontrolled glaucoma	6 (27.3)
Persistent epithelial defect	3 (13.6)
Wound separation	2 (9.0)
Postoperative retinal detachment	1 (4.5)
Epithelial downgrowth	1 (4.5)
Unknown	1 (4.5)

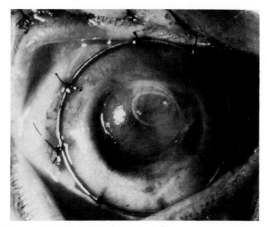

Figure 26–10. Thick organ-cultured donor corneal button (arrow) in recipient bed at time of transplantation.

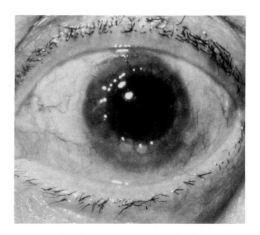

Figure 26–11. Same cornea as in Figure 26–10 2 weeks after operation. Corneal thickness is 0.62. Cornea is clear.

aphakic transplants for the first 4 postoperative months.

The postoperative complications encountered with 37° C organ-cultured donor material are similar to those reported using donor material stored by other methods except for the suspicion that organ-cultured donors may yield a higher incidence of wound separation (Table 26–6).

SUMMARY

Organ culture at 37° C is a complicated and expensive method of donor cornea storage requiring a well-trained technician and a microbiology laboratory staff experienced in sterility check procedures. The major advantage of this system is the long-term storage it makes possible. Our experience demonstrates that it is an efficacious method of long-term donor corneal storage prior to penetrating keratoplasty and that it is safe when used with the appropriate personnel and safeguards. Results to date using organ-cultured stored corneal material are as good as those obtained with corneas stored by 4° C moist-chamber refrigeration, in M-K medium, or by cryopreservation.

Table 26–6. ORGAN-CULTURED CORNEA: POSTOPERATIVE COMPLICATIONS

Type	Number	Per Cent
Glaucoma	39/114	34.2
Aphakic	35/39	89.7
Phakic	4/39	10.3
Immune rejection	33/114	28.9
Synechia to graft	24/114	21.1
Successful	18/92	19.6
Failed	6/22	27.3
Immune reaction	7/31	22.6
Aphakic grafts	20/70	28.6
Phakic grafts	4/42	9.5
Cataract	5/42*	11.9
Wound separation	11/114	9.6
Epithelial defect	10/114	8.8
Infections	6/114	5.3
Herpes simplex	4/10†	40.0
Stitch abscess	2/114	1.8
Endophthalmitis	1/114	0.9

*Total phakic cases.
†Total herpes simplex cases.

REFERENCES

1. Stocker, F. W.: The endothelium of the cornea and its clinical implications. Trans Amer Ophthalmol Soc 51:669, 1953.
2. Hassard, D. T. R.: Selection of donor material for corneal grafting. In King, J. H., Jr., and McTigue, J. W. (eds.): *The Cornea: World Congress.* London, Butterworth, 1965, pp. 370–383.
3. Burki, E.: Über ein neues Verfahren zur Konservierung von Hornhautgewebe. Ophthalmologica (Basel) 114:233, 1947.
4. Burki, E.: Weitere Ergebnisse zur Keratoplastik mit Paraffin-Material. Ophthalmologica (Basel) 115:241, 1948.
5. Rycroft, B. W.: The corneal grafting act. Brit J Ophthalmol 37:549, 1953.
6. Magitot, A.: Recherches experimentales sur la survie impossible de la cornée en dehors de l'organisme et sur la keratoplastic différée. Ann Oculist (Paris) 146:1, 1911.
7. Stocker, F. W.: Preservation of donor cornea in autologous serum. Amer J Ophthalmol 60:21, 1965.
8. Geeraets, W. J., Lederman, I. R., Woo, H., and Guerry, D.: In vivo corneal graft reaction after short term storage. Amer J Ophthalmol 60:28, 1965.
9. Kuwabara, T.: Studies of heterokeratoplasty. Jpn J Ophthalmol 5:243, 1961.
10. Sachs, A.: A new medium for storage of donor eyes for corneal grafts. Brit J Ophthalmol 41:558, 1957.
11. Pakarinen, P.: Preservation of the cornea for penetrating keratoplasty. Acta Ophthalmol 106 (Suppl):9, 1969.
12. Fjordbotten, A. L.: Preservation of the cornea by dehydration. In King, J. H., Jr., and McTigue, J. W. (eds.): *The Cornea: World Congress.* London, Butterworth, 1965, p. 398.
13. Archer, C. B., and Trevor-Roper, P. D.: Organization and administration of Westminster Moorfield's Eye Bank. Brit J Ophthalmol 51:1, 1967.
14. Smith, A. U.: The problems of prolonged storage of rabbit cornea at low temperature. In King, J. H., Jr., and McTigue, J. W. (eds.): *The Cornea: World Congress.* London, Butterworth, 1965, p. 384.
15. O'Neill, P.: The measurement of viability. In Casey, T. A. (ed.): *Corneal Grafting.* London, Butterworth, 1972, p. 81.
16. Kuming, B. S.: The assessment of endothelial viability. S Afr Med J 43:1083, 1969.
17. Messier, T. E., and Haufman, R. F.: Mechanisms of corneal graft healing. Arch Ophthalmol 42:148, 1949.
18. Summerlin, W. T., Miller, G. E., Harris, J. E., and Good, R. A.: The organ cultured cornea: An in vitro study. Invest Ophthalmol 12:176, 1973.
19. Doughman, D. J., Van Horn, D. L., Harris, J. E., Miller, G. E., Lindstrom, R. L., and Good, R. A.: The ultrastructure of human organ cultured cornea. I. Endothelium. Arch Ophthalmol 92:516, 1974.
20. Doughman, D. J., Van Horn, D. L., Harris, J. E., Miller, G. E., Lindstrom, R. L., Summerlin, W., and Good, R. A.: Endothelium of the organ cultured cornea: An electron microscopic study. Trans Amer Ophthalmol Soc 71:304, 1973.
21. Lindstrom, R. L., Doughman, D. J., Van Horn, D. L., Dancil, D., and Harris, J. E.: A metabolic and electron microscopic study of human organ-cultured cornea. Amer J Ophthalmol 82:72, 1976.
22. Van Horn, D. L., Doughman, D. J., Harris, J. E., Miller, G. E., Lindstrom, R. L., and Good, R. A.: The ultrastructure of human organ cultured cornea. II. Stroma and epithelium. Arch Ophthalmol 93:275, 1975.
23. Doughman, D. J., Van Horn, D. L., Rodman, W., Byrnes, P., and Lindstrom, R. L.: Human corneal endothelial layer repair during organ culture. Arch Ophthalmol 94:1791, 1976.
24. Lindstrom, R. L., Doughman, D. J., Van Horn, D. L., Schmitt, M. K., and Byrnes, P.: Organ culture corneal storage at ambient room temperature. Arch Ophthalmol 95:869, 1977.
25. Jacobs, B. D., and Uphoff, D. E.: Immunologic modification: A basic survival mechanism. Science 185:582, 1974.
26. Opelz, G., and Terasaki, P. I.: Lymphocyte antigenicity loss with retention of responsiveness. Science 184:464, 1974.
27. Lafferty, K. J., Cooley, M. A., Woolnough, J., and Walker, K. Z.: Thyroid allograft immunogenicity is reduced after a period in organ culture. Science 188:259, 1975.
28. Doughman, D. J., Miller, G. E., Mindrup, E. A., Schmitt, M. K., Harris, J. E., and Good, R. A.: The fate of experimental organ cultured corneal xenografts. Transplantation 22:132, 1976.
29. Hall, J. M., Smolin, G., Doughman, D. J., and Krasnobrod, H.: Changes in the antigenic composition of cultured bovine corneas. Invest Ophthalmol 14:295, 1975.
30. Doughman, D. J., Harris, J. E., and Schmitt, M. K.: Penetrating keratoplasty using 37° C organ cultured corneas. Trans Amer Acad Ophthalmol Otolaryngol 81:OP788, 1976.
31. Doughman, D. J.: Prolonged donor cornea preservation in organ culture: Long term clinical evaluation. Trans Amer Ophthalmol Soc 78:567, 1980.
32. McCarey, B. E.: Corneal storage and handling. In Kaufman, H. E., and Zimmerman, T. (eds.): *Current Concepts in Ophthalmology.* Vol. 5. St. Louis, C. V. Mosby Co., 1976, p. 156.
33. Larson, P. A., Lindstrom, R. L., and Doughman, D. J.: *Torulopsis glabrata* endophthalmitis after keratoplasty with an organ cultured cornea. Arch Ophthalmol 96:1019, 1978.
34. Polack, F. M.: *Corneal Transplantation.* New York, Grune & Stratton, 1977, pp. 153–175.
35. Bourne, W. M., Doughman, D. J., and Lindstrom, R. L.: Organ cultured corneal endothelium in vivo. Arch Ophthalmol 95:1818, 1977.
36. Bourne, W., and Kaufman, H. E.: The endothelium of clear corneal transplants. Arch Ophthalmol 94:1730, 1976.

Donor Material for Penetrating Keratoplasty: Long-Term Cryopreservation

27

RICHARD S. SMITH, M.D.
LINDA A. SMITH, B.A.

The first successful cryopreserved corneal graft was reported in 1954,[1] but the results of a large series of cases were not published until 1966.[2] Using ideas suggested by earlier corneal workers and information from other areas of tissue banking, Kaufman and Capella developed the principles of the corneal cryopreservation technique described in this chapter.[3, 4] In clinical studies[5-7] Kaufman and others went on to prove that the surgical results obtained with cryopreserved material were equivalent to those achieved with fresh eye bank tissue. Morphologic and functional viability of cryopreserved tissue was demonstrated by histochemical, ultrastructural, and physiologic studies[8-17] as well as by the observation in humans of clear grafts achieved by this technique.

Although some eye banks have an abundance of donor tissue, others suffer from chronic shortages. Under the latter circumstance optimum utilization of tissue is essential. Corneal cryopreservation allows all suitable tissue to be used for transplantation, largely eliminating the problems arising from the requirement that the patient and the physician be available on short notice. It permits surgical scheduling at the convenience of the patient and the operative team, thereby optimizing the conditions of surgery. The constant availability of excellent quality donor tissue is an additional advantage in dealing with corneal trauma, corneal perforations, and other emergency situations. Rarely can comparable availability of donor material be assured by short-term preservation techniques.

Corneal cryopreservation is a safe and effective eye bank method with a number of advantages and some disadvantages. In addition to providing constant availability of donor tissue, the most important advantage of this technique lies in the degree of bacteriologic control it allows. When donor material stored by the moist-chamber technique or in a modified tissue-culture medium is used, transplantation surgery often is performed before the results of microbiologic studies are available. Although antibiotics are applied to the donor eye and are added to intermediate-term storage media, they do not guarantee sterility of the donor corneas, and occasionally the outcome is tragic.[18, 19] This is dramatically illustrated by the following case. Prior to our use of cryopreservation, a seemingly perfect pair of eyes from an 18-year-old accident victim were removed less than 1 hour after death. Both corneas were used within 6 hours of enucleation and both recipients developed an antibiotic-resistant streptococcal endophthalmitis. The two recipient eyes were lost.

The ability to perform careful bacteriologic screening on donor tissue that is cryopreserved is of inestimable value. Our eye bank recently received a pair of eyes similar to those described above from a 17-year-old donor. The eyes were enucleated and the corneas cryopre-

583

served. A heavy growth of coagulase-positive *Staphylococcus aureus* was identified in the culture taken from the limbus prior to removal of the corneas from the enucleated globes, and the tissue was discarded. The absence of urgency for use of the donor tissue provided by the cryopreservation technique may well have averted a recurrence of the earlier tragedy.

Despite its advantages, cryopreservation has not been widely used in recent years. Where donor material is abundant, its storage for 48 to 72 hours often is satisfactory. Although this has undoubtedly contributed to the lack of popularity of the cryopreservation technique, it is likely that its complexity is an even more significant cause of the failure of the technique to be adopted universally. Corneal cryopreservation is a complicated procedure that requires considerably more time per donor eye than moist-chamber storage or storage in modified tissue culture medium. Expensive equipment is needed and highly trained technical personnel must be available 24 hours a day. The potential for serious error, which renders the tissue unsuitable for transplantation, is great, and the error may not be recognized prior to surgery. There is no routine procedure for assessing the viability of the donor cornea immediately prior to its use.

TECHNIQUE

From the beginning Kaufman stressed that scrupulous adherence to technique was important. Small procedural variations may produce large changes in tissue quality. As an example, a few years ago glass vials of the depth and diameter used by Capella ceased to be commercially available. The closest substitute produced an altered freezing curve, which necessitated recalibration of the

rate freezer. As important as the method used is the availability of an intellectually honest, reliable, and careful technician who removes and freezes the corneas. This person must understand that *any* break in technique mandates that the cornea be discarded. Factors that disqualify a cornea will be discussed in subsequent paragraphs.

When living tissue is frozen in uncontrolled fashion, large ice crystals form within the cell and cell membranes are disrupted, resulting in cellular death. These events are avoided in successful cryopreservation by several techniques. Removal of water prior to freezing reduces the free water available for crystal formation. This is accomplished by dehydrating the corneas in a series of solutions of increasing concentrations of dimethyl sulfoxide (DMSO) and sucrose at 4° C (Table 27–1).

The DMSO acts as a membrane stabilizer. During the freezing process ice crystals form as the solution passes through its freezing point. The rate freezer controls the temperature drop at this crucial point and minimizes ice crystal formation. Since small alterations in technique are important, the paragraphs that follow detail the steps taken in our eye bank. This technique is similar to that originally described by Kaufman and Capella.[4]

Preparation of Solutions

Four consecutively numbered 50-ml. multidose bottles each containing the appropriate amount of sucrose for solutions 1 to 4 are covered with aluminum foil and sterilized for 10 minutes at 350° F in a hot air oven along with rubber stoppers, metal sealant caps, and a small glass beaker. After cooling, the rubber stoppers and metal caps are clamped onto the bottles and the appropriate amount of salt-poor human albu-

Table 27–1. SOLUTIONS FOR CORNEAL DEHYDRATION

	Solution 1	Solution 2	Solution 3	Solution 4
Albumin	39.2 ml.	38.4 ml.	37.6 ml.	37.0 ml.
DMSO	0.8 ml.	1.6 ml.	2.4 ml.	3.0 ml.
Sucrose	1.0 g.	2.0 g.	3.0 g.	4.0 g.

min (available through the American Red Cross) is added. These bottles are chilled overnight in the refrigerator. On the following day the DMSO is sterilized by filtration through a Nalgene filter unit with a 0.45-micron grid membrane (catalog number 245) and then decanted into a sterile glass beaker. Regular Millipore filters are not suitable since they are dissolved by the DMSO. The appropriate amount of DMSO is then added drop by drop, with constant agitation, to each bottle. If the DMSO is added too rapidly, it precipitates and denatures the albumin. Each time a cornea is preserved, a small amount of each of the four solutions is cultured. After 3 to 4 months any remaining solution is discarded as a safeguard against contamination due to multiple insertions of a 19-gauge needle to withdraw the solutions.

Removal of Corneas

While still in the eye bank bottle, the globes are irrigated with Neosporin solution applied every 30 seconds for 10 minutes. After irrigation the limbal area is swabbed and cultured. To avoid epithelial damage, the cornea is not touched. While the eyes are irrigated with antibiotics, a sterile field is arranged with drapes, instruments, and sutures. The technician then dons sterile gloves and removes the globes from the eye bank container using sterile forceps. Each globe is placed on a separate piece of sterile gauze and partially wrapped in the gauze to facilitate handling. Neosporin irrigation continues every minute until the actual removal of the cornea and scleral rim from the globe.

Using a sterile knife, an incision is made through the sclera 3 mm. behind the limbus to the level of the lamina fusca. A 6-0 silk suture is passed through the edge of the scleral rim for ease in handling. Using ball-tipped, angled scissors, this incision is extended for a full 360°. While traction is exerted with the suture and the uvea is depressed with a blunt instrument, the cornea and scleral rim are detached from the globe. This must be done with great care to avoid

collapse of the anterior chamber with resultant iris-endothelial touch. If this occurs, the cornea is discarded. All of the above steps are performed in a laminar air flow hood.

The isolated cornea is then placed in a sterile glass vial (19 by 48 mm., Kimble Company) and 2.0 ml. of solution 1 are added. Care is taken not to squirt the solution onto the endothelial surface. The corneas in their respective vials are then placed in a covered tray and kept in a 4° C refrigerator for 10 minutes between each of the solution changes. The portion of the suture that lies outside the vial is considered unsterile, and care is taken not to allow the unsterile portion to contaminate the inner wall of the sterile vial. Once the corneas are placed in their individual vials, they are not removed and placed in new vials for solution changes. To minimize manipulation of the tissue, the solutions are decanted after each 10-minute interval, and the next fresh solution is placed in the vials by the technique described above.

Freezing of Corneas

While the corneas are in solution 2, the rate freezer is filled with liquid nitrogen. When the corneas reach solution 4 (only 1.5 ml. of solution 4 is used to match the amount in the control vial), the temperature probes are placed in the rate freezer for precooling with the lid closed. While the tissue is in solution 4, a control vial containing 1.5-ml. of solution 4 is also chilled at 4° C for 10 minutes.

When ready for freezing, the corneas in solution 4 are placed in the rate freezer in a clean screw-cap plastic vial 7/8 by 2 1/2 in., 20-ml. capacity (Lermer Packing Corp.) adjacent to the control vial. The temperature probes are placed in the control vial, the lid is closed, and freezing ensues. The freezing curve (Fig. 27–1) is monitored to be certain that the rate of freezing follows the proper calibrated curve. If this does not occur, the corneas are discarded. When the freezing process has gone to completion at −80° C, the frozen vials are removed

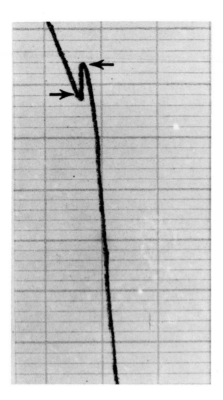

Figure 27–1. Temperature curve recorded during corneal freezing. The start of the curve is at 4° C. The end of the curve is approximately −80° C. The arrows indicate the phase change that occurs as freezing of the tissue takes place.

Figure 27–2. A, Postoperative appearance of a successful corneal graft using a cryopreserved donor cornea. B, Specular photomicrograph illustrating the endothelial morphology of a successful graft from a cryopreserved donor eleven years after surgery.

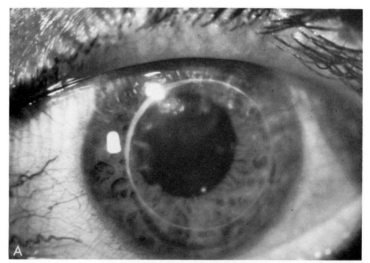

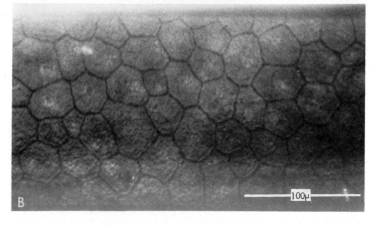

from the rate freezer and are placed in the liquid nitrogen holding tank.

Thawing of Corneas

Thawing is as critical as freezing if thermal damage to the preserved cornea is to be avoided. In the operating room the cornea is removed from the liquid nitrogen transport container and the screw-top plastic vial is thawed in a 60° C water bath for exactly 50 seconds. When the cornea is removed from the water bath, an ice ball remains on the endothelial surface. This is allowed to melt at room temperature, which occurs within 15 to 30 seconds. Care must be taken not to agitate the container or the endothelium will be damaged by the ice ball. When thawing is complete, solution 4 is decanted and a portion is reserved for bacteriologic studies. Fresh, chilled, salt-poor human albumin is added (2 ml.), again with care taken not to damage the endothelium. The technician brings the thawed cornea to the surgeon, grasps the unsterile portion of the suture, and brings the preserved cornea to the upper portion of the glass vial. This enables the surgeon to grasp a sterile portion of the suture with sterile forceps, cut off the unsterile portion of the suture, and transfer the cornea to a sterile work area for trephining. After the corneal button is cut, a portion of the sclerocorneal rim also is cultured.

It must be re-emphasized that any break in technique requires that the cornea in question be discarded. Of particular importance are the following: (1) inadvertent breaks in sterile technique, (2) loss of the anterior chamber with iris-endothelial touch, (3) improper freezing curve, and (4) incorrect thawing. With careful attention to technique, we rarely find it necessary to discard a cornea.

This technique provides corneas that, in our opinion, are equal to those preserved by short-term techniques and superior to fresh tissue (Fig. 27–2). In 7 years of using cryopreservation, we have had no primary donor failures attributable to the technique and no postoperative infections. Although cryopreservation requires a larger initial investment and careful attention to technique, it offers important advantages in the bacteriologic control of donor tissue that are superior to other techniques. In addition, the maximum utilization of donor material in areas where corneas are in short supply is an important consideration.

REFERENCES

1. Eastcott, H. H. G., Cross, A. G., Leigh, A. G., and North, D. P.: Preservation of corneal grafts by freezing. Lancet 1:237, 1954.
2. Kaufman, H. E., Escapini, H., Capella, J. A., Robbins, J. E., and Kaplan, M.: Living preserved corneal tissue for penetrating keratoplasty: Clinical trial. Arch Ophthalmol 76:471, 1966.
3. Capella, J. A., Kaufman, H. E., and Robbins, J. E.: Preservation of viable corneal tissue. Arch Ophthalmol 74:669, 1965.
4. Kaufman, H. E., and Capella, J. A.: Preserved corneal tissue for transplantation. J Cryosurg 1:125, 1968.
5. Aquavella, J. V.: Cryopreserved tissue in corneal transplantation. Sight Sav Rev 42:151, 1972.
6. Capella, J. A., Kaufman, H. E., and Polack, F. M.: Prognosis of keratoplasty in phakic and aphakic patients and use of cryopreserved donor tissue. Trans Amer Acad Ophthalmol Otolaryngol 76:1275, 1972.
7. Mathieu, M.: Further results obtained with cryopreserved corneas. In Capella, J. A., Edelhauser, H. F., and Van Horn, D. L. (eds.): Corneal Preservation. Springfield, Ill., Charles C Thomas, 1973, pp. 172–178.
8. Keates, R. H.: Results of evaluation of cryopreserved corneal tissue with trypan blue. In Capella, J. A., Edelhauser, H. F., and Van Horn, D. L. (eds.): Corneal Preservation. Springfield, Ill., Charles C Thomas, 1973, pp. 270–279.
9. Sperling, S.: Corneal cryopreservation evaluated by trypan blue staining. Ophthalmol Res 6:23, 1974.
10. McCarey, B. E., Edelhauser, H. F., and Van Horn, D. L.: The effect of cryoprotection and cryodamage on corneal rehydration and endothelial structure. Cryobiology 10:298, 1973.
11. Schultz, R. O.: Laboratory evaluation of cryopreserved corneal tissue. Trans Amer Ophthalmol Soc 69:563, 1971.
12. Taillebourg, O., Payrau, P., Pouliquen, Y., and Faure, J. P.: Corneal cryopreservation. Ophthalmol Res 5:342, 1973.

13. Van Horn, D. L., Edelhauser, H. F., and De Bruin, J.: Functional and ultrastructural changes in cryopreserved corneas. Arch Ophthalmol 90:312, 1973.

14. Van Horn, D. L., Edelhauser, H. F., Gallun, A. B., and Schultz, R. O.: Reversibility of ultrastructural freeze-thaw–induced injury. Arch Ophthalmol 87:422, 1972.

15. Van Horn, D. L., and Schultz, R. O.: Endothelial survival in cryopreserved human corneas: A scanning electron microscopic study. Invest Ophthalmol 13:7, 1974.

16. Waller, W., and Van Horn, D. L.: Electron microscopic study of the endothelium of stored and cryopreserved monkey corneas. Albrecht von Graefes Arch Klin Ophthalmol 187:79, 1973.

17. Bourne, W. M.: In vitro survival of cryopreserved endothelial cells in primates. Arch Ophthalmol 92:146, 1974.

18. Le Francois, M., and Baum, J. L.: Flavobacterium endophthalmitis following keratoplasty. Use of a tissue culture medium–stored cornea. Arch Ophthalmol 94:1907, 1976.

19. Shaw, E. L. and Aquavella, J. V.: Pneumococcal endophthalmitis following grafting of corneal tissue from a (cadaver) kidney donor. Ann Ophthalmol 9:435, 1977.

Operative Procedures in Penetrating Keratoplasty

28

HOWARD M. LEIBOWITZ, M.D.
GEORGE O. WARING, III, M.D.

This chapter presents a practical discussion of the techniques used in penetrating keratoplasty. To accomplish this goal, we have divided the operation into a series of steps, and we shall discuss each step individually. Twelve of the contributors to this book (Aquavella, Doughman, Krachmer, Laibson, Leibowitz, McCulley, Moore, O'Day, Poirier, Raber, Smith, and Waring) provided data describing the manner in which they perform each step. This information was collated and forms the basis for our discussion. The technique recommended for each step of the operation is the approach used by the majority of the contributing authorities. Whenever an alternative method was used by more than a single contributor, it is also presented. Wherever there was no consensus, this, too, is pointed out.

PREOPERATIVE REGULATION OF THE INTRAOCULAR PRESSURE

Goal: To soften the eye in order to prevent the intraoperative expulsion of the intraocular contents through the trephine opening and to assure a formed anterior chamber at the completion of surgery.

Half of our authorities administer 20 per cent mannitol intravenously prior to surgery on a more or less routine basis (Fig. 28–1). Another uses it occasionally, and still another confines its use to children. Only two authorities use oral hyperosmolar agents such as glycerol, and similarly, only three include oral acetazolamide in their preoperative regimen. Thus, when medications are required to lower the intraocular pressure prior to penetrating keratoplasty, the consensus recommendation is for 20 per cent mannitol administered intravenously over 30 to 45 minutes (1.5 to 2.0 gm./kg.), 45 minutes prior to surgery.

All but two authorities stress the importance of the routine preoperative application of pressure on the globe (in addition to medications when they are used). In the majority of instances, intermittent pressure (e.g., 20 seconds on, 10 seconds off) is applied to the eye manually for 5 to 10 minutes (Fig. 28–2). Two of the authorities use a machine (Honan balloon) in some of their cases. One of the two surgeons who does not apply pressure to the globe preoperatively performs a paracentesis at the outset of surgery to soften the globe (as described in Chapter 23).

DRAPING

Goal: To prevent contamination of the surgical field.

In addition to being a source of bacterial contamination, the lashes may be a mechanical impediment during surgery. A loose eyelash also has the potential to become an unnoticed intraocular foreign body. Therefore, virtually all of our surgeons either isolate the lashes

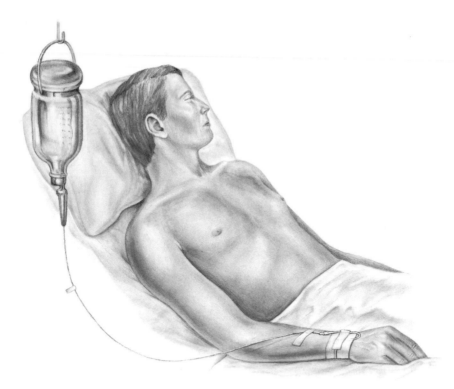

Figure 28–1. Preoperative intravenous administration of 20 per cent mannitol to lower intraocular pressure.

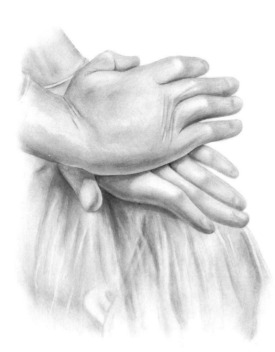

Figure 28–2. Following injection of local anesthesia or administration of general anesthesia, intermittent pressure is applied to soften the globe.

beneath the adhesive plastic drape or have them clipped preoperatively (Fig. 28–3). In the latter group there is a strong preference that the lashes be clipped before the patient arrives in the operating room suite.

The majority of surgeons use a commercially available adherent plastic fenestrated drape and apply it carefully to the prepared periocular skin (Fig. 28–4). Several of our contributors recommend that the lashes and meibomian orifices be isolated under the sterile drape. To accomplish this they place a non-fenestrated plastic adherent drape over the eye, slit the drape over the palpebral fissure, and wrap the adhesive-backed cut edge around the lid margin (Fig. 28–5). Variations of this approach can be accomplished with a fenestrated drape and isolated Steristrips (Fig. 28–6) placed at or around the lid margin.

LID POSITION

Goal: To maintain the lids in an open position without pressure on the globe.

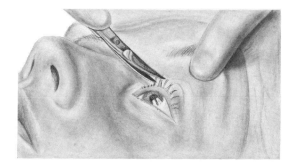

Figure 28–3. Lashes are clipped preoperatively, before the patient is brought to the surgical suite.

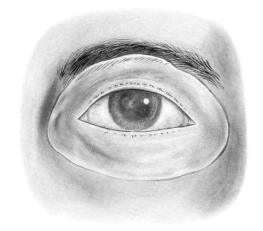

Figure 28–4. Commercially available adherent plastic fenestrated drape in position.

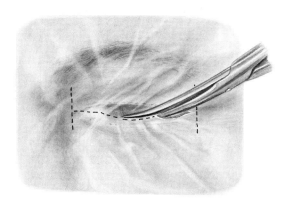

Figure 28–5. Slitting a non-fenestrated plastic drape to form flaps that isolate the lashes and lid margins.

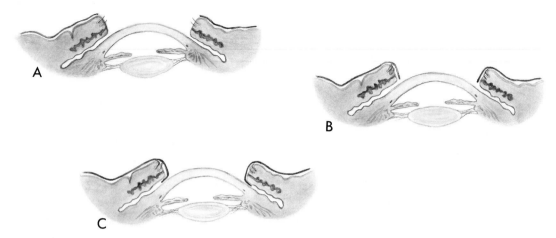

Figure 28–6. Variations in draping. The surface of the lids *(A)*, the lashes and meibomian orifices *(B)*, or the entire lid margin *(C)* can be isolated beneath Steristrips used in combination with a fenestrated drape or beneath flaps cut in a non-fenestrated plastic drape.

The majority of contributing surgeons use a simple wire speculum, most commonly some variation of the Barraquer speculum (Fig. 28–7). The remainder express a wide range of personal preferences, including the Guyton-Park or Maumenee-Park speculum, lid sutures, flexible lid retractors, a scleral ring with sutures, or a scleral ring with attached blepharostat (Goldmann-McNeill ring).

SCLERAL SUPPORT

Goal: To prevent the globe from collapsing and to maintain a round corneal opening after trephination.

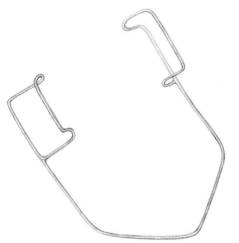

Figure 28–7. A wire lid speculum, the most common device used to maintain lids in proper position intraoperatively.

Virtually all of the contributing surgeons place a scleral ring on the recipient eye prior to trephination to prevent the globe from collapsing and in an attempt to maintain a round corneal opening. Both of the authors of this chapter favor a double ring, but all of their colleagues use a single ring. The majority use a relatively large ring (approximately 16 to 18 mm.) that when sutured in place lies 3 to 4 mm. posterior to the limbus. However, a minority recommend the use of a smaller ring that is sutured to the globe closer to the limbus.

The recipient eye is fixated, using either a scleral twist grip placed near the limbus or a toothed forceps, for placement of the first two sutures; thereafter the ring generally can be grasped for proper fixation and positioning of the globe (Fig. 28–8). The needle is passed through conjunctiva and a bite is taken in the superficial sclera (Fig. 28–9). Sutures passed only through conjunctiva will not allow the ring to support the globe. Our contributors stress the importance of a spatula needle to prevent inadvertent scleral perforation. Short bites should be taken and the suture should not be tied tightly; long, tight bites will pucker the trephine opening. Opinion concerning the optimal number of bites (four to eight) and the optimal suture material varies. Our

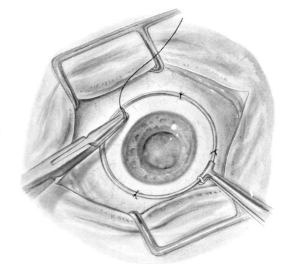

Figure 28–8. Suturing a supporting ring to the sclera of the recipient eye.

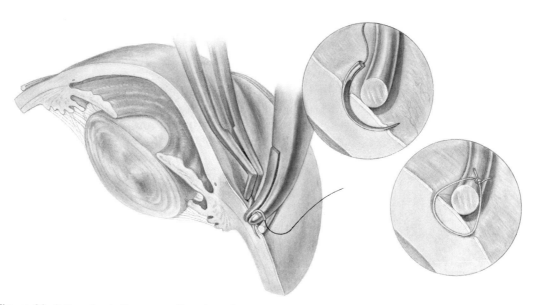

Figure 28–9. To attach the supporting ring, short suture bites are passed through the superficial sclera using a spatula needle. Care is taken not to tie the sutures too tightly.

contributors use 6-0 and 7-0 silk, 7-0 and 8-0 vicryl, 5-0 dacron, and 4-0 and 6-0 mersilene to secure the ring.

TREPHINATION OF THE DONOR EYE

Goal: To prepare donor corneal tissue with round, uniform margins and without damage to its endothelium.

Most of the contributing surgeons obtain the donor corneal material from a corneoscleral button that consists of the entire cornea and a 2-mm. rim of sclera that has been excised from the donor eye. Usually the corneoscleral button has been stored in McCarey-Kaufman medium (Fig. 28–10). Techniques for removing the corneoscleral button from the storage medium vary. Generally, the McCarey-Kaufman medium is slowly decanted into a sterile container by the circulating nurse, allowing the corneoscleral button to float to the orifice of the bottle (Fig. 28–11). Here it is grasped by its scleral rim, most often with a 0.12-mm. toothed forceps, and transferred to a concave cutting block (Fig. 28–12). A minority of the contributing surgeons gently pour the McCarey-Kaufman medium and the corneoscleral button from the storage bottle into an easily accessi-

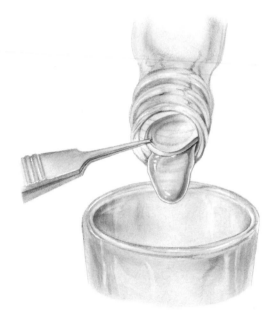

Figure 28–11. The McCarey-Kaufman medium is decanted slowly, allowing the corneoscleral button to float to the opening of the storage container, where it is grasped by forceps.

ble container before grasping the tissue. Others reach into the storage bottle with alligator forceps and remove the button for transfer to the cutting block. In all cases the tissue is placed on the block endothelial side up, and the trephine cut is made from the endothelial side.

The cutting block, constructed of Teflon, silicone, polycarbonate, and so forth, provides a firm base upon which to punch out a donor button with the trephine. Since the radius of curvature of the depression in the cutting block should approximate that of the donor epithelial surface, a block containing multiple depressions of varying curvature is advantageous. A majority of our authorities prefer an independent block and use a disposable, hollow trephine without a guard (Fig. 28–13). If a guard is present in the trephine, it should be retracted to avoid contact with the donor endothelium. Three contributors use a punch device that maintains the disposable trephine in a vertical position and incorporates the cutting block in its base (Fig. 28–14). There is a two-to-one preference that the block be dry rather than wet during trephination of the donor button. Most of the contributing sur-

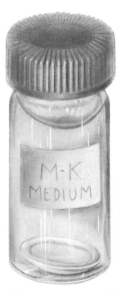

Figure 28–10. Donor cornea with scleral rim stored in sterile McCarey-Kaufman medium.

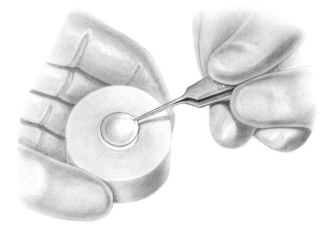

Figure 28–12. The corneoscleral button is transferred to a concave cutting block.

geons using corneoscleral material (in contradistinction to a whole eye) cut the donor button 0.2 to 0.5 mm. larger than the recipient opening. Among those surgeons favoring a donor button of the same size as the recipient opening, some use a larger donor button in aphakic cases. All attempt to obtain a uniformly perpendicular wound edge around the circumference of the donor button. The surgeon must take great care to visually center the trephine over the endothelial surface of the corneoscleral button prior to punching, since this technique permits only a single attempt at trephination. Markings in the base of the depression of the punching block such as a

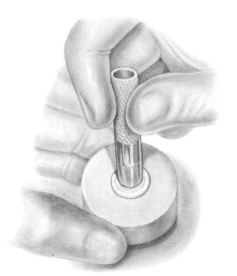

Figure 28–13. A hollow, disposable trephine is used to punch out the donor corneal button from its endothelial side on a cutting block.

colored disk, an etched circle, or a central hole help center the button and trephine during punching.

The majority of contributing surgeons do not remove the epithelium from the donor cornea. However, when the donor cornea has been maintained in organ culture, it becomes edematous and the epithelium is difficult to maintain. The donor button invariably is prepared prior to trephination of the recipient eye. During the interval before it is transferred to the recipient bed its endothelial surface is covered with McCarey-Kaufman medium or Balanced Salt Solution (Fig. 28–15A) and stored endothelial side up beneath a protective cover (Fig. 28–15B).

Only two of the contributing surgeons routinely obtain the donor corneal button from a whole eye. A third surgeon obtains his donor material from the whole eye approximately 50 per cent of the time. In each case the donor eye is wrapped in a sterile 4 in. × 4 in. gauze sponge and fixated by hand (Fig. 28–16). Prior to trephination, copious amounts of a broad spectrum antibiotic (e.g., tobramycin, gentamicin, or a neomycin-polymyxin B formulation) are applied to the corneal surface of the donor eye (Fig. 28–16). Each of the surgeons who prefers this approach stresses the importance of avoiding the application of excessive pressure to the donor eye with the fixating hand during trephination (Fig. 28–17A). Two of these surgeons use a trephine equal in size to that used on the

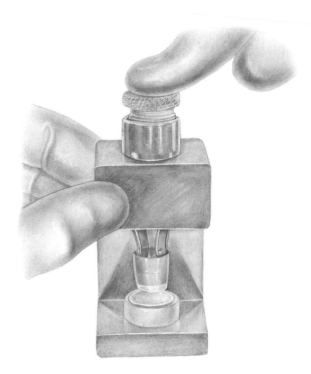

Figure 28–14. Use of a punch device to prepare the donor corneal button.

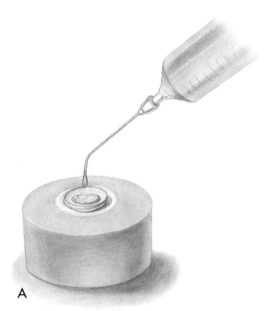
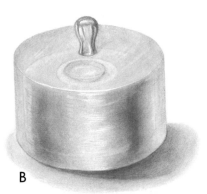

A   B

Figure 28–15. Before transfer to the recipient bed, the endothelial surface of the donor corneal button is covered with McCarey-Kaufman medium or Balanced Salt Solution *(A)* and stored beneath a protective cover *(B)*.

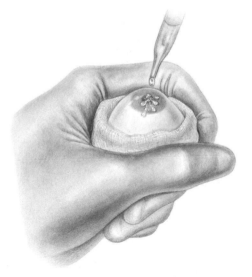

Figure 28–16. When the donor corneal button is obtained from a whole eye, the globe is wrapped in a sterile gauze sponge and is fixated, and copious amounts of an antibiotic solution are applied to the corneal surface prior to trephination.

The edge of the donor button is grasped with fine-toothed (0.12 mm.) forceps, avoiding contact with the endothelial surface, and lifted gently. The lower blade of the scissors is carefully inserted into the anterior chamber, avoiding contact with the corneal endothelium, and the circular incision is completed by cutting in the trephine groove. During this maneuver the tip of the scissors within the anterior chamber is lifted slightly to avoid the iris.

TREPHINATION OF THE RECIPIENT EYE

Goal: To prepare a round bed with uniform edges in the recipient cornea.

recipient cornea; the third uses a trephine 0.5 mm. larger. Each prefers to penetrate the donor eye with the trephine (Fig. 28–17B), although this is not mandatory, and to excise the donor button with corneal scissors (Fig. 28–17C).

During trephination of the recipient eye it is necessary to stabilize and prevent rotary motion of the globe. This can be accomplished by several techniques, and we could identify no particular pattern of preference among our contributing authorities. Some prefer to obtain three points of fixation, using superior and inferior rectus bridle sutures (Fig. 28–18A) or, if a scleral ring was in place,

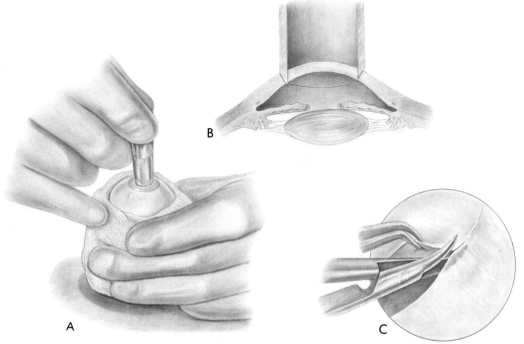

Figure 28–17. Trephination of the donor corneal button from a whole eye (A). Perforation initially is accomplished with the trephine (B) and the donor button is excised with scissors (C).

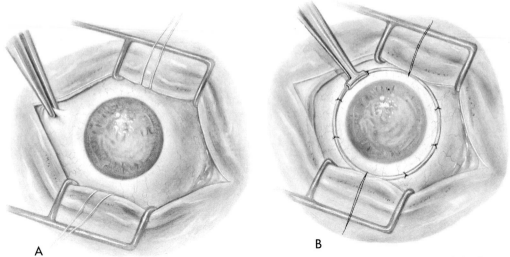

A   B

Figure 28–18. Fixation of the globe must be obtained prior to trephination of the recipient cornea. Bridle sutures can be attached to the superior and inferior recti *(A)* or to the superior and inferior poles of a scleral ring *(B)*. A third fixation point is obtained by grasping a horizontal rectus muscle *(A)*, a point adjacent to the limbus (not shown), or the scleral ring *(B)*.

bridle sutures attached to the superior and inferior poles of the ring (Fig. 28–18B) to establish two of the fixation points. The third point of fixation is obtained by grasping a horizontal rectus muscle with toothed forceps (Fig. 28–18A), by holding a point adjacent to the limbus with either toothed forceps or a scleral twist grip, or by fixating the scleral ring (Fig. 28–18B).

Virtually all of the authorities use a hollow disposable trephine. Two surgeons use non-disposable trephines with a central guard, one a Grieshaber trephine, the other a King trephine with a right-angle handle. The size of the recipient bed is determined by the extent and location of the corneal abnormality, but in the majority of cases the incision is 7.5 to 8.5 mm. in diameter. The surgeon visually centers the trephine over the cornea, unless an eccentric button is to be removed, and lightly marks the epithelium with the trephine (Fig. 28–19). Fluorescein enhances visualization of the mark. If the mark is not in the desired location, the trephine is moved and another mark is made.

Most of the contributing authorities then reinsert the trephine in the superficial mark and use it to make a partially penetrating wound in the host cornea (Fig. 28–20) by grasping the trephine between thumb and forefinger and rotating it back and forth with gentle pressure on the globe. Few of the contributing authorities perforate the recipient cornea with the trephine by design. The trephine wound is deepened and the anterior chamber is entered with a disposable miniblade, a razor blade chip, or a diamond knife (Fig. 28–21A). The

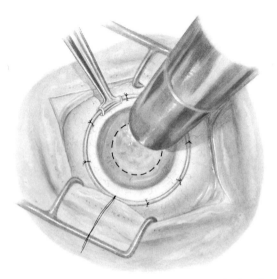

Figure 28–19. The trephine is centered visually over the cornea and used to mark the epithelium lightly.

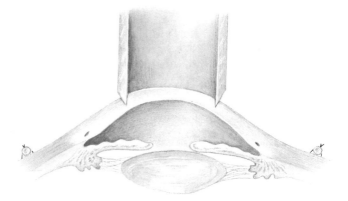

Figure 28–20. When the superficial mark is properly centered, the trephine is reinserted in the mark and a partially penetrating wound is made in the recipient cornea.

initial perforating incision is extended one to two clock hours with the knife (Fig. 28–21B) to allow smooth insertion of the scissor blade into the anterior chamber (Fig. 28–22A). The host corneal button then is excised with a corneal scissors of the surgeon's choice. The scissors is inserted with its tip directed toward the periphery of the anterior chamber. The edge of the host corneal button is fixated with fine-toothed forceps while the tip of the inner blade is tilted slightly superiorly, away from the iris, and the outer blade is closed slowly into the trephine groove (Fig. 28–22B).

During each bite, the scissors is not closed completely so that they may be advanced without removing them intermittently from the anterior chamber. Most contributing surgeons prefer a host wound with a slight posterior bevel, while a minority recommend a vertical wound; in either case the angle of the scissors must be changed during cutting to create a uniformly shaped wound. Most trim a significant irregularity in the host wound with a Vannas scissors or comparable instrument. The configuration of the opening in the recipient cornea is carefully inspected; if a suture

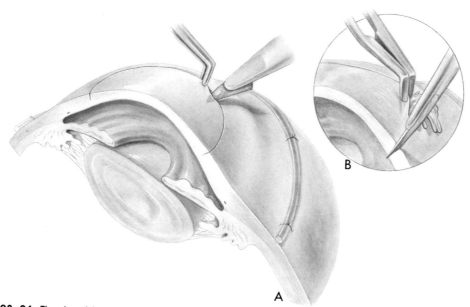

Figure 28–21. The trephine wound is deepened and the anterior chamber is entered with a knife blade *(A)*. The initial perforating incision is extended approximately two clock hours with the knife blade *(B)*.

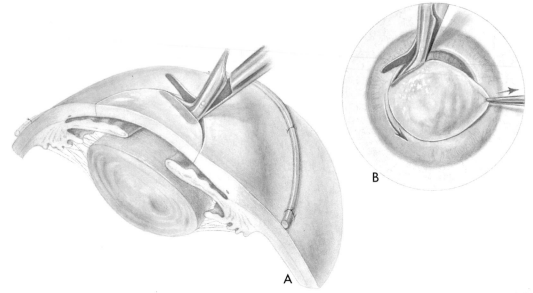

Figure 28–22. A scissor blade is inserted into the anterior chamber *(A)* and, while the edge of the host corneal button is fixated with forceps, the button is excised by closing the outer blade into the trephine groove *(B)*.

securing the scleral ring produces sufficient tension to distort the circular opening, it is cut and removed. The goal of all of these maneuvers is to create a host bed that is uniform around its entire circumference.

USE OF VISCOUS MATERIAL IN THE ANTERIOR CHAMBER

Goal: To maintain the anterior chamber and to protect the donor corneal endothelium from mechanical trauma.

At the time this chapter was written Healon was the only viscous material approved for use in the anterior chamber of the eye. Virtually all of the contributing surgeons favor its use as an adjunct to penetrating keratoplasty under some circumstances (Fig. 28–23), but there is little uniformity among these authorities in defining the indications for its use. Some confine the use of Healon to phakic eyes, whereas others recommend its use in both phakic and aphakic eyes. There was fairly uniform agreement that this material should be used whenever an intraocular lens implant is present and is to remain in place or is to be

implanted as part of a combined procedure at the time of penetrating keratoplasty. Most contributors use only small quantities, since large amounts of Healon can be accompanied by a transient but extreme elevation of the intraocular pressure postoperatively. Several surgeons also inject a small quantity into the anterior chamber angle to help prevent the postoperative re-formation of peripheral anterior synechiae whenever they had been broken during the penetrating keratoplasty procedure. Healon is packaged in a convenient syringe to which a blunt cannula can be fitted for direct use.

INTRAOPERATIVE MANAGEMENT OF THE IRIS

Iridectomy

Goal: To promote the flow of aqueous humor from the posterior to the anterior chamber and to prevent pupillary block.

Half the contributing surgeons routinely perform an iridotomy or iridectomy in phakic eyes. However, all agree that it is indicated if the eye has been

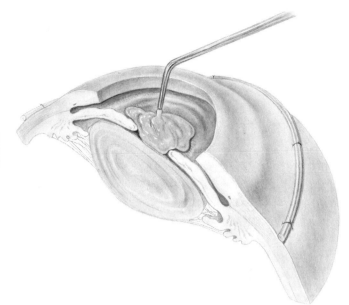

Figure 28–23. Instillation of Healon into the anterior chamber to help maintain the chamber and to protect the donor endothelium.

inflamed. When the procedure is performed, all recommend a single iris opening. There is no strong feeling about the relative superiority of an iridotomy versus an iridectomy, although most of the contributing surgeons indicate that they do an iridotomy. With minor variations, the iris is grasped superiorly at or slightly peripheral to the corneal trephine opening, elevated and positioned with a forceps of the surgeon's choice (e.g., jeweler's, McPherson's, Bonn, Colibri), and cut with a Vannas or De-Wecker scissors (Fig. 28–24). Care must

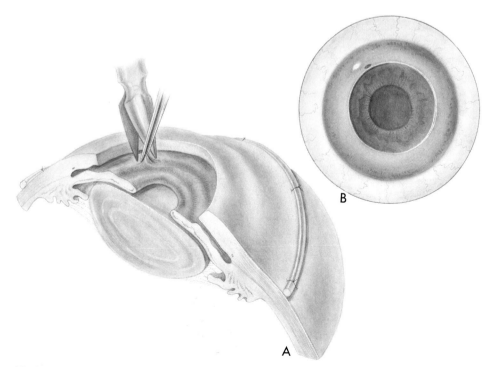

Figure 28–24. Performance of an iridotomy through the corneal trephine opening *(A)*; final appearance and position of the iridotomy *(B)*.

be exercised in carrying out this maneuver; if the iris is pulled excessively, an iridodialysis and bleeding may result.

An iridectomy is almost invariably present in an aphakic eye. If an acceptable iris opening is not present, it is created unless an anterior vitrectomy is performed. A proper vitrectomy usually eliminates the potential for pupillary block.

Peripheral Anterior Synechiae

Goal: To restore the normal anatomic configuration of the anterior chamber, to prevent glaucoma, and to prevent iris adhesion to the wound.

There is uniform agreement that peripheral anterior synechiae should be severed before the donor cornea is sutured in place. Most contributing surgeons use a fine cyclodialysis spatula to gently sweep the periphery of the anterior chamber and bluntly dissect the adhesions (Fig. 28–25). Two contributors think that injection of Healon into the anterior chamber angle is helpful in defining the synechiae and protecting the peripheral corneal endothelium. If sweeping of the angle is unsuccessful, several surgeons recommend that the synechiae be cut with a Vannas scissors. However, an equal number indicate that if the synechiae cannot be severed by sweeping with a fine spatula, they would not resort to sharp dissection and would simply leave the synechiae intact. When superior peripheral anterior synechiae result in an updrawn pupil, an inferior radial sphincterotomy is recommended.

Central Anterior Synechiae

Goal: To allow removal of the central host cornea after trephination, to attempt to restore the normal anatomic configuration of the anterior chamber, to prevent adhesion of the iris to the keratoplasty wound, and, if possible, to maintain pupillary function.

If the central anterior synechiae are not extensive and if anterior chamber visualization is adequate, then the pro-

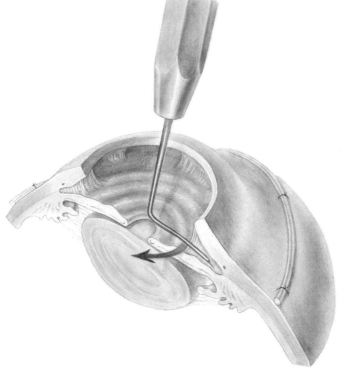

Figure 28–25. Severing peripheral anterior synechiae through the trephine opening by blunt dissection with a fine spatula.

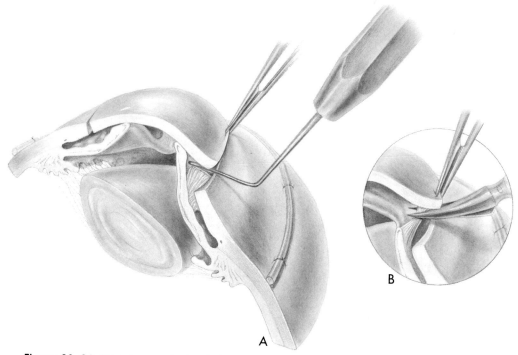

Figure 28–26. Severing central anterior synechiae by blunt *(A)* and sharp *(B)* dissection.

cedures for handling them are similar to those used to sever peripheral anterior synechiae. Following trephination and completion of the circular wound with scissors, the edge of the host corneal button is grasped with 0.12 mm. Colibri or Castroviejo forceps and elevated slightly. An attempt is made to break the synechial attachments with a gentle sweeping motion of a fine cyclodialysis spatula (Fig. 28–26A). If this fails to sever the synechiae or if it seems likely to induce significant tearing of the iris, the attachment is cut with Vannas scissors (Fig. 28–26B) in a manner that is most apt to preserve iris tissue and pupillary function. Phakic and aphakic eyes are approached similarly.

In the case of extensive central anterior synechiae and/or poor anterior chamber visualization, a more cautious approach is required. The trephine groove in one area is deepened progressively with a knife until the anterior chamber is entered by the ab externo incision (Fig. 28–27A). If the iris is encountered, the trephine wound is cautiously extended with the knife around its circumference (Fig. 28–27B) while the iris is maintained as a protective shield in front of the lens or vitreous humor. Healon is then introduced into the anterior chamber to better define tissue planes, and iridocorneal adhesions are broken by blunt or sharp dissection (Fig. 28–27C).

Posterior Synechiae

Goal: To restore, insofar as possible, the physiologic status of the iris and pupil and to prevent pupillary block.

In a phakic eye with posterior synechiae the iris is grasped near the pupil with any fine smooth forceps and gently elevated. An attempt is made to break the attachments between the posterior iris and the anterior lens capsule by a gentle to-and-fro motion of the iris (Fig. 28–28A). Alternatively, as the iris is elevated, a smooth, fine spatula is inserted behind the iris through a portion of the pupil not involved by posterior synechiae and, while the iris is lifted, the spatula is carefully swept around the circumference of the pupil (Fig. 28–28B).

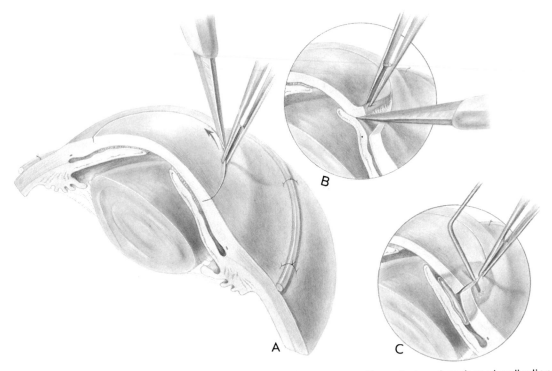

Figure 28–27. When central anterior synechiae are extensive and/or anterior chamber visualization is poor, the anterior chamber is entered by an ab externo incision with a knife blade *(A)*, the trephine wound is extended around its circumference with the blade *(B)*, and Healon is introduced into the anterior chamber periphery to better define tissue planes *(C)*.

In cases of total pupillary seclusion, in which no area of the posterior synechial attachment can be broken by elevation and gentle movement of the iris, a small iridotomy can be performed with Vannas scissors adjacent to the pupil (Fig. 28–28C). This will permit passage of a fine spatula posterior to the iris for an attempt at synechiolysis (Fig. 28–28D). Several of the contributing surgeons suggest that, if the lens is clear and the posterior synechia is small, it be left alone. If during attempts to lyse posterior synechiae the lens capsule ruptures, extracapsular lens extraction must be performed.

Posterior synechiae in aphakic eyes involve the attachment of the posterior iris to a pupillary membrane. Initially the iris may be grasped with smooth forceps and elevated, so that an attempt can be made to sever the attachments by sweeping with a fine spatula (Fig. 28–29A) or cutting with fine scissors. In any event the membrane is excised with fine scissors (Fig. 28–29B) or with a vitrec-

tomy instrument (Fig. 28–29C) and a vitrectomy is then performed, removing the central, anterior third of the vitreous humor. One preserves as much iris as possible.

Pupil

Goal: To regulate pupillary size as necessary for surgical manipulations.

Should mydriasis be required after excision of the recipient corneal button has been completed, several drops of epinephrine may be applied to the surface of the iris. Non-preserved epinephrine hydrochloride for intracardiac injection (Parke-Davis and others) is preferred. The contents of a single ampule (1 mg. in 1 ml. [1:1000]) are added to 500 ml. of BSS Plus so that a final concentration of 1:500,000 is used. Intraoperative miosis is obtained by application of several drops of acetylcholine chloride 1:100 or carbachol 0.01 per cent (Miochol, Miostat) to the iris surface.

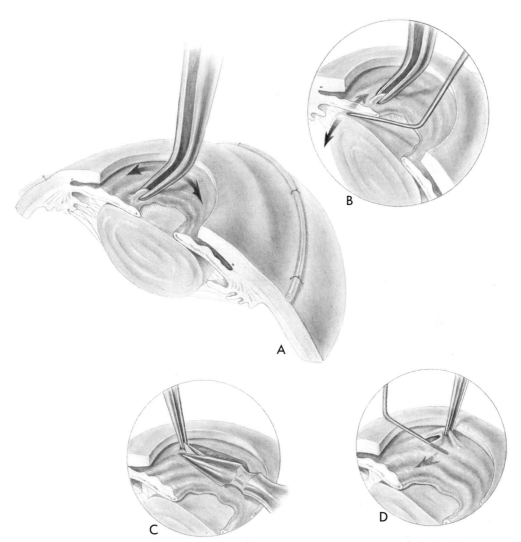

Figure 28–28. In a phakic eye with posterior synechiae, the iris is grasped near the pupil and attachments are broken by gentle to-and-fro motions *(A)*. Alternatively, a fine spatula is inserted through the pupil beneath the elevated iris and posterior synechiae are broken by blunt dissection *(B)*. In the face of total pupillary seclusion, a small iridotomy is made *(C)* through which the spatula is inserted for an attempt at synechiolysis *(D)*.

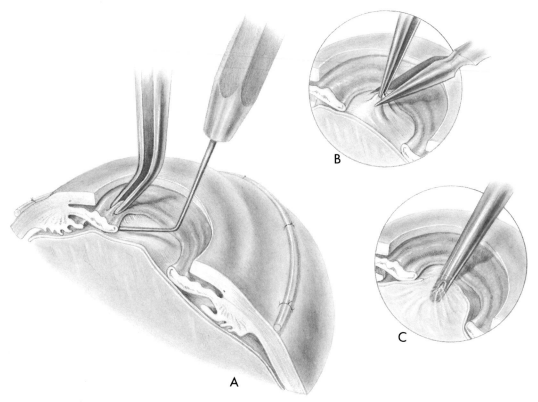

Figure 28–29. In an aphakic eye, the iris is grasped and elevated and attachments between posterior iris and pupillary membrane are severed with a spatula (A) or Vannas scissors (not shown). The membrane is excised with fine scissors (B) or a vitrectomy instrument (C) and a vitrectomy is performed.

In phakic eyes the pupil is constricted preoperatively with 1 per cent pilocarpine to obtain whatever protection the iris might offer a clear lens during surgery. If a combined penetrating keratoplasty and cataract extraction are to be performed, mydriasis is induced preoperatively with phenylephrine 2.5 per cent and a short-acting parasympatholytic agent such as tropicamide 1 per cent or cyclopentolate 1 per cent.

Following penetrating keratoplasty in an aphakic eye with a sector iridectomy, the iris may come forward and progressively "zipper up" the angle. The anterior chamber initially is deep, intraocular pressure initially is normal, and there is no evidence of relative pupillary block. Nonetheless, the peripheral anterior chamber progressively shallows and closes, generally within 4 to 6 months after surgery. The cause of this phenomenon is unknown, but it is rarely seen in eyes with an intact pupillary sphinc-ter. In an effort prevent the postoperative formation of peripheral anterior synechiae, a minority of contributing surgeons recommend that iris colobomas be sutured closed. Three or four interrupted 10-0 polypropylene sutures on a round needle are loosely tied with the knot moved into or behind the stroma to accomplish this (Fig. 28–30). While this maneuver may help to prevent the postoperative formation of peripheral anterior synechiae, the majority of contributing surgeons seldom close iris colobomas.

INTRAOPERATIVE EVALUATION OF THE LENS

Goal: To evaluate the transparency of the lens in order to determine whether or not cataract extraction is indicated.

There is agreement among contributing surgeons that the status of the lens

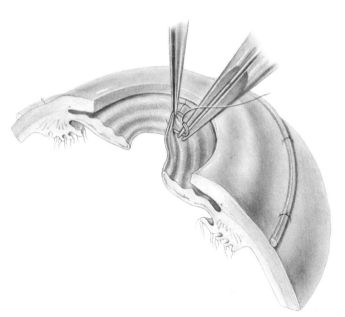

Figure 28–30. An iris coloboma may be closed with interrupted 10-0 polypropylene sutures on a round needle.

and the decision regarding its removal is best made preoperatively at the slit lamp biomicroscope. In some cases, however, the corneal opacity prevents satisfactory preoperative evaluation of the lens and its transparency must be evaluated intraoperatively after removal of the recipient cornea. Unfortunately, assessment of lens transparency through the operating microscope is an inexact procedure. General inspection of the lens at high magnification is carried out.

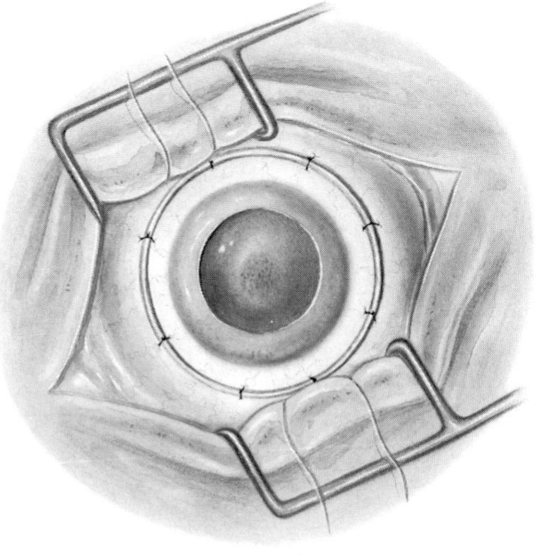

The slit lamp attachment of the operating microscope is of little value, and only a minority of contributing surgeons indicate that they use it at all. Perhaps the best approach is to darken the operating room and, using only the coaxial illumination source of the microscope, to study the lens against the red fundus reflection (Fig. 28–31).

TECHNIQUE FOR LENS EXTRACTION

Goal: To remove the opaque lens without vitreous loss.

When, in addition to a corneal opacity, an opaque lens is present, the cataract is removed during the corneal transplantation operation. Half the surgeons indicate that their procedure of choice is a planned extracapsular cataract extraction, three prefer intracapsular cataract extraction, and three state that they perform both types of lens extraction with roughly equal frequency.

The technique for intracapsular cataract extraction requires preoperative dilatation of the pupil. Mydriasis can be supplemented intraoperatively after trephination of the cornea by application of non-preserved epinephrine to the iris surface. A cryoprobe is applied to the anterior lens surface and "open-sky"

Figure 28–31. When the corneal opacity prevents preoperative evaluation of the lens, its transparency can be evaluated through the trephine opening using coaxial illumination to study the lens against the red fundus reflection.

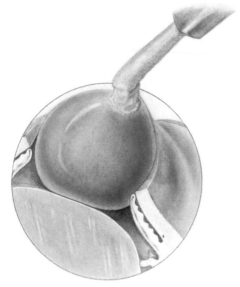

Figure 28–32. Intracapsular cataract extraction is carried out by applying a cryoprobe to the anterior lens surface and effecting an "open-sky" delivery through the trephine opening.

lens delivery is effected by gentle upward and to-and-fro motions (Fig. 28–32). If necessary, α-chymotrypsin may be instilled, or the zonules may be stripped with a cyclodialysis spatula or similar instrument. There is no difficulty delivering the lens through a 7.5-mm. or larger trephine opening in the cornea.

Planned extracapsular cataract extraction similarly is performed through the corneal trephine opening. Maximum mydriasis is obtained as above; if necessary, it may be maintained during surgical manipulation of the lens by repeated anterior chamber instillation of non-preserved epinephrine 1:500,000 through the trephine opening or by adding the epinephrine to the irrigating solution.

An anterior capsulotomy is performed (Fig. 28–33A), and the anterior capsule is removed from the anterior chamber (Fig. 28–33B). There is a wide variety of instruments used by our contributing surgeons to perform the capsulotomy. They include a bent hypodermic needle, an irrigating cystotome, a diamond knife, a disposable miniblade, and a Vannas scissors. The nucleus is then dislodged into the anterior chamber by external pressure directed behind the lens with a lens loop or other instrument placed 2 mm. posterior to the limbus (Fig. 28–34A), by direct manipulation with an instrument such as a cystitome (Fig. 28–34B), or by irrigation into the cortex behind the nucleus with a blunt-tipped cannula or irrigating vectis (Fig. 28–34C), and delivered.

The cortex is aspirated using a mechanical irrigation/aspiration apparatus (Fig. 28–35A) or a manual double-bore needle. Peripheral cortex is engaged in the aspiration port, drawn centrally, stripping it from the capsule, and aspir-

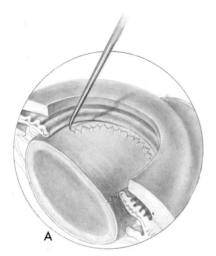

A

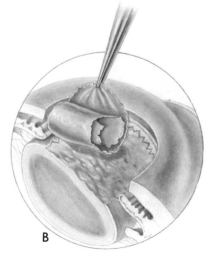

B

Figure 28–33. Extracapsular cataract extraction is initiated through the trephine opening by performing an anterior capsulotomy with a bent needle or other instrument (A) and removing the central anterior capsule from the anterior chamber (B).

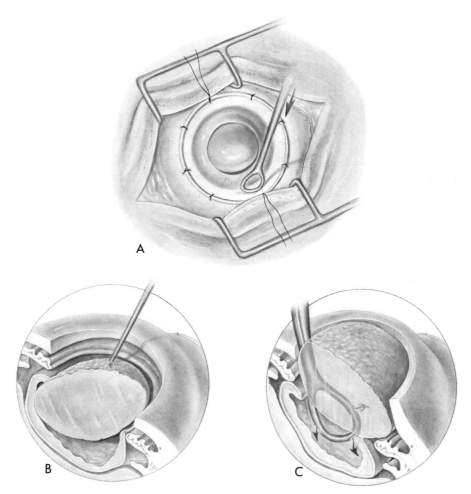

Figure 28–34. After completion of the capsulotomy, the nucleus is dislodged into the anterior chamber by external pressure directed behind the lens with a lens loop *(A)*, by direct manipulation with a cystitome or similar instrument *(B)*, or by irrigation behind the nucleus with an irrigating vectis *(C)*, and delivered.

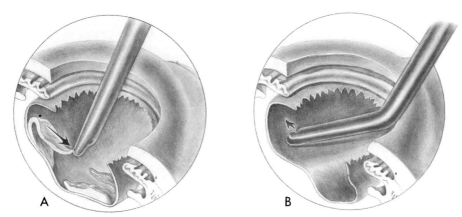

Figure 28–35. The cortex is aspirated *(A)* and the posterior capsule is left intact and polished with one of a variety of instruments *(B)*.

ated. Approximately two thirds of the contributing surgeons polish the posterior capsule (Fig. 28–35B) using a variety of instruments. Most leave the capsule intact; if a posterior capsulotomy is done, most use a bent hypodermic needle.

INTRAOCULAR LENS IMPLANTATION IN CONJUNCTION WITH PENETRATING KERATOPLASTY

Goal: To provide optical correction of aphakia, when possible, with an intraocular lens implant.

Implant Removal

The contributing surgeons agree that if an intraocular lens implant is in place at the time of penetrating keratoplasty, the decision about whether to leave it in place or to remove it must be based on the individual circumstances present in each case. Most think that the implant should be left in place if possible. However, various types of implants tend to be treated differently. Most of the contributing authorities tend to remove iris-fixated implants, particularly those with metal haptics. They think that this type of implant is unstable and is likely to compromise the corneal transplant. The negative feeling against anterior chamber implants is somewhat less strong, but three of the contributing surgeons indicate that they would remove all anterior chamber implants and a substantial percentage are removed by other contributors. A posterior chamber implant is most likely to be left in place.

The following preoperative criteria serve as a guide for the removal of an intraocular lens implant at the time of penetrating keratoplasty: (1) a poorly fixed, dislocated, or tilted implant; (2) distortion of the iris; (3) intraocular inflammation; (4) hyphema; (5) glaucoma; (6) pupillary membrane; (7) vitreous humor in the anterior chamber; (8) shallow anterior chamber; (9) endothelial contact; (10) pain; (11) implant of incorrect power; or (12) the patient wishes to have it removed.

If the implant presents a technical problem for proper execution of the corneal surgery, it is removed. Alternatively, if the intraocular lens implant is held firmly in place by fibrotic tissue and attempts to remove it require excessive manipulation, it should be left in place. This will avoid vitreous traction intraocular hemorrhage, iridodialysis, and large iris colobomas. A membranectomy/vitrectomy may be performed behind the implant with a mechanical vitrectomy instrument to create a clear pupillary opening.

If an implant is to be removed, all of the contributing surgeons advise that initially the surgeon should attempt to simply slide it out using the forceps of the surgeon's choice. Should a large quantity of vitreous be present in the anterior chamber and adherent to the implant, the surgeon may perform a shallow vitrectomy behind the implant with a vitrectomy instrument or with cellulose sponges and scissors prior to removing the implant from the globe. Alternatively, if the surgeon observes vitreous adhering to the implant as he begins to lift it from the eye, he may cut these vitreous adhesions concurrently

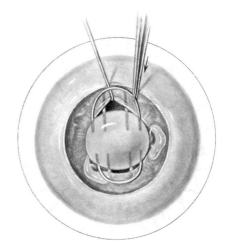

Figure 28–36. To remove an iris-fixated lens implant, the anterior haptic is grasped and, concurrently, the iris is retracted. Adhesions are broken by blunt or sharp dissection under observation.

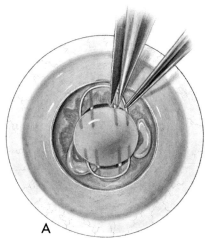
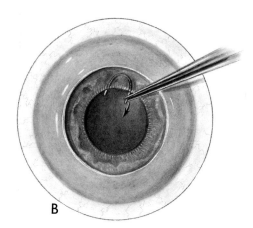

A   B

Figure 28–37. Posterior haptics encapsulated by fibrotic tissue may be amputated and left in place *(A)*. Since the fibrotic tissue encapsulates but does not adhere to the haptic, the haptic can, at times, be removed by sliding it in a circular direction *(B)*.

with implant removal. In either case the goal is to minimize vitreous traction.

To remove an iris-fixated lens, the surgeon grasps one of the haptics of the implant and concurrently retracts the iris (Fig. 28–36). Adhesions can be broken by blunt or sharp dissection under direct observation. If the posterior haptics are encapsulated by dense fibrotic tissue, they may be amputated with scissors (Figs. 28–37A) and left in place while the optic is lifted from the anterior chamber. Since the fibrotic tissue generally does not adhere to the haptics but rather forms an encapsulating envelope around them, the amputated posterior haptics often may be slid in a circular

direction from their fibrotic capsule (Fig. 28–37B). Whenever it is present, an iris-fixation suture is removed.

To remove an anterior chamber implant, initial attempts are directed to simply sliding the implant from the eye without creating a cyclodialysis. The implant is grasped with a smooth angled forceps and gently slid peripherally while the opposite edge of the trephine opening is grasped with fine-toothed forceps and elongated (Fig. 28–38). If this is not successful, the optic is grasped with smooth angled forceps and tilted, and one haptic is amputated with scissors (Fig. 28–39). The two pieces of the implant can be removed from the ante-

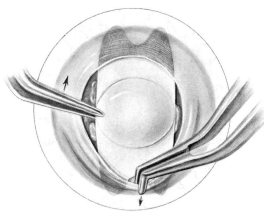
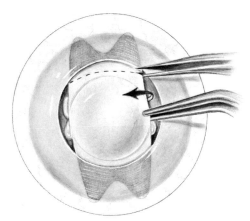

Figure 28–38. Initial attempts to remove an anterior chamber lens implant involve sliding it peripherally while elongating the opposite edge of the trephine opening.

Figure 28–39. If necessary, one haptic of an anterior chamber implant can be amputated to effect its removal.

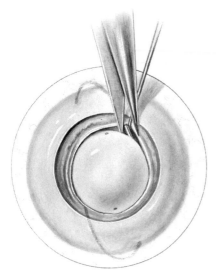

Figure 28–40. To remove a posterior chamber lens implant, the haptics generally are amputated and left in place.

rior chamber without difficulty. A vitrectomy is required in most cases.

To remove a posterior chamber implant, the haptics are generally amputated (Fig. 28–40) and left in place. The optic is lifted from the eye and a vitrectomy is performed.

Implant Insertion

When performing a combined penetrating keratoplasty and cataract extraction in an eye free of other pathology, three of the contributing surgeons indicate that they would not insert an intraocular lens implant, and two additional surgeons indicate they do so only occasionally. The remaining seven authorities state that they do so regularly based on their criteria for primary placement of an implant after cataract extraction. Almost invariably a planned extracapsular cataract extraction is performed and a posterior chamber implant is inserted. The intraocular lens power generally is calculated using ultrasonography and standard formulas, recognizing the limitations imposed by the unavailability of preoperative keratometry readings in most cases and by the unpredictability of postoperative keratometry readings.

The implant is grasped with a smooth angled forceps at the edge of the optic and the inferior loop is slid into the inferior capsular bag or ciliary sulcus (Fig. 28–41A). The superior loop is

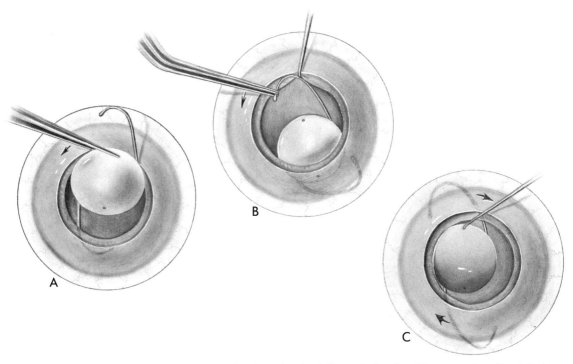

Figure 28–41. To insert a posterior chamber lens implant through the trephine opening, the inferior loop is slid into the inferior capsular bag or ciliary sulcus *(A)*, the superior pupillary margin is retracted while the superior loop is inserted behind the iris *(B)*, and the implant is rotated to avoid iris tuck and to center the optic *(C)*.

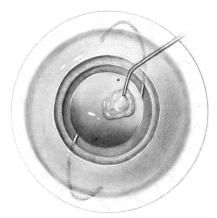

Figure 28–42. Healon is applied to the anterior surface of the implant and the peripupillary iris surface.

grasped at its tip and bent toward the optic, the superior pupillary margin is retracted with a small hook, and the superior loop is inserted behind the iris (Fig. 28–41B). The implant is rotated by inserting a lens guide into a guide hole in the implant (Fig. 28–41C) to avoid iris tuck and to center the optic. Acetylcholine is instilled to induce miosis and Healon is applied to the anterior surface of the implant and on the peripupillary iris surface (Fig. 28–42).

In contrast, in regard to performing a penetrating keratoplasty on an aphakic eye free of other pathology, there appears to be little enthusiasm for placement of an intraocular lens implant. Seven of the twelve contributing surgeons state that they do not do this

procedure. The others indicate that they do it rarely or occasionally. When intraocular lens implantation is performed under these circumstances, a flexible-loop, anterior chamber implant generally is used (Fig. 28–43).

A vitrectomy generally is performed before insertion of an anterior chamber lens unless the posterior capsule is intact. To avoid tucking the iris, Healon is injected into the angle or a lens glide is used. The anterior chamber implant is grasped by the superior haptic and the inferior haptic is slid through the trephine opening into the inferior angle (Fig. 28–43A). The optic is grasped with a smooth angled forceps and maintained in position while the superior haptic is grasped at its free end, bent toward the optic, and lowered through the trephine opening into the superior angle. The surgeon should avoid pushing the implant towards the inferior angle with enough force to create a cyclodialysis. Healon is spread over the anterior surface of the implant (Fig. 28–43B). A donor button slightly larger than the trephine opening is helpful in avoiding contact between the graft endothelium and the anterior surface of the implant.

INTRAOPERATIVE MANAGEMENT OF A PUPILLARY MEMBRANE

Goal: To remove opaque tissue from the visual axis.

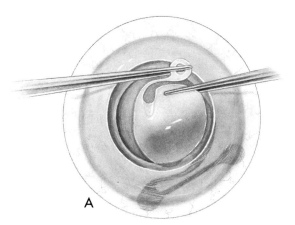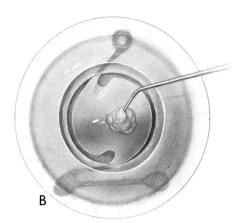

A   B

Figure 28–43. To insert an anterior chamber lens implant through the trephine opening, the inferior haptic is slid into the inferior angle and the superior haptic is then bent toward the optic and lowered into the superior angle (A). The anterior surface of the optic is coated with Healon (B).

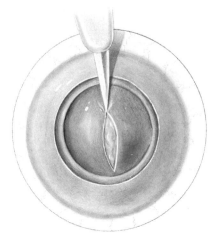

Figure 28–44. A thin elastic pupillary membrane is incised to create a clear pupillary opening.

In the case of a thin, elastic membrane that retracts readily and leaves a large pupillary opening, the majority of contributing surgeons simply incise the membrane (Fig. 28–44). In an attempt to spare a potentially intact hyaloid face, the tip of the blade is drawn lightly across the face of the membrane; the knife is not plunged deeply through the membrane. If the membrane is thicker or fails to retract, it is excised. While performing this maneuver, the surgeon should strive to preserve iris and pupillary function. Adhesions between iris and the membrane are severed by blunt dissection where possible; otherwise they are cut with fine scissors. The membrane initially is incised with scissors and forceps (Fig. 28–45A) and then excised either with the scissors and forceps or with a vitrectomy instrument (Fig. 28–45B). When the latter is used, the cut edge of the membrane initially is incised in multiple locations with scissors, creating small flaps that can easily be drawn into the port of the vitrectomy instrument. Whenever the surgeon is cutting in proximity to the pupillary margin, attempts are made to maintain the port away from the pupillary margin to avoid inadvertent excision of the iris.

Most surgeons create a large central opening to reduce the potential for contraction or recurrence of the membrane. The iris can be retracted to facilitate membranectomy. Sufficient membrane must be excised to prevent recurrence of adhesions between the pupil and residual membrane, but excision of the peripheral membrane in the area of the zonules and vitreous base is to be avoided.

INTRAOPERATIVE MANAGEMENT OF VITREOUS HUMOR

Goal: To prevent postoperative contact of the vitreous humor with the corneal endothelium and its entrapment in the corneal wound.

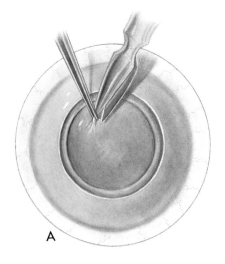

A

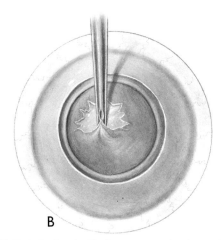

B

Figure 28–45. A thick inelastic pupillary membrane initially is incised with forceps and scissors *(A)* and then excised either with forceps and scissors or with a vitrectomy instrument *(B)*.

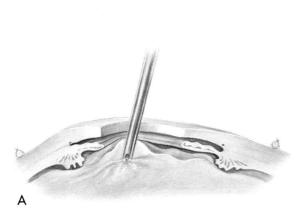

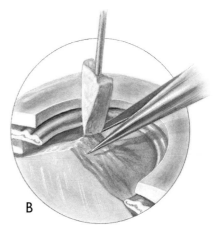

A

B

Figure 28–46. In penetrating keratoplasty on an aphakic eye, a vitrectomy often is performed using a vitrectomy instrument (A); cellulose sponges and scissors can be used if a vitrectomy unit is unavailable (B).

Four of the contributing surgeons perform a vitrectomy as part of the penetrating keratoplasty operation in all aphakic cases. Two additional surgeons do so in the majority of such cases. The remaining six contributors list the following criteria for doing a vitrectomy: (1) intraoperative loss of vitreous humor; (2) vitreous humor in the anterior chamber; (3) broken anterior hyaloid face; (4) positive vitreous pressure, bulging vitreous with intact anterior hyaloid face, or persistent convexity of the iris; and (5) vitreous humor occluding the iridectomy.

Most contributing surgeons use a vitrectomy instrument (Fig. 28–46A); cellulose sponges and scissors (Fig. 28–46B) are used if a vitrectomy unit is not available. Irrespective of technique, traction on the vitreous must be minimized. This can be accomplished with the vitrectomy instrument by submerging its cutting port in the vitreous humor while using moderate suction and a high cutting rate. The use of cellulose sponges and scissors is facilitated by application of gentle pressure on the scleral ring. This prolapses the vitreous humor into the pupil and avoids the necessity of working in the vitreous cavity. Upon completion of the vitrectomy, the surgeon applies a cellulose sponge to the iris surface, pupillary margin, and iridectomy to ensure the absence of residual vitreous strands. The eye may be refilled with Balanced Salt Solution prior to placement of the corneal graft.

The goal of the vitrectomy procedure is the elimination of all vitreous humor from the anterior chamber and from the central one third to one half of the vitreous cavity so that the iris surface is free of vitreous, the iridectomy sites are open, and the iris is well back and concave (Fig. 28–47).

MANAGEMENT OF INTRAOPERATIVE HEMORRHAGE

Goal: To control intraocular bleeding.

Almost all of the contributing surgeons initially manage an intraoperative

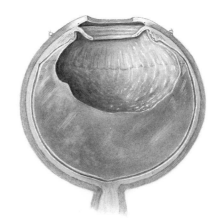

Figure 28–47. The vitrectomy procedure eliminates the vitreous humor from the anterior chamber and from the central one third to one half of the vitreous cavity.

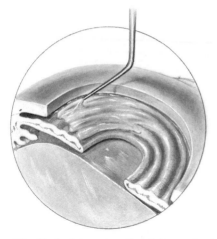

Figure 28–48. An intraoperative intraocular hemorrhage initially is managed by irrigation to wash out the blood and maintain visibility.

INTRAOPERATIVE MANAGEMENT OF THE DONOR CORNEAL BUTTON

Goal: To transport the donor corneal button to the recipient eye and to secure it in the trephine opening of the recipient cornea with a watertight wound without endothelial trauma.

The contributing surgeons are evenly divided in the method they use to transport the donor corneal button from the table on which it has been prepared to the recipient eye. Half bring the block on which the donor button is resting in proximity to the recipient eye, lift the button from the block with fine-toothed forceps (Fig. 28–50), and transfer it to the recipient site. The remaining surgeons bring the donor button adjacent to the recipient eye on a Castroviejo spoon (Fig. 28–51) and place it in the trephine opening with fine-toothed forceps.

Similarly, the contributing surgeons are equally divided on the type of forceps they prefer to grasp the donor corneal button while placing the first suture. Half use a single-pronged forceps with 0.12-mm. teeth, while half prefer a double-pronged forceps (Fig. 28–52).

The majority of contributing surgeons place four cardinal sutures at the 12, 6, 9, and 3 o'clock meridians to initially

intraocular hemorrhage by irrigating to wash out the blood and maintain visibility (Fig. 28–48). If the hemorrhage does not stop spontaneously, most contributors use a bipolar cautery if they are able to identify the source of the bleeding. The Mentor wet-field coagulator is the instrument most commonly used (Fig. 28–49). Use of an appropriate intraocular diathermy probe also may be helpful. If this is unsuccessful, there is little to do but to suture the donor cornea in place and allow the elevated intraocular pressure to tamponade the bleeding.

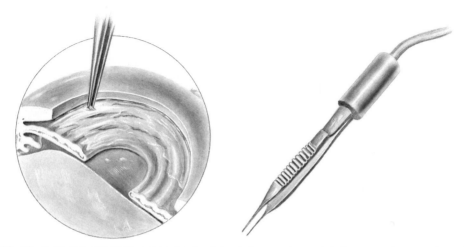

Figure 28–49. If an intraoperative intraocular hemorrhage does not stop spontaneously, a bipolar cautery is used if the source of the bleeding can be identified.

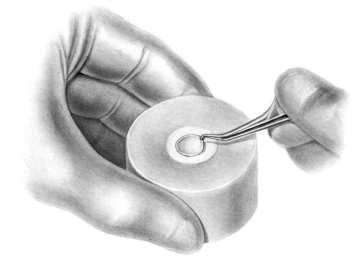

Figure 28–50. The donor corneal button can be transported to the recipient eye on the cutting block on which it was prepared.

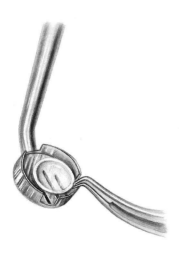

Figure 28–51. Alternatively, the donor corneal button can be transported to the recipient eye on a Castroviejo spoon.

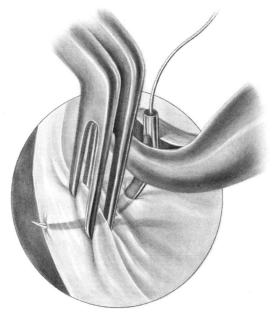

Figure 28–52. A double-pronged forceps can be helpful in placing the first cardinal suture.

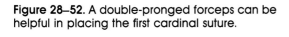

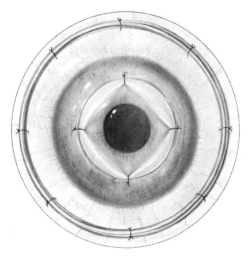

Figure 28–53. The donor corneal button initially is secured in the recipient bed with four cardinal sutures of 10-0 nylon placed at the 12, 6, 3, and 9 o'clock meridians.

secure the donor button (Fig. 28–53). Two surgeons indicate that they place eight cardinal sutures. With only one exception these authorities use 10-0 nylon for the cardinal sutures. The lone dissenter prefers 9-0 silk.

There is great variability in the suturing pattern used to secure the donor button and form a watertight wound. Following the principles discussed earlier in this text (see Chapter 24), a running suture or interrupted sutures or a combination of both may be used in any individual case as the circumstances re-

quire. However, in general the contributing surgeons prefer a running suture to interrupted sutures and tend to use a single running suture (Fig. 28–54) more often than a double running suture. On the average a total of five to seven bites per quadrant is placed (including the cardinal sutures). All surgeons use 10-0 monofilament nylon for the running suture, although several indicated that they prefer 11-0 suture material for the second stitch of a double running suture.

Almost all of the contributors agree that an optimally placed suture should incorporate seven eighths of the corneal thickness and believe that they can place most suture bites through three quarters to seven eighths of the cornea. Most contributors believe that 1.0 mm. represents an optimal size bite in donor cornea and that the bite in recipient cornea should be slightly longer, 1.5 mm. (Fig. 28–55). With one exception, all surgeons orient the needle perpendicular to the edge of the donor cornea and place individual bites radially across the wound. Also with one exception, when placing interrupted sutures, the surgeon places them sequentially on opposite sides of

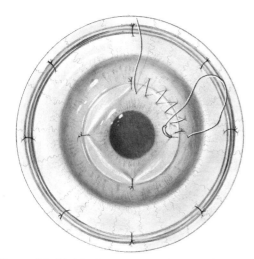

Figure 28–54. Most commonly, the donor cornea is secured with a single running suture of 10-0 nylon.

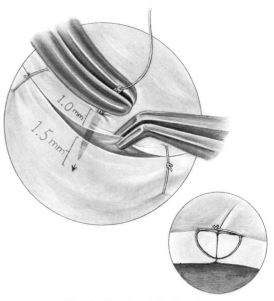

Figure 28–55. Ideally, the bite in donor cornea should be 1.0 mm.; the bite in the recipient cornea should be slightly longer, 1.5 mm. An optimally placed suture should incorporate seven eighths of the corneal thickness (inset).

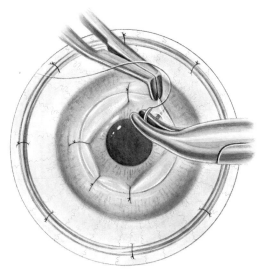

Figure 28–56. Interrupted sutures are placed sequentially on opposite sides of the donor button.

the donor button (Fig. 28–56). Only one surgeon indicated that he completely sutures one quadrant at a time.

Irrespective of the suturing technique for securing the donor button, most contributing surgeons place each bite beneath the tip of the forceps. Only two surgeons place each suture bite beside the tip of the forceps. All contributors initially place the tip of the needle perpendicularly into donor tissue, and most tend to visualize the needle tip as it emerges from the tissue edge in the wound in order to judge the depth of placement. Similarly, during each bite all of the contributing surgeons grasp the recipient tissue with the forceps. Only half of the surgeons use the forceps as a fulcrum over which to push the needle.

The contributors are equally divided over their preferred method for using the needle holder. Half turn the needle holder so that the needle is pulled through host tissue in sewing position and is ready for placement of the next bite. The other half reposition the needle in the needle holder after each bite. Similarly, while placing a running suture, half the surgeons tend to pull each bite snugly while suturing; the other half leave each loop loose and tighten them all later.

Most of the contributing surgeons maintain a formed anterior chamber during suturing by refilling the chamber with Balanced Salt Solution as necessary to keep it deep, introducing the solution through the wound with a 30-gauge cannula. Several surgeons maintain the anterior chamber with Healon while suturing, particularly in phakic cases. Use of this viscous material eliminates the need to refill the chamber during suture placement. All of the contributing surgeons use Healon if an intraocular lens implant is in place. Upon completion of wound closure most contributors deepen the anterior chamber with Balanced Salt Solution or, if an intraocular lens implant is in place, with Healon. Since Healon can cause a postoperative elevation of intraocular pressure, the smallest quantity necessary to protect the corneal endothelium is instilled.

Before the running suture is tightened, three or four loops are taken in the two suture ends, beginning the final knot and closing the wound at that point (Fig. 28–57A). These initial throws are used to take up the resulting slack each time all of the individual loops are tightened. Most of the contributing surgeons tighten the running suture by grasping a middle loop initially and tightening each successive loop around 180 degrees of the wound toward the free end, then repeating the process for the second half of the running suture (Fig. 28–57B to E). Only three of the contributors prefer to begin at one end and tighten successive loops around the entire circumference of the wound. To tighten each loop, it is grasped with fine tying forceps and pulled radially, parallel to the jaws of the forceps. Care must be exercised to avoid drawing the suture over the edge of the forcep tips, where it might be broken. The process may be repeated until the wound edges are approximated with slight tissue compression and the knot then is secured.

The technique for tying knots varies among surgeons and is influenced by such factors as whether or not the wound edges are easily juxtaposed and

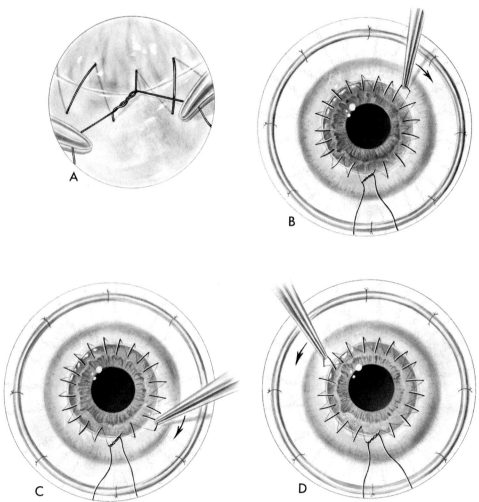

Figure 28–57. Prior to tightening the running suture, three or four loops are taken in the two suture ends *(A)*; these initial throws begin the final knot and are used to take up the resulting slack each time the individual loops are tightened. Then, a middle loop is grasped and each successive loop around 180 degrees of the wound is tightened toward the free end; the process is repeated for the second half of the running suture *(B to E)*. A common pattern for tying the final knot in the running suture is four loops followed by three individual single loops thrown in opposite directions to form a series of square knots *(F)*. Sutures are tightened to approximate the wound edges with slight tissue compression *(G)*. The tied suture is cut, leaving short ends at the knots *(H, I)*.

Illustration continued on opposite page

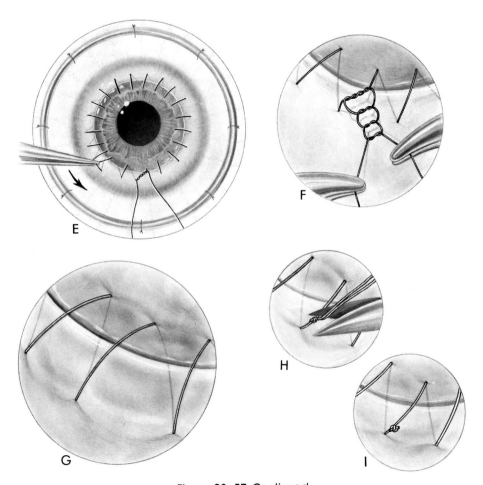

Figure 28–57 *Continued.*

whether one is dealing with an interrupted or a running suture. The most common patterns are four loops followed by three individual, single loops (Fig. 28–57F), four loops followed by two single loops, and three loops followed by two single loops. In each case, successive loops are thrown in opposite directions to form a series of square knots. Most contributing surgeons tie the knot firmly, approximating the wound edges so that slight tissue compression is visible (Fig. 28–57G). Few contributors tie sutures so as to only barely approximate the wound edges or sufficiently tightly to compress opposing wound edges enough to create a barrel-top configuration. Most cut the tied suture leaving short ends; a blade or scissors is used with equal frequency for this maneuver (Fig. 28–57H and I). A minority of contributing surgeons attempt to cut the tied suture flush with the knot; all use a blade for this purpose.

Virtually all contributing surgeons bury knots (Fig. 28–58A) on the recipient side of the wound though a minority bury them in donor tissue. For the most part, knots are buried in the anterior stroma, but several surgeons attempt to bury them at the level of Bowman's layer. None of the contributors enlarge the entrance of the suture track to facilitate burying of the knot. The conventional technique for burying a knot leaves the suture ends in the configuration of an arrowhead type of barb (Fig. 28–58A), which can interfere considerably with later suture removal. Therefore, after burying the knot, some surgeons reverse its direction slightly, causing the tip of the arrowhead configuration of the suture ends to point toward the corneal surface (Fig. 28–58B), which it is hoped will facilitate subsequent suture removal.

When the suturing technique involves placement of four cardinal sutures followed by a running suture, two thirds of the contributors remove the cardinal sutures at the end of the procedure. The remaining third leave the cardinal sutures in place at the close of surgery.

Corneal surgeons select specific sutures and needles to meet the peculiar needs of keratoplasty.

Sutures

All of the surgeons surveyed use 10-0 monofilament nylon suture approximately 23 to 27 microns in diameter. The nylon has the advantages of familiarity to the surgeon, induction of minimal inflammation in the tissue, and an acceptable tensile strength of 32 gm. Its elasticity allows it to stretch about 28 per cent before breaking. Since the nylon polymer contains water, the suture biodegrades at about 15 to 20 per cent annually, losing its color 12 to 24

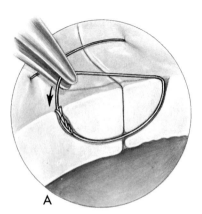

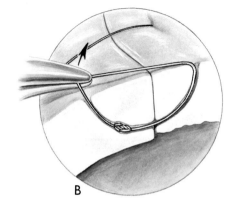

Figure 28–58. Knots are buried in the anterior stroma on the recipient side of the wound. This can cause the suture ends to form an arrowhead type of barb *(A)*, which may interfere with subsequent suture removal. After the knot is buried, its direction is reversed slightly, causing the tip of the arrowhead configuration of the suture ends to point toward the corneal surface *(B)*.

months postoperatively and developing focal breaks 24 to 48 months postoperatively, so that the free ends work their way to the surface, poke through the epithelium, and create a foreign body sensation and nidus for mucus accumulation and vascularization.

Polypropylene suture is both stronger than nylon, the 10-0 size having a tensile strength of 37 gm., and more elastic than nylon, with a stretch elongation of about 38 per cent. These characteristics produce more tissue compression. Since the polymer does not contain water, it is not biodegradable, as demonstrated by decades of use to secure cardiac valves and vascular grafts. In the eye, however, it may degrade very slowly under the impact of light. Polypropylene also ties differently from nylon: the suture flattens out in the knot when pulled tightly, whereas nylon remains round.

Nylon sutures of 9-0 and 11-0 diameter also are used in corneal surgery: 9-0 for closing corneal wounds where extra suture strength is needed, such as repair of corneal lacerations and placement of cardinal sutures in penetrating keratoplasty; the 11-0, which appears as tenuous as angel hair, as a second running suture intended to remain in the cornea indefinitely, because it buries easily in the tissue and compresses the wound less than larger diameter sutures.

Most surgeons avoid silk suture in the cornea because it induces greater inflammation and buries poorly in the tissue. New suture materials such as polyester are being developed for corneal surgery.

Needles

The corneal surgeon requires a needle that passes through the tissue with minimal resistance, has a curvature that creates a natural arc for a small, deep bite, and does not bend during surgery. Current needle design and sharpness are so good that many needles pass through corneal tissue without fixation by forceps.

All the surgeons use a spatula-shaped, side-cutting needle that penetrates the cornea easily, even though the sharpness varies among manufacturers. Surgeons must be alert to changes in needle quality and test samples of new products from suture company representatives.

The tensile strength of needles is important to surgeons who use running sutures, taking 12 to 20 bites to secure a penetrating keratoplasty. A needle that bends halfway around the graft complicates the rest of the suturing. Harder and stronger alloys are improving sharpness and durability of needles. The smaller the wire diameter of the needle, the easier it passes through the tissue—all other factors being equal. Needles usually used for corneal surgery have diameters of approximately 0.10 mm. (4 mil.), 0.15 mm. (6 mil.), and 0.20 mm. (8 mil.), the strength of the needle decreasing as the diameter decreases.

Needles are available in two configurations: single curve and compound curve. Single curve needles are the standard ones with a curvature of 140 to 160 degrees, the radius of curvature varying from approximately 2.5 to 2.0 mm. Most corneal surgeons prefer to take small, deep suture bites in an attempt to reduce astigmatism and enhance wound approximation. A needle with a greater curvature (160 to 175 degrees, radius 2.0 mm.) allows the surgeon to take a small, deep bite easily.

The compound curve needles are shaped like a fishhook, an appropriate appellation, since the needle tenaciously hooks drapes and lid specula during surgery. It has a greater curvature near the tip (about 190 degrees, radius 1.4 mm.) and a lesser curve in the middle and posterior parts (approximately 160 degrees, radius 2.50 mm.). Manufacturers have needles of different compound configuration, so the surgeon can select the one that suits him best. The compound curve needle enables the surgeon to make a shorter, deeper, squarer bite: using a straight needleholder and holding the needle so that the tip is perpendicular to the plane of the cornea, the surgeon passes the needle vertically toward Descemet's membrane, changes direction in the deep stroma and pushes the needle parallel to Descemet's membrane across the wound, and brings the needle out vertically on the opposite side of the wound, using the tip of the forceps for counterpressure.

The length of the needle is important, especially for placement of running sutures, since many surgeons bring the needle out far enough on the host side of the incision to grasp it in the center with the needle holder so it is ready for the next suture bite without repositioning. Needle length varies from approximately 4.8 to 7.0 mm., a length of 6.0 mm. being standard.

Sutures for Iris and Intraocular Lens

For suturing the iris, surgeons usually select a round needle that does not cut or tear the iris tissue. Needles used for vascular suturing are ideal for this purpose since they have a small diameter, a sharp curve, and a length similar to those used in corneal surgery. Alternatively long flat needles designed for suturing intraocular lenses are also available. The surgeon should tie iris sutures loosely, because the tight suture will often tear through the iris months to years after the surgery.

EVALUATION AND MANAGEMENT OF PROBLEMS AFTER WOUND CLOSURE

Goal: To detect and correct problems present after the donor button has been sutured in place.

Problems in the anterior chamber noted after wound closure are managed through the wound by eight of the contributing surgeons and through a preplaced limbal paracentesis by the remaining four. Ten of the twelve contributors evaluate the eye at the close of surgery for the presence of anterior synechiae simply by general inspection at high magnification through the operating microscope. Only two surgeons believe the slit lamp attachment on the operating microscope is of value. One surgeon finds careful observation of the dynamics of posterior movement of the iris as BSS is injected into the anterior chamber to be helpful in the diagnosis of anterior synechiae. Two other surgeons fill the anterior chamber with air while evaluating the eye for the presence of synechiae (Fig. 28–59); the air is subsequently removed.

These maneuvers sometimes cause iris attachments to the wound to break free. Should they persist, a small adhe-

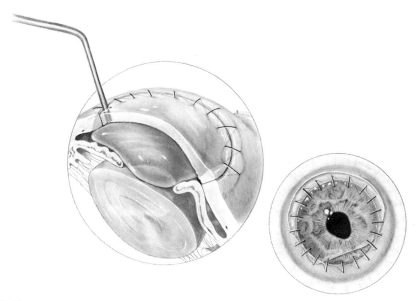

Figure 28–59. Upon completion of wound closure, the anterior chamber may be filled with air to aid in the detection of anterior synechiae; the air subsequently is removed.

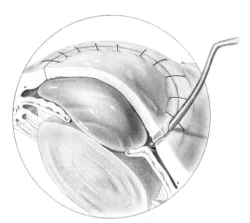

Figure 28–60. Small adhesions to the back of the wound often can be separated by passing a fine cyclodialysis spatula or by gently irrigating through the wound at the point of attachment.

sion to the back of the wound often can be separated by passing a fine cyclodialysis spatula (Fig. 28–60) or by gently irrigating through the wound at the point of attachment. More extensive and tenacious attachments may be separated by introducing a fine iris sweep through the wound approximately two clock hours away from the adhesion, passing it behind the host cornea, and gently sweeping toward the pupil to break the adhesion (Fig. 28–61). Use of an irrigating sweep or Healon facilitates this maneuver by maintaining the anterior chamber.

Peripheral anterior synechiae may lead to progressive angle closure ("zip-

pering of the angle") postoperatively. The surgeon should, therefore, make every attempt to ensure that they are not present at the conclusion of the procedure by careful inspection under high magnification. Often peripheral anterior synechiae are concealed by an opaque peripheral host cornea, but their presence should be suspected in eyes with a preoperative narrow angle, with a sector iridectomy, or with a history of intraocular inflammation. Attempts to separate them by sweeping with a fine spatula are fraught with danger; tearing of the iris, iridodialysis and hemorrhage may occur. Peripheral anterior synechiae are better and more safely approached by injection of Healon in an attempt to break the adhesion. If a large quantity of Healon is used, it is aspirated and replaced with Balanced Salt Solution to avoid postoperative elevation of intraocular pressure. If this technique fails, the synechial attachment is best left alone.

The presence of vitreous adhesion to the wound is difficult to see intraoperatively. Peaking or distortion of the pupil generally is the only clinical sign signaling its existence. If suspected, its presence may occasionally be confirmed by touching the tip of a cellulose sponge to the wound and observing adherent strands of vitreous humor as the sponge is gently elevated. Most of the contributors stress that this complication should not occur if a vitrecotmy is properly performed before the donor button is sutured in place.

There is a spectrum of opinion about the management of an irregular pupil observed at the close of surgery. Several surgeons do nothing if the anterior chamber is deep, particularly if a vitrectomy has been performed. However, the majority favor sweeping the involved area with a fine spatula. If this is ineffective, a minority favor the injection of acetylcholine into the anterior chamber and, if the pupil still is not round, an attempt may be made to cut the adherent vitreous strand by inserting an intraocular scissors blade through the wound between sutures.

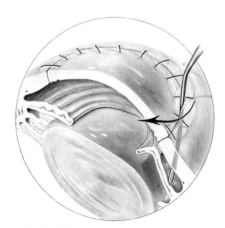

Figure 28–61. Extensive or tenacious attachments of the iris to the wound are separated by blunt dissection with a fine iris sweep.

With modern sutures and microsurgical techniques, wound leaks are infrequent. Nonetheless, the wound should be inspected under high magnification after it has been dried with a cellulose sponge. Gentle pressure is applied to the host cornea in each quadrant and the wound is observed for leaks. Any area exhibiting a leak is reinforced with an interrupted 10-0 nylon suture.

FACTORS THAT AFFECT POSTOPERATIVE ASTIGMATISM

Goal: To minimize corneal astigmatism after final suture removal.

Among the most difficult problems confronting the corneal surgeon is postoperative astigmatism. Factors that may contribute to astigmatism of a successful corneal graft include: (1) an eccentric trephine wound in the host cornea, (2) an oval trephine wound in the host or donor cornea, (3) a tight suture around the scleral supporting ring that distorts the host trephine opening, (4) an irregular margin in the host or donor trephine wound, (5) malposition of the donor button in the host trephine opening, and (6) improper suture placement.

The contributing surgeons share the belief that if meticulous surgical technique is exercised, little else can be done intraoperatively to reduce postoperative astigmatism. Only two of the twelve use an operating keratometer to check for it. Several trim the wound in areas where there seems to be less than optimal apposition of the wound edges. All replace and retie any interrupted sutures that are tied too tightly (Fig. 28–62) or too loosely or that are obviously malpositioned. Many attempt to distribute the tension of the running suture evenly after it has been tied. However, even if proper control of these variables produces a spherical graft at the conclusion of surgery, a large degree of astigmatism may appear months later following suture removal.

MEDICATIONS USED AT THE CONCLUSION OF SURGERY

Goal: To prevent infection, reduce inflammation, and induce mydriasis postoperatively.

There is little agreement among the contributing surgeons concerning the medications to be used at the conclusion of a penetrating keratoplasty. All but one surgeon instill an antibiotic topically, but a wide variety of antibiotics are used. They include chloramphenicol, gentamicin, tobramycin, erythromycin, a neomycin–polymyxin B–gramicidin combination, a neomycin–polymyxin B combination, and a bacitracin–polymyxin B combination. Five of the twelve contributors instill a corticosteroid topically. The drugs used are prednisolone acetate, dexamethasone alcohol, and dexamethasone phosphate. Nine of the twelve instill a mydriatic-cycloplegic agent at the conclusion of surgery. Most use a strong parasympatholytic agent such as atropine 1 per cent or scopolamine 0.25 per cent except in cases of keratoconus, in which cyclopentolate 1 per cent, tropicamide 1 per cent, or no mydriatic is employed.

Eight of the twelve contributing surgeons inject an antibiotic subconjunctivally at the conclusion of surgery (Fig. 28–63); all administer 0.5 ml. of genta-

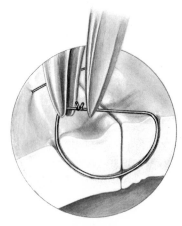

Figure 28–62. Any sutures that are tied too tightly or too loosely or that are obviously malpositioned are removed and replaced.

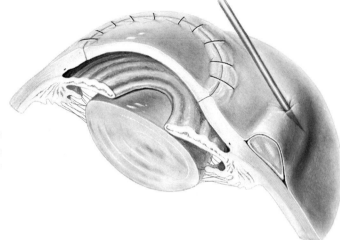

Figure 28–63. At the conclusion of penetrating keratoplasty an antibiotic or a corticosteroid or both may be injected subconjunctivally.

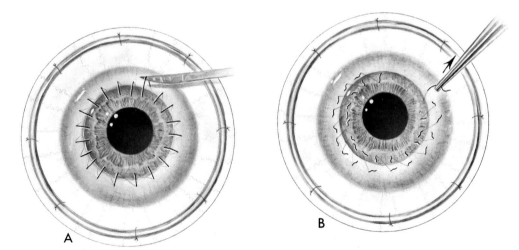

A

B

Figure 28–64. Sutures can be removed by inserting a fine knife blade beneath each suture loop on the host side of the wound, gently lifting and cutting each loop *(A)*, and then grasping the cut ends with jeweler's forceps *(B)*.

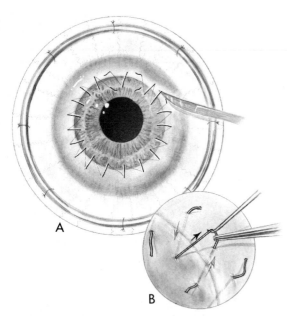

A

B

Figure 28-65. Alternatively, sutures can be removed by cutting every other loop on the host side of the wound *(A)*, and inserting the bent tip of a 22-gauge needle beneath the uncut loops to lift the suture fragments, which are then removed with jeweler's forceps *(B)*.

micin (20 mg). One surgeon injects 0.5 ml. of cefazolin (100 mg.) in addition. Eight surgeons also inject a corticosteroid subconjunctivally at the end of surgery. Six administer 0.5 ml. of betamethasone sodium phosphate (2 mg.), and two inject 0.5 ml. of dexamethasone sodium phosphate (2 mg.). In all instances the eye is covered with a sterile dressing, but a single or double patch may be used and it may be applied loosely or firmly.

TECHNIQUE OF SUTURE REMOVAL FROM CORNEAL GRAFTS

Goal: To remove sutures with minimal disruption of the corneal wound and the corneal epithelium.

The timing of suture removal varies among surgeons and is in part dependent on the suturing technique and the pathology for which the graft was performed. There is also great variability in the methods used to remove corneal sutures, but they include the following general techniques. A fine knife blade (e.g., Beaver 59s, razor blade fragment) is inserted beneath each suture loop on the host side of the wound; the loop is lifted gently and cut (Fig. 28–64A). The cut ends are then grasped with jeweler's forceps and removed (Fig. 28–64B). Alternatively, the surgeon may cut down on every other loop on the host side of the wound (Fig. 28–65A), insert the bent tip of a 22-gauge needle (or similar instrument) beneath the alternating uncut loops, and lift the suture fragments (Fig. 28–65B). They are then removed from the cornea with a jeweler's forceps. A topical antibiotic and corticosteroid generally are instilled and a patch is applied if necessary. Patients must be examined 24 hours after suture removal to ascertain that separation or shifting of the wound margins has not occurred.

Altering the Contour of the Cornea: Keratorefractive Surgery

29

STEVEN P. DUNN, M.D.

JAY H. KRACHMER, M.D.

It has long been appreciated that spectacles, and more recently contact lenses, may fail to provide satisfactory functional vision for many patients. This has prompted attempts at the controlled modification of the anterior corneal curvature to correct or alter refractive errors. The Chinese applied small bags of sand on their eyelids overnight in an attempt to alter the refractive status of the eye. Thermal cautery was used in Europe during the second half of the 1800s in an effort to flatten the cornea and reduce corneal astigmatism in patients with keratoconus. In 1949 Barraquer introduced the concept of implanting synthetic and alloplastic intrastromal lenticules as a means of correcting aphakia.[1] From these initial studies the field of hydrogel and lamellar refractive keratoplasty has emerged, with the goal of providing an alternative to the correction of myopia, hyperopia, and aphakia. Sato[2] in the 1930s and more recently Fyodorov and Durnev[3] have advocated the use of radial corneal incisions as a means of reducing and correcting myopia and astigmatism. High postoperative astigmatism, the bane of all ophthalmic surgeons, has received greater attention during recent years. Selective suture removal, relaxing incisions, and wedge resections have added much to our ability to manage this problem.

Technologic advances have played a key role in the development of many of these procedures. Sandbags have been replaced by contact lenses, bare electrical wires by machines that regulate and monitor temperature, and steel scalpels by diamond blades. Computers with sophisticated programs and lathing instruments are now an integral part of numerous refractive procedures. At times it seems that the technology itself may limit the use of many of these procedures by the general ophthalmologist. This is particularly true of keratomileusis, keratophakia, and epikeratophakia. The development of a feasible technique for storage of prelathed lenticules may reverse this trend and in the future allow for more general utilization of these techniques. In contrast, the relative simplicity of selective postoperative suture removal, relaxing incisions, and radial keratotomy has undoubtedly influenced their appeal and growing popularity.

The past four decades have seen significant advances in all of the keratorefractive procedures. However, large gaps in our knowledge still remain. This chapter will review the current status of many of these procedures. Research in most of these areas centers on predictability of the outcome of a procedure and the factors that influence it, stability of the ensuing surgical result, and identification of potential, immediate, and long-term complications. All are exciting evolving techniques whose final roles have not yet been determined.

ORTHOKERATOLOGY

Orthokeratology is the sole nonsurgical method of corneal refractive modification practiced today. This procedure has been defined by the American Optometric Association as the reduction, modification, or elimination of refractive anomalies by the programmed application of contact lenses or other related procedures.[4] It is the outgrowth of observations made by contact lens practitioners regarding alterations in the corneal surface, particularly flattening, induced by contact lenses. Since its introduction in 1962 the procedure has been surrounded by controversy. Much of the early information on this subject was empirical and conflicting. Different fitting techniques, incomplete data collection and reporting, poor controls, and inadequate follow-up and data analysis are but a few of the problems that characterize the early literature.

Kerns in 1976[5, 6] and Binder and coworkers in 1980[7] were the first to publish well-controlled statistical studies dealing with the predictability, stability, and safety of orthokeratology. A variety of fitting techniques and procedures have been advocated by orthokeratologists, and this has made it difficult to compare the results of different investigators. The technique of Grant and May[8, 9] described below appears to be one of the more popular approaches.

A large diameter (8.5 mm to 10.2 mm) hard contact lens fitted on K or 0.37 to 0.50 diopter flatter is prescribed. The power is adjusted to provide good vision. Following an adaptation period, re-evaluation is performed at four- to six-week intervals with successive lenses, fitted in the original fashion, being prescribed when flattening of the corneal curvature has occurred. This procedure is continued until a plano refraction is achieved or stabilization takes place. A plano or low plus retainer lens is then worn for a period of six months to facilitate further stabilization. When this has been accomplished, a slow, systematic reduction in the wearing time of the retainer lens takes place until lens wear reaches a minimum or becomes unnecessary. Though the need for a retainer lens varies from patient to patient, many require intermittent use of the lens to maintain the induced effect.[8]

A question that arises with orthokeratology is not whether corneal topography and refraction can be modified by the programmed application of contact lenses, for this has been well demonstrated, but whether it can be done in a predictable fashion. It was originally believed that myopia, hyperopia, and astigmatism could be treated with this technique. Grant suggested that the practical limits of the procedure beyond which full correction cannot be expected are 4 diopters of myopia, 2 diopters of hyperopia, and 2.5 diopters of astigmatism.[10] Binder found that the procedure was capable of reducing an average of 1.5 diopters of myopia in a group with a pretreatment mean refraction of −3.78 diopters. A second group with an average initial refraction of −1.87 diopters averaged an improvement of only 0.39 diopter. Twenty-eight per cent of this group developed more myopia during the course of the study. It was his impression that orthokeratology was capable of reducing myopia in eyes with moderate but not low refractive errors.[7] Kerns, using a slightly different technique, looked at 36 eyes with a mean spherical equivalent of −2.11 diopters[11] and noted a reduction of 0.77 diopter of myopia in this group. Both Kerns and Binder observed that nearly maximal reduction of myopia occurred by the ninth to tenth month with only gradual reduction occurring beyond that point.

Topographic evaluation of the central cornea has shown a significant flattening of the horizontal meridian but no significant predictable effect on the vertical meridian.[7, 11] The central cornea tends to become spherical, emulating the posterior surface of the contact lens. No significant alteration in the peripheral cornea, as measured with a Wesley-Jessen photokeratometer, was observed.

Kerns was able to make a number of general statements about the visual improvement in his patient group that have since then been confirmed by Binder. Orthokeratology can definitely change unaided visual acuity. Binder noted 70 per cent of the eyes in his study achieved 20/40 vision unaided and 55 per cent were able to obtain 20/25 vision at some time during the course of the study. In this same group of patients 35 per cent reached 20/20 visual acuity in the first 15 months, but only 20 per cent of the group was at this level after 15 months. Fluctuation in unaided visual acuity seemed to occur both during the course of the study and during any given day. Some individuals in Binder's study were able to predict when their best unaided visual acuity would occur. The quality of unaided vision was uniformly poorer than with contact lenses or spectacles. Though patients with less than 4 diopters of myopia tended to make up the bulk of patients achieving a good visual response, they still suffered from the same unpredictability and fluctuations in unaided visual acuity.

The permanence of benefits from orthokeratology remains questionable. The difficulty in getting a study group to relinquish their contact lenses is underscored by the number of researchers who have attempted to answer this question. Many patients, but not all, tended to approach their pretreatment levels of myopia and visual acuity when lens wear was discontinued. In Kerns' study two of 12 eyes followed to the end of the recovery period (56 days) were found to have an unaided visual acuity of 20/20. Sixty-seven per cent of the eyes (eight eyes) had some improvement in unaided visual acuity over prefitting levels at the end of the 56-day recovery period. Eighteen eyes could not be followed to the end of the recovery period, and it is speculated that many of these patients were unable to tolerate the poor visual acuity that resulted from cessation of contact lens wear. Six of eight eyes that reached the retainer lens stage in Binder's study were followed for 6 months after lens wear was discontinued. The average visual acuity in these patients prior to discontinuing the retainer lens was 20/35. At the end of the 6-month recovery period the average was 20/90. The average spherical equivalent increased over the same period of time in two of three patients. The cornea demonstrated a tendency to revert to the pretreatment keratometric values in both the horizontal and vertical meridians. The influence of long-term retainer lens use on the permanence of the orthokeratologic effect has not been evaluated.

Few adverse effects have been reported as a result of orthokeratology. Binder assessed various functional and structural corneal parameters and found no evidence of corneal warpage, scars, endothelial damage, or increased incidence of epithelial defects or abrasions during the course of his study. He did, however, report the finding of permanent corneal warpage in two patients referred for evaluation 18 months after orthokeratology was discontinued. Tredici reported seeing three patients who developed keratoconus-like changes following orthokeratology.[12] Long-term follow-up of this group of patients is definitely needed to determine the true incidence of complications. Slight reduction in corneal sensitivity similar to that seen in patients wearing conventional contact lenses has been observed. Distortion of the keratometric mires was noted in both Kerns' and Binder's studies and probably contributed to the objective observation of a decreased quality of unaided vision as compared to vision with hard contact lenses or spectacles reported by Binder. A number of his patients reported an inability to read with their lenses in place and required reading glasses.

Kerns noted the development of excessive amounts of induced astigmatism in two patients.[6] All patients had a tendency for increases in corneal curvature in the vertical meridian. The average astigmatism at the beginning of the study was 0.31 diopter and gradually increased throughout the study period and recovery period to a value of 0.69 diopter.

It would appear that orthokeratology can alter the corneal curvature in such a way as to provide good unaided visual acuity in some patients. Others, however, gain only a small measure of benefit or no benefit. Myopia is the only factor known so far to influence the predictability of the procedure. Kerns found a poor correlation between lens curvature and corneal curvature and the amount of corneal flattening and felt that corneal or ocular rigidity might be an important determinant.

The overall picture is clouded by the fact that it appears to take at least 24 months before the patient reaches the retainer lens stage. A large investment of time and money is usually made by patients involved in this procedure. Binder showed that if the refractive error was less than 4 diopters at the start of the procedure, the patient had approximately a 50 per cent chance to achieve better than 20/25 unaided visual acuity at some point during the first 30 months. However, the presence of fluctuating visual acuity and diminished overall quality of vision limits the value of this procedure to a small number of patients. The excellent tolerance of extended wear contact lenses by myopic patients would seem to be a more predictable and less time-consuming alternative method of providing stable, high-quality vision. Additional short- and long-term studies will be needed to determine the future role of orthokeratology.

THERMOKERATOPLASTY

Thermal cauterization of the cornea as a means of altering its curvature dates back to at least 1879. In that year Gayet reported his use of cautery in the treatment of keratoconus.[13] The cautery was applied to the apex of the cone until it perforated. Abadie, in an effort to avoid a central opacity, attempted to flatten the cornea by applying cautery to the base of the cone.[14] In 1900 Terrien reported on the use of cautery to reduce high astigmatism in patients with marginal thinning.[15]

Knapp described a series of 14 patients with keratoconus treated with a 2-mm. round cautery applied to the corneal apex.[16] The burn extended to the deepest stromal layers and perforation was effected with a fine point cautery. A firm monocular patch then was applied for 5 or 6 weeks. Although final corrected vision improved in 13 of the 14 reported cases, infection and secon-

dary glaucoma complicated the course of a number of the patients. Cauterization remained the treatment of choice for modifying the corneal curvature in keratoconus until 1936, when Castroviejo introduced his technique for penetrating keratoplasty.

Thermal keratoplasty, as we think of it today, was reintroduced by Gasset and coworkers in 1973.[17] Using data on the collagen shrinkage temperature of normal human cadaver corneas,[18] they developed an instrument that was capable of producing a graded flattening of the cornea. This technique, modified only slightly by those using thermokeratoplasty today, consisted of the application of the heat probe to the desired area for a few seconds. The temperature of the probe was 90° C and the procedure was generally performed with a topical anesthetic. Subsequent investigators have varied the temperature from 90 to 120° C and favor the use of multiple "instantaneous applications" under microscopic control. The procedure is viewed as a noninvasive means of altering the corneal curvature, and, therefore, its refractive status. It is touted as an alternative to corneal transplantation in patients with keratoconus, allowing the problems of long-term postoperative care, irregular astigmatism, graft rejection, and the inherent risks of the surgery itself to be avoided in selected patients.

Gasset and Kaufman in 1975 reported on a series of 59 keratoconus cases in whom visual acuity could not be corrected with either spectacles or contact lenses.[19] All were treated with thermokeratoplasty. Most demonstrated improvement in vision when fitted with a hard contact lens, with less than 5 per cent requiring subsequent penetrating keratoplasty. Other investigators, however, have since reported less successful results, with 50 to 78 per cent of patients failing to reach an acceptable visual acuity.[20, 21] Unfortunately only Keates and Dingle make note of the best pretreatment vision obtained by pinhole or poorly tolerated contact lenses.[20] The two patients in this series who avoided penetrating keratoplasty realized their best pretreatment vision with contact lenses after thermokeratoplasty, which is the most one can realistically expect from the procedure. The fact that most of Gasset's patients obtained a post-treatment visual acuity of 20/30 or better with contact lenses suggests that the density of the central scarring was less in his patient series. The gradual resteepening of the cornea observed by many investigators minimally influenced the course of events.[20]

Thermokeratoplasty, though initially considered a simple and safe procedure, has since been shown to have its share of problems. Arentsen and colleagues[22] and Fogle and coworkers[23] demonstrated destruction of the epithelial basement membrane by transmission electron microscopy. Damage to the basement membrane complexes persists for many months after thermokeratoplasty and correlates well with clinically observed, persistent epithelial defects and recurrent erosions. A possible neurotrophic component may also exist. Stromal haze is a uniform feature that may last from 1 to 15 months, occasionally becoming a chronic problem. Superficial stromal scarring is not uncommon. A number of cases of corneal thinning with and without melting have been observed. Two cases of anterior stromal vascularization have been reported.

The role of thermokeratoplasty in the treatment of keratoconus remains disputed, and the original enthusiasm for this mode of corneal modification has unquestionably lessened. Evidence seems to suggest improved contact lens tolerance regardless of the amount of keratometric change. Those patients with central scarring do not usually achieve a satisfactory visual result. Treatment of thin corneas is a contraindication because of the risk of perforation. Aquavella and coworkers reported accelerated recovery and healing of persistent corneal hydrops treated with thermokeratoplasty.[24] The use of thermokeratoplasty has not precluded or been shown to alter the outlook of eyes later undergoing penetrating kerato-

plasty,[25] and many investigators have advocated its use in patients who may be mentally unstable and do not require excellent vision. It is also a modality to be considered in patients who are unwilling or unable to undergo surgery for religious or medical reasons.

Other approaches to the use of thermal energy to modify the corneal curvature have been proposed. Rowsey reported the use of a radio frequency probe that permits quantitative electrothermal application to the cornea.[26] The probe has been designed to selectively heat the midstromal collagen to its contraction temperature without disturbing the epithelium and endothelium. This is contrasted with standard conductive thermokeratoplasty, in which the temperature peak and maximal structural effect are at the anterior corneal surface.

INTRASTROMAL HYDROGEL IMPLANTS

The concept of using an alloplastic intrastromal implant to modify refraction is one of the oldest in the field of refractive keratoplasty. Introduced in 1949 by Barraquer,[1] it was soon abandoned by him after a series of disappointing experiments. His attention turned to the new, more promising keratomileusis and keratophakia procedures. A slow trickle of experimental data did, however, find its way into the literature over the next three decades.

Flint glass, plexiglass, and semihydrated celluloidin were the materials originally studied by Barraquer.[1, 27] Lenticules were introduced into a central midstromal pocket. Initially lenses were well tolerated, modifying the anterior corneal curvature in proportion to their own anterior curvature. Unfortunately, however, all cases eventually failed as a result of the development of either an opaque, occasionally vascularized anterior stromal scar or anterior stromal necrosis with elimination of the lenticule. The retrolenticular stromal layers remained transparent in most cases. Barraquer believed that the poor tolerance of these lenses was due to their barrier effect on metabolic exchange between the posterior and anterior layers of the cornea.

Stone and Herbert, in an attempt to develop an artificial corneal graft, devised a two-stage procedure, the first stage involving the placement of a methyl methacrylate implant intrastromally.[28] Holes were drilled in the implant peripherally to allow for tissue ingrowth and fixation. Two of the nine interlamellar discs extruded at the end of 19 months, but the remaining seven were well tolerated by the rabbit eye for a period of 24 months.

The first reports of human studies were by Krwawicz in 1961.[29] These investigations stemmed from a series of rabbit experiments that had drawn three conclusions: (1) intrastromal lenticules change the refraction of the eye; (2) early corneal clarity is maintained, but there is a danger of late stromal opacification if the implants remain in place; and (3) the refractive effect of the lenticule continues even if the implant is removed after 8 to 10 days.[30] Eight aphakic human eyes underwent implantation of a plastic lens in a central, deep stromal pocket. The lens was removed after 8 to 10 days and the pocket allowed to close and heal unimpeded. Krwawicz claimed that the gap left in the corneal stroma did not collapse but was filled with optically clear stromal tissue. Partial correction of the refractive error was obtained and was stable over the limited period of observation (2 to 7 months). Krwawicz unfortunately never reported the keratometric or refractive changes in his patients. Visual results without overcorrection were reported as 20/60 in four cases, 20/80 in one case, and 20/120 in the other three cases. No long-term follow-up was ever reported. As judged by the absence of other studies or reports, the approach apparently never caught on.

The search for a suitable implant material and surgical technique continued with Bowen,[31] Belau and coworkers[32] and Henderson[33] conducting animal studies using coated and uncoated polymethyl methacrylate, silicone, and glass. Henderson and Belau in 1964 reported

the successful midstromal implantation of a polymethyl methacrylate lenticule in a human aphakic eye.[33] At 1 year the cornea was clear, but unfortunately the lens had migrated superiorly out of the visual axis, and the patient had to resort to the use of aphakic spectacles for visual correction.

Concurrently knowledge of corneal physiology was being advanced by a number of investigators who were using interlamellar plastic membranes as a research rather than a therapeutic tool. Knowles,[34] using a technique originated by Bock and Maumenee,[35] placed water-impermeable membranes intrastromally in rabbits. He observed thinning of the external lamella with eventual ulceration in many of the corneas. Brown and Dohlman attributed this to dehydration and were able to prevent it with tarsorrhaphies.[36] Brown and Mishima noted that evaporation of tears between blinks resulted in an increase in the tear tonicity that is in part responsible for an aqueous-to-tear movement of water within the cornea.[37] A nonpermeable interlamellar membrane disrupts this movement, and, if large enough and left in place for a long enough period, will lead to anterior stromal dehydration, thinning, and desiccation with attendant tissue loss. In a similar fashion the glucose concentration of the epithelium and stroma were found to be derived from the aqueous. Thoft and colleagues observed that the glucose concentration present at the anterior stromal surface is not in great excess of the epithelium's metabolic requirements[38] and suggested that a barrier to glucose permeability might easily lead to epithelial defects.

These observations led to the use of water permeable acrylic hydrogels as lenticular interlamellar implants. Glyceryl methacrylate (88 per cent water) was the first to be tried. Dohlman and coworkers, using flat implants ranging from 0.19 to 0.57 mm. in thickness, found anterior stromal thinning and extrusion in many of their rabbit corneas.[39] The implants were well tolerated, however, by cat corneas for the 11-month study period. The poor results in the rabbit model were thought to be due to the infrequent blink rate of this animal and the reduced permeability of glyceryl methacrylate in vivo. The role of thickness was not investigated. Mester and colleagues reported on the successful use of hydroxyethyl methacrylate (38 per cent water) intrastromal implants of 0.2 mm. thickness,[40] which were well tolerated by the rabbit cornea for the duration of their 18-month study. These implants were generally thinner than those used by Dohlman and coworkers and had an anterior base curve that matched the rabbit cornea.

The most recent studies are those of McCarey and Andrews,[41] who implanted lenticules trephined from perfilcon-A contact lenses within an interlamellar corneal pocket. These investigators were able to demonstrate a correlation between epithelial glycogen content and perfilcon-A thickness in the range evaluated (0.15 to 0.34 mm.). Their data showed a glucose flux across the hydrogel lenticule that was in excess of its epithelial consumption, suggesting the feasibility of using this material for refractive keratoplasty. The lenticules were extremely well tolerated with only slight dehydration of the stroma anterior to the peripheral edge of the hydrogel implant. It was postulated that this thinning was related to mechanical stress produced by the thick-edged implant and might be relieved with the use of thinner-edged lenticules. Subsequent experiments with thinner-edged lenticules have confirmed this impression, and long-term primate studies are currently underway.[42]

The appeal of heteroplastic intrastromal implants, particularly the newer hydrogel lenticules, stems from the relative simplicity of the surgical procedure. Although careful microscopic technique and instrumentation are a feature of all forms of refractive corneal surgery, the need for the surgeon to employ sophisticated lathes and complex computer programs is circumvented with this approach. Commercial production could provide both an ample supply and a wide range of standardized implant sizes, powers, and shapes. In the event that the patient's refractive status shifts, the lenticule can be removed or replaced. Minimal interface scarring has been observed in animal studies to date.

Thus, large strides have been made since Barraquer first introduced the concept of intrastromal implants. Hydrogel materials offer the greatest promise of the materials studied to date. Results of long-term animal studies currently underway will have a strong impact on the future of intrastromal lenticular implantation as a method of altering the anterior corneal curvature.

KERATOPHAKIA

Barraquer's disappointing results with synthetic intrastromal lenticules led to his investigation of cadaver corneal tissue as an optical intrastromal insert.[1] The benefits of alloplastic tissue were quickly appreciated, since its use averted the dissolution of the overlying epithelium and stroma and vascular ingrowth. The production of a predictable refractive correction then became the challenge. The procedure that Barraquer developed and has advanced with the help of many investigators is known as keratophakia (Fig 29–1).

Technically, keratophakia is a three-step procedure: (1) lathing of the donor tissue, (2) lamellar dissection, and (3) suturing of the anterior cap with the lenticule centered beneath it back into its original position. A modified contact lens lathe is used to carve lyophilized[45] or fresh frozen donor tissue according to a set of computer-determined parameters. These settings are based on the patient's flattest keratometry readings, desired dioptic correction, estimated thickness of the patient's anterior lamellar section, thickness of the donor's posterior corneal layers and, when freezing is used, the unfrozen and frozen thickness of the prelathed donor tissue. Once lathing is completed, the lenticule may be thawed, rehydrated, and immediately used, or it may be stored in liquid nitrogen[46] or in its lyophilized state until the time of surgery.

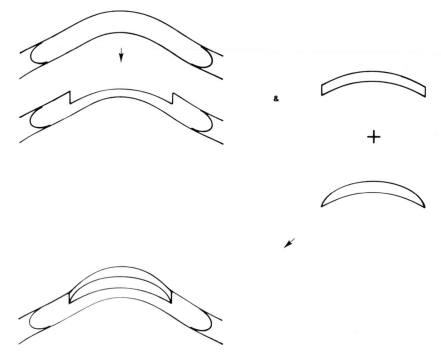

Figure 29–1. Keratophakia. A cryolathed donor lenticule is sandwiched between a lamellar piece of host cornea and the underlying stroma.

Surgery may be performed with the patient under general or retrobulbar anesthesia. A specially designed, grooved suction ring centered about the optical axis provides fixation of the globe and a means of raising and lowering the intraocular pressure. It also serves as a guide and template for the microkeratome, which is used to perform a superficial lamellar keratectomy. The keratectomized lamellae are sutured back into their original position with a continuous 10-0 nylon suture. The pre-lathed lenticule is inserted beneath this anterior cap, centered, and secured in position when the running suture is tied.

Various problems and complications may occur during each stage of the procedure. The lathe must be carefully calibrated and care must be taken to dial the proper settings lest a misshaped or incorrectly powered lenticule result. Since lathing is performed on donor tissue, abnormalities can be discarded. Improper placement of the suction ring results in eccentric anterior lamellae, or, worse, the ring may release during the keratectomy, causing an irregular cut or perforation. A dull blade will produce an irregular interface and optical interference. It is imperative that the donor lenticule be centered beneath the anterior lamellar cap to prevent induced distortion and aberration. Although dust and lint particles in the interface remain a common problem, these foreign bodies do not incite an inflammatory reaction or seem to interfere with the patient's visual result. Epithelial inclusions have been noted clinically and reported pathologically.[47] Once in place, the lenticules are extremely well tolerated; no immunologic reaction has been reported, which is not surprising since the keratocytes of the donor tissue are destroyed during cryopreservation[48] or lyophilization.

Visual recovery following keratophakia is usually delayed. Though most patients achieve 20/40 to 20/50 vision at 3 to 6 months postoperatively, improvement often continues for a year or more.[46, 49, 50] Various explanations for this delayed recovery have been proposed. Most surgeons feel that the lenticule must be repopulated by recipient keratocytes before visual recovery is maximal. Resolution of irregular astigmatism and corneal edema in the anterior cap and lenticule also seems to lead to improved vision. Troutman and coworkers felt there was a correlation between the final corneal thickness and visual acuity.[51] One also might speculate that the corneal endothelium might be incapable of completely deturgescing the cornea if corneal thickness exceeds a yet undetermined value.

The accuracy of keratophakia has steadily improved, with most surgeons able to achieve a result that is within 1.50 to 2.00 diopters of the desired correction. Troutman and colleagues recently reported a series of keratophakic cases that were corrected to within 6.5 per cent of the values calculated to correct their aphakia.[52] In this group of 32 patients 41.7 per cent were corrected to within 1 diopter of their calculated refractive error and 75 per cent to within 3 diopters. Twenty-five per cent required greater than 3 diopters of correction. Binder reviewed the visual results of more than 130 cases performed by different surgeons and noted that 70 per cent achieved a best corrected visual acuity with spectacles or contact lenses of 20/40 or greater. The best corrected visual acuity was 20/80 or better for 92 per cent of these patients. Overall, a predictability of 80 to 100 per cent was achieved by this group of surgeons.[50] Astigmatism tends to increase following keratophakia surgery; an average increase of approximately 1.50 diopters has been reported by both Troutman and Friedlander.[52, 53]

Keratophakia is primarily a secondary surgical procedure to be considered for patients who have undergone unilateral cataract extraction and, in addition, are unable or unwilling to function monocularly. Occasionally it may be considered in patients with bilateral aphakia who refuse to wear spectacles and in whom contact lenses have failed. Under these conditions keratophakia is an alternative to secondary intraocular lens implantation. Most investigators feel that a thorough trial of daily- and continuous-wear contact lenses is necessary before considering this mode of therapy. The advantage of keratophakia lies in its extraocular nature. Its disadvantages lie in the complexity of the procedure itself and the equipment used, the delayed visual recovery, and the limited accuracy of results.

An understanding of the complex mathematics required to determine lathing parameters and calibration and use of the lathe, as well as the cost of the instrumentation, have limited keratophakia's appeal. However, the introduction of clinically feasible methods of lenticular storage may dramatically advance the popularity of keratophakia. A ready supply of standardized, prelathed donor lenticules would remove the major obstacles to the use of keratophakia by many surgeons. The performance of a careful lamellar keratectomy with the microkeratome would be the only new procedure required of the surgeon. Although the present limited supply of donor tissue in most eye banks precludes the immediate "mass" production of prelathed keratophakia lenticules, the growth of eye banking and greater donor recruitment may make this practical in the future.

KERATOMILEUSIS

Keratomileusis is a term coined by Barraquer in 1963 to describe a lamellar refractive procedure aimed at reducing myopia and hyperopia.[54] In contrast to keratophakia and epikeratophakia, in which donor tissue is lathed to produce a positive lenticule, keratomileusis involves the cryolathing of the anterior lamellae to produce either a negative (Fig. 29–2) or positive cap. The actual procedure and potential complications are otherwise similar to keratophakia.

Swinger and Barraquer reported on the clinical results of 85 eyes undergoing myopic keratomileusis and 32 eyes undergoing hyperopic keratomileusis at the Instituto Barraquer in Bogota, Colombia.[49] They achieved a mean decrease in corneal power after myopic

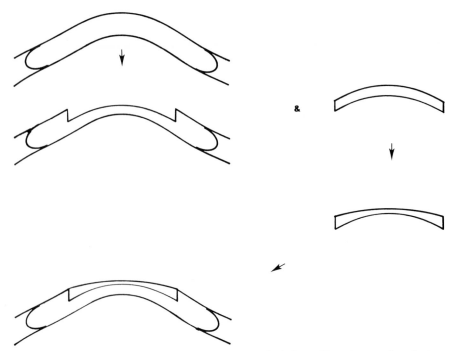

Figure 29–2. Keratomileusis. Patient's own cornea used. A lamellar piece of anterior cornea is removed and cryolathed to form a negative lens (myopic keratomileusis, shown in this figure) or a positive lens (hyperopic keratomileusis), then sutured back.

keratomileusis of 4.09 diopters and a decrease in the average spherical equivalent of 5.92 diopters. An increase in astigmatism of approximately 0.75 diopter was noted. Although a maximal keratometric change of 10.93 diopters was obtainable, the final mean correction after a follow-up period of 1.5 to 9.5 years was only 51.33 per cent with a standard deviation of 27.8 per cent. Visual stabilization required 2 to 3 months; a small but insignificant increase in myopia was noted in each subsequent year. The best corrected visual acuity was improved following myopic keratomileusis in 67.1 per cent of patients, unchanged in 24.7 per cent, and decreased in 8.2 per cent. Postoperative uncorrected visual acuities were not reported.

The 32 eyes that underwent hyperopic keratomileusis achieved a mean increase in corneal curvature of 8.04 diopters and an increase in the average spherical equivalent of 5.46 diopters. Astigmatism also increased. Undercorrection was common, with a mean correction after a follow-up period of 3 to 33 months of 61.4 per cent. The standard deviation

was 25.6 per cent. Visual stabilization was thought to be complete by 3 months. A best corrected vision of 20/40 or better was achieved in 87.5 per cent of patients without amblyopia. Again, postoperative uncorrected visual acuities were not reported.

Keratomileusis has attracted limited interest in the United States. Friedlander and coworkers reported on the results of seven cases of hyperopic keratomileusis and 11 cases of myopic keratomileusis that were performed using preserved corneal tissue.[53] The average overcorrection in the former group was 3.86 ± 0.63 diopters as compared with 4.35 ± 1.28 diopters in the latter group. Eleven of 18 patients achieved a best corrected visual acuity of 20/40 or better. Again, uncorrected visual acuities were not reported. Based on the results of these 18 cases, the investigators felt that hyperopic keratomileusis using preserved corneal tissue was less predictable than myopic keratomileusis.

Barraquer suggested a possible role for keratomileusis in healthy eyes in which glasses or contact lenses do not satisfactorily improve an ametropia.[55] Whether for myopia or hyperopia, the procedure currently lacks the predictability necessary to completely eliminate the refractive problem, and a moderate overcorrection is still required in most eyes to achieve optimal visual acuity. The popularity of keratomileusis will most likely remain limited until greater accuracy and simplification of the instrumentation and procedure are achieved.

EPIKERATOPHAKIA

Epikeratophakia is the newest approach to the surgical correction of refractive errors. Initially perceived as a means of correcting aphakia in patients unable to tolerate spectacles who are not candidates for or who are unable to cope with contact and intraocular lenses,[56] it has now also been used in the treatment of certain cases of keratoconus[57] and myopia.[58] A role in the rehabilitation of children with either congenital or acquired monocular cataracts has been proposed as well.

The concept of a "living contact lens" was introduced in 1979 by Kaufman in his Jackson Memorial Lecture on the correction of aphakia.[56] Developed by Werblin and colleagues, the technique requires that the recipient corneal epithelium first be denuded with absolute alcohol.[59-61] A 7.0 to 8.0 mm. diameter trephine then is used to cut through Bowman's membrane to a depth of 0.2 mm. The inner edge of the trephine mark is excised, leaving a circumferential groove 0.5 mm. wide. A positive lenticule composed of a central optical zone and peripheral wing is lathed from cryopreserved corneal tissue and then is sutured in place with interrupted 10-0 nylon sutures (Fig. 29–3). A 0.3 mm. thick plano lamellar graft has been used in patients treated for keratoconus.[57] The use of negative power lenticules as treatment for myopia has also been reported.[58]

Complications, though uncommon, may occur at any stage of the procedure. Technically, the most exacting portion of the procedure involves lathing the

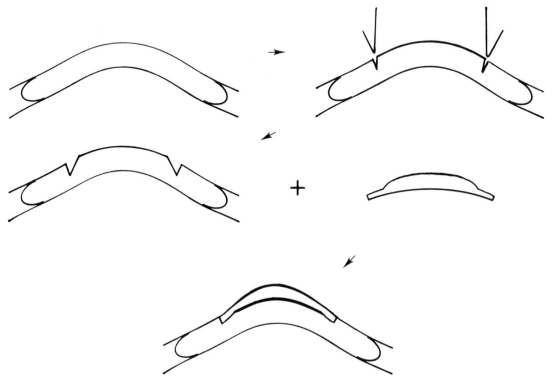

Figure 29–3. Epikeratophakia. Epithelium removed and a 360-degree groove formed. A cryolathed lenticule of donor tissue is then sutured into place.

donor tissue. Errors in computing the lathing parameters or in the calibration of the lathe will result in the production of an incorrectly powered lenticule. If a lathing mistake is recognized prior to surgery, the tissue can be discarded and a new donor lenticule produced. A distinct advantage of epikeratophakia over other refractive procedures is that most of the surgery is superficial and performed outside the visual axis. If the procedure is aborted or if the graft is lost secondary to trauma or infection or is intentionally removed, a peripheral, superficial scar is all that will remain, and the patient will still be able to wear a contact lens or spectacles. Interface opacities may result from dust and lint or residual nests of epithelial cells. Although persistent epithelial defects were initially a problem during the postoperative period, the use of a bandage soft contact lens worn for 3 to 4 weeks postoperatively has eliminated this problem. Preliminary results have been reported by Werblin and coworkers.[61] Although the follow-up period for the group was only 1 to 8 months, a best corrected visual acuity of 20/50 or better was observed in the eight eyes followed for 3 months or longer. However, only two of the eight eyes had vision equal to their preoperative acuity. A delay in lenticular deturgescence of 6 to 12 months has been noted and is one of the current drawbacks to the procedure.[62] McDonald suggested that the use of a tissue press, as discussed below, may result in more rapid clearing of the lenticule,[63] and further study of this approach is underway.

The question of whether epikeratophakia is applicable to the young pediatric population also is being investigated.[64-66] Delayed lenticular deturgescence and difficulty in producing clinically feasible high-powered lenticules are problems of particular concern in this group. In 1982 Morgan and coworkers reported the results in 28 aphakic children between the ages of 2 months and 6.6 years;[64] the longest follow-up was 17 months. Early in the course of their study they averaged an increase in corneal curvature of approx-

imately 12 diopters. The use of a tissue press in later cases led to an average improvement of approximately 16 diopters, but undercorrection remained a problem in most cases. Spectacle overcorrection usually was provided 2 months postoperatively, and intensive monocular patching was begun as soon as sutures were removed (5 weeks). Pattern visual evoked potentials were used to monitor amblyopia and visual acuity in the younger, preverbal patients. The epikeratophakia grafts were clear in 85 per cent of eyes, but it will take a number of years before a complete visual evaluation of the group as a whole can be performed.

Barraquer pointed out that, at least in theory, any amount of correction is obtainable by varying the thickness of the tissue, the diameter of the optical zone, or both.[55] Werblin reported that epikeratophakia could theoretically increase the power of the anterior corneal surface by as much as 37 diopters.[59] From a practical standpoint both biologic and mechanical limitations currently exist. McDonald noted difficult in creating human tissue lenticules of greater than 15 diopters with acceptably large optical zones.[67]

In Werblin's series, undercorrection was a major problem, averaging 4.66 ± 2.67 diopters.[61] Safir speculated that the poor predictability might be due to an inability to control corneal swelling or deturgescence at various stages of the epikeratophakic procedure. Therefore, a centripetal corneal press was designed that mechanically dehydrates the donor tissue prior to cryolathing. Preliminary data on the use of this device suggest greater agreement between the predicted and actual results.[68]

Epikeratophakia is an evolving technique that offers considerable promise in the management of large degrees of hyperopia and aphakia, but it is too early to determine its value in the future treatment of myopia and keratoconus. The problems of delayed deturgescence, undercorrection, and limited lenticular power are already being tackled by a number of investigators. Solutions to these problems, coupled with the perfection of a technique for storage of prelathed lenticules, would enable most ophthalmic surgeons to perform this procedure.

RADIAL KERATOTOMY

The use of radial incisions as a means of altering the corneal curvature was introduced by Sato in 1939.[2] Initially it was conceived as a treatment for keratoconus, but subsequent studies showed that a decrease in myopia and corneal astigmatism could also be obtained with this technique. Sato's procedure involved making five to nine posterior corneal incisions per quadrant through the endothelium, Descemet's membrane, and the posterior two thirds of the corneal stroma. Forty anterior radial incisions extending from the peripupillary zone to the limbus to a depth just short of perforation also were performed.[69] These procedures reduced myopia by 1.5 to 7.0 diopters in a small series of patients. A slight modification of this technique was used to reduce astigmatism, and a greater reduction was noted in the meridian of maximum curvature in these cases.[69, 70] Follow-up, however, revealed that an extremely high percentage of patients developed bullous keratopathy in their forties.

Interest in Sato's technique decreased but did not disappear. In the early 1970s Fyodorov and coworkers began experimenting with anterior surface radial keratotomy.[3] The present version of this technique involves making either eight (Fig. 29–4) or 16 radial incisions from a predetermined optical zone to the limbus. The current trend is to perform

Figure 29–4. Radial keratotomy. Sixteen or eight (now most popular) incisions, 90 + per cent depth, to the limbus, leaving an uncut 3- to 4-mm. optical zone.

these incisions with a diamond blade to a depth of at least 90 per cent of corneal thickness, as shown by pachymetry. Some surgeons perform peripheral deepening incisions. The incisions are irrigated of debris, an antibiotic is instilled, and the eye is patched. The role of postoperative steroids remains uncertain.

Many investigators have confirmed Fyodorov's findings of a reduction in myopia with radial keratotomy, but questions concerning the predictability of the procedure, its stability, and its potential immediate and long-term complications persist. To date only two large clinical series have been published (Fyodorov and Durnev in 1979[3] and Rowsey and Balyeat in 1982[71]), but they are not completely comparable since different techniques were used and different data were reported. However, certain trends and correlations seem to exist.

In the series by Fyodorov and Durnev published in 1979,[3] 676 patients who underwent radial keratotomy for myopia with a follow-up of more than 1 year were studied. The only preoperative information published from this study was the preoperative refraction. These procedures employed a 16-incision technique with varying optical zones, and the depth of the cuts visually approached three quarters of corneal thickness. Group A contained 130 patients with myopia of 3 diopters or less. Of these patients, 77.7 per cent reached emmetropia, 12.3 per cent were left with myopia of less than 1 diopter, and 10 per cent were overcorrected and made hyperopic. All patients had a visual acuity of 20/50 or better postoperatively, with 85.4 per cent of patients achieving 20/20 to 20/25. Group B consisted of 546 patients with myopia of 3.25 to 6.00 diopters. In this group only 20.8 per cent reached emmetropia, while 35 per cent were left with less than 1 diopter of myopia and 32.0 per cent had a residual myopia of 1.00 to 1.75 diopters. Approximately 80 per cent of these patients achieved a visual acuity of 20/50 or better, including 37.2 per cent who achieved 20/20 or 20/25.

A preliminary report by these investigators of 60 eyes suggested an inverse relationship between the diameter of the central optical zone and the effect obtained in patients with less than 3 diopters of myopia.[3] Therefore, it is assumed that the optical zones chosen in the series of 676 eyes were based on these data. Whether a correlation also existed for patients with greater than 3 diopters of myopia cannot be determined from the limited data reported, and no statistical analysis was made of data derived from either group of patients.

In 1982 Rowsey and Balyeat reported a study of radial keratotomy performed on 126 eyes.[71] In this study multivariant analysis was performed in an effort to determine the predictive value of such factors as the patient's age, diopters of myopia, corneal diameter, corneal thickness, anterior chamber depth, axial length, scleral rigidity, initial keratometry readings, size of the optical zone, and the final amount of correction. No single factor allowed for accurate predictability, but they were able to confirm statistically Fyodorov's earlier observation that the smaller the optical zone is, the larger the refractive change will be.

Patients were divided into 11 groups according to the number of radial incisions performed, the size of the optical zone, and whether or not the incisions extended across the limbus. The choice of optical zone size depended on the degree of myopia. Incisional depth extended to 90 per cent of the corneal thickness shown by pachymetry. Although patient follow-up was good, at the time of publication only 20 of the 126 eyes had been followed for 1 year, an additional 31 eyes had been followed for 6 to 11 months. Only five patients in the eight-incision group had reached a 6-month follow-up and none had reached 1 year. This relatively short follow-up time for all patients has placed some limitations on the assessment and interpretation of the resulting data.

Eyes with a preoperative refractive error of less than 4.00 diopters achieved an uncorrected visual acuity at 6 months of 20/20 or better in 70 per cent and 20/25 to 20/40 in 18 per cent of cases. However, 21 per cent were overcorrected. Those with a preoperative refraction of greater than 4.00 diopters realized a visual acuity at 6 months of 20/20 or better in 23 per cent and 20/25 to 20/40 in 23 per cent of cases. Only 4 per cent of patients in this group were overcorrected. Overall, 97 per cent of patients in this study showed some improvement in their uncorrected visual acuity.

A wide range of refractive change was observed in all groups studied. As noted earlier, multivariant analysis found the size of the optical zone to be a useful predictor of the amount of refractive change achievable. A 4-mm. optical zone resulted in a mean refractive change of 1.72 diopters at 6 months as compared with 4.46 diopters when a 3-mm. optical zone was used. The amount of correction achieved 1 year postoperatively in any single patient ranged from 29 to 134 per cent of the preoperative refractive error.

A partial loss of the initial power change occurred in all patients between the first and fourth week. Though Fyodorov reported stabilization of the corneal curvature by 3 months,[3] subsequent studies suggest instability for at least 6 months. Rowsey and Balyeat noted a postoperative variation in the refractive change from the sixth to the twelfth month of as much as 18 per cent.[71] Whether the cornea undergoes further change after 12 months has not been clearly determined.

The complications of radial keratotomy are varied but generally fall into two groups: those that are purely anatomic in character and those related to visual function.

Endothelial cell damage is the structural alteration that is of greatest long-term concern. Studies in nonhuman primates demonstrated a mean central endothelial cell loss of 6 to 10 per cent 1 month after 8- and 16-incision radial keratotomies to a depth of 90 per cent of corneal thickness were performed.[72]

A 14 to 15 per cent mean cell loss was observed in this same group of eyes at 6 months—a statistically significant difference. Hoffer and coworkers observed mean central and peripheral endothelial cell losses of 10 per cent and 9 per cent respectively.[73] No significant increase was observed in those eyes with perforations. Rowsey and Balyeat noted at 1, 6, and 12 months mean central endothelial cell losses of 5.6, 6.9, and 4.5 per cent respectively, suggesting that endothelial cell loss was not progressive.[71] Although those patients with fluctuation in their central curvature of greater than 1 diopter had slightly greater cell loss (9.4 per cent at 1 month and 15.7 per cent at 6 months), progressive loss was not observed at 1 year (7.3 per cent). Villasenor reported an increased cell loss with reincision.[74] Cowden and Sultana observed no significant difference between central mean preoperative endothelial cell density and postoperative cell density at 1 year.[75]

Alterations of the monkey posterior corneal surface 3 months postoperatively were observed with the electron microscope by Yamaguchi and colleagues.[76, 77] These alterations included linear protrusions on the posterior cornea beneath and parallel to the radial keratotomy incisions, foci of enlarged and degenerated endothelial cells at the central margin of the radial incisions and between adjacent incisions, and areas of exposed Descemet's membrane. Whether a greater degree of damage occurred at the time of surgery itself or whether corneal endothelial cells migrated and multiplied to cover these defects is not known. Immediately following radial keratotomy in their monkey model, Jester and coworkers found no histopathologic or transmission electron microscopic evidence of endothelial damage.[72] However, they did note an inflammatory cell infiltrate on and between endothelial cells beneath the incisions 48 hours postoperatively. They also found electron microscopic evidence of intercellular vacuoles and occasional abnormal-appearing endothelial cells, suggestive of cell degeneration and death, after 7 to 14 days. Following resolution of these changes, no additional damage was observed up to 6 months postoperatively. No linear ridges were observed in this study.

The long-term effects of radial keratotomy on either primate or human endothelial function are not known. However, the effects of radial keratotomy on the endothelial barrier in the rabbit were studied by Hull and coworkers using fluorophotometry.[78] Their preliminary findings indicated no alteration in endothelial permeability during the 6 weeks following this procedure.

Ingrowth of epithelium into the incisions, corneal vascularization, and perforation are well-recognized complications of radial keratotomy. Also, secondary traumatic cataracts may result from lens injury at the time of perforation, and one case of endophthalmitis has been noted.[79] Published reports of these complications are few thus far. The Rowsey and Balyeat study of 126 eyes[71] reported epithelial ingrowth in 14 per cent of these eyes, corneal vascularization in 1 per cent, and perforation in 10 per cent; but, as stated previously, these data were reported after a relatively short follow-up period.

The problem of fluctuating vision has been reported postoperatively in a high percentage of patients. An increase in anterior corneal curvature occurs in these patients as the day progresses. This problem seems to persist for an average of 3 to 6 months. Some patients require glasses or contact lenses in the afternoon or evening for satisfactory vision. Rowsey and Balyeat noted that most patients eventually stabilized at a point close to their evening refractive status, but they were unable to determine if the problem itself and stabilization of visual acuity were related to the number of incisions made.[71] It has been speculated that corneal hydration and intraocular pressure play a role in this problem.

Increased sensitivity to glare and difficulty with night vision are common problems that seem to correlate with the size of the optical zone and the width of the incisional scar. Objective assessment of these complaints has been aided by a new clinical glare tester.[80]

Overcorrection is a problem in 4.4 to 14 per cent of patients, its incidence being inversely related to the magnitude of the preoperative refractive status.[3, 71] Undercorrection has been more frequently encountered. This problem either has been left untreated or has been treated with repeat radial keratotomy or with spectacle or contact lens overcorrection. As mentioned previously, repeat surgery entails the risk of further endothelial cell loss. In addition, an increased incidence of corneal neovascularization in rabbit eyes fitted with cellulose-acetate-butyrate contact lenses has been reported.[81] However, despite some difficulties with fitting contact lenses on these patients, an increased incidence of neovascularization has not yet been reported. As more patients undergo radial keratotomy, it will become apparent whether or not this is a problem.

Since its introduction in the United States, radial keratotomy has caused excitement, doubt, and opposition among ophthalmologists and the public alike. This procedure does reduce physiologic myopia in most eyes, and clinical and laboratory research currently is being carried out to determine its effectiveness, predictability, and short- and long-term safety. Only when this information is known will an accurate therapeutic comparison be possible between spectacles, contact lenses, and radial keratotomy.

SURGICAL REDUCTION OF HIGH POST–CATARACT EXTRACTION ASTIGMATISM

Older literature recognized that astigmatism "against the rule" was a common finding following cataract extraction, presumably the result of loose wound closure, eroded or premature suture removal or absorption, or wound rupture. Improvements in surgical techniques, instrumentation, and materials have made possible tighter, less shiftable wound closures. The result of these improvements is an increased incidence of "with the rule" astigmatism. This condition may be a temporary one, depending on the type of suture used and the inclination of the surgeon toward suture removal.

Although much has been written about the effects of various sutures, types of incisions, and incisional closures on postoperative cataract astigmatism, no single reproducible technique yet exists to prevent the occasional occurrence of high postoperative corneal astigmatism.

Sequential keratometric evaluation of the cornea following cataract extraction demonstrates a change in corneal topography for up to 6 months, with most of the change occurring by the sixth to twelfth postoperative week.[82] Knowing this, it would seem feasible to intervene in those cases with high postoperative astigmatism at a point where keratometry readings have stabilized, that is, after 6 to 8 weeks.

Various surgical techniques have been proposed to eliminate corneal astigmatism following cataract surgery. These fall roughly into five groups, as follows.

Suture Removal

Nonabsorbable sutures facilitate the modification of the corneal curvature in cases of high postoperative astigmatism. A suture corresponding to the steepest meridian measured with the keratometer can be removed (Fig. 29–5). Although

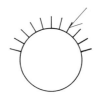

42.50 × 150°   +9.25 +3.00 × 60°
46.50 × 60°

Figure 29–5. Cutting sutures to reduce high postcataract extraction astigmatism. Cut sutures in steep meridian (in this example, 60 degrees).

an effect of this technique may be observed immediately, its full effect may be delayed.

Incisions Related to the Corneal or Scleral Wound

An incision is made with a razor blade fragment or diamond knife, either in the original cataract incision or concentric with it, and running perpendicular to the steepest meridian to a depth of half the cornea or sclera. This procedure is similar to the relaxing incisions performed for high astigmatism following penetrating keratoplasty.

Thermal Cauterization

Many surgeons have experimented with this modality, which unquestionably has the desired result of steepening the treated meridian. However, the technique has lost its appeal because of its unpredictability.

Corneal Resection

Single and double corneal wedge resections have been employed successfully in the management of large degrees of corneal astigmatism following cataract extraction and penetrating keratoplasty. This technique involves the incision of a partial-thickness crescentic wedge 1 to 2 mm. wide and three clock hours long at one end of the flatter meridian. The resulting gap is then closed with non-absorbable sutures.[83, 84] Troutman suggested the use of this procedure at the time of surgery if "against the rule" astigmatism in excess of 4 or 5 diopters is noted preoperatively.[85] In these cases a small wedge of tissue is removed from the anterior lip of the incision and closure is made in the usual fashion.

Anterior or Posterior Nonperforating Corneal Incisions

Sato was one of the first to suggest the use of corneal incisions to reduce astigmatism.[69] He devised a tangential form and a radial form of posterior half-corneal incisions, and his initial results were good. However, many of his patients developed endothelial decompensation in later years. Anterior corneal incisions either tangential to the steep meridian or parallel to it have been proposed by Fyodorov and have been considered successful in many cases.[3] Further information regarding this method should be forthcoming as experience with radial keratotomy and its application to postoperative corneal astigmatism increases.

WEDGE RESECTION AND RELAXING INCISIONS FOR HIGH POSTKERATOPLASTY ASTIGMATISM

Improvements in microsurgical techniques and instrumentation, surgical training, eye banking procedures, and the management of postoperative complications have enabled corneal surgeons to expect a very high rate of clear grafts after penetrating keratoplasty. Although the graft may be clear the patient may not regain good vision because of residual high astigmatism. In an attempt to correct the problem, contact lenses or even spectacles with a high cylindrical power often are tried, but in some cases they fail to restore useful vision. This forces the physician to choose between doing nothing to correct the refractive problem or performing an additional surgical procedure to reduce the astigmatism.

The simplest procedure to reduce postkeratoplasty astigmatism is to remove selected sutures when still in place. Slit-lamp examination often reveals tight sutures in the steep meridian. Once the keratoplasty wound has healed and all sutures have been removed, the modification of postkeratoplasty astigmatism must be done by other methods.

It is a simple matter to remove interrupted sutures. Figure 29–6 illustrates the removal of selected interrupted sutures or portions of a running suture. Since the patient has astigmatism with

RUNNING

INTERRUPTED

steep × 90°

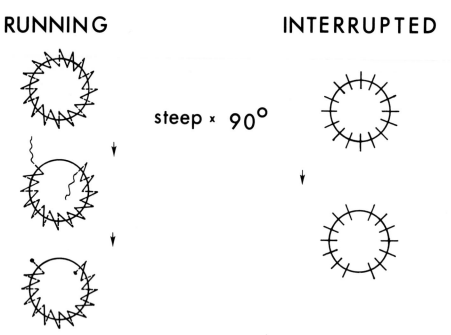

Figure 29–6. Selective suture removal to reduce high postkeratoplasty astigmatism. Remove suture segment(s), or individual suture(s) at one or both ends of the steep meridian (90 degrees in this example).

the steep meridian at 90 degrees, sutures in the 90-degree and/or 270-degree meridian are removed.

Removal of a segment of running suture is more difficult but can be performed either at the slit lamp or under an operating microscope. Usually one must operate on both ends of the steep meridian. The suture is first cut in the steep meridian, and one or two loops are loosened to provide enough material to tie a knot. The points of one tying forceps grasp the loose end of the suture, which is then wrapped around the tips of another forceps. The suture is then pulled gently away from the cornea and down into a knot which, when released, will retract slightly into the tissue. A microscissors is then used to trim the loop and free end as close to the cornea as possible.

Surgical attempts to reduce high astigmatism after corneal transplantation are aimed at steepening the flatter meridian or flattening the steeper meridian. Troutman was the first to describe the wedge resection to steepen the flatter meridian and relaxing incisions to flatten the steeper meridian.[85, 86] Although both procedures are effective,[83] they differ sub-

stantially in level of difficulty, inconvenience to the patient, length of time before satisfactory visual acuity is reached, and expense. With regard to all of these factors, a relaxing incision is a better procedure than a wedge resection.

The wedge resection is an operating room procedure. All examinations required before penetrating keratoplasty are performed, retrobulbar anesthesia is administered, and an operating microscope is used. The first incision is made to three-quarters depth into the transplant wound for slightly less than three clock hours at one end of the flatter meridian. A second incision is made either in the host tissue or the donor tissue to form a crescentic wedge with the widest central portion between 1 and 2 mm. wide. (The exact width is determined grossly by the amount of astigmatism rather than by mathematic calibration.) A paracentesis is performed to facilitate wound closure. Usually seven to nine interrupted 10-0 nylon sutures are used to close the wound, the knots are buried, and the steeper meridian should then be in the meridian of the wedge resection. A keratometer or keratoscope can be used to confirm the shift

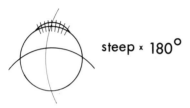

Figure 29–7. Wedge resection to reduce high postkeratoplasty astigmatism. Wedge used to steepen the flatter meridian (90 degrees in example shown).

of the steeper meridian to that of the wedge resection.

The patient can be discharged on the first or second day after surgery. Antibiotics and topical steroids are instilled, and after a week the antibiotics are stopped and the steroids tapered. Since the interrupted sutures are in the steeper meridian, they can gradually be removed to reduce the astigmatism to as close to zero as possible. However, the sutures must not be removed for 4 to 6 weeks to preserve the effect of the wedge resection. Figure 29–7 is a diagram of a patient with astigmatism in which the steep meridian is at 180 degrees. A wedge resection would therefore be performed in the flatter meridian, which places the wedge either at 90 or 270 degrees. In this case there was enough distance between the transplant wound and the limbus to place the second incision in the host tissue rather than the donor tissue.

In contrast to the wedge resection, which must be performed in the operating room, relaxing incisions can be done at the slit lamp on an outpatient basis with the patient under topical anesthesia. A sterile razor blade in a blade holder or possibly the new instruments that are used for radial keratotomy can be used. Relaxing incisions are made directly in the corneal transplant wound, from one-half to two-thirds its depth, at both ends of the steep meridian for approximately two clock hours. The surgeon must examine the posterior wound with a slit lamp in order to identify defects so as not to make the incisions too deep. Extra care must be taken in aphakic patients to avoid the

potential of vitreous coming to a site of perforation, and minor operating room facilities should be available for closure of a perforation, if it occurs, with an interrupted 10-0 nylon suture.

The patient instills antibiotic drops four times daily at home and returns in 1 week, at which time the wounds have usually re-epithelialized and antibiotic drops can be stopped. A refraction can be planned for 4 to 6 weeks postoperatively, when keratometry readings are usually stable. Sometimes, however, immediately after relaxing incisions have been performed, patients experience greatly improved vision because of dramatically reduced corneal astigmatism.

It must be emphasized that relaxing incisions will have little or no effect if they are performed a long time after sutures have been removed. Therefore, it is advisable to examine the patient 1 month after suture removal, at which time a plan of management can be instituted if high astigmatism exists. If relaxing incisions are decided upon, they can be made at that time. Figure 29–8 illustrates high corneal astigmatism with the steep axis at 180 degrees and relaxing incisions would be made in this case at both ends of the horizontal meridian.

Relaxing incisions are probably the procedure of choice for high postkeratoplasty astigmatism because results are achieved within 4 to 6 weeks rather than a year or longer and because it is an outpatient procedure rather than a major eye operation requiring hospitalization. Because relaxing incisions are easy to perform and have not been associated with significant complications, patients

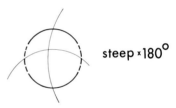

Figure 29–8. Relaxing incisions to reduce high postkeratoplasty astigmatism. Incisions placed in the graft wound to flatten the steeper meridian (180 degrees in example shown).

with as little as 4 to 5 diopters of corneal astigmatism can benefit from the procedure. A patient with 5 diopters of corneal astigmatism would require approximately 3.5 diopters of refractive cylinder in spectacles. Relaxing incisions usually would reduce the astigmatism to no more than 2 diopters, in which case the refractive cylindric requirement would be about 1.5 diopters and therefore more acceptable. If adequate reduction of astigmatism is not achieved from relaxing incisions, a wedge resection can be performed later.

REFERENCES

1. Barraquer, J. I.: Queratoplastia refractiva. Estudias e Informaciones Oftalmologiaces 2:10, 1949.
2. Sato, T.: Treatment of conical cornea (incision of Descemet's membrane). Acta Soc Ophthalmol Jpn 43:541, 1939.
3. Fyodorov, S. N., and Durnev, V. V.: Operation of dosaged dissection of corneal circular ligament in cases of myopia of mild degree. Ann Ophthalmol 11:1885, 1979.
4. American Optometric Association—Project Team on Orthokeratology (Activity No. 62530).
5. Kerns, R. L.: Research in orthokeratology. Part II: Experimental design, protocol and method. J Amer Optom Assoc 47:1275, 1976.
6. Kerns, R. L.: Research in orthokeratology. Part III: Results and observations. J Amer Optom Assoc 47:1505, 1976.
7. Binder, P. S., May, C. H., and Grant, S. C.: An evaluation of orthokeratology. Ophthalmology 87:729, 1980.
8. Grant, S. C. and May, C. H.: Orthokeratology—Control of refractive errors through contact lenses. J Amer Optom Assoc 42:1277, 1971.
9. Orthokeratology Fitting Sets Educational Bulletin. AO Contact Lens Division, 1973.
10. Grant, S. C.: Orthokeratology: A safe and effective treatment for a disabling problem. Surv Ophthalmol 24:291, 1980.
11. Kerns, R. L.: Research in orthokeratology. Part VIII: Results, conclusions, and discussion of techniques. J Amer Optom Assoc 49:308, 1978.
12. Tredici, T. J.: Role of orthokeratology: A perspective. Trans Amer Acad Ophthalmol 86:698, 1979.
13. Gayet: Lyon medicale XXX, 1879.
14. Abadie, C.: These de Guot, 1887.
15. Terrien: Dystrophie marginale symétrique des deux cornées avec astigmatisme régular consécutif et guérison par la cautérisation ignée. Arch Ophthalmol (Paris) 20:12, 1900.
16. Knapp, A.: Keratoconus: Etiology and treatment. Arch Ophthalmol 2:658, 1929.
17. Gasset, A. R., Shaw, E. L., Kaufman, H. E., et al.: Thermokeratoplasty. Trans Amer Acad Ophthalmol Otolaryngol 77:441, 1973.
18. Stringer, H., and Parr, J.: Shrinkage temperature of eye collagen. Nature 204:107, 1964.
19. Gasset, A. R., and Kaufman, H. E.: Thermokeratoplasty in the treatment of keratoconus. Amer J Ophthalmol 79:226, 1975.
20. Keates, R. H., and Dingle, J.: Thermokeratoplasty for keratoconus. Ophthalmic Surg 6:89, 1975.
21. Stark, W. J.: Keratoconus. Audio-Digest 13:15, 1975.
22. Arentsen, J. J., Rodrigues, M. M., and Laibson, P. R.: Histopathologic changes after thermokeratoplasty for keratoconus. Invest Ophthalmol Vis Sci 16:32, 1977.
23. Fogle, J. A., Kenyon, K. R., and Stark, W. J.: Damage to epithelial basement membrane by thermokeratoplasty. Amer J Ophthalmol 83:392, 1977.
24. Aquavella, J. V., Buxton, J. N., and Shaw, E. L.: Thermokeratoplasty in the treatment of persistent cornea hydrops. Arch Ophthalmol 95:81, 1977.
25. Mandelberg, A. I., Rao, G., and Aquavella, J. V.: Penetrating keratoplasty following thermokeratoplasty. Ophthalmology 87:750, 1980.
26. Rowsey, J. J.: Radiofrequency probe keratoplasty. In Schachar, R. A., Levy, N. S., and Schachar, L. (eds.): Keratorefraction. Denison, Texas, LAL Publishing, 1980, p. 65.
27. Barraquer, J. I.: Modification of refraction by means of intracorneal inclusions. Int Ophthalmol Clin 6:53, 1966.
28. Stone, W., and Herbert, E.: Experimental study of plastic material as replacement for the cornea: A preliminary report. Amer J Ophthalmol 36:168, 1953.
29. Krwawicz, T.: New plastic operation for correcting the refractive error of aphakic eyes by changing the corneal curvature. Preliminary report. Brit J Ophthalmol 45:59, 1961.
30. Krwawicz, T.: Attempted modification of corneal curvature by means of experimental plastic surgery. Klin Oczna 30:229, 1960.
31. Bowen, S. F.: Intracorneal lens: Experimental study. Proc Mayo Clin 36:627, 1961.
32. Belau, P. G., Dyer, J. A., Ogle, K. N., and Henderson, J. W.: Correction of ametropia with intracorneal lenses: An experimental study. Arch Ophthalmol 72:541, 1964.
33. Henderson, J. W., and Belau, P. G.: Insertion of a plastic intracorneal lens: Report of case. Proc Mayo Clin 39:772, 1964.
34. Knowles, W. F.: Effect of intralamellar plastic membranes on corneal physiology. Amer J Ophthalmol 51:274, 1961.
35. Bock, R., and Maumenee, A. E.: Corneal fluid metabolism: Experiments and observations. Arch Ophthalmol 50:282, 1953.
36. Brown, S. I., and Dohlman, C. H.: A buried corneal implant serving as a barrier to fluid. Arch Ophthalmol 73:635, 1965.
37. Brown, S. I., and Mishima, S.: The effect of intralamellar water-impermeable membranes on corneal hydration. Arch Ophthalmol 76:702, 1966.
38. Thoft, R. A., Friend, J., and Dohlman, C. H.: Corneal glucose concentration: Flux in the presence and absence of epithelium. Arch Ophthalmol 85:467, 1971.
39. Dohlman, C. H., Refojo, M. F., and Rose, J.: Synthetic polymers in corneal surgery. I. Glyceryl methacrylate. Arch Ophthalmol 77:252, 1967.
40. Mester, V., Roth, K., and Dardenne, M. V.: Versuche mit 2–hydroxyaethylmethacrylat Linsen als Keratophakie-material. Ber Dtsch Ophthalmol Ges 72:326, 1972.

41. McCarey, B. E., and Andrews, D. M.: Refractive keratoplasty with intrastromal hydrogel lenticular implants. Invest Ophthalmol Vis Sci 21:107, 1981.

42. McCarey, B. E.: Personal communication

43. Mester, V., Heimig, D., and Dardenne, M. V.: Measurement and calculation of refraction in experimental keratophakia with hydrophilic lenses. Ophthalmol Res 8:111, 1976.

44. Gillette, T. E., Udell, I. J., and Abelson, M. B.: Hydrogel keratophakia. In Schachar, R. A., Levy, N. S., and Schachar, L. (eds.): Keratorefraction. Denison, Texas, LAL Publishing, 1980, p. 127.

45. Maguen, E., and Nesburn, A. B.: A new technique for lathing lyophilized cornea for refractive keratoplasty. Arch Ophthalmol 100:119, 1982.

46. Friedlander, M. H., Rich, L. F., Werblin, T. P., Kaufman, H. E., and Granet, N.: Keratophakia using preserved lenticules. Ophthalmology 88:687, 1980.

47. Binder, P. S., Beale, J. P., and Zavala, E. Y.: The histopathology of a case of keratophakia. Arch Ophthalmol 100:101, 1982.

48. Rich, L. F., Friedlander, M. H., Kaufman, H. E., and Granet, N.: Keratocyte survival in keratophakia lenticules. Arch Ophthalmol 99:677, 1981.

49. Swinger, C. A., and Barraquer, J. I.: Keratophakia and keratomileusis: Clinical results. Ophthalmology 88:709, 1981.

50. Binder, P. S.: Refractive surgery for aphakia. Symposium CLAO, Las Vegas, 1982.

51. Troutman, R. C., Swinger, C. A., and Kelley, R. J.: Keratophakia: A preliminary evaluation. Ophthalmology 86:523, 1979.

52. Troutman, R. C., Swinger, C. A., and Goldstein, M.: Keratophakia update. Ophthalmology 88:36, 1981.

53. Friedlander, M. H., Werblin, T. P., Kaufman, H. E., and Granet, N. S.: Clinical results of keratophakia and keratomileusis. Ophthalmology 88:716, 1981.

54. Barraquer, J. I.: Queratomileusis para la correccion de la miopia. An Inst Barraquer 5:209:2, 1964.

55. Barraquer, J. I.: Keratomileusis for myopia and aphakia. Ophthalmology 88:701, 1981.

56. Kaufman, H. E.: The correction of aphakia: XXXVI Edward Jackson memorial lecture. Amer J Ophthalmol 89:1, 1980.

57. Kaufman, H. E., and Werblin, T. P.: Epikeratophakia for the treatment of keratoconus. Amer J Ophthalmol 93:324, 1982.

58. Berkowitz, R. A., McDonald, M. B., Werblin, T. P., Safir, A., and Kaufman, H. E.: Epikeratophakia for myopia. Invest Ophthalmol Vis Sci 22(Suppl):201, 1982.

59. Werblin, T. P., and Klyce, S. D.: Epikeratophakia: The surgical correction of aphakia. I. Lathing of corneal tissue. Curr Eye Res 1:123, 1981.

60. Werblin, T. P., and Kaufman, H. E.: Epikeratophakia: The surgical correction of aphakia. II. Preliminary results in a non-human primate model. Curr Eye Res 1:131, 1981.

61. Werblin, T. P., Kaufman, H. E., Friedlander, M. H., and Granet, N.: Epikeratophakia: The surgical correction of aphakia. III. Preliminary results of a prospective clinical trial. Arch Ophthalmol 99:1957, 1981.

62. Werblin, T. P.: Refractive surgery for aphakia: Symposium CLAO, Las Vegas, 1982.

63. McDonald, M. B.: Refractive surgery for aphakia: Symposium CLAO, Las Vegas, 1982.

64. Morgan, K. S., Asbell, P. A., May, J. G., Loupe, D. N., and Kaufman, H. E.: Surgical and functional results of pediatric epikeratophakia. Invest Ophthalmol Vis Sci 22:(Suppl):201, 1982.

65. Morgan, K. S., Werblin, T. P., Friedlander, M. H., and Kaufman, H. E.: Epikeratophakia in the pedi-

atric patient: A case report. J Ocular Ther Surg 1:198, 1982.

66. Morgan, K. S., Werblin, T. P., Asbell, P. A., Loupe, D. N., Friedlander, M. H., and Kaufman, H. E.: The use of epikeratophakia grafts in pediatric monocular aphakia. J Pediatr Ophthalmol 18:23, 1981.

67. McDonald, M. B., Friedlander, M. H., Koenig, S., and Kaufman, H. E.: Alloplastic epikeratophakia in monkeys. Invest Ophthalmol Vis Sci 22(Suppl):26, 1982.

68. Safir, A.: Refractive surgery for aphakia: Symposium CLAO, Las Vegas, 1982.

69. Sato, T., Akiyama, K., and Shibata, H.: A new surgical approach to myopia. Amer J Ophthalmol 36:823, 1953.

70. Sato, T.: Posterior half-incision of cornea for astigmatism. Amer J Ophthalmol 36:462, 1953.

71. Rowsey, J. J., and Balyeat, H. D.: Preliminary results and complications of radial keratotomy. Amer J Ophthalmol 93:437, 1982.

72. Jester, J. V., Steel, D., Salz, J., Miyashiro, J., Rife, L., Schanzlin, D. J., and Smith, R. E.: Radial keratotomy in non-human primate eyes. Amer J Ophthalmol 92:153, 1981.

73. Hoffer, K. J., Darin, J. J., Pettit, T. H., Hofbauer, J. D., Elander, R., and Levenson, J. E.: UCLA clinical trial of radial keratotomy: Preliminary report. Ophthalmology 88:729, 1981.

74. Villasenor, R. A.: Radial keratotomy: Symposium CLAO, Las Vegas, 1982.

75. Cowden, J. W., and Sultana, M.: Corneal endothelial cell density following radial keratotomy. Invest Ophthalmol Vis Sci 22(Suppl):30, 1982.

76. Yamaguchi, T., Kaufman, H., Fukushima, A., Safir, A., and Asbell, P.: Histologic and electron microscopic assessment of endothelial damage produced by anterior radial keratotomy in the monkey cornea. Amer J Ophthalmol 92:313, 1981.

77. Yamaguchi, T., Asbell, P., Yasuu, I., Fukushima, A., Safir, A., Kaufman, H. E., and Ostrick, M.: Electron microscopic and thymidine autoradiographic studies on monkeys after anterior radial keratotomy using a diamond blade. Invest Ophthalmol Vis Sci 22(Suppl):27, 1982.

78. Hull, D. S., Farkas, S., Laughter, L., Elijah, R. D., Bowman, K., and Green, K.: Rabbit corneal endothelial permeability following radial keratotomy. Invest Ophthalmol Vis Sci 22(Suppl):239, 1982.

79. Gelender, H.: Personal communication.

80. Miller, D., and Miller, R.: Glare sensitivity in simulated radial keratotomy. Arch Ophthalmol 99:1961, 1981.

81. Katz, H. R., Duffin, M., Glasser, D. A., and Pettit, T. H.: Complications of contact lens wear after radial keratotomy in an animal model. Invest Ophthalmol Vis Sci 22(Suppl):27, 1982.

82. Thygeson, J., Reersted, P., Fledelius, H., and Corydon, L.: Corneal astigmatism after cataract extraction: A comparison of corneal and corneoscleral incisions. Acta Ophthalmol 57:243, 1979.

83. Krachmer, J. H., and Fenzl, R. E.: Surgical correction of high post keratoplasty astigmatism: Relaxing incisions vs wedge resection. Arch Ophthalmol 98:1400, 1980.

84. Troutman, R. C.: Astigmatic considerations in corneal graft. Ophthalmic Surg 10:21, 1979.

85. Troutman, R. C. (ed.): Proceedings of the Third International Symposium Microsurgery Study Group, Merida, Yucatan. Basel, Switzerland, S. Karger AG, 1972.

86. Troutman, R. C.: Microsurgery of the Anterior Segment of the Eye. St. Louis, C. V. Mosby Co., 1977, p. 286.

XI

CONTACT LENSES AND THE ABNORMAL CORNEA

30 Therapeutic Uses of Hydrophilic Contact Lenses in Corneal Disease

JAMES V. AQUAVELLA, M.D.

The concept of binding or applying a bandage in cases of injury or disease probably dates to prehistoric times. The first recorded instance of a specific eye bandage is that of Celsus,[1] who applied a dressing of honey-soaked linen directly into the inferior fornix to prevent the development of symblepharon.

In more recent years the technique of applying a true "ocular bandage" was revived by Ridley[2] and his associates working in England. Primarily as a result of meticulous fitting, they were able to fit hard methyl methacrylate "shells" as protective devices in a variety of corneal conditions. The lenses were difficult for the patient to tolerate, and their use was characterized by short wearing time, discomfort, and a high incidence of secondary infection. Moreover, the initial fitting process was sufficiently involved to preclude its routine use. Nevertheless, a modicum of success was achieved with these lenses.

Wichterle and Lim[3] reported the use of a cross-linked hydrophilic polymer for contact lenses in 1960. Utilizing a different hydrophilic polymer, Gasset and Kaufman[4] reported on the use of "bandage lens" therapy in a variety of corneal conditions. Subsequently a number of investigators using additional types of hydrophilic material contributed to our present concept of "bandage lens" therapy. This form of therapy represents a significant addition to the ophthalmologist's armamentarium for the treatment of corneal disease.

CHEMICAL AND PHYSICAL PROPERTIES

The plastic shells utilized by Ridley and his associates were composed of simple polymethyl methacrylate (PMMA), the substance utilized for the manufacture of traditional "hard" contact lenses. PMMA is a synthetic polymer formed by the linear addition of small units (monomer) that are condensed to produce a very high molecular weight polymeric chain. The chemical reaction involved is termed polymerization, and it is often initiated by the addition of a small amount of free radical–forming reagent in the form of a catalyst.

The process in which more than one monomer is involved in the polymerization reaction has been termed copolymerization. Following copolymerization the two monomers may appear in the polymeric chain on a completely random basis, or they may be structured so that the resultant frequency of component monomer units as well as their sequence of distribution is deliberate.[5] The practical significance of such matters is that random copolymers generally tend to have physical properties intermediate between those of their parent homopolymers, whereas nonrandom copolymers may possess some or all of the properties of either of their parent homopolymers. In every case there is a close relationship between the inherent chemical composition of the polymer and its physical properties. The ultimate clinical performance of the bandage lens may be directly related to one or more specific polymer properties.

Hydrophilic contact lenses are made of polymers capable of absorbing substantial quantities of water. The first hydrophilic material used as a contact lens was synthesized by copolymerization of 2-hydroxyethyl methacrylate (HEMA) with ethylene glycol dimethacrylate (EGDMA).[3] Most hydrophilic lenses are made of chemically cross-linked acrylic polymers; the cross-links add stability to the lens. The cross-linked polymer swells in a solvent (usually physiologic saline) to form a gel whose water content at saturation depends on a variety of factors. These include the water solubility of the noncross-linked polymer, the number of cross-links, and the nature of the aqueous solution in which the gel is equilibrated as well as temperature, pH, and osmotic and hydrostatic pressures. When all these variables are constant, the degree of swelling of the hydrogel is consistent and reproducible.

It is apparent, therefore, that the hydrogels from which hydrophilic contact lenses are constructed are comprised of two components, a permanent, solid polymer network and a variable aqueous component that can undergo exchange with the surrounding environment. All such hydrogels are inherently relatively weak materials because their polymeric chains are diluted by the solvent. Water-soluble substances can enter the interstices of a hydrogel if their molecular size is smaller than the interconnecting spaces within the hydrogel. These spaces contain water and are open to the surfaces of the hydrophilic contact lens. In general, the average diameter of the spaces within the lens increases as water content of the hydrogel increases. Resistance to diffusion within the hydrogel is inversely proportional to the size of the resisting molecule. Most water-soluble drugs, such as steroids and antibiotics as well as preservatives and metabolites, can easily diffuse in and out of a hydrogel lens, an important factor when medications are used in patients who are wearing bandage lenses. Larger substances, such as proteins, viruses, and bacteria, cannot penetrate an intact hydrogel contact lens. Contamination by proteinaceous deposits and pathogens usually occurs only on the surface of the lens. Pathogens can, however, penetrate into defects in hydrogel lenses that have deteriorated.

Theoretically, certain clinically desirable physical properties can be incorporated into a polymer by altering its chemical composition (e.g., water content). The performance of a hydrophilic material as a bandage lens is therefore potentially directly related to its composition. Unfortunately, the actual situation is more complex, largely because of difficulties in controlling the polymerization process. A host of variables resulting from specific manufacturing techniques can affect the performance of the hydrophilic polymer. Ultimately, however, the design of the finished bandage lens and its architectural configuration result in a specific fitting relationship when it is placed on a cornea.[6, 7] The fitting relationship is determined in part by lens diameter, curvature, thickness, and sagittal depth, and it markedly affects the performance of the lens.

One of the most important characteristics of a good bandage lens is its ability to transport fluid and oxygen to the underlying diseased cornea and to allow removal of carbon dioxide and other metabolic wastes. Most hydrophilic polymers have, in themselves, a relatively low degree of gas permeability. Indeed, it is considerably lower than the high gas permeability of silicone rubber or the more rigid cellulose acetate butyrate (CAB) material. Nonetheless, hydrophilic contact lenses do allow oxygen to move from the air (or from the palpebral conjunctiva when the eye is closed) through the lens material to the cornea. The property of oxygen transmissibility of a hydrophilic contact lens is due to the high water content of the polymer.

Fluid content varies from approximately 38 per cent with polymacon to 55 per cent for the vifilcon and bufilcon materials to an upper limit of approximately 85 per cent in other materials. Gases do not flow through the polymers of which hydrophilic contact lenses are made; there are no pores within the contact lens material filled with a gaseous phase. Instead the gas is dissolved in the water component of the soft contact lens material. Fatt has presented the analogy that gas is carried in the lens material just as it is in an unopened bottle of beer.[8] Thus, the oxygen transmissibility of hydrogel lenses is largely a function of the amount of water incorporated into the hydrogel structure. Although water content is not the sole determinant of oxygen transmissibility (the chemical nature of the polymeric material also has some effect), oxygen transmissibility does appear to be linearly related to the hydration (grams of water per gram of dry material) of a gel. Carbon dioxide transmissibility of hydrogel materials is about 20 times greater than oxygen transmissibility;[8] therefore, there is no significant accumulation of carbon dioxide beneath any contact lens that allows sufficient oxygen to reach the cornea.

Oxygen transmission is related not only to the water content of a hydrogel but also to its thickness. For any given hydrophilic material, oxygen transmission is greater as the thickness of the lens decreases. Thus, in their present form the Bausch & Lomb "T" lens of approximately 0.18 mm. thickness (water content 38 per cent) and a Softcon lens of approximately 0.35 mm. thickness (water content 55 per cent) can be expected to deliver comparable amounts of oxygen to the cornea.[9]

MANUFACTURING TECHNIQUES

Spin-Cast Lenses

The spin-cast process is used by Bausch & Lomb for manufacture of its Soflens (Fig. 30–1).[10, 11] This is a process of centrifugal casting in which a monomer solution containing a mixture of HEMA,

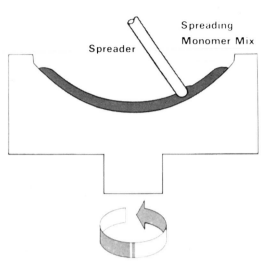

Figure 30–1. Schematic illustration of the spin casting manufacturing process. The monomer is spread over the mold, which is then rotated. Polymerization occurs during the spinning process.

a small amount of cross-linking agent, and a polymerization initiator is poured into a mold that is spinning about its central axis while polymerization occurs. Only a concave mold is used, and the posterior or ocular surface of the lens assumes a shape that varies according to the speed of rotation, the viscosity of the material, and the rate of polymerization. To design the actual contact lens, a combination of chord diameter and radius of curvature for the mold is selected. Spin speeds and volume of the polymer injected are calculated to give the desired values of the finished back vertex power and lens thickness.[11]

The volume of liquid utilized and the sagittal depth of the mold control the thickness of the finished Soflens. Low spin speeds of the mold produce flat lenses with long radii of curvature (oblate), whereas higher spin speeds result in steeper lenses of relatively short radii of curvature (prolate).

The advantages of this form of construction lie in the fact that the spin-casting process is totally automated, and consequently the cost of the finished contact lens to the manufacturer is less than that incurred with the lathe process. In addition, the quality of the product is not related to the skill of any one

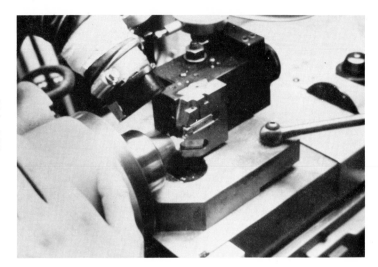

Figure 30–2. Precision lathe used to fashion a hydrophilic contact lens from a dry rod of the polymer. The finished lens is allowed to hydrate.

particular operator. The molding process produces a convex surface of excellent optical quality, and the quality of the concave (ocular) surface is far superior to that cut on a lathe. Manufacturers also claim a high degree of reproducibility with this method.

Lathe-Cut Lenses

Lathe cutting is the method of manufacture utilized by the majority of hydrophilic and silicone lens manufacturers (Fig. 30–2). The hydrophilic material is polymerized and kept dry, and the resulting plastic resembles rods of ordinary polymethyl methacrylate (PMMA). In this state it can be cut into buttons, machined, and polished (only oil-based polishing compounds should be utilized for this). After the lens manufacturing process is complete, the finished lens is

allowed to hydrate. Hydration is accompanied by a dimensional change that proceeds according to a fixed formula. The finished product is then stored in buffered 0.9 per cent saline solution.

Lathe cutting makes it possible to produce a large variety of lens designs.[12] The method does have the drawback of being a labor-intensive system. Considerable improvement has been made in the past few years in the methods of precision lathe cutting. The lathes must be precisely balanced even with respect to the electrical windings of the motor. Experience has shown that with precision cutting and a reduction in the length of time required for subsequent polishing, the resultant button is considerably more durable than that formerly obtained. With attention to detail and with a greatly purified polymer, reproducibility and yield are currently at very high ratios. The proponents of this

Figure 30–3. Schematic illustration showing the relationship of lens diameter, base curve of the lens, and sagittal depth.

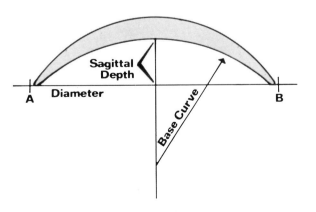

method feel that the ultimate acuity obtained with a lathe-cut lens is inherently superior to that obtained with a spin-cast material.

In considering the lathe-cut lens, it is necessary to understand the interrelationship of various lens parameters.[6, 13] There is a specific relationship between the diameter, the base curve, and the sagittal depth (Fig. 30–3). All lenses of 8.4 mm. curvature and 14.0 mm. diameter will have the same sagittal depth. One can conserve the sagittal depth relationship by altering both the base curvature and diameter. Altering either curvature or diameter alone changes the sagittal depth.

LENS CHARACTERISTICS

Currently in the United States a number of hydrophilic lenses are available for use as bandage lenses (Table 30–1). The Bausch & Lomb Soflens and the American Optical Softcon lens were the first. The former is based on the polymer originally developed by Wichterle and consists of a homopolymer of hydroxyethyl methacrylate (HEMA) that is lightly cross-linked with ethylene glycol dimethacrylate (EGDMA). The finished polymer is known as polymacon and consists of approximately 38 per cent water by weight.

The Bausch & Lomb "T" lens has a 14.7 mm. diameter, 8.1 mm. curvature, and 0.18 mm. central thickness. The lens was originally designed as a wholly therapeutic lens. Currently it has been largely replaced by the "U-4" lens, which has a 14.5 mm. diameter, 8.6 mm. curvature, and 0.7 mm. central thickness, and the "O-4" lens, which has a 14.5 mm. diameter, 8.5 mm. curvature, and 0.035 mm. central thickness.

The Softcon polymer, vifilcon A, is formed by polymerizing HEMA and poly-n-vinyl pyrrolidone (PVP), with the resultant graft copolymer containing about 55 per cent water by weight.

The Permalens polymer, perfilcon A, is formed by polymerizing hydroxyethyl methacrylate (containing about 1 per cent EGDMA and 3 per cent methacrylic acid) and polyvinyl pyrrolidone.[14] When fully hydrated in normal saline, the resultant copolymer contains approximately 72 per cent water by weight.

The Sauflon polymers are lidofilcon A and lidofilcon B. They are cross-linked copolymers of a hydrophilic polymer, poly vinyl pyrrolidone (PVP), and a relatively hydrophobic monomer, methyl methacrylate (MMA). Different proportions of PVP to MMA exposed to different radiation doses from a cobalt 60 gamma radiation source (which determines the degree of linking between PVP and MMA) yields hydrogels with a hydration range of 70 to 85 per cent by weight.[14]

The various lathe-cut bandage lenses are available in a range of diameters from 13.5 to 15.0 mm. and a range of posterior base curves from 7.8 to 9.4 mm.

FITTING THE LENS

In fitting the bandage lens, one should be concerned primarily with the stability, curvature, thickness, and refractive power of the lens selected. Stability is largely a function of diameter with the lathe-cut lens; the larger the diameter, the greater the adherence or stability. The stability of the spin-cast plano "T" lens is derived partially from its large diameter but also from the thinness of the lens and its reduced weight. The curvature of the lens also affects stability. With a smaller radius of curvature (steeper) the lens will exhibit more adherence and stability, whereas with a larger radius of curvature (flatter) it will exhibit less adherence and less stability. By varying these parameters and consequently by varying the geometric relationship between the lens and the underlying cornea, one can achieve great differences in therapeutic effect.

An important factor in obtaining a desired therapeutic result with bandage lens therapy relates to the architectural relationship between the lens utilized and the underlying cornea. Thus, there

Table 30–1. HYDROPHILIC LENSES AVAILABLE FOR THERAPY OF CORNEAL DISORDERS

Lens Designation	Chemical Name of Polymer	Manufacturer	Trade Name	H_2O Content (Per Cent)	Thickness (mm.)	Base Curve	Diameter (mm.)	Power Range
Plano T	Polymacon	Bausch & Lomb	Soflens	38.6	0.18	—	14.8	Plano
U-4	Polymacon	Bausch & Lomb	Soflens	38.6	0.7	—	14.5	−0.25D to −9.00D
O-4	Polymacon	Bausch & Lomb	Soflens	38.6	0.035	—	14.5	−1.00D to −9.00D
Softcon HBL	Vifilcon A	American Optical	Softcon	55	0.3	7.8–8.7	13.5–14.5	−8.00D to +18.00D
Permalens HBL	Perfilcon A	Cooper Vision	Permalens	71	0.24	7.7–9.0	13.5–15.0	Plano
Permalens STD	Perfilcon A	Cooper Vision	Permalens	71	0.1–0.43	7.7–8.3	13.5	−20.00 to +35.00
CSI HBL	Crofilcon A	Syntex	CSI	38.5	0.035	8.6–9.4	14.8	−20.00D to +20.00D
Sauflon HBL	Lidofilcon B	American Hospital	Sauflon PW	79	0.24	8.7–9.0	15.5	Plano

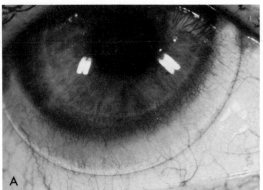 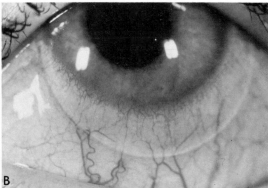

Figure 30–4. Centration of a therapeutic hydrophilic contact lens. *A,* Satisfactory fit; lens is sufficiently steep and does not decenter on upward gaze. *B,* Unsatisfactory fit; lens is excessively flat and decenters on upward gaze.

are certain basic guidelines for good hydrophilic bandage lens fitting regardless of the specific nature of the underlying corneal disease or the type of lens used to treat the disorder. Paramount is the fact that the lens must center well on the cornea and not tend to decenter with blinking or ocular rotations (Fig. 30–4). Secondly, the lens selected must be comfortable. Thus, in many instances we discourage the use of topical anesthetics during the fitting process because they may mask a basically uncomfortable fit of a lens. The edges of the lens should be examined with the slit lamp. Edges that tend to flare may cause increased sensation with blinking. Edges that adhere too tightly may produce an aching sensation.

A large, flat-fitting lens that centers well will probably do the job in most instances. If a painful epithelial defect is present, a steeper-fitting lens with a large interface area may be indicated, at

least for the first few days until the epithelium has begun to heal. The lens can then be changed. These large, steep lenses are very versatile, but they can cause edema. This usually does not interfere with therapy and will subside when a flatter lens is applied or when lens wear is discontinued.

INDICATIONS FOR BANDAGE LENS THERAPY

The medical indications for bandage lens therapy are summarized in Table 30–2 and the surgical indications in Table 30–3. Certain specific types of corneal pathology that cause pain or reduced visual acuity may be amenable to treatment with this device. The pain is caused by devitalization or edema of the corneal epithelium and/or by a persistent defect of the corneal epithelium, resulting in abnormal stimulation of the sensory nerve endings. Reduced visual acuity generally is due to irregular astigmatism related to the abnormal epithe-

Table 30–2. MEDICAL INDICATIONS FOR HYDROPHILIC BANDAGE LENSES

Chronic corneal edema
Abrasions, erosions, ulcerations
Filamentary keratitis
Chemical keratitis
Neurotrophic keratitis
Neuroparalytic keratitis
Herpes simplex keratitis (persistent epithelial defect after stromal involvement)
Dry eye syndromes
Ectatic dystrophies
Anterior membrane corneal dystrophies
Entropion, trichiasis, lid defects

Table 30–3. SURGICAL INDICATIONS FOR HYDROPHILIC BANDAGE LENSES

Postoperative discomfort
Lacerations
Perforations
Persistent epithelial defect following:
    Penetrating keratoplasty
    Lamellar keratoplasty
    Lamellar keratectomy
    Thermokeratoplasty

lial surface and/or an associated abnormality of the precorneal tear film. Relief of pain is afforded in 70 to 90 per cent of cases treated with a bandage lens.[15–17] In those cases in which bandage lens therapy can be maintained, the great majority also show improvement in the appearance of the corneal lesion. Success in improving visual acuity is more variable; this depends on the nature of the corneal pathology and on its location.

Bullous keratopathy is a major indication for bandage lens therapy, and a hydrophilic contact lens can be extremely effective in this entity.[16, 18, 19] This disorder produces symptoms of pain, epiphora, photophobia, and blepharospasm as well as a decrease in vision. When concomitant pathology in the involved eye precludes a satisfactory visual result, when the clinical situation does not warrant a surgical procedure of the magnitude of penetrating keratoplasty, or when the patient is awaiting the availability of donor tissue, relief of discomfort becomes the prime therapeutic goal. Prior to the advent of the hydrophilic contact lens, failure of traditional therapy (e.g., topically administered hypertonic agents) to control pain made surgical intervention necessary in the form of a tarsorrhaphy, conjunctival flap, or cauterization of Bowman's membrane. However, the experience of many now indicates that these patients can be fitted with a hydrophilic contact lens and that more than 90 per cent will experience symptomatic relief (Fig. 30–5). The lens does little to alter the pathophysiology of the disease process itself. Therefore, symptomatic relief is directly dependent upon the lens remaining in place on the diseased cornea. Its removal usually results in a rapid recurrence of symptoms.

Simple acute corneal abrasions are best treated by application of a pressure patch. However, in instances in which the epithelial defect persists and in which pain is a significant problem, the application of a hydrophilic bandage lens should be considered.[20] The lens is worn continuously, 24 hours a day, until

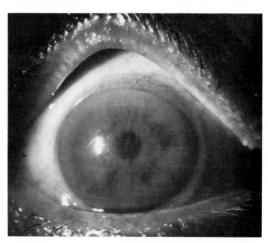

Figure 30–5. A hydrophilic contact lens used to treat bullous keratopathy. (Courtesy of Howard M. Leibowitz, M.D.)

the defect heals (Fig. 30–6). Usually it is left in place for at least a week after complete regeneration appears to have occurred, to ensure that adequate adherence to the underlying basement membrane occurs. In recurrent erosion and other syndromes involving a deficiency in the basal epithelium–basement membrane complex the bandage lens should be worn continuously for a minimum of 8 to 12 weeks to afford sufficient time for complete epithelial healing with the production of new basement membrane.[21] Frequent instillation of artificial tear solutions should be continued. When bandage lens therapy is discontinued, it is wise to prepare the patient for the possibility of recurrence of the dis-

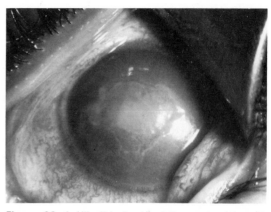

Figure 30–6. Ultrathin hydrophilic contact lens in place over an indolent epithelial defect. (Courtesy of Howard M. Leibowitz, M.D.)

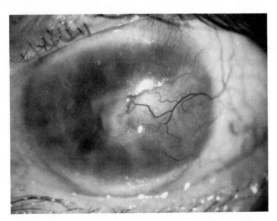

Figure 30–7. Ultrathin hydrophilic contact lens in place over an indolent herpes simplex stromal ulcer. (Courtesy of Howard M. Leibowitz, M.D.)

ease. Topical instillation of artificial tear solutions and nighttime use of emollients or hypertonic saline ointment should be maintained for several days following removal of the bandage lens. When finally the lens is removed, it should be at a time convenient for both patient and physician, in anticipation of a possible recurrence.

In filamentary keratitis, whether primary or secondary to ocular surgery or a dry eye, the application of a hydrophilic bandage lens can afford rapid relief and effect a lasting cure. In herpes simplex keratitis, the use of the lens is usually associated with recurrent stromal disease and persistent epithelial defects (Fig. 30–7). In the dry eye syndromes the use of hydrophilic bandage

lens is not without risk. The incidence of success with the use of these lenses in any of the dry eye syndromes is relatively low when compared with that evidenced in bullous keratopathy. Nevertheless, when the bandage lens is utilized as part of a comprehensive therapeutic regimen, it can be an important adjunct (Fig. 30–8). The bandage lens does not eliminate the necessity for frequent application of artificial tear solutions; indeed, there are those who feel that bandage lenses may even require additional amounts of topical medication to maintain their hydration. Moist-chamber goggles, punctum occlusion, and solid tear substitutes are important aspects of a comprehensive therapeutic regimen for dry eye syndromes.

In neurotrophic or neuroparalytic keratitis (Fig. 30–9) it is sometimes necessary to reduce the size of the interpalpebral fissure by partial tarsorrhaphy in order to prevent excessive evaporation and repeated loss of the lens. These cases also show a high incidence of "lensopathy," which is discussed in the section on Complications later in this chapter.

Hydrophilic contact lenses should be readily available in every institution performing ophthalmic surgery. A descemetocele (Fig. 30–10) or a small corneal perforation without incarceration of uveal tissue (Fig. 30–11) can be treated primarily by application of a bandage lens.[22, 23] A relatively tight-fitting band-

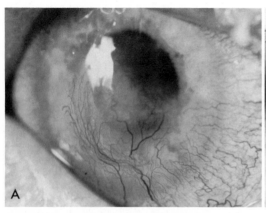
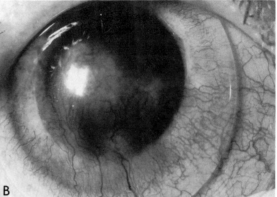

Figure 30–8. Keratitis sicca. *A,* Irregularity and roughening of corneal surface, scarring, and neovascularization. *B,* Same patient fitted with a hydrophilic bandage lens. The pathology has improved, but intensive topical medication is needed to maintain the hydration of the lens and the cornea.

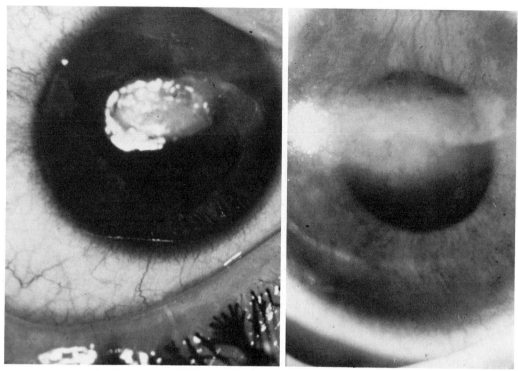

Figure 30–9. Neurotrophic corneal ulcer in a dry eye. *Left:* Appearance of cornea prior to treatment. *Right:* Appearance after 3 years of lens wear. (This patient has now worn a hydrophilic contact lens continuously for 12 years.)

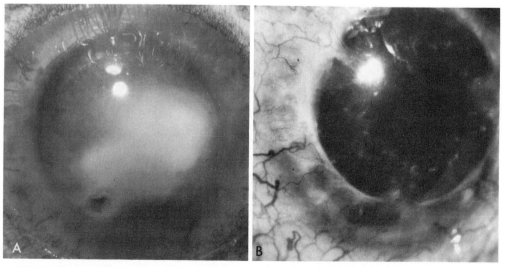

Figure 30–10. Stromal herpes simplex keratitis with secondary staphylococcal infection and descemetocele; *A,* Integrity of the globe is maintained with a hydrophilic contact lens during initial topical therapy with antimicrobial and antiinflammatory agents. *B,* Subsequently, definitive therapy in the form of penetrating keratoplasty is carried out. (Courtesy of Howard M. Leibowitz, M.D.)

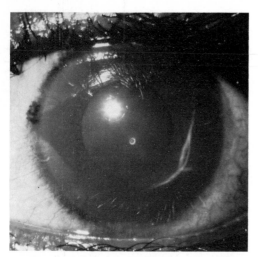

Figure 30–11. Appearance of a healed perforating corneal laceration that was treated only with a hydrophilic contact lens. (Courtesy of Howard M. Leibowitz, M.D.)

age lens often results in rapid reformation of the anterior chamber (Fig. 30–12), and on occasion no further therapy is necessary. The application of the lens is followed by swelling and coaptation of the wound margins, and ultimately healing ensues. Even when surgical in-

tervention is necessary, the initial application of a lens enables surgery to be delayed, converting an emergency procedure into a scheduled one. Should discomfort be caused by the suture knots following surgical repair of a corneal laceration, a therapeutic hydrogel lens can easily be inserted postoperatively to relieve the discomfort. Similarly, if a cyanoacrylate adhesive is used to repair the laceration, it may cause discomfort after it polymerizes and hardens. If a hydrophilic lens can be successfully fitted over the elevated, hardened glue, it can dramatically relieve the symptoms.

In infants and young children undergoing penetrating keratoplasty or other forms of anterior segment surgery, the application of a hydrogel lens while the patient is on the operating table immediately after completion of surgery can improve the prognosis of the surgical procedure.[24] Discomfort, blepharospasm, and excessive lacrimation are all reduced, and postoperative observation and examination of the child are greatly simplified. Immediate application of a bandage lens following pene-

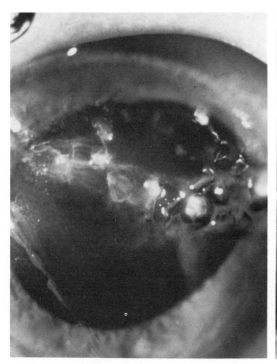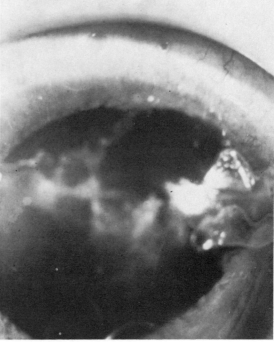

Figure 30–12. Split illustration showing the appearance of a perforating corneal laceration prior to (left) and after (right) fitting of a hydrophilic contact lens.

trating keratoplasty for chemical keratitis also appears to be quite useful. The lens seemingly protects the epithelium, enhances surface lubrication, and improves the early postoperative course, perhaps also improving the ultimate prognosis of the graft. Following lamellar keratoplasty or keratectomy, application of a lens rapidly makes the eye comfortable. Thus, the hydrophilic bandage lens has proved to be a useful surgical adjunct, particularly for corneal surgery. Postoperative epithelial defects are protected and a moist corneal surface is maintained.

CONTRAINDICATIONS

The contraindications to hydrophilic bandage lens therapy are (1) the presence of active bacterial or fungal infection, (2) the lack of adequate follow-up capability, and (3) the inability of the patient to manage lens therapy. Obvious poor general hygiene is a strong relative contraindication. High corneal infection rates have been reported in dry eye patients,[25, 26] and the use of a hydrophilic lens in this group must be approached with extreme caution.

MECHANISMS OF THERAPEUTIC EFFICACY

A variety of properties of hydrophilic bandage lenses are thought to be responsible for the therapeutic benefits derived.[13, 27]

Permeability

The relationship of fluid permeability and oxygen transport has been alluded to, but it is important to recall that exchange of drugs and metabolites is not wholly dependent on the permeability of the lens. A pumping action, initiated by the blink reflex, has been described. The pressure of the upper lid during the blink tends to collapse the lens and disrupt the lens-cornea interface, with an active expulsion of its fluid contents. Secondarily, there is a relaxation of the upper lid and active reformation of the interface. In very flat-fitting lenses the exchange can also occur via a process of capillarity.

Topical medication applied over the surface of the lens does not result in concentration of the drug in the lens. In order for concentration to occur, the lens must be presoaked in the drug. When protein debris binds to the lens surface, concentration of commonly used solution preservatives may occur and result in epithelial toxicity and irritation. The routine instillation of standard ophthalmic preparations containing preservatives has not resulted in irreversible epithelial damage. A far greater danger exists when one dispenses topical medications without preservatives, increasing the risk of secondary infection and permanent corneal damage.

Wetting

The application of a hydrophilic bandage lens tends to trap the interface fluid and to assure the constant wetting of the entire corneal epithelium (Fig. 30–13). Although the contents of the interface are exchanged during blinking, a constant and uniform wetting of the entire corneal surface ensues. This is particularly important in cases of instability of the tear film and in the presence of surface corneal irregularities. Both abnormalities are encountered in dry eye syndromes. In such cases, prior to application of the lens, pre-existing sym-

Figure 30–13. Schematic illustration showing that when a hydrophilic contact lens is fitted over a corneal ulcer, the lens-cornea interface is filled with tears and metabolic products, assuring the constant wetting of the entire corneal surface.

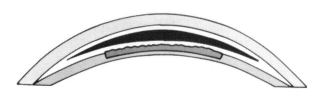

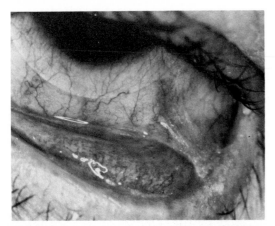

Figure 30–14. In dry eye cases with symblepharon the conjunctival fornices must be expanded sufficiently to allow for proper seating of the hydrophilic contact lens.

blepharon must be severed and the conjunctival fornices expanded sufficiently to allow for proper seating of the bandage lens (Fig. 30–14). Lid defects should be corrected surgically and consideration given to reduction of the palpebral aperture.

Concomitant blepharitis should be treated vigorously and topical artificial tear substitutes instilled as frequently as necessary to maintain hydration of the bandage lens. This may be at 15-minute intervals when therapy is initiated. However, after an equilibrium has been reached, it may be possible to reduce the frequency of instillation. The use of long-term prophylactic antibiotics has been criticized, but many authorities agree that prophylactic therapy is indicated in long-term treatment of dry eye syndromes, particularly when hydrophilic bandage lenses are utilized. If the lenses are to be worn 24 hours a day, removal followed by thorough cleaning and disinfection every week or every 2 weeks also is advisable. Two lenses are often prescribed so that this process may be performed on one lens while the second lens is in the eye. Superficial sterile infiltrates have been noted to develop under bandage lenses utilized in the treatment of dry eye syndromes. The etiology of these infiltrates is obscure, but the presence of an active infection must always be suspected. Every occurrence of an infiltrate or ulceration developing under a bandage lens must be examined immediately and treated as an infection until proved otherwise (see Fig. 15–1B).

Visual Acuity

When a bandage lens is applied in a case of Fuchs' dystrophy, improvement in visual acuity may be related to deturgescence of the edematous corneal epithelium (Fig. 30–15) or to replacement of the irregular surface with the smooth, uniform refracting surface provided by the bandage lens (Fig. 30–16).[28] Topical instillation of hypertonic saline solution

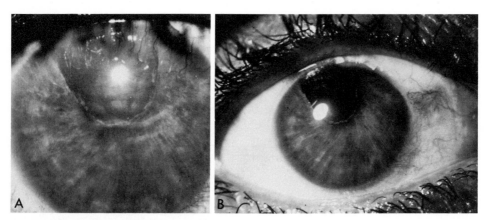

Figure 30–15. Early endothelial decompensation secondary to chronic glaucoma and the trauma of intraocular surgery. *A,* Corneal edema prior to therapy. *B,* Appearance of cornea 6 weeks after therapy with a hydrophilic contact lens and 5 per cent sodium chloride drops. (Courtesy of Howard M. Leibowitz, M.D.)

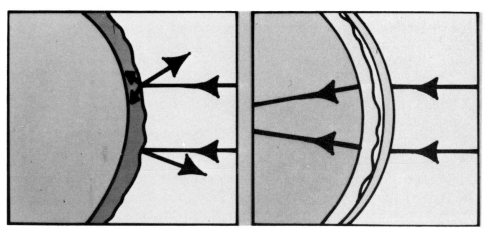

Figure 30–16. Illustration showing that when poor visual acuity is the result of an irregular corneal surface and the resulting irregular astigmatism, a hydrophilic contact lens may improve vision by providing a smooth anterior refracting surface.

over the lens can result in corneal deturgescence.[29] With the control of discomfort, the elimination of glare, and the reduction in epiphora and photophobia provided by the lens, the tendency is for further improvement in visual acuity while therapy is progressing. Visual acuity can be assisted even with an ordinary plano lens without regard to the refractive error or by fitting a lens with the appropriate power to provide optimal acuity. If optimal acuity is sought, it can often be obtained by fitting a large diameter, flat-fitting bandage lens. Improvement in visual acuity often is limited since many such eyes are afflicted with deep stromal scarring and stromal edema with Descemet's folds, as well as with glaucoma and a variety of macular and posterior segment disorders. However, dramatic improvements are possible at times in cases in which the media and the posterior pole are relatively normal and in which the bandage lens is fitted for optimal acuity. In monocular patients the importance of the ability of the patient to see reasonably well and to function while his therapy progresses cannot be overestimated.

In treating painful aphakic bullous keratopathy, the first consideration should be toward amelioration of pain with a thin bandage lens. Once the condition has stabilized and the patient is comfortable, an attempt can be made to fit a lens that will provide optimal acu-ity. The lens should be fit as flat as possible to allow for virtual contact between the posterior surface of the lens and the anterior surface of the cornea in the optical zone. If such a lens is comfortable, the patient may be instructed to remove the lens at night and insert it in the morning. Overrefraction can be performed and any residual spherical or astigmatic error corrected with spectacles. A bifocal reading addition may be indicated as well.

Protection

The application of a hydrophilic bandage lens protects the underlying cornea not only from desiccation and noxious environmental agents but also from any traumatic effects of the lids and the lashes (Fig. 30–17). Damaged epithelium is permitted to heal under the protection afforded by the lens (Fig. 30–18). Even in the event of rapid re-epithelialization, however, a prolonged interval may be necessary to allow a strong bond to form between adjacent epithelial cells and between the basal epithelial cells and the newly formed basement membrane. During this period the cells are particularly vulnerable to minor trauma, and the continued protection afforded by the hydrophilic lens, particularly in disorders such as recurrent erosion, is a helpful therapeutic adjunct.

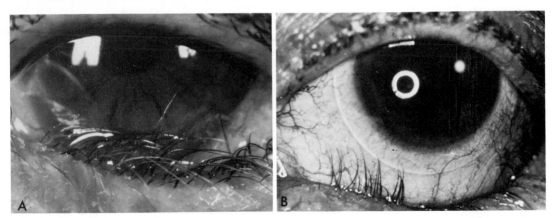

Figure 30–17. Spastic entropion of lower lid. *A,* Secondary corneal erosion with pain and excessive lacrimation; *B,* Immediate relief and protection of cornea afforded by a hydrophilic contact lens prior to definitive surgical correction of lid.

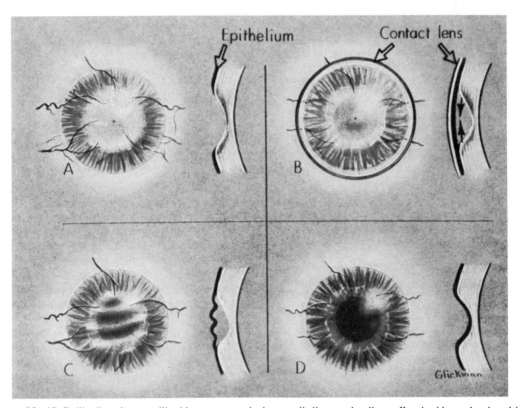

Figure 30–18. Epithelium is permitted to regenerate beneath the protection afforded by a hydrophilic contact lens. The presumed sequence of events is depicted in these illustrations. *A,* Indolent central stromal ulcer. *B,* With lens in place, epithelial regeneration occurs. It is believed that the lens acts as a scaffolding, promoting epithelial growth while protecting it from the lid margins during blinking. *C,* After removal of lens, epithelium may appear as a flaccid bulla not yet tightly adherent to the underlying stroma. *D,* In successful cases the new epithelium ultimately becomes tightly adherent to the underlying tissue. (From Leibowitz, H. M., and Rosenthal, P. R.: Hydrophilic contact lenses in corneal disease. I. Superficial, sterile, indolent ulcers. Arch Ophthalmol 85:163, 1971. Copyright 1971, American Medical Association.)

The protective effects of hydrophilic bandage lenses are utilized in a number of other situations. They are a requisite in the postoperative management of penetrating keratoplasty in the alkali-burned cornea for maintenance of the graft epithelium,[30] and they are regularly applied, when necessary, to protect the surfaces of corneal grafts performed for other disorders. Hydrogel lenses are particularly useful when postoperative tear secretion is marginal or tear distribution over the surface of the graft is abnormal. Large-diameter bandage lenses are of value in protecting the cornea during the course of surgical procedures for the correction of ptosis and lid defects. They also may be utilized in cases of spastic entropion as a temporary measure to obtain comfort prior to surgical repair. In cases of exposure keratitis and filamentary keratitis protection of the cornea can result in rapid healing.

Splinting

In some cases of full-thickness corneal laceration or perforation and in deep ulcerations a hydrophilic bandage lens can function as a splint (Fig. 30–12).[23] The body of the lens prevents buckling and distortion of the cornea in the presence of blinking and blepharospasm. A certain amount of splinting of a surgical wound also can be provided by the use of a bandage lens following penetrating keratoplasty or cataract extraction. The device often can tamponade a wound leak with a shallow anterior chamber. For these purposes slightly thicker lenses are utilized.

When the lenses are applied in cases of perforation, a large, tight-fitting lens is advisable. Prophylactic antibiotics, mydriatics, and carbonic anhydrase inhibitors are also indicated as part of the comprehensive therapy. The tight-fitting lens impedes the flow of aqueous through the lesion. Secondary swelling of stromal tissues seals off the leak with subsequent reformation of the anterior chamber. If the anterior chamber has not reformed within a reasonable period of time, adhesives or appositional sutures may be employed.

Pain Relief

Bullous keratopathy, recurrent erosion, and filamentary keratitis are instances in which the richly innervated epithelium has been disrupted. In these situations the application of a bandage lens can afford truly dramatic relief. Generally speaking, a steeper fitting lens is desirable, although any of the high-water-content thin lenses will work well provided the fit is adequate. Regardless of the specific lens that is used, it is important to select one that centers well over the eye and does not move excessively with ocular rotation and blinking. Motion of the lens can further abrade the epithelial surface and can cause a secondary anterior uveitis. The combination of minimal lens movement, a relatively steep lens-cornea interface, and prevention of apical touch is particularly suitable for relief of pain in the short term. The addition of a cycloplegic during the first few days of therapy will further ameliorate the situation by reducing ciliary spasm. If the lens selected is too steep, stromal edema with an increase in the number of folds in Descemet's membrane may result. In any event, following resolution of the pain it is often advisable to fit a flatter lens. For long-term use, a lens that does not move on the surface of the eye can result in a tight lens syndrome.

When initiating bandage lens therapy, the lens should be worn continuously 24 hours a day. If it is properly fitted and if the patient is comfortable, there is no necessity for either the patient or the physician to remove the lens. Healing can be monitored with the slit-lamp biomicroscope without removing the lens. The process of insertion and removal is an open invitation to secondary contamination and the introduction of bacterial elements into the system. Even intraocular pressure can be measured reasonably well by pneumotonometry with a thin bandage lens in place, or the lens can be rotated off the central cornea to permit measurement of the intraocular pressure.

When the painful episode has stabilized, it may be advisable to switch to an intermittent form of contact lens wear. Depending on the cause of the pain, modifications of the wearing schedule should be instituted when indicated. Arbitrary insistence on full-time wear is often not in the best interests of the patient.

DRUG DELIVERY

The presence of a hydrogel bandage lens is not a contraindication to the use of topical drugs, but it does represent a physical barrier to the delivery of medication to the underlying diseased cornea. Hydrophilic materials with a high water content may constitute a lesser barrier to the delivery of water-soluble medications. In any event, the rate of entry of the drug into the polymer and its subsequent passage into the cornea will depend on the physical properties of the drug and of the polymer as well as the characteristics of the lens–tear film interface, the thickness of the lens, and the state of the lens surface at the time of instillation. It is important to recall that although no specific pore structure exists in the hydrophilic polymer, generally speaking, particles with a molecular weight in excess of 500 may have a difficult time entering the substance of the polymer. Large molecules, such as viruses and bacteria, cannot enter the undamaged surface of the hydrophilic bandage lens, but topically applied substances as well as bacteria, viruses, and debris may enter the lens-cornea interface by virtue of the pumping action of the lens.

Podos[31] and others have demonstrated that soaking hydrophilic bandages in pilocarpine can result in an increased therapeutic effect that lasts for prolonged periods. Even in the absence of presoaking, a hydrophilic lens might accumulate a drug, subsequently presenting a uniform surface from which the medication might be pulsed into the cornea. Although hydrogel lenses might exhibit fundamental properties suitable for a versatile ocular drug delivery system, they have not proved practical for this function and are not at present being widely utilized for this purpose.

ANCILLARY THERAPY

The presence of a therapeutic hydrophilic contact lens does not prevent treatment of the underlying corneal pathology with appropriate medications. Thus, antibiotics, steroids, antivirals, and glaucoma medications can be employed as indicated in each particular case. Blepharitis may create a hostile environment for the bandage lens, and, when present, it should be treated vigorously, both prior to and subsequent to lens fitting.

If there is inadequate tear formation, a hydrophilic bandage lens will tend to dry out. In this instance artificial tears or saline solution must be instilled as frequently as necessary to maintain the hydration of the lens and the underlying cornea. In cases of lid or conjunctival defects adequate surgical correction must precede lens fitting if the lens is to be maintained. Thus, symblepharon, if present, must be severed if it will interfere with proper lens wear. If the palpebral fissure is too wide, a partial tarsorrhaphy may be necessary to support lens therapy.

Most of the cases treated with this modality will have some anterior chamber reaction, although it may be difficult to observe through the diseased cornea. Thus, cycloplegics should be utilized at the onset of therapy and should be continued for several days. Attention to small degrees of blepharitis and iritis will minimize the number of patients who do not respond well to bandage lens therapy.

Standard ophthalmic preparations containing preservatives should be utilized.[15, 27] The use of medications without preservatives bears an unacceptable risk of secondary infection.

In most cases the bandage lens will be worn continuously, day and night, until the desired therapeutic goal has been achieved. Although healing often can be adequately monitored with the slit lamp without removing the lens, it may be desirable and at times necessary to remove the lens during therapy. This is usually done for purposes of cleaning, replacement, or refitting of the lens, for more precise evaluation of the cornea, or for the performance of various diagnostic tests. Alternatively, a regimen of insertion and removal may be more desirable and is employed particularly in the case of neovascularization.

If the epithelium is fragile, one should take great care to float the lens off by directing a stream of irrigating fluid at the lens margin. The lens may then be easily lifted from the cornea without injury to underlying tissues. The lens should be disinfected before being reapplied. In cases of poor tear formation or in the process of active infection it may be advisable to disinfect the lens periodically. In bullous keratopathy, however, the lenses are usually worn for long periods of time, and routine cleaning and disinfection are carried out at 3- to 6-month intervals.

A prophylactic antibiotic generally is indicated along with periodic disinfection of the lens, especially in cases of poor tear formation. Lid scrubs and overall good hygiene are important adjuncts. The bandage lens is not a substitute for routine therapy, but, rather, it should be a focal point of a comprehensive therapeutic regimen.

DISINFECTION OF HYDROPHILIC BANDAGE LENSES

When bandage lenses are shipped from the manufacturer, they have been autoclaved and are sterile, as mandated by the Food and Drug Administration. Following their initial introduction into the pharmacopoeia, there was considerable concern voiced about the necessity for frequent disinfection; indeed, this was responsible for creating a bias within the FDA that persisted for more than a decade. Initially boiling was the only method of approved disinfection. Subsequently dry heat was introduced in an attempt to maintain the standards of heat disinfection set up by the FDA and yet eliminate many of the problems involved with boiling. Although both boiling and dry heat are effective disinfection systems, they are cumbersome for both practitioner and patient.

To many authorities perhaps the most important consideration in this area is proper surface cleaning of the lens. This can be accomplished by a number of commercially available surfacing cleaners and by hydrogen peroxide. Use of the latter requires that both surfaces of the lens first be cleaned with a surfacing lubricant. The lubricant then is flushed from the lens under running tap water, and the lens is maintained in a solution of 3 per cent hydrogen peroxide for 10 minutes. Finally the hydrogen peroxide is eluted from the lens by rinsing it with preserved buffered normal saline solution. Usually three or four rinses of a few minutes each in normal saline solution are sufficient to eliminate the hydrogen peroxide from the lens. Return of the fluid within the lens to a neutral pH eliminates the sensation of stinging and irritation upon reinsertion. If the saline solution is warm, the process will be accelerated. With the hydrogen peroxide system lenses can be completely disinfected and reinserted within 30 minutes.

Proponents of the hydrogen peroxide system claim that it also flexes the structure of the polymer and assists in flushing of the pore structure. Internal cleaning of the lens as well as surface disinfection are thus accomplished. In order to eliminate some spores and fungi completely, much longer periods of H_2O_2 treatment are necessary. However, if the lens has been surface cleaned and flushed with running water, the potential number of organisms is greatly reduced and limited exposure to H_2O_2 (in the absence of protein debris) will be sufficient.

A number of so-called cold systems require surface cleaning and storage in a solution containing thimerosal, EDTA, and chlorhexidine as preservatives. The lens is then rinsed with preserved, buffered normal saline solution before it is inserted into the eye. In chronically inflamed and debilitated eyes, we have found that the thimerosal/chlorhexidine systems are excessively toxic. Currently the toxicity of preservative systems has come under close observation, and an effort is being made to reduce the concentration of these toxic drugs. Regardless of which system is used, however, it is important to note that fingers (patient's or physician's) are the best vehicles for introduction of contamination into the system. The hands should be washed well, rinsed, and dried before lens insertion. As an additional precaution the eye is routinely flooded with gentamicin sulfate 0.3 per cent following the insertion of the bandage lens.

COMPLICATIONS

A discussion of the complications arising from the use of hydrophilic contact lenses must differentiate between their use to correct a refractive error and their use as a therapeutic bandage. Hundreds of thousands of patients have been fitted with hydrophilic contact lenses for the correction of ametropia. These patients insert their lenses in the morning, wear the lenses essentially all waking hours, and remove them in the evening. Large numbers of even the relatively new extended-wear lenses have now been worn. Among those using hydrophilic contact lenses to correct refractive errors, there have been few cases of irreversible corneal damage. Nevertheless, it is well documented that misuse of any contact lens, primarily through infrequent disinfection, faulty personal hygiene, or overwear, can result in an increased incidence of minor corneal and conjunctival inflammatory episodes.

When fitting normal healthy eyes, we must insist that products and systems be of low risk. However, in dealing with possible complications resulting from the therapeutic use of hydrophilic bandages, it is important to consider the concept of risk versus benefit. In the treatment of severe debilitating corneal disease the benefits of hydrophilic bandage lens therapy may far outweigh the potential risks. Therefore, certain risks might be acceptable here that would not be acceptable in a normal eye with a refractive error.

In addition, one must differentiate between true complications and therapeutic failure.[32] Confusion between these concepts has resulted in controversy concerning the efficacy of hydrophilic bandage lenses and their relative indications and contraindications. Thus, in a case of severe herpetic keratitis with deep ulceration or in a severe alkali burn a hydrophilic bandage lens may be applied to the cornea. If within 24 hours a perforation occurs beneath the lens, in all probability we are dealing with a case of therapeutic failure—the application of the hydrophilic bandage lens was inadequate to prevent continued ulceration and perforation. The perforation in these cases was not directly related to or caused by the application of the hydrophilic bandage lens. It occurred because of the severity of the disease process in spite of attempted therapeutic measures.

Severe cases of neurotrophic keratitis and Stevens-Johnson syndrome are characterized by frequent secondary infections, the result of inadequate ocular defenses. These include breaks in the corneal epithelium and a deficiency of tears. When a hydrophilic bandage lens is fitted in such an eye and an infection occurs, the lens may well have contributed to the infectious process. However, in assessing the incidence of the lens-related complication, one must bear in mind that a certain number of infections would undoubtedly have occurred had the lens not been fitted.

True complications of bandage lens therapy include discomfort, intolerance, secondary infection, and neovascularization. The patient with corneal pathology who is successfully wearing a hydrophilic bandage lens may develop discomfort as a result of the deposition of insoluble material on the lens (Figs. 30–19 and 30–20). Deposits on the posterior surface or toward the lens periphery may be particularly annoying. Dis-

comfort also occurs in cases of bullous keratopathy in which a bulla has ruptured beneath the lens. This can be controlled by refitting the patient with a steeper lens until the epithelial defect has healed.

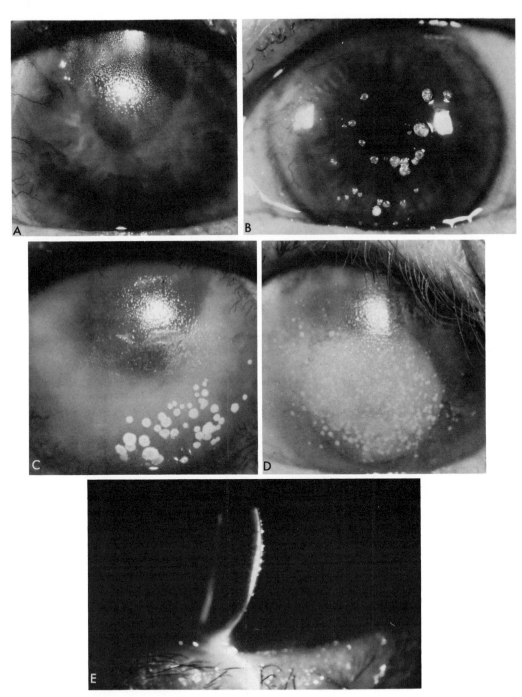

Figure 30–19. Deposits on the hydrophilic lens. These are not toxic or otherwise harmful to the eye but may produce discomfort and interfere with vision. *A,* Oil film on lens surface. *B,* Localized deposits. *C,* Localized deposits and diffuse oily film. *D,* Coalescence of the localized deposits to form an opaque plaque. *E,* Slit-lamp photo showing anterior surface location of the deposits. (*A, C, D,* and *E* courtesy of Howard M. Leibowitz, M.D.)

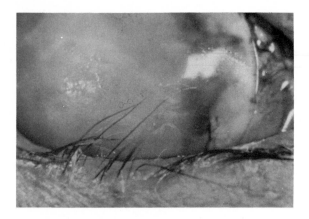

Figure 30–20. Patient with trichiasis who had been comfortably wearing a hydrophilic contact lens to protect the cornea. Marked deposition of insoluble material on the lens surface resulted in sufficient discomfort to necessitate fitting of a new lens.

Although it is true that some patients cannot be made comfortable with a hydrophilic bandage lens regardless of the pathology involved, the number of such cases decreases as the experience of the physician increases. Patient intolerance can be minimized by the use of cycloplegics and anti-inflammatory medications. If the lens selected is in effect too flat, it may increase irritation by rubbing against a corneal ulcer. On occasion a true intolerance is manifest by a sterile hypopyon and increased ocular inflammation (Fig. 30–21). Such cases are extremely rapid in onset and should not be confused with secondary infection. Removal of the lens and treatment with topically instilled steroids will reverse the process. Intolerance of hydrogel lenses also is associated with the appearance of a giant papillary conjunctivitis.[33] However, this seems to be primarily a problem when the lens is used to correct a refractive error; it is uncommon in therapeutic cases.

In my experience no irreversible corneal damage has occurred from the routine use of topical medications containing preservatives in conjunction with bandage lens therapy. To the contrary, there is a far greater risk of contamination when preservatives are omitted. Thus, standard ophthalmic medications are preferred for the treatment of corneal pathology in conjunction with hydrogel lenses.

Neovascularization associated with bandage lens wear may be superficial or deep. Most authorities believe that it is the result of decreased oxygen tension resulting from constant wear of the hydrogel lens. Others implicate the direct traumatic effects of wearing the lens. In normal ametropic eyes fitted with hydrophilic lenses I have seen few cases of corneal neovascularization when the lens is inserted and removed daily. Therefore, if the beginnings of neovascularization are observed, it may be advisable to shift from continuous to intermittent wear; patients should remove their lenses at bedtime if the disorder under treatment permits. It may be possible to discontinue the use of lenses altogether after a period of time without recurrence of pain or ulceration. A clinical decision must be made in each case individually.

Typically, thinner, high-water-content lenses cause fewer instances of neovas-

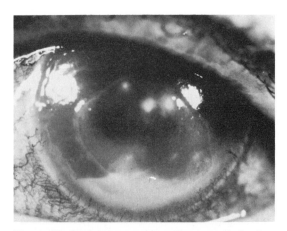

Figure 30–21. Intolerance to a therapeutic hydrophilic contact lens characterized by the sudden onset of increased hyperemia of the bulbar conjunctiva, sterile anterior stromal infiltrates, and a sterile hypopyon.

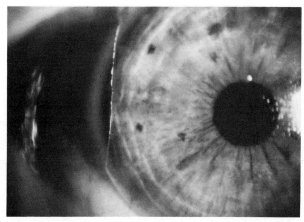

Figure 30–22. Therapeutic hydrophilic contact lens that tore during wear. The rough edge of the torn lens was uncomfortable and the lens had to be replaced.

cularization. When present, it does not necessarily imply that continued use of the bandage lens is contraindicated. Quite the contrary, in severe debilitating corneal disease neovascularization may be helpful. The continued use of the hydrophilic bandage lens, although not a panacea, is often the only method of preventing the complete, irreversible loss of visual function.

Complications must be differentiated from untoward lens events. The latter include loss, tearing (Fig. 30–22), or discoloration of a lens and coating of the lens surface by insoluble debris. Untoward lens events usually require a replacement lens, which increases the cost of therapy, but in most instances they do not adversely affect the eye.

A variety of medications are utilized with hydrophilic bandage lenses and may cause hardening or discoloration. Fluorescein and epinephrine (Fig. 30–23) products are well known to discolor

the lenses. Long-term administration of a variety of topical medications ultimately will result in slight brown discoloration of the lens. Particularly in the dry eye syndromes there is an increased tendency for the development of "lensopathies."[34] These are caused by deposition of insoluble material on the lens. Depending on the individual case, the material has been identified as calcium, mucin, bacteria, or a combination of lipoproteinaceous debris. The deposit is in part related to the surface characteristics of the lens–tear film interface as well as to the tendency for heavier particulate matter to plug the structure of the hydrophilic polymer.

In instances of demonstrated "lensopathy" or debris formation the lenses should be subjected to periodic cleaning with a good surfacing cleaner. Enzyme cleaning solutions are available, and the use of 3 per cent hydrogen peroxide can have a beneficial effect in retarding the

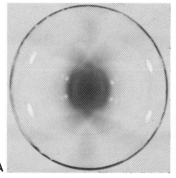
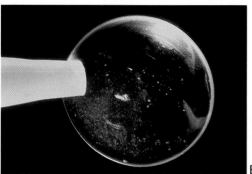

Figure 30–23. Discoloration of hydrophilic contact lens resulting from the use of topical epinephrine compounds for the treatment of glaucoma. *A,* Brown discoloration; *B,* Black discoloration.

development of such formations. If the debris is relatively minor and is not associated with disturbances in visual acuity or with discomfort, the deposits may be allowed to remain. In cases in which prophylactic measures do not retard the development of debris and the debris causes discomfort or reduction in visual acuity, the simplest approach is to change the lens.

Primarily because of their large diameter, hydrophilic bandage lenses, when fitted properly, are not readily lost. However, the lenses do have a limited life span. The life span of the average hydrophilic bandage lens used for treating dry eye conditions might be as short as several weeks to a few months, whereas in the presence of relatively normal tear flow a life span of a year or more may be anticipated. Other factors that affect the durability of the lenses relate to damage as a result of handling. A lens can be damaged by contact with improper lens cases, long fingernails, or instrumentation.

AVOIDANCE OF COMPLICATIONS

To avoid complications, we recommend the following routine.

1. Preliminary Steps

A. Attempt to determine the visual potential of the eye prior to fitting the bandage lens. An accurate refraction, fundus examination, and estimation of the degree of corneal irregularity, opacity, and scarring should be made.

B. Elevation of intraocular pressure should be ruled out (an electronic tonometer usually will be required). If present, it should be treated with the appropriate topical and systemic medications. If epinephrine is being used to control the intraocular pressure, an alternative means of glaucoma control must be used in conjunction with hydrogel lens therapy because the oxidative products of epinephrine will stain the lens.

C. Chronic iritis is often a component of chronic corneal disease. In many cases the degree of corneal opacity precludes an accurate diagnosis. These cases should be treated with cycloplegics and topical steroids when necessary.

D. An estimation of corneal sensation is important. Use of a lens in neurotrophic keratitis carries an increased risk.

E. Treat pre-existing blepharitis.

2. Lens Insertion

An attempt should be made to select an initial lens that has great potential for being the definitive lens used in therapy.

A. No anesthetic should be instilled prior to fitting the lens. The presence of a topical anesthetic precludes an accurate assessment of the comfort afforded by the bandage lens. If a patient is discharged before the effects of the anesthetic have worn off, discomfort subsequently may develop.

B. Evaluation of lens fitting should be made after an interval of at least 20 minutes has elapsed to allow for the lens to stabilize. Initial lacrimation may cause a lens to move excessively.

C. A relatively thin, high-water-content lens should be used for initial therapy even if an aphakic lens is indicated at a later date. Initially the patient is more easily stabilized with a thin, high-water-content lens.

D. Before actually inserting the lens, the physician should wash, rinse, and dry his hands.

E. The patient should be optimally positioned to facilitate lens insertion. If he is supine and the lens inadvertently falls from the physician's fingers, it will tend to land in the eye rather than on the floor.

F. A steep-fitting lens should generally be avoided unless specifically indicated. Such a lens will demonstrate very little or no movement on the eye. Although it may be comfortable initially, it is apt to become uncomfortable in time. In contrast, if the lens fits too loosely, excessive movement (several millimeters) will occur and the lens will not tend to center after each blink or after ocular movements. This type of lens will be uncomfortable in the long run.

3. Patient Instruction

A number of complications can be avoided by accurately explaining to the patient what is expected of him in caring for his lens and what he should anticipate while wearing the lens.

A. Written instruction should be provided, in booklet form if possible, stating how to remove the lens. Specific instruction in insertion and removal should be given to the patient or to a member of his family even if the lens is to be worn on a full-time basis.

B. The patient must have a telephone number of an ophthalmologist or another individual who can be contacted should difficulties arise.

C. The comprehensive medical regimen should be fully explained to the patient and written down if possible. One should address blepharitis, iritis, and glaucoma as well as the specific therapy indicated for the corneal disease.

D. The patient must have an appointment (date and time) for a return visit to the ophthalmologist.

E. In the event of pain, increased redness, reduced vision, corneal opacity, or corneal infiltrates, the patient must be seen as soon as possible.

4. Evaluation and Refitting of the Lens

When the situation has stabilized, an attempt should be made to refit the contact lens in those cases in which there is a possibility of improving visual acuity.

A. Generally speaking, a flatter-fitting contact lens will afford the best vision.

B. Overrefraction is often facilitated with the aid of a keratometer. A reading is taken over the anterior surface of the lens.

C. When corneal edema and irregularity have stabilized, a trial of a high-water-content aphakic contact lens should be considered in aphakic eyes thought capable of visual improvement.

D. If at all possible, the patient should insert and remove a thicker, aphakic contact lens on a daily basis. Extended wear may be indicated, but corneas that are marginally compensated or decompensated will do better with daily insertion and removal.

E. The patient should again be instructed on the principles of good long-term hygiene.

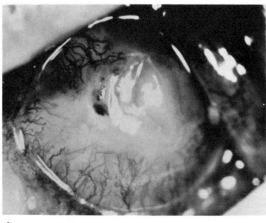 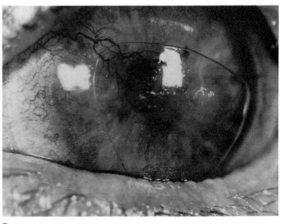

A   B

Figure 30–24. Corneal ulcer with descemetocele secondary to Stevens-Johnson syndrome. *A,* Corneal ulcer has been unresponsive to conventional therapy. *B,* Appearance of cornea after 2 years of bandage lens therapy. Neovascularization and fibroplasia have occurred and filled in the deep ulcer. (An air bubble is present in the lens-cornea interface.)

5. Ultimate Re-evaluation of Therapy

If the patient has been made comfortable, further decisions concerning his therapy may be deferred. Similarly, if an ulcer heals beneath a contact lens (Fig. 30–24), further therapeutic decisions may be deferred. However, each case should be re-evaluated at periodic intervals. If relief of pain is inadequate, the therapy may be discontinued, and perhaps one should consider conjunctival flap or penetrating keratoplasty. If the vision is inadequate for the patient's needs, keratoplasty may be specifically indicated.

SUMMARY

Theoretically, an infinite number of hydrophilic polymers can be constructed, each with a specific set of inherent physical properties. Because of high research and development costs, the same materials utilized for cosmetic fitting are available for bandage purposes. Differences in manufacturing techniques as well as in specific polymeric constitution make direct comparisons difficult.

Bandage lens therapy, while not a panacea, has been a significant addition to our therapeutic armamentarium for the treatment of severe corneal disease.

REFERENCES

1. Arrington, G. E.: A History of Ophthalmology. New York, M. D. Publications, 1959.
2. Ridley, F.: Therapeutic uses of scleral contact lenses. Int Ophthalmol Clin 2:687, 1969.
3. Wichterle, O., and Lim, D.: Hydrophilic gels for biological usage. Nature 185:117, 1960.
4. Gasset, A. R., and Kaufman, H. E.: Therapeutic uses of hydrophilic contact lenses. Amer J Ophthalmol 69:252, 1970.
5. O'Driscoll, K. F.: Polymeric aspects of soft contact lenses. In Gasset, A. R., and Kaufman, H. E. (eds.): Soft Contact Lens. St. Louis, C. V. Mosby Co., 1972, pp. 3–15.
6. Aquavella, J. V., Jackson, G. K., and Guy, L. F.: Therapeutic effects of bionite lenses: Mechanism of action. Ann Ophthalmol 3:1341, 1971.
7. Dorman-Brailsford, M. I.: The importance of sag heights when fitting bionite lenses. Ophthalmol Opt 12:1047, 1972.
8. Fatt, I.: Gas transmission properties of soft contact lenses. In Ruben, M. (ed.): Soft Contact Lenses: Clinical and Applied Technology. New York, John Wiley and Sons, 1978, pp. 83–110.
9. Mobilia, E. F., Dohlman, C. H., and Holly, F. J.: A comparison of various soft contact lenses for therapeutic purposes. Contact Intraocul Lens Med J 3:9, 1977.
10. Uotila, M. H., and Gasset, A. R.: Fitting manual for the Bausch and Lomb and Griffin lenses. In Gasset, A. R., and Kaufman, H. E. (eds.): Soft Contact Lens. St. Louis, C. V. Mosby Co., 1972, pp. 285–313.
11. Clements, L. D.: Spin casting Bausch and Lomb Soflens (polymacon) contact lenses. In Ruben, M. (ed.): Soft Contact Lenses: Clinical and Applied Technology. New York, John Wiley and Sons, 1978, pp. 435–442.
12. Aquavella, J. V.: Lathe cut versus spin cast lenses. Ophthalmol Times 2:5, 1977.
13. Aquavella, J. V.: Bionite hydrophilic bandage lenses in the treatment of corneal disease. In Gasset, A. R., and Kaufman, H. E. (eds.): Soft Contact Lens. St. Louis, C. V. Mosby Co., 1972, pp. 190–198.
14. Refojo, M. F.: The chemistry of soft hydrogel lens materials. In Ruben, M. (ed.): Soft Contact Lens: Clinical and Applied Technology. New York, John Wiley and Sons, 1978, pp. 19–39.
15. Leibowitz, H. M.: The soft contact lens. II. Therapeutic experience with the Soflens. Int Ophthalmol Clin 13:179, 1973.
16. Aquavella, J. V.: Chronic corneal edema. Amer J Ophthalmol 76:201, 1973.
17. Aquavella, J. V.: New aspects of contact lenses in ophthalmology. Adv Ophthalmol 32:2, 1976.
18. Leibowitz, H. M., and Rosenthal, P. R.: Hydrophilic contact lenses in corneal disease. II. Bullous keratopathy. Arch Ophthalmol 85:283, 1971.
19. Gasset, A. R., and Kaufman, H. E.: Bandage lenses in the treatment of bullous keratopathy. Amer J Ophthalmol 72:376, 1971.
20. Leibowitz, H. M., and Rosenthal, P. R.: Hydrophilic contact lenses in corneal disease. I. Superficial, sterile, indolent ulcers. Arch Ophthalmol 85:163, 1971.
21. Stark, W. J., Fogle, J. A., and Kenyon, K. R.: Damage to epithelial basement membrane by thermokeratoplasty. Amer J Ophthalmol 83:392, 1977.
22. Leibowitz, H. M., and Berrospi, A. R.: Initial treatment of descemetocele with hydrophilic contact lenses. Ann Ophthalmol 7:1161, 1975.
23. Leibowitz, H. M.: Hydrophilic contact lenses in corneal disease. IV. Penetrating corneal wounds. Arch Ophthalmol 88:602, 1972.
24. Aquavella, J. V., and Shaw, E. L.: Hydrophilic bandages in penetrating keratoplasty. Ann Ophthalmol 8:1207, 1976.
25. Dohlman, C. H., Boruchoff, S. A., and Mobilia, E.

F.: Complications in the use of soft contact lenses in corneal disease. Arch Ophthalmol 90:367, 1973.

26. Brown, S. I., Bloomfield, S., Pearce, D. B., and Tragakis, M.: Infections with the therapeutic soft lens. Arch Ophthalmol 91:275, 1974.

27. Aquavella, J. V.: The soft contact lens. I. Therapeutic experience with the Softcon lens. Int Ophthalmol Clin 13:167, 1973.

28. Aquavella, J. V.: Treatment of Chronic Corneal Edema. New York, Medcom Publications, 1973.

29. Takahashi, G., and Leibowitz, H. M.: Hydrophilic contact lenses in corneal disease. III. Topical hypertonic saline in bullous keratopathy. Arch Ophthalmol 86:133, 1971.

30. Brown, S. I., Bloomfield, S. E., and Pearce, D. B.: A follow-up report on transplantation of the alkali-burned cornea. Amer J Ophthalmol 77:538, 1974.

31. Podos, S. M., Becker, B., Asseff, C., and Hartstein, J.: Pilocarpine therapy with soft contact lenses. Amer J Ophthalmol 73:336, 1972.

32. Aquavella, J. V.: Therapeutic uses of hydrophilic lenses. Invest Ophthalmol 13:484, 1974.

33. Allansmith, M. R., Korb, D. R., Greiner, J. V., Henriquez, A. S., Simon, M. A., and Finnemore, V. M.: Giant papillary conjunctivitis. Amer J Ophthalmol 83:697, 1977.

34. Tripathi, R. C., Tripathi, B. J., and Ruben, M.: The pathology of soft contact lens spoilage. Ophthalmology 87:365, 1980.

Contact Lens Fitting in Keratoconus and Following Keratoplasty

GEORGE E. GARCIA, M.D.

KERATOCONUS

Management of patients with keratoconus is perhaps the greatest challenge to the contact lens practitioner. The formulas generally used to fit contact lenses simply do not apply to keratoconus patients; any attempt to apply them in these cases is met with failure. On the other hand, it is the keratoconus patients for whom the stakes are highest. Since their vision cannot be corrected with glasses, failure with contact lenses usually requires penetrating keratoplasty. Although keratoconus patients represent one of the most favorable groups for keratoplasty, the surgical procedure is not without considerable risk and economic impact. Even when the graft is successful, the patient frequently requires contact lenses for full visual rehabilitation postoperatively—and these lenses also are very often difficult to fit.

To achieve success with keratoconus patients, one must adopt a different approach to fitting and a new set of criteria for success. Most importantly, one must develop the ability to interpret the topography of the individual conical cornea. The contact lens practitioner who is accustomed to fitting lenses by some formula related to keratometry readings has no basis for proceeding in the keratoconus patient; the mires are irregular and frequently the curvature cannot be measured with any validity. One must develop the capacity to interpret fluorescein patterns and learn how to modify the parameters of the lens to effect

proper centration, venting, and movement. It is frequently impossible to fit keratoconus patients without some central bearing, intermediate pooling, an increased sense of awareness, corneal staining, or other residual problems. The successful fitter must be able to assess the steepness and extent of the cone, the degree and direction of its eccentricity, and the nature of the transitional zone between the area of coning and the normal cornea.

Patients with minimal keratoconus and satisfactory vision with spectacles need not be fitted with contact lenses. Despite claims that contact lenses retard the progression of keratoconus, there is no valid scientific evidence, such as a controlled study of matched groups of patients, for this claim. Many patients develop mild degrees of keratoconus (at least in one eye) and remain stable for years. We have also seen many patients progress to the point where they can no longer be fitted with contact lenses satisfactorily while wearing contact lenses full time. Since most of these patients require contact lenses for satisfactory correction of their vision, a controlled study to resolve this question is impractical.

In a patient with early keratoconus, initial attempts at fitting should be made with conventional polymethyl methacrylate (PMMA) lenses or semirigid gas-permeable lenses (cellulose acetate butyrate [CAB] or silicone-PMMA polymers) using a trial set. If possible, these patients should be fitted with the flattest

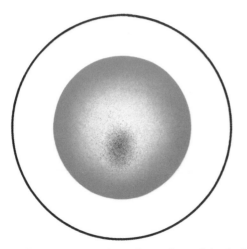

Figure 31–1. Fluorescein pattern of a satisfactorily fit contact lens on an early keratoconic cornea.

lens of conventional diameter that will provide minimal clearance of the apex of the cornea and an adequate exchange of tears. This goal is accomplished if one observes a thin film of fluorescein centrally (Fig. 31–1) and "washing out" of the fluorescein under the contact lens in less than 3 to 4 minutes, especially with PMMA lenses. The increased permeability of gas-permeable lenses to oxygen and carbon dioxide allows slightly more leeway in the rate of exchange of tears, but the fitter cannot disregard the rate of tear exchange; this material is not sufficiently permeable to these gases to permit total dependence on their exchange through the lens to support corneal metabolism. The advantage of using lenses of conventional diameters (approximately 8.5 to 9.5 mm.) is that they provide more stable vision should eccentricity of the cone result in eccentric centration of the contact lens. Contact with the upper lid also helps to elevate a low-riding lens, a frequent problem when the cone is inferior to the center of the cornea, as it is in most keratoconus patients.

Most keratoconus patients are myopes. In contrast to conventional cosmetic contact lens fitting, keratoconus contact lenses have to be fitted steeper than "K." Additional minus power must be prescribed in the lens to compensate for the convex lacrimal lens. High minus lenses frequently result in excessive

edge thickness and less comfort, so that a compromise has to be reached with regard to size to minimize this effect. Often a smaller lens than that used in an ordinary myope is fitted. Only with experience and through trial and error can the correct size for a particular patient be determined.

In treating patients with moderate degrees of keratoconus, one generally has to resort to small PMMA or gas-permeable lenses (approximately 6.8 to 8.2 mm.). It is often impossible to obtain minimal clearance of the apex of the cone. In such cases some degree of touch or bearing on the cone cannot be avoided (Fig. 31–2). This is surprisingly well tolerated by most keratoconus patients and frequently does not result in central staining with fluorescein. These lenses have rather steep central posterior curves. The transitional zone to the peripheral curves of the contact lens must be rather abrupt to conform to the topography of the cornea and to allow for sufficient exchange of tears. Corneal curvature beyond the area of coning is more or less normal. Unless this is borne in mind, it is impossible to obtain proper tear exchange under the lens. The cornea will not tolerate the lens for more than a few hours if adequate tear exchange is not maintained. Attempts to correct this deficit by flattening the central posterior

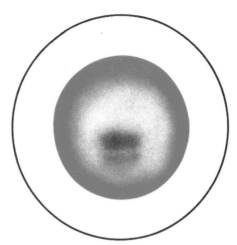

Figure 31–2. Fluorescein pattern showing acceptable touch or bearing of a contact lens on the apex of the cone. This is often well tolerated by keratoconus patients.

curve result in excessive central bearing. This, in turn, leads to central abrasions and staining, pain, and injection, especially following removal of the contact lens. Excessive bearing for extended periods of time can also result in stromal scarring and an increased risk of infection. In cases of excessive central bearing, the contact lens fitter begins to observe "bull's-eye" patterns after instillation of fluorescein (Fig. 31–3). This consists of a bright intermediate zone of pooled fluorescein between dark central and peripheral zones. Fortunately the cone is usually somewhat elliptical and irregular. As a result, the intermediate zone or "doughnut shaped" fluorescein pattern is irregular, allowing an exchange of tears with the adjoining areas. The exchange of tears, as evidenced by "washout" of the fluorescein, must take place, ideally in no more than 5 minutes. A small amount of central stippling after several hours of wear frequently must be accepted in these patients, but a confluent area of central staining is not acceptable.

Eyes with high degrees of keratoconus are fitted in a manner similar to that used for eyes with moderate degrees of the disorder, using small lenses. Because the central posterior curve must be very steep, the fitting is generally compli-

cated by the fact that very high minus lenses of 7 to 15 diopters usually are required. Proper fabrication of these lenses by a skilled technician becomes increasingly important in the successful fitting of these patients. Satisfactory blending of peripheral curves with smooth transitional zones and thin comfortable anterior bevels must be obtained. In some cases, gas-permeable lenses become too unstable in this high minus range, and the fitter must rely on PMMA lenses to avoid excessively frequent lens replacements. The doughnut-shaped band of pooling becomes more pronounced, but fortunately at least one corneal meridian usually is relatively steep and serves as a channel for tear exchange (Fig. 31–3). This channel is especially helpful if it is oriented between the 45- and 135-degree meridians with its axis in a more or less vertical direction; this seems to provide better exchange than a channel oriented in a generally horizontal direction. In occasional cases one can achieve surprisingly good vision and reasonable comfort with a lens as small as 6.5 mm. if the cone is not too eccentric.

Relatively small, slightly eccentric and slightly elliptical or circular cones are generally easier to fit than larger cones. This is especially true for those corneas that have progressed beyond the earlier stages of keratoconus. Some patients who develop keratoconus early in life are in the habit of squinting to improve their vision. They may develop small interpalpebral spaces with excessive lid tone. Generally these patients tolerate small lenses better than large ones, even when only moderate degrees of coning are present. The advent of gas-permeable materials, such as CAB and Polycon, has resulted in greater success in the management of keratoconus. Lenses made of these materials generally are tolerated for longer intervals, from both objective and subjective points of view.

Soft lenses have not had a significant impact on the management of keratoconus, since they rarely provide satisfactory visual acuity in these patients. Nonetheless, a trial of soft lenses in mild

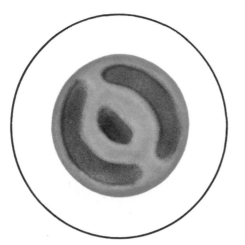

Figure 31–3. Bull's-eye fluorescein pattern indicative of substantial touch or bearing of a contact lens on a keratoconic cornea. Note the communication at the 11 o'clock to 5 o'clock meridian providing a channel for tear exchange.

cases of keratoconus with a relatively broad cone will be rewarded wth an occasional success. Occasional successes also have been reported using hydroxyethyl methacrylate as a carrier for a PMMA lens. At present, the criteria for appropriate selection of cases for this combined approach are not clear, however. It requires a great deal of technical skill on the part of the contact lens practitioner and a similar amount of patience on the part of the patient. The role of other new materials, such as silicone, in the management of keratoconus patients also is not clear at this time.

It is apparent that the major goal of contact lens fitting in keratoconus patients is proper vaulting of the conical portion of the cornea. Vaulting is the distance between a flat or a curved surface, such as the cornea, and the back surface of a steeper curvature passing over it, such as a contact lens. Soper has introduced the helpful concept of sagittal depth in the fitting of keratoconic patients to achieve this goal.[1] Sagittal depth is the distance between the apex of a contact lens and the chord of the optical zone of that lens (Fig. 31–4A). The vaulting effect of contact lenses varies among lenses with a constant optical zone diameter but different radii of curvature. Similarly, the vaulting effect varies among contact lenses with a constant radius of curvature but with optical zones of different diameter. It is apparent that if two lenses have the same optical zone diameter but different curvatures, the steeper lens will produce a greater vaulting of the cornea than the flatter lens (Fig. 31–4B). Perhaps not so obvious is the fact that sagittal depth also changes when the optical zone diameter is increased or decreased (Fig. 31–4C). If two lenses have the same posterior central curvature, the lens with the central optical zone of larger diameter will have a greater sagittal depth than the smaller lens.

The lenses advocated by Soper[2] are designed with a steep posterior central curve to fit the cone and a flatter peripheral area to conform to the normal pe-

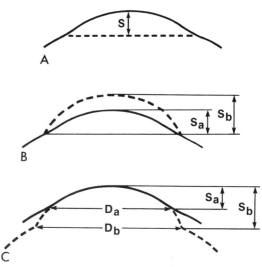

Figure 31–4. The concept of sagittal depth in fitting contact lenses in keratoconus. (S = sagittal depth; D = diameter of the optical zone). *A,* Sagittal depth is the distance between the apex of a contact lens and the chord of the optical zone of that lens. *B,* If two lenses have the same optical zone diameter, the steeper lens (smaller radius of curvature) will have a greater sagittal depth (S_b) than the flatter lens (S_a). *C,* If two lenses have the same posterior central curve, the lens with the optical zone of larger diameter (D_b) will have a greater sagittal depth (S_b) than the lens with the optical zone of smaller diameter (D_a).

ripheral areas of the cornea. As stated above, the larger the diameter of the central posterior curve (the central, steeper, optical zone), the greater the sagittal value or vaulting effect of the lens. For example, if two lenses are of the same overall diameter and have the same central posterior curve but one lens has a larger diameter of the optical zone (or central posterior curve) than the other, it will result in greater vaulting or sagittal depth. Employing the principles cited above, these lenses provide a very satisfactory approach to the fitting of keratoconus patients. Only a modest number of trial lenses are required. Excessive vaulting over the apex of the cone results in an air bubble, which is readily seen beneath the lens. In such a case, lenses with lesser sagittal depth would be tried until the bubble no longer was present. Conversely, if a lens produced gross apical touch (readily evident as a dark spot in the fluorescein pattern), a lens with greater sagittal depth would be tried. The optimal fit is one in which the lens moves over the cornea and clears the apex of the cone.

PENETRATING KERATOPLASTY

Fitting a contact lens on an eye that has undergone a penetrating keratoplasty similarly can present a significant challenge. Many such patients see well without any correction or with a spectacle correction, and contact lenses are not required for those patients. However, even in the hands of the most skilled surgeon using the most modern techniques, there are successful cases with a clear graft that have high degrees of ametropia, especially high astigmatism or irregular astigmatism. These cases often require a contact lens for satisfactory correction of their vision.

In some cases, the irregular zone may be limited and a soft lens may provide central vision that satisfies the patient's visual needs. If the astigmatism occurs because the margin of the donor button is depressed at the wound edge, a rigid lens, slightly larger than the graft, can be fitted; this will center well and provide satisfactory venting and good vision. If the astigmatism occurs because the margin of the donor button flattens and slightly overrides the incision, achieving a good fit is much more difficult. This is due to the fact that a much flatter central posterior curve must be used and the lens tends to be displaced much more readily. Since the amount of astigmatism in these cases is generally quite high, even a small lens tends to rock excessively and is easily displaced, resulting in constantly varying vision. These are the most challenging cases of all, and frequently the fitter must resort to toric or double toric lenses or possibly

a soft lens with a piggyback hard lens. Fitting these lenses requires skill and patience and, most of all, an understanding and highly motivated patient.

Although I am not aware of any objective evidence that irritation from a contact lens can precipitate a graft reaction, I am much less tolerant of any sign of irritation, bearing, edema, or chronic staining in a postkeratoplasty eye than in other postoperative situations (e.g., aphakia) or in the unoperated eye. Every effort must be made to fashion a lens that is well tolerated with minimal signs of any type of irritation. It is also important to remember the advantages of gas-permeable materials when dealing with postkeratoplasty patients in order to minimize the physiologic insult to the graft.

Another complicating factor in fitting both keratoconus patients and postoperative graft patients is that many of them exhibit excessive lacrimation, which causes excessive mobility of the lens. In addition, as noted above, occasional patients who developed their poor vision very early in life have increased orbicularis tone and slitlike interpalpebral fissures, which make it more difficult to find a comfortable lens with a stable fit.

In conclusion, the problems encountered in fitting patients with keratoconus and those who have had successful penetrating keratoplasty are much greater than those of fitting the usual refractive errors. The effort required to arrive at a successful fit is much greater, but the degree of satisfaction when one has achieved a successful fit also is correspondingly greater. It is most helpful to advise these patients at the outset that theirs is not a routine problem and that the procedure will be considerably more complicated than the conventional contact lens fitting.

REFERENCES

1. Soper, J. W., and Jarrett, A.: Results of a systematic approach to fitting keratoconus and corneal transplants. Cont Lens J 9:12, 1975.
2. Soper, J. W., and Girard, L. J.: Designing the corneal lens. In: Girard, L. J., Soper, J. W., and Sampson, W. G. (eds.): Corneal Contact Lenses. 2nd ed. St. Louis, C. V. Mosby Co., 1970, pp. 120–124.

INDEX

Page numbers in *italics* indicate illustrations;
page numbers followed by t indicate tables.